Textbook of Hemodynamic Monitoring & Therapy in the Critically Ill

Textbook of Hemodynamic Monitoring & Therapy in the Critically Ill

Second Edition

Editors

Atul Prabhakar Kulkarni
MD FISCCM PGDHHM FICCM
Professor and Head
Division of Critical Care Medicine
Department of Anesthesiology, Critical Care and Pain
Tata Memorial Hospital
Homi Bhabha National Institute
Mumbai, Maharashtra, India
Editor-in-Chief, Indian Journal of Critical Care Medicine
President, Asia Pacific Association of Critical Care Medicine
Past President, Indian Society of Critical Care Medicine
Past Chancellor, Indian College of Critical Care Medicine
Past President, Association of SAARC Critical Care Societies

Amol Trimbakrao Kothekar
MD IDCCM
Professor
Division of Intensive Care Medicine
Department of Anesthesia, Critical Care and Pain
Tata Memorial Center
Homi Bhabha National Institute
Mumbai, Maharashtra, India

Jigeeshu Vasistha Divatia
MD FICCM FCCM
Professor and Head
Department of Anesthesia, Critical Care and Pain
Tata Memorial Hospital
Homi Bhabha National Institute
Mumbai, Maharashtra, India

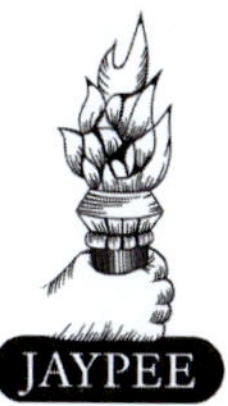

JAYPEE BROTHERS MEDICAL PUBLISHERS

The Health Sciences Publisher

New Delhi | London

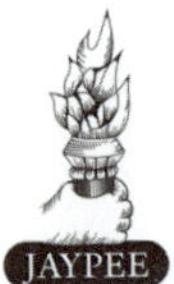

Jaypee Brothers Medical Publishers (P) Ltd

Headquarters
EMCA House, 23/23-B
Ansari Road, Daryaganj
New Delhi 110 002, India
Landline: +91-11-23272143, +91-11-23272703
+91-11-23282021, +91-11-23245672
e-mail: jaypee@jaypeebrothers.com

Overseas Office
JP Medical Ltd.
83, Victoria Street, London
SW1H 0HW (UK)
Phone: +44-20 3170 8910
e-mail: info@jpmedpub.com

Corporate Office
4838/24, Ansari Road, Daryaganj
New Delhi 110 002, India
Phone: +91-11-43574357
Fax: +91-11-43574314
e-mail: jaypee@jaypeebrothers.com

EU GPSR Authorised Representative
Logos Europe, 9 rue Nicolas Poussin
17000, La Rochelle, France
Phone: +33 (0) 6 67 93 73 78
e-mail: contact@logoseurope.eu

Website: www.jaypeebrothers.com
Website: www.jaypeedigital.com

Inquiries for bulk sales may be solicited at: jaypee@jaypeebrothers.com

Textbook of Hemodynamic Monitoring & Therapy in the Critically Ill

First Edition: 2020
Second Edition: **2025**

Reprint : **2026**

ISBN: 978-93-6616-420-5

Printed at: Sterling Graphics Pvt. Ltd.

Dedicated to

The intensivists, the warriors who are vigilant in patient monitoring to anticipate, prevent, and treat disasters, keeping the sickest safe all the time!

Contributors

Ajmer Singh MD
Director
Medanta Institute of Critical Care
and Anesthesiology
Medanta —The Medicity
Gurugram, Haryana, India

Alexandra Beurton MD
Research Fellow
Medical Resuscitation Service
Department
Bicêtre Hospital
(University Hospitals Paris-Sud)
Paris, France

Amol Trimbakrao Kothekar
MD IDCCM
Professor
Division of Critical Care Medicine
Department of Anesthesia
Critical Care and Pain
Tata Memorial Center
Homi Bhabha National Institute
Mumbai, Maharashtra, India

Anand Vinaykumar Joshi
MBBS DNB (GenMed) FRCP (Lon) FNB (Crit Care)
EDIC FCICM (Aus&Nz)
Consultant Intensivist
Department of Intensive Care Unit
Campbelltown Hospital
Sydney, NSW, Australia

Armand Mekontso Dessap
Faculty of Medicine of Créteil
AP-HP, Henri Mondor University
Hospitals DHU A-TVB
Créteil Medical Intensive Care Unit
94010 France
University of Paris Est Créteil
IMRB, GRC CARMAS, Créteil, 94010,
France

Ashish Kumar Srivastava
DA DNB FNB
Consultant
Department of Critical Care Medicine
Manipal Hospital
Bengaluru, Karnataka, India

Atul Prabhakar Kulkarni
MD FISCCM PGDHHM FICCM
Professor and Head
Division of Critical Care Medicine
Department of Anesthesiology
Critical Care and Pain
Tata Memorial Hospital
Homi Bhabha National Institute
Mumbai, Maharashtra, India
Editor-in-Chief, Indian Journal of Critical
Care Medicine
President, Asia Pacific Association of
Critical Care Medicine
Past President, Indian Society of Critical
Care Medicine
Past Chancellor, Indian College of
Critical Care Medicine
Past President, Association of SAARC
Critical Care Societies

Babu Abraham
MD (General Medicine) MRCP (UK)
Fellowship in Critical Care Medicine
(University of Toronto) FICCM
Senior Consultant
Department of Critical Care Medicine
Apollo Hospitals
Chennai, Tamil Nadu, India

Bindiya Salunke MA (Anesthesiology)
Professor
Department of Anesthesiology,
Critical Care and Pain
Tata Memorial Center and
Homi Bhabha National Institute
Mumbai, Maharashtra, India

Can Ince
Professor
Translational Physiology; Intensive Care
Med Academic Medical Center; Erasmus
MC Rotterdam
Netherlands

Daniel De Backer MD PhD
Head
Department of Intensive Care
CHIREC Hospitals
Université Libre de Bruxelles
Brussels, Belgium

Deeksha Singh Tomar
DA IDCCM IFCCM EDIC
Senior Consultant
Department of Critical Care
Narayana Super specialty Hospital
Gurugram, Haryana, India

Deepak Govil MD EDIC FCCM FICCM
Vice Chairman
Department of Critical Care Medicine
Institute of Critical Care and Anesthesia
Medanta—The Medicity
Gurugram, Haryana, India

Divya Pal
MD (Anesthesiology) IDCCM
FNB (Critical Care Medicine)
Senior Consultant
Department of Critical Care Medicine
Institute of Critical Care and Anesthesia
Medanta—The Medicity
Gurugram, Haryana, India

Ebenezer Rabindrajan
DNB IFCCM EDIC
Senior Consultant
Department of Critical Care Medicine
Apollo Hospitals
Chennai, Tamil Nadu, India

Gurudas Sadanand Pundpal
MD (Medicine/Chest/Anaesthesia)
DNB (Medicine/Chest/Anaesthesia)
Consultant Critical Care
Wockhardt Hospital
Mumbai, Maharashtra, India

Guruprasad N MBBS DA FCCCM EDIC
Consultant
Department of Critical Care Medicine
Chirayu Critical Care
Gadag, Karnataka, India

Harish MM
MBBS MD DM (Critical Care Medicine) DNB IDCCM EDIC (Dublin) Fellowship in Infectious Diseases FIARC MBA (Hospital Management)
Director
Institute of Critical Care Medicine
Kauvery Hospital
Bengaluru, Karnataka, India

Ian Seppelt
MB BS BSc(Med) FANZCA FJFICM
Clinical Professor
Department of Intensive Care Medicine
Nepean Hospital
Macquarie University
Professional Fellow
The George Institute for Global Health
Sydney, New South Wales, Australia

Jacob George Pulinilkunnathil
MBBS MD (Respiratory Medicine)
IDCCM EDIC DM (Critical Care) FCCP
Consultant
Department of Critical Care
Mar Sleeva Medicity Palai
Pandalam, Kerala, India

Jayant Shelgaonkar
MBBS DA MD FRCA FICCM
Head
Department of Critical Care
Jupiter Hospital
Pune, Maharashtra, India

Jean-Louis Teboul MD PhD
Service de Médecine Intensive-réanimation
Hôpital de Bicêtre, GHU APHP
Université Paris-Saclay, France
Université Paris-Sud
Faculté de médecine Paris-Sud
France

Jigeeshu Vasistha Divatia
MD FICCM FCCM
Professor and Head
Department of Anesthesia, Critical Care and Pain
Tata Memorial Hospital
Homi Bhabha National Institute
Mumbai, Maharashtra, India

Jitendra Choudhary
MD (Anesthesia) IDCCM FNB (Critical Care) EDIC
Consultant
Department of Critical Care
Fortis Hospital
Mumbai, Maharashtra, India

Kandaswamy N
MD DNB (Anesthesiology)
DM (Critical Care Medicine)
Assistant Professor
Department of Anesthesiology and Critical Care
Jawaharlal Institute of Postgraduate Medical Education and Research
Puducherry, India

Mirza Alamdar Ali Baig
MBBS MD (Internal Medicine) IDCCM
Fellow
Department of Critical Care Medicine
Kauvery Hospital
Bengaluru, Karnataka, India

Muralikrishna T
MD DM (Cardiac Anesthesia)
Consultant
Department of Cardiac Anesthesia and Cardiac Critical Care
Fortis Malar Hospital
Chennai, Tamil Nadu, India

Natesh Prabu R
DM (Critical Care Medicine) MD DNB (Anesthesiology) EDIC
Associate Professor
Department of Critical Care Medicine
St John's Medical College and Hospital
Bengaluru, Karnataka, India

Nishanth Baliga MD DM EDIC
Assistant Professor
Department of Critical Care Medicine
Father Muller Medical College
Mangaluru, Karnataka, India

Olcay Dilken
Department of Intensive Care
Erasmus MC, University Medical Center
Rotterdam, Netherlands

Prasad Padwal
MD (Pulmonary Medicine)
FNB (Critical Care Medicine)
Associate Consultant
Department of Critical Care
Fortis Hospital
Mumbai, Maharashtra, India

Rahul Pandit
MD FJFICM FCICM FCCP EDIC IFCCM DA
Chair, Critical Care
Sir HN Reliance Foundation Hospital and all Reliance Health Care Initiatives
Mumbai, Maharashtra, India

Ruchira Wasudeo Khasne
MBBS DA DNB IDCCM
EDAIC & EDIC Fellowship in Critical Care Ultrasound (FCCU)
Consultant and Head
Department of Critical Care Medicine
SMBT Institute of Medical Sciences and Research Centre
Nasik, Maharashtra, India

Rui Shi MD
Service de Médecine Intensive-réanimation
Hôpital de Bicêtre, GHU APHP
Université Paris-Saclay, France
Université Paris-Sud
Faculté de médecine Paris-Sud
France

Sachin Gupta
MD IDCCM IFCCM EDIC FCCM FICCM
Director
Department of Critical Care
Narayana Superspeciality Hospital
Gurugram, Haryana, India

Sheila Nainan Myatra
MD FCCM FICCM
Professor
Department of Anesthesiology, Critical Care and Pain
Tata Memorial Hospital
Mumbai, Maharashtra, India

Shilpushp Jagannath Bhosale
DM (Critical Care Medicine) Fellowship Ped Crit Care (University of Toronto)
Professor and Head
Division of Critical Care Medicine
Advanced Centre for Training
Research and Education in Cancer
Tata Memorial Centre
Homi Bhabha National Institute
Mumbai, Maharashtra, India

Shivshankar Biradar
MBBS MD (Anesthesiology)
IDCCM Fellow
Department of Critical Care Medicine
Kauvery Hospital
Bengaluru, Karnataka, India

Shrikanth Srinivasan
MD DNB FNB EDIC FICCM
Consultant and Head
Department of Critical Care Medicine
Manipal Hospital
New Delhi, India

Shweta Ram Chandankhede
MBBS MD (Anesthesiology) IDCCM IFCCM (Critical Care)
Consultant Intensivist
Department of Critical Care Medicine
CARE Hospitals
Hyderabad, Telangana, India

Simone Giglioli MD
Department of Intensive Care
CHIREC Hospitals
Université Libre de Bruxelles
Brussels, Belgium

Srinivas Samavedam
MD DNB FRCP FNB EDIC FICCM DMLE MBA
Chief Intensivist
Department of Critical Care
Ramdev Rao Hospital
Hyderabad, Telangana, India
President Elect, ISCCM (2024–2025)
Associate Editor, IJCCM

Suhail S Siddiqui
MD (Anesthesiology) DM (Critical Care Medicine) EDIC
Additional Professor
Department of Critical Care Medicine
King George's Medical University
Lucknow, Uttar Pradesh, India

Sumalatha A MBBS MD DM (PhD) EDIC
Consultant and Head, PhD Scholar, Assistant Professor
Department of Critical Care Medicine
ClearMedi Multispeciality Hospital
Mysuru
JSS Medical College, Mysuru
Adichunchanagiri Institute of Medical Sciences
Mysuru, Karnataka, India

Suresh Ramasubban
AB-Int-Medicine, Pulmonary & CCM
Senior Consultant
Department of Critical Care
Apollo Gleneagles Hospital
Kolkata, West Bengal, India

Suresh Rao KG MD MBA
Head
Department of Cardiac Anesthesia and Cardiac Critical Care
Fortis Malar Hospital
Chennai, Tamil Nadu, India

Tineesh Mathew MBBS MD Anaesthesia
Senior Clinical Fellow
Anaesthesia, Critical Care and Pain
Norfolk and Norwich University Hospital
Norwich, United Kingdom

TWL Scheeren MD PhD
Professor
Department of Anesthesiology
University Medical Center Groningen
Groningen, Netherlands

Vijaya Prakash Patil MD
Professor and Head
Department of Anesthesia, Critical Care and Pain
Tata Memorial Center
Mumbai, Maharashtra, India

VR Srivats
MD (Anesthesiology) DM (Critical Care Medicine)
Assistant Professor
Department of Critical Care Medicine
King George's Medical University
Lucknow, Uttar Pradesh, India

Xavier Monnet MD PhD
Service de Médecine Intensive-réanimation
Hôpital de Bicêtre, GHU APHP
Université Paris-Saclay, France
Université Paris-Sud
Faculté de médecine Paris-Sud
France

Yatin Mehta MD MNAMS FRCA FAMS FIACTA FICCM FTEE
Chairman
Department of Critical Care and Anesthesia
Medanta Institute of Critical Care and Anesthesiology
Medanta—The Medicity
Gurugram, Haryana, India

Preface to the Second Edition

स्वगृहे पूज्यते मूर्खः स्वग्रामे पूज्यते प्रभुः। स्वदेशे पूज्यते राजा विद्वान् सर्वत्र पूज्यते।।

[A fool is honored in his own house, a landlord is honored in his own village, a king is honored in his own country (but not beyond its boundaries), however, a scholar is honored everywhere]

It has been our constant endeavor at the Department of Anesthesiology, Critical Care, and Pain, Tata Memorial Hospital, to spread the spark of curiosity throughout India. We have a storied reputation for bringing out books which encourage curiosity leading to quest for knowing the *why* behind all physiological, pathophysiological, and pathological processes confronting the budding clinicians and even the veterans. This effort leads to deep reflection, and thereby better understanding of the processes which lead to manifestations of diseases in the form of the clinical presentation, the behavior when the organism is sick and how it may impact the outcomes. A better understanding of why a patient behaves in a certain way and why he/she responds or does not respond to the therapy hopefully points to the correct choice of therapy.

We are very happy to present to you the second edition of the *Textbook of Hemodynamic Monitoring & Therapy in the Critically Ill* on the happy occasion of the 20th CME on hemodynamics, the well-known Tutorials in Hemodynamic Monitoring and Therapy in Critical Care (THEMATICC 2024). After the second edition of *Case-based Review in Critical Care Medicine* for the students of Critical Care Medicine, and before the forthcoming 6th edition of the *Objective Anesthesia Review* it seems to be an opportune moment. We hope that you like the effort put in by all the masters, old and new, to make this edition better than the first one, though some chapters have remained almost the same. As usual, we hope that we receive constructive criticism from all of you as usual so that the next edition will be even better.

We wish you a pleasant reading.

Atul Prabhakar Kulkarni
Amol Trimbakrao Kothekar
Jigeeshu Vasistha Divatia

Preface to the First Edition

विद्या ददाति विनयं विनयाद्याति पात्रताम्।
पात्रत्वाद्धनमाप्नोति धनाद्धर्मं ततः सुखम्

[(True/complete) knowledge gives discipline, from discipline comes worthiness, from worthiness one gets wealth, from wealth (one does) good deeds, from that (comes) joy]

It is a joyous occasion for our team from the Department of Anesthesia, Critical Care and Pain, at Tata Memorial Hospital, Mumbai. This year's workshop plus CME, the famed *Tutorials in Hemodynamic Monitoring and Therapy in Critical Care (THEMATICC 2019)*, is 15th in the series of CMEs, we have held annually starting in 2005. As such, this seemed an appropriate occasion to bring out the *Textbook of Hemodynamic Monitoring and Therapy in the Critically Ill*. The Department of Anesthesia, Critical Care and Pain, at Tata Memorial Hospital, Mumbai, has a strong tradition of publishing books which are of great use, in particular to the students of the subject; and the experienced practitioners in general, as well. The previous books, *Objective Anesthesia Review* published for the Anesthesiology postgraduate students, which is in the 4th edition (and we are about to come out with the 5th edition soon), and *Case-based Review in Critical Care Medicine* for the students of Critical Care Medicine, have proved to be immensely popular.

We hope that the current book *Textbook of Hemodynamic Monitoring and Therapy in the Critically Ill* will prove to be equally successful. It will be useful to all for understanding the intricacies of the bewildering array of monitors available today. We also hope that it will make their task of managing critically ill patients suffering from complex illnesses easier, and will improve their patient outcomes.

The topics in this book have been authored by experts in their own field of monitoring, from India and abroad. We hope their experience and application of their knowledge in writing these chapters will lend an authentic aura to the discussion.

Finally the core ICU team from the department has poured their sweat and blood in the making of this book, we would like to believe that the effort proves its worth, by pleasing the only critics that matter to us, you, the readers.

We wish you a pleasant reading.

Atul Prabhakar Kulkarni
Amol Trimbakrao Kothekar
Jigeeshu Vasistha Divatia

Acknowledgments

We wish to thank all our authors for continuing to work with us as we grow along with the book which has turned out to be a high-quality, authoritative reference book for hemodynamic monitoring systems and therapy for those with compromised circulation. We dare to believe that this book will teach the newbies as well as the experts a few new things. We hope to provoke and stimulate discussion on various topics and hear from you, the discerning leader.

Many thanks to our families who tolerate our mental absence and whimsical behavior (when stressed) while we are working to bring out this book.

We are especially thankful to Shri Jitendar P Vij (Group Chairman), Mr Ankit Vij (Managing Director), Mr MS Mani (Group President), Mr Sabyasachi Hazra (Associate Director—Publishing and Digital Sales), and Mr Naman Singh (Development Editor) of M/s Jaypee Brothers Medical Publishers (P) Ltd, New Delhi, India, for helping us in every way possible to bring out this book.

Last but most important, our prayers and thanks to the Almighty for blessing us in this task.

Contents

SECTION 3: DOWNSTREAM PARAMETERS AND OTHERS

SECTION 4: TYPES OF SHOCK

SECTION 5: ASSESSING CARDIAC FUNCTION

SECTION 6: SUPPORTING THE CARDIOVASCULAR SYSTEM

SECTION 7: ULTRASONOGRAPHY AND ECHOCARDIOGRAPHY IN THE CRITICALLY ILL

Plate 1

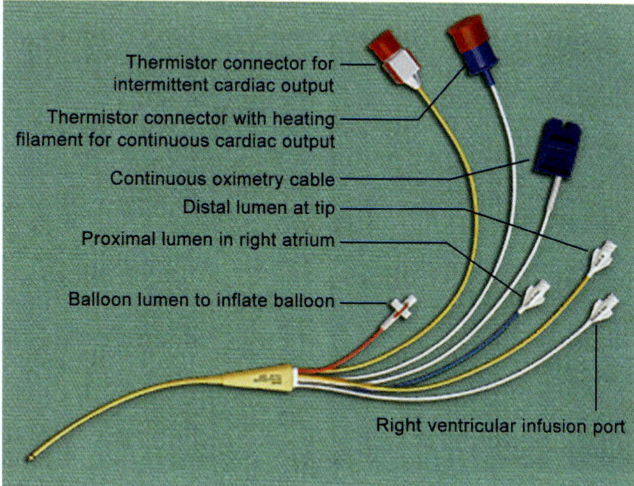

Fig. 1: Pulmonary artery catheter *(Chapter 8)*.

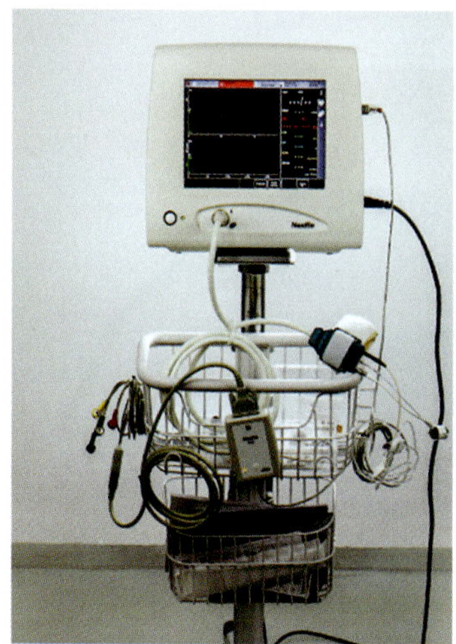

Fig. 1: Nexfin monitor *(Chapter 17)*.

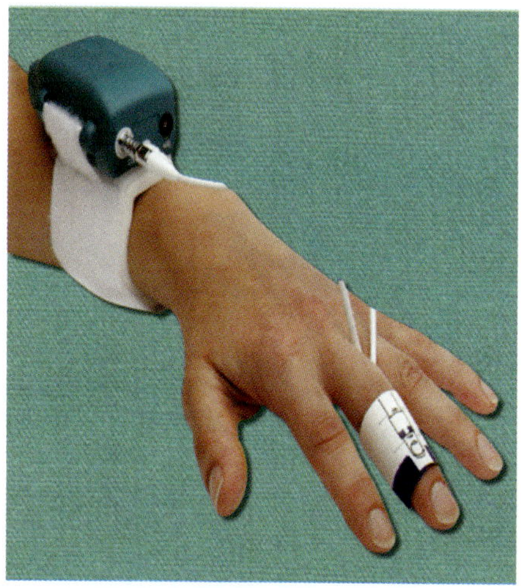

Fig. 2: Finger cuff *(Chapter 17)*.

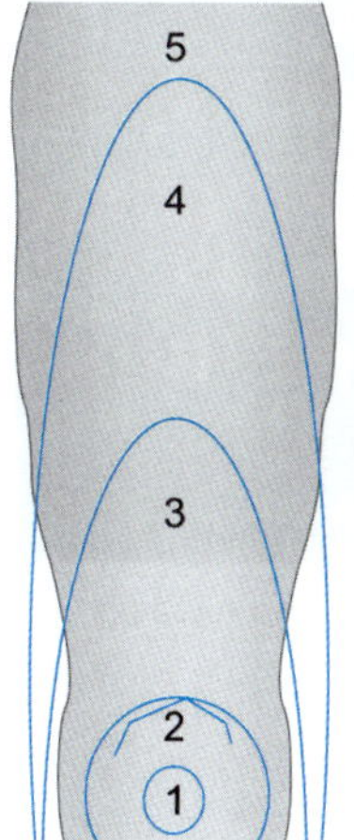

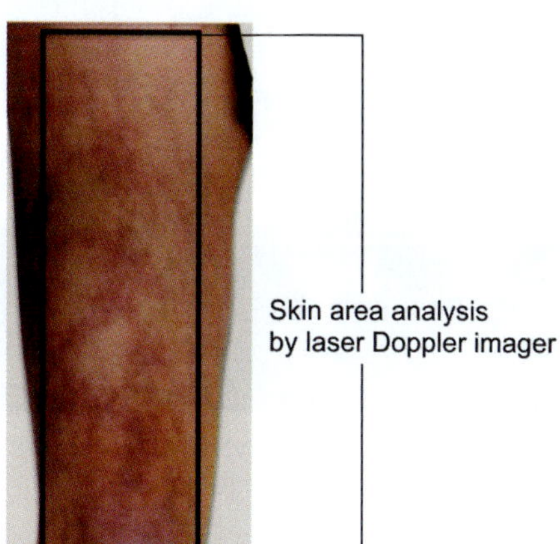

Fig. 3: Mottling score based on mottling area extension on legs. [Score 0: No mottling; Score 1: Modest mottling area (coin size) localized to the center of the knee; Score 2: Moderate mottling area that does not exceed the superior edge of the kneecap; Score 3: Mild mottling area that does not exceed the middle thigh; Score 4: Severe mottling area that does not exceed the fold of the groin; and Score 5: Extremely severe mottling area that exceeds the fold of the groin] *(Chapter 18)*.

Plate 2

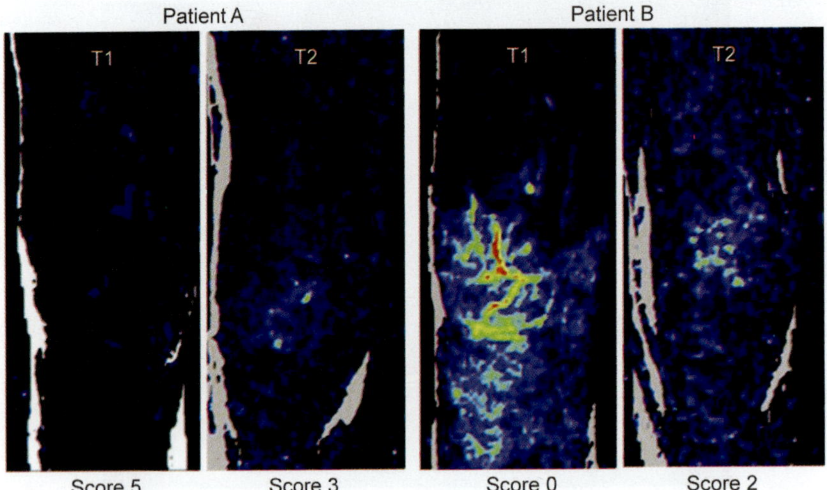

Fig. 4: Examples of laser Doppler images. In patient A, the mottling score decreased from 5 to 3 (improved), whereas in patient B mottling score increased (worsened) from 0 to 2 ***(Chapter 18)***.

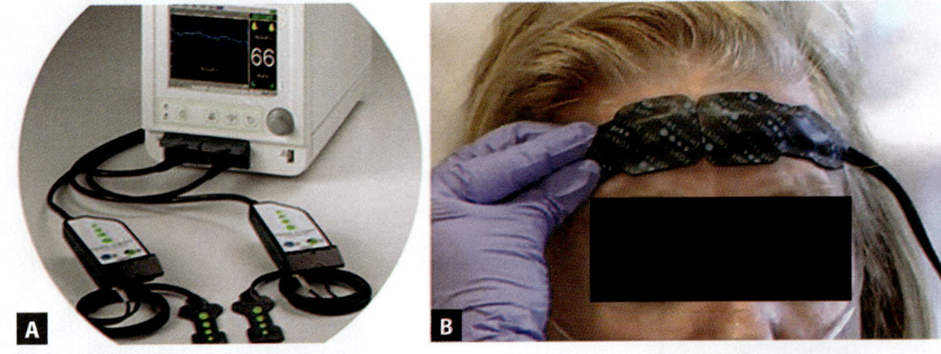

Figs. 1A and B: Equipment used for near-infrared spectroscopy ***(Chapter 22)***.

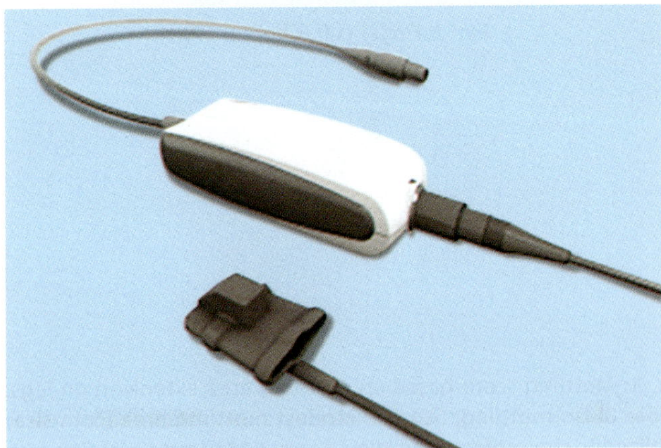

Fig. 5: LiMON probe ***(Chapter 22)***.

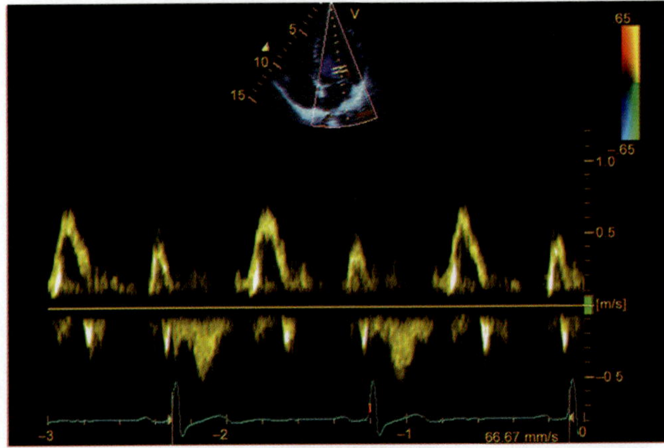

Fig. 1: Normal mitral valve inflow showing E and A waves ***(Chapter 29)***.

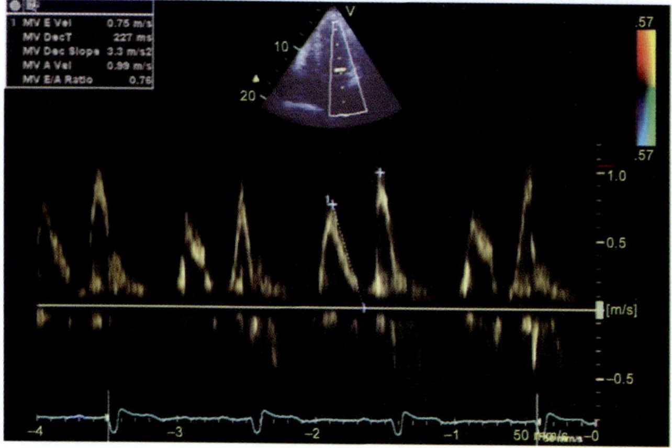

Fig. 2: E and A reversal—grade I dysfunction *(Chapter 29)*.

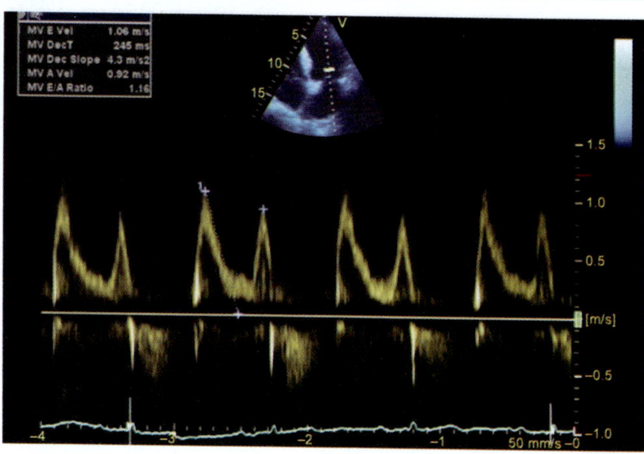

Fig. 3: Pseudonormal pattern grade II dysfunction *(Chapter 29)*.

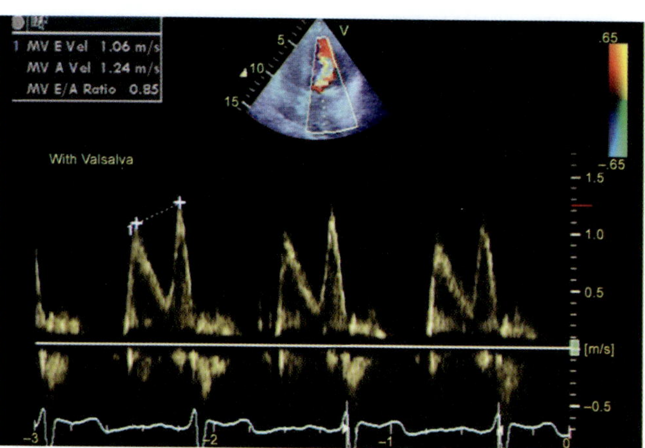

Fig. 4: Unmasking pseudonormal with Valsalva *(Chapter 29)*.

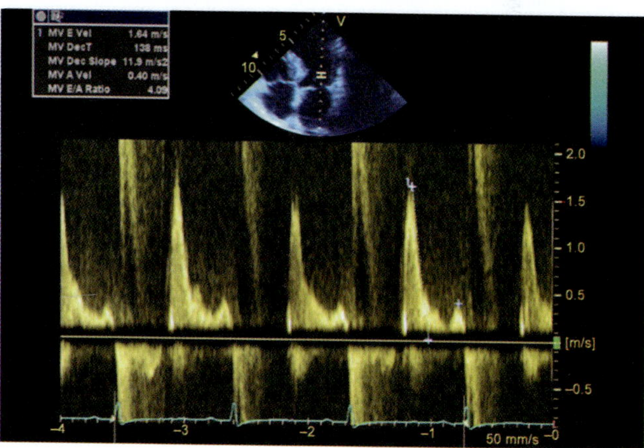

Fig. 5: Grade III diastolic dysfunction *(Chapter 29)*.

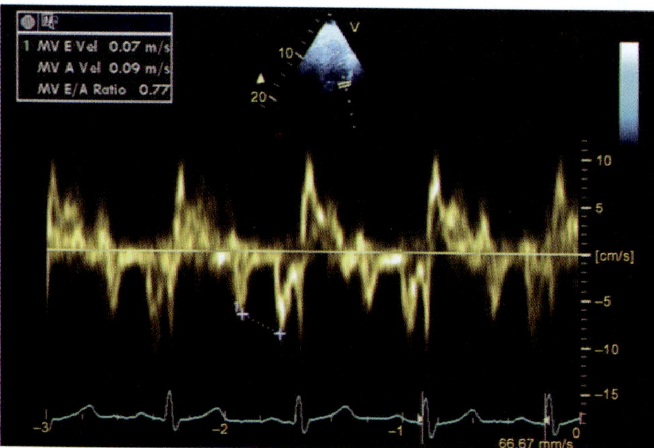

Fig. 6: Abnormal relaxation *(Chapter 29)*.

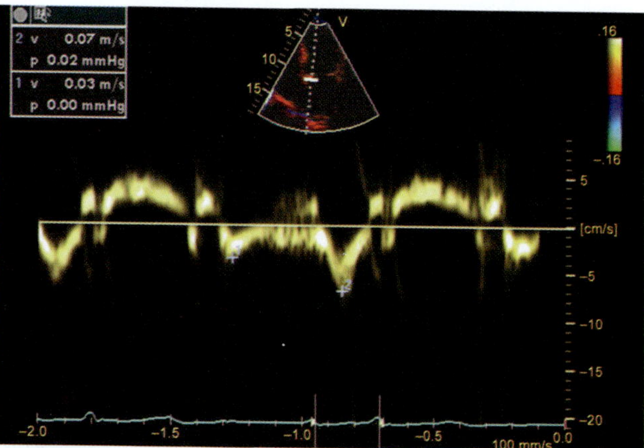

Fig. 7: Pseudonormal *(Chapter 29)*.

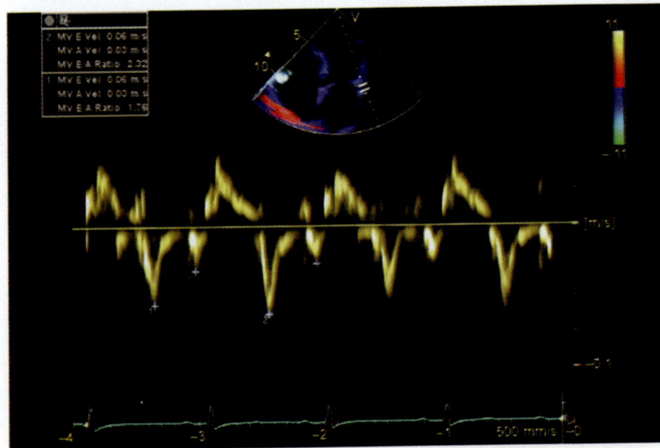

Fig. 8: Restrictive pattern *(Chapter 29)*.

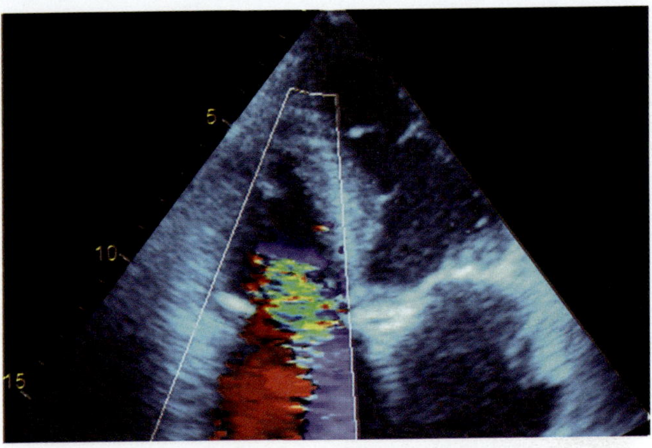

Fig. 9: Tricuspid regurgitation *(Chapter 29)*.

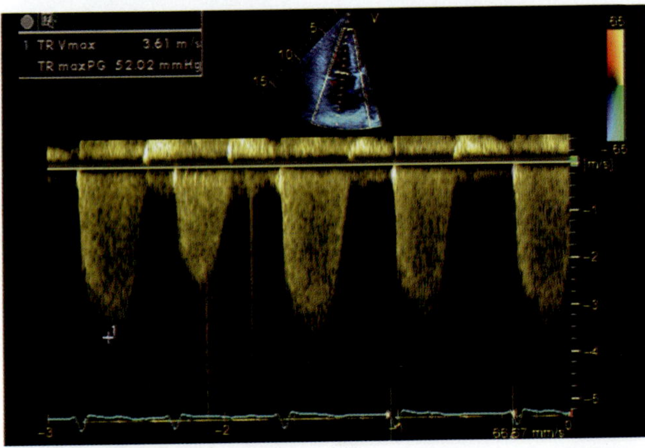

Fig. 10: Tricuspid regurgitation (TR) peak velocity *(Chapter 29)*.

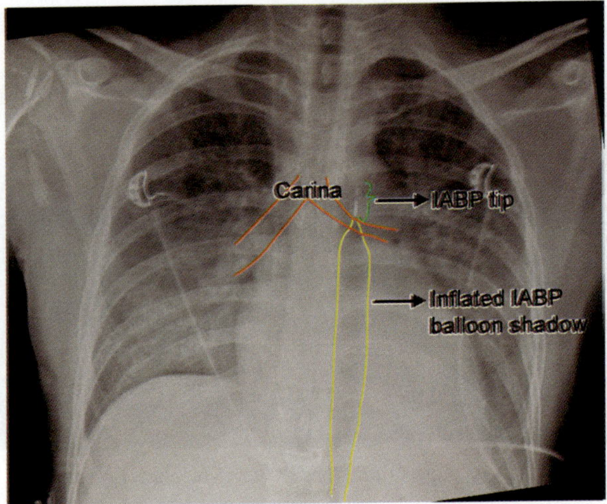

Fig. 5: Position of distal tip of intra-aortic balloon pump (IABP) placed through femoral access *(Chapter 34)*.

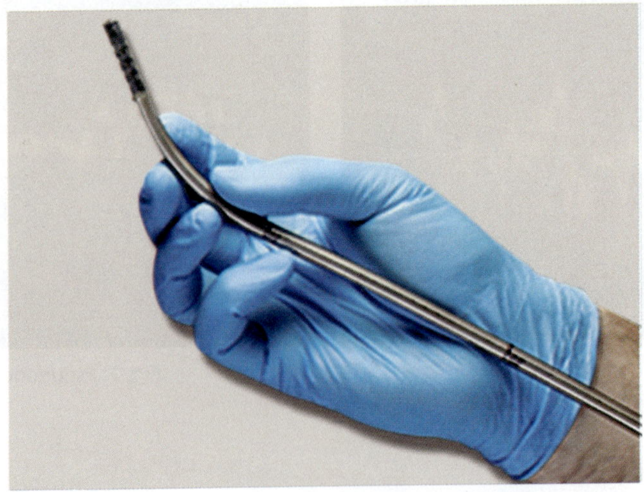

Fig. 4: TandemHeart kit component, Protek Solo transseptal cannula: The curved distal tip enables placement in the left atrium (LA) and has 14 side holes for draining blood from LA *(Chapter 35)*.

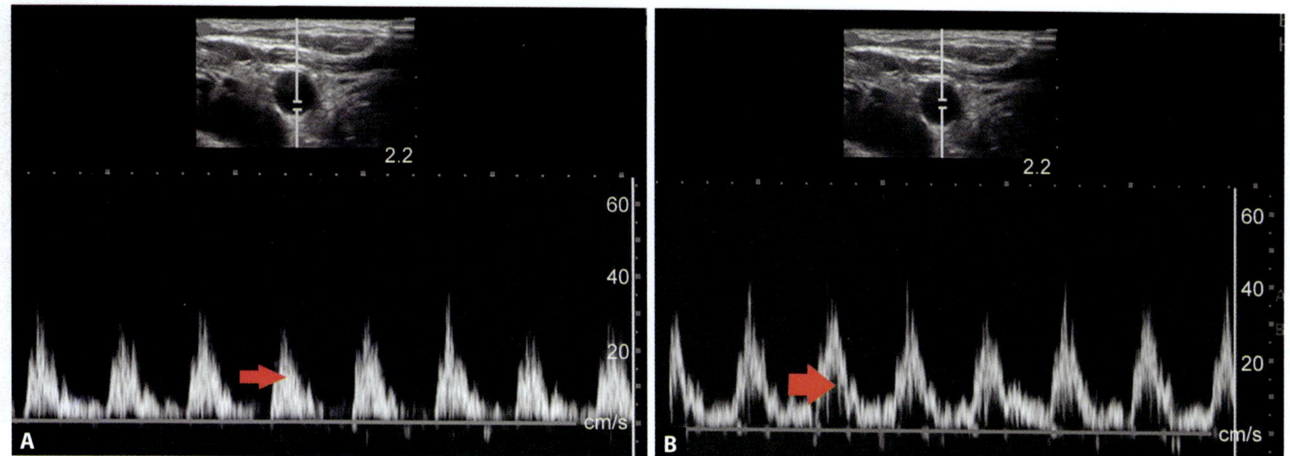

Figs. 9A and B: (A) Incorrect sample gate causing spectral broadening artifact; (B) Correct sample gate with no spectral broadening artifact *(Chapter 38)*.

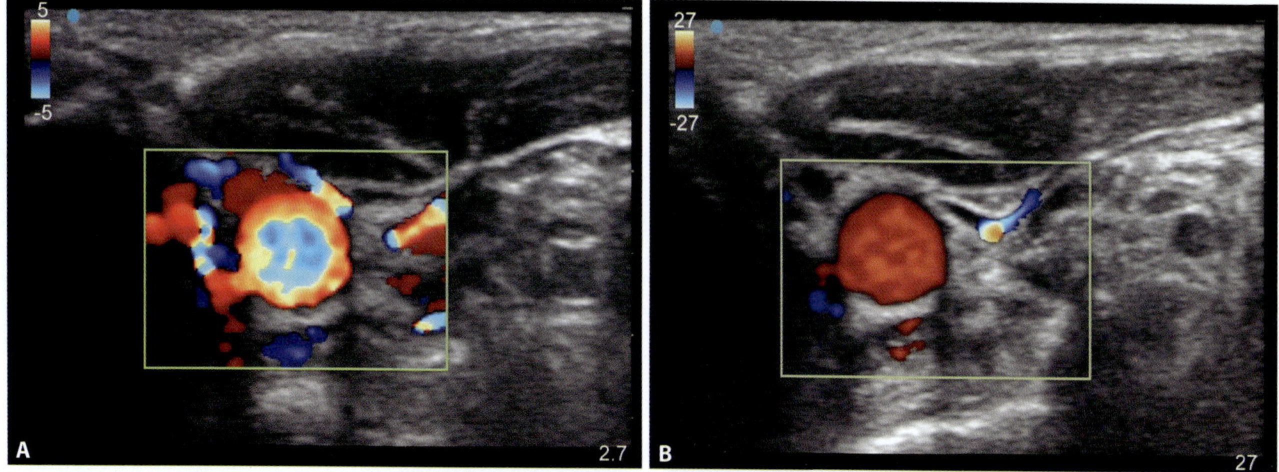

Figs. 10A and B: (A) Excessively high Doppler gain causing blooming artifact; (B) Optimal Doppler gain setting causing disappearance of blooming artifact *(Chapter 38)*.

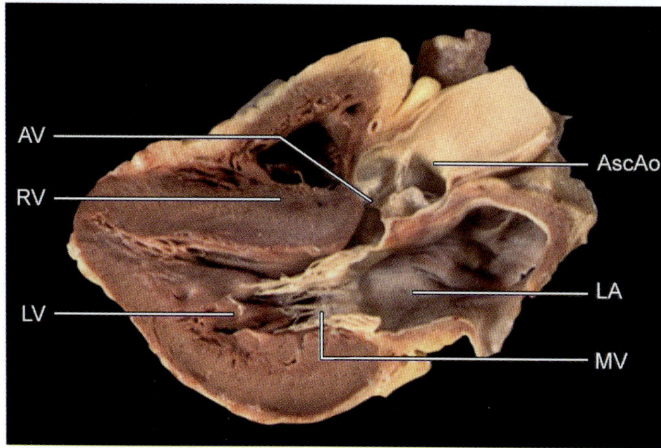

Fig. 8C: Parasternal long-axis (PLAX) view *(Chapter 40)*.

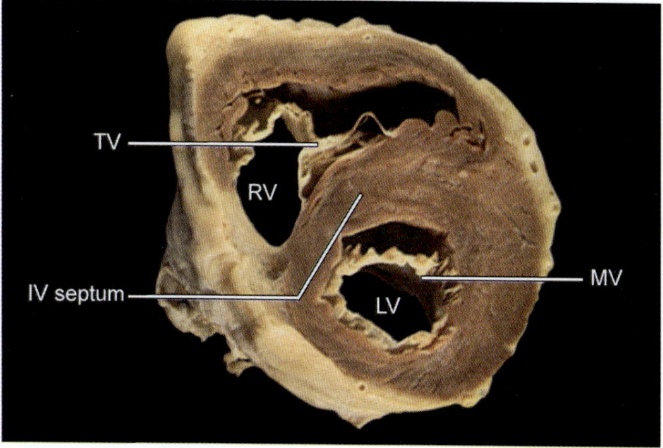

Fig. 11A: Parasternal short-axis mitral valve view *(Chapter 40)*.

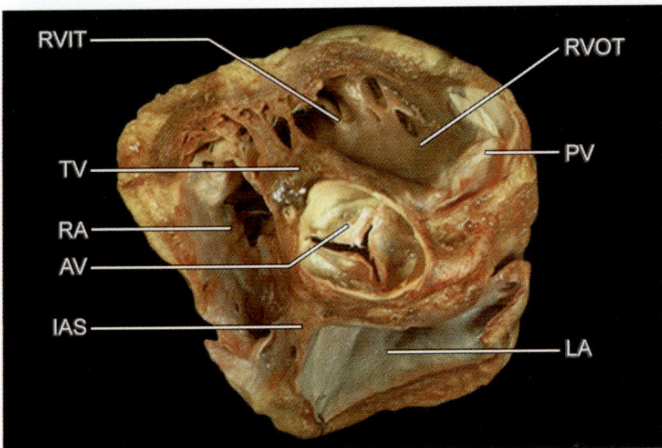

Fig. 12C: Parasternal short-axis base view *(Chapter 40)*.

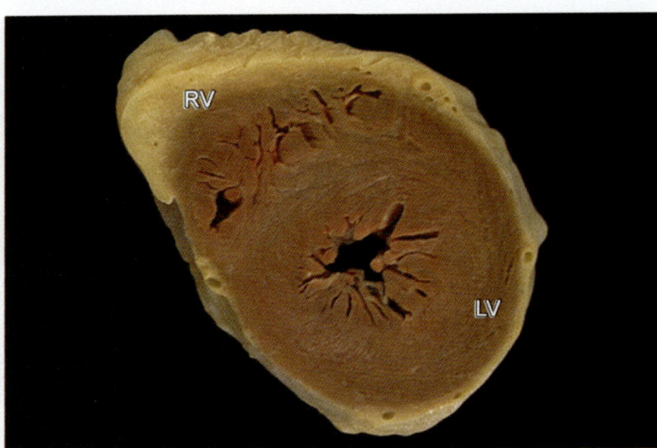

Fig. 13B: Parasternal short-axis apex view *(Chapter 40)*.

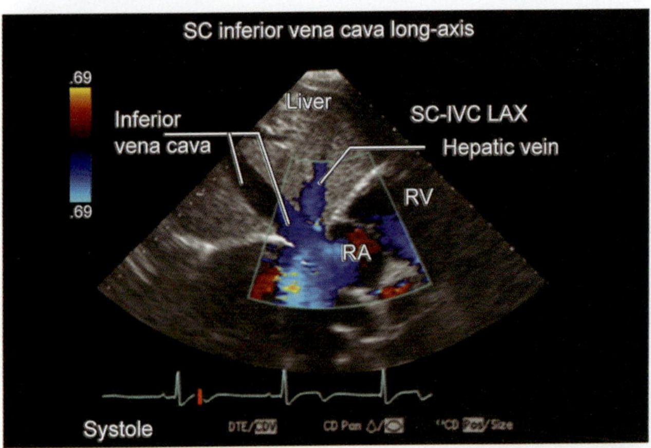

Fig. 17: Subcostal inferior vena cava view *(Chapter 40)*.

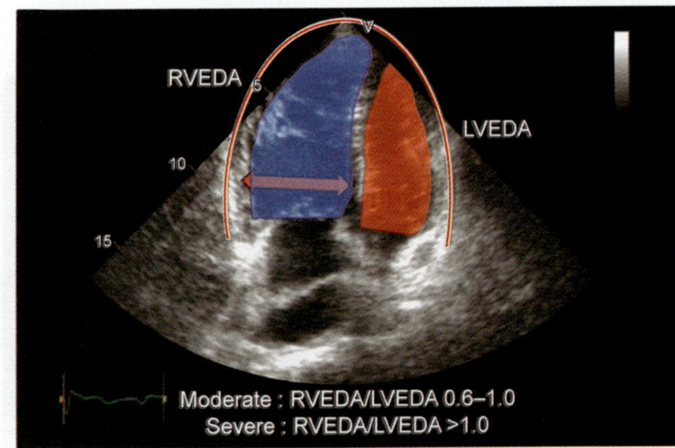

Fig. 20: RV/LV ratio *(Chapter 40)*.

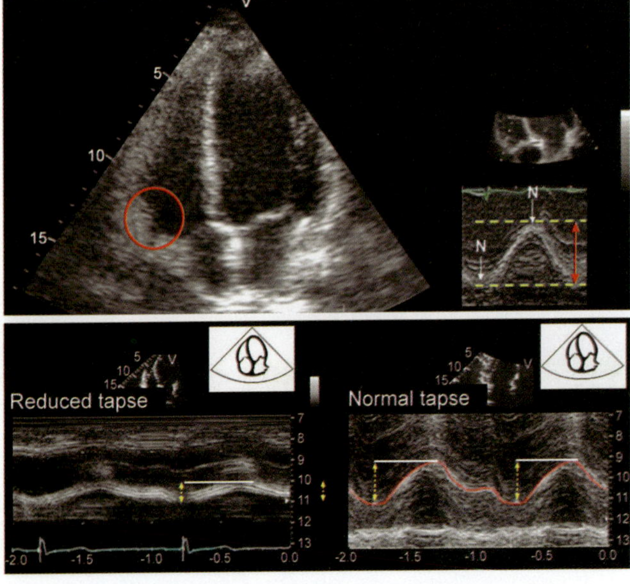

Fig. 22: RV systolic function (TAPSE) *(Chapter 40)*.

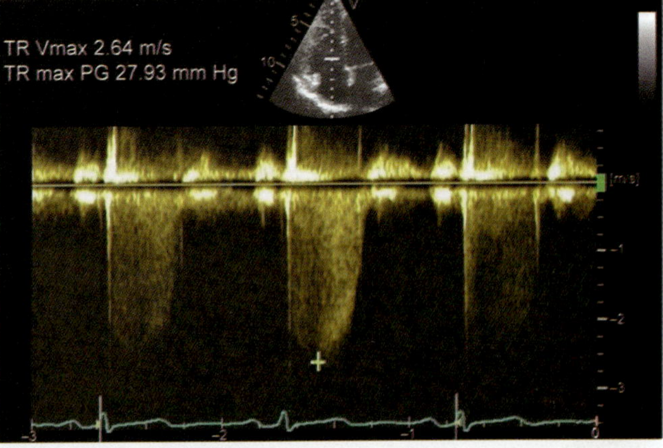

Fig. 23: Tricuspid regurgitation (TR) tracing for pulmonary artery systolic pressure (PASP) *(Chapter 40)*.

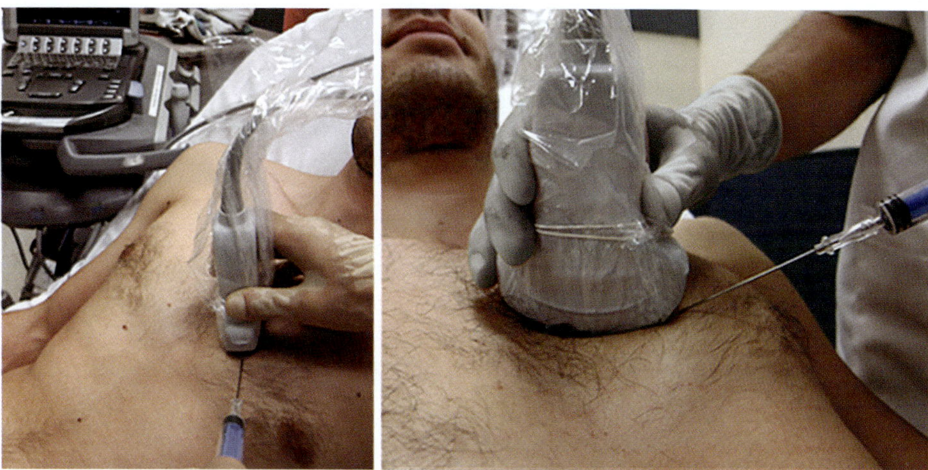

Fig. 28: Parasternal approach for pericardiocentesis *(Chapter 40)*.

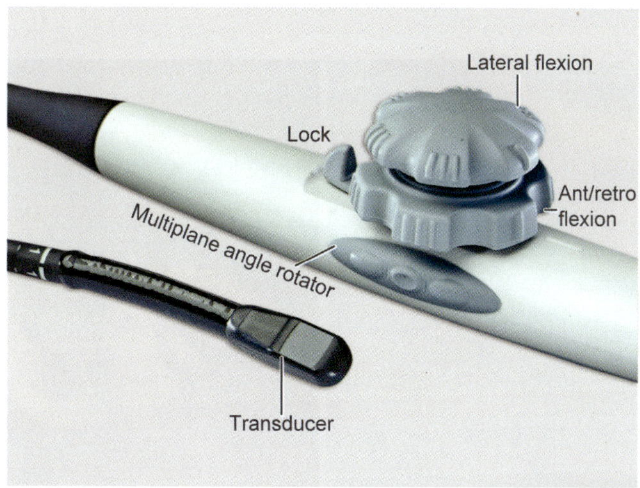

Fig. 1: Transesophageal echocardiography probe showing the transducer at the tip and the dual controls *(Chapter 41)*.

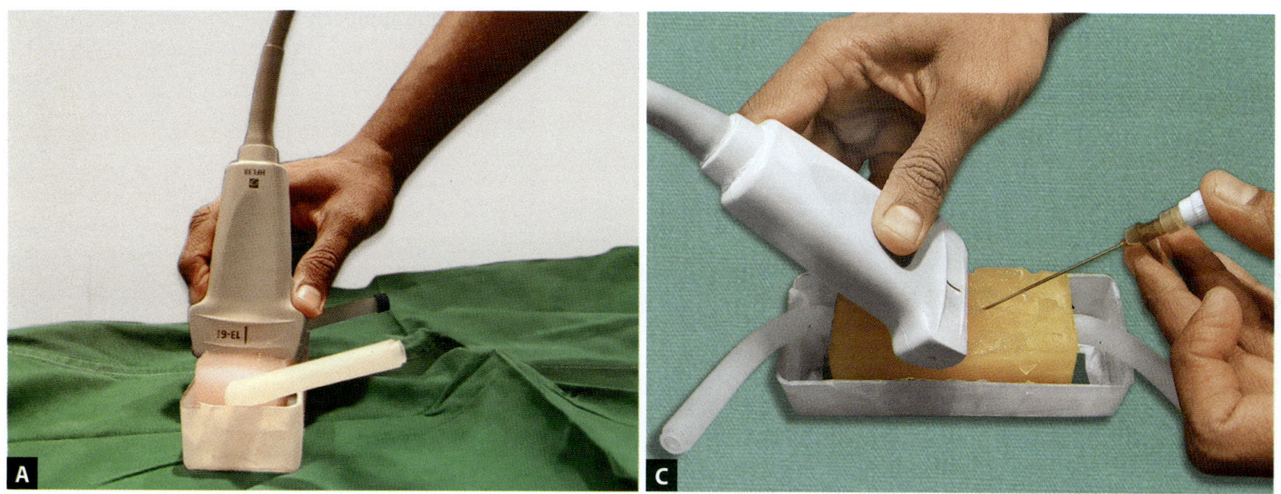

Figs. 7A and C: Images of short-axis view *(Chapter 45)*: (A) Relationship of the probe and the vessel; (C) Relationship of liner probe, vessel, and needle.

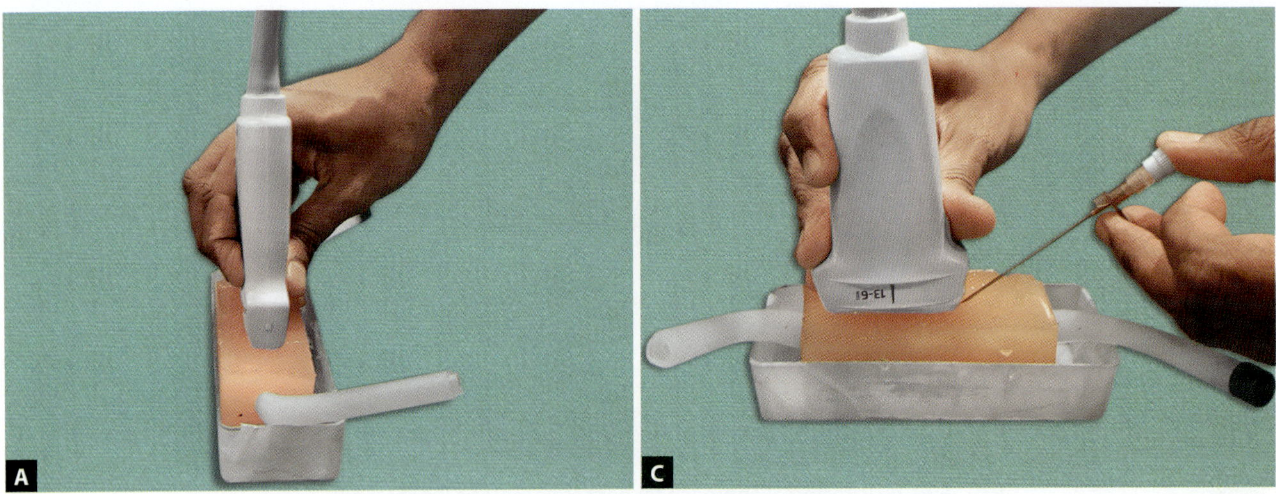

Figs. 9A and D: Images of long-axis view *(Chapter 45)*: (A) Relationship of the probe and the vessel; (C) Relationship of liner probe, vessel, and needle.

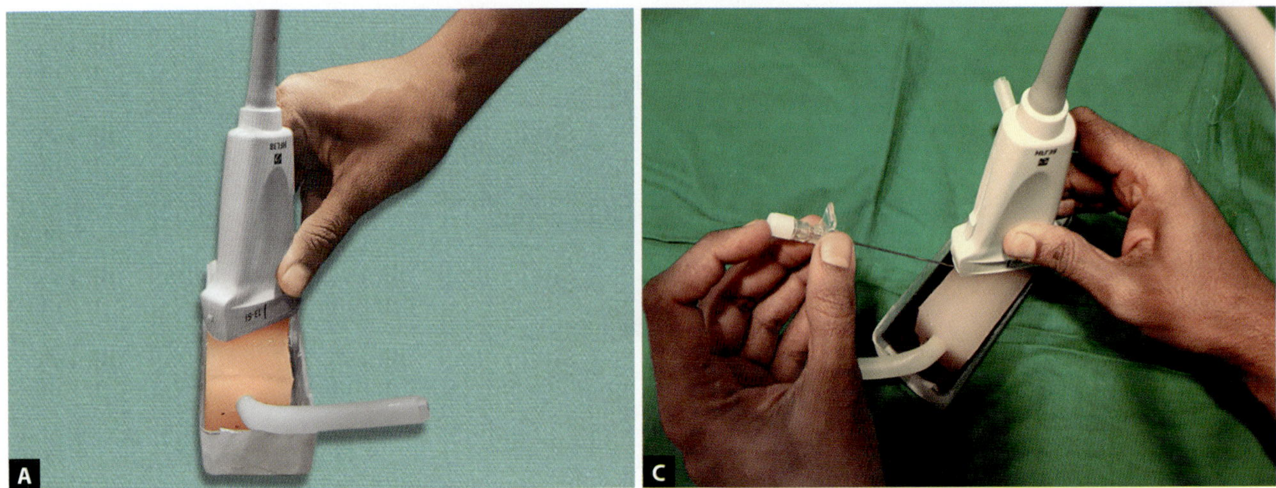

Figs. 14A and C: Images of oblique-axis view *(Chapter 45)*: (A) Relationship of the probe and the vessel; (C) Relationship of liner probe, vessel, and vessel in oblique approach

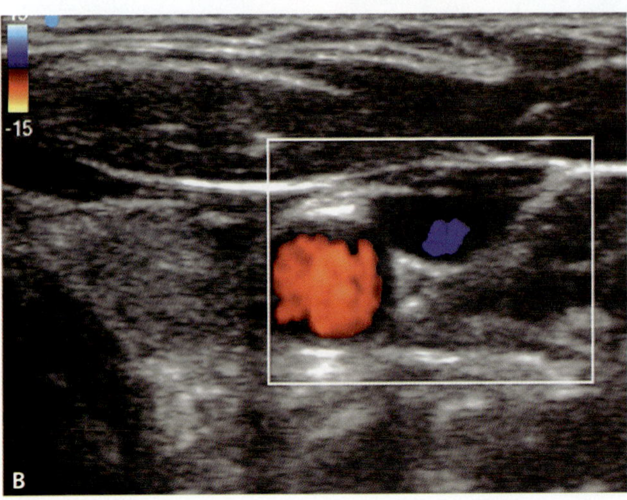

Fig. 16B: Ultrasound images demonstrating the anatomic relationship of the internal jugular vein *(Chapter 45)*: (B) Color mode ultrasound image of the internal jugular vein and carotid artery.

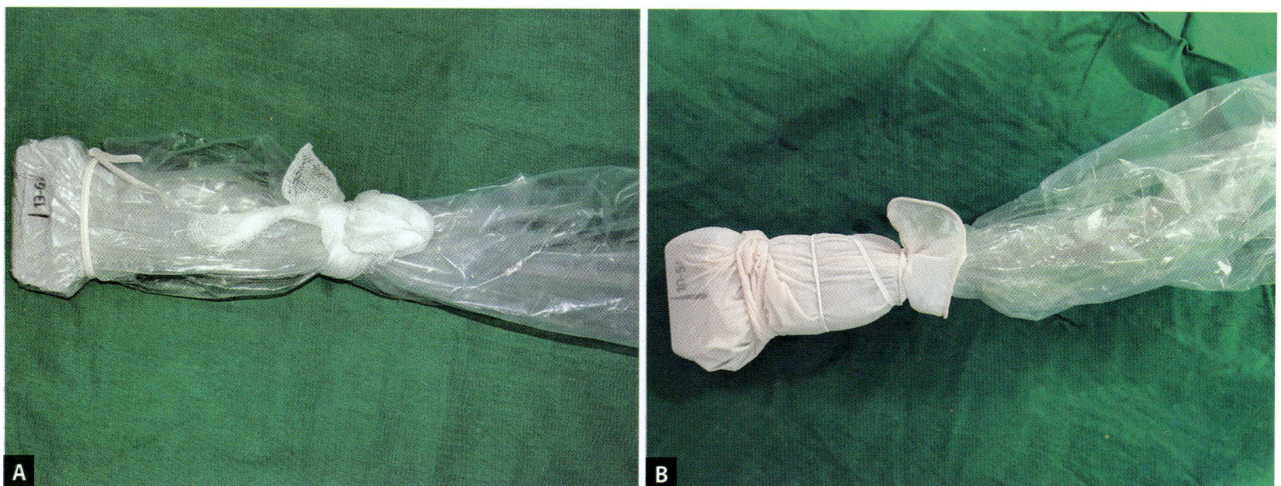

Figs. 17A and B: Image of ultrasound probe covered with (A) sterile camera cover and (B) sterile gloves *(Chapter 45)*.

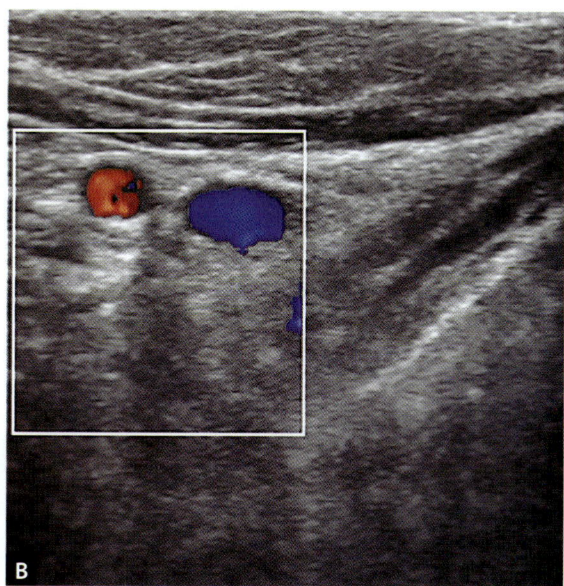

Fig. 20B: Ultrasound images demonstrating the anatomic relationship of the subclavian vein *(Chapter 45)*: (B) Color mode ultrasound image of subclavian vein and artery.

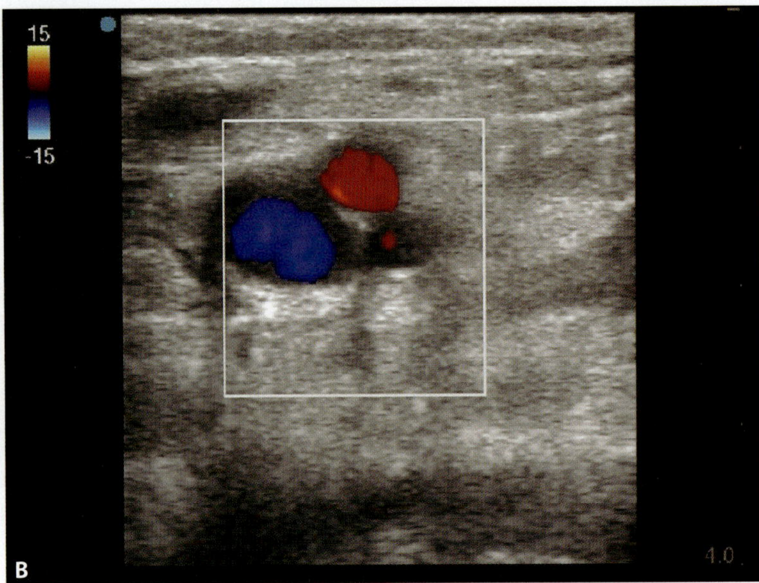

Fig. 22B: Ultrasound images demonstrating the anatomic relationship of femoral vessels ***(Chapter 45)***: (B) Color mode ultrasound image of femoral vessels.

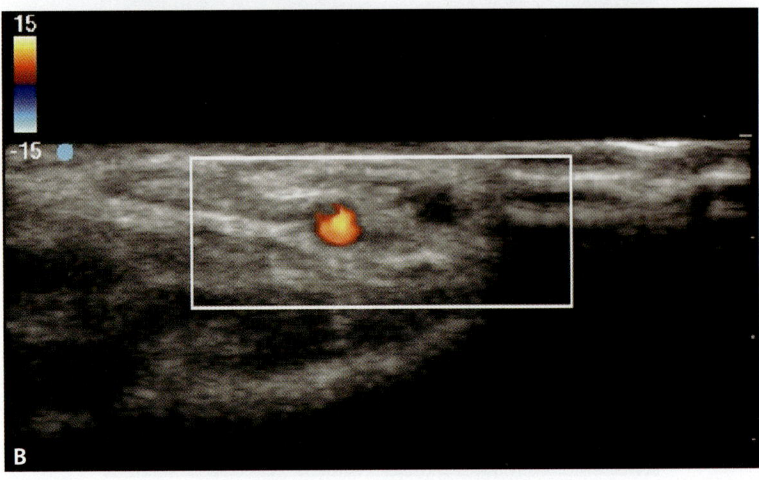

Fig. 23B: Ultrasound images of the radial artery ***(Chapter 45)***; (B) Color mode ultrasound image of the radial artery.

SECTION

Physics and Physiology

CHAPTER

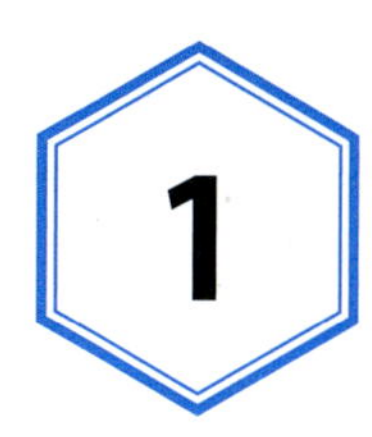

Physical Principles and Sources of Error in Invasive Blood Pressure Measurement in the Critically Ill

Atul Prabhakar Kulkarni

"The discovery of the blood pressure was more important than the discovery of the blood"

—Johannes Muller[1]

This is how Stephan Hale described his first attempt at the measurement of blood pressure in a horse.[1]

> *"In December I caused a mare to be tied down alive on her back; she was 14 hands high, and about 15 years of age; had a fistula of her withers, was neither very lean nor yet lusty; having laid open the left crural artery about three inches from her belly, I inserted into it a brass pipe whose bore was one-sixth of an inch in diameter. I fixed a glass tube of nearly the same diameter, which was 9 feet in length: Then untying the ligature of the artery, the blood rose in the tube 8 feet 3 inches perpendicular above the level of the left ventricle of the heart; when it was at its full height, it would rise and fall at and after each pulse 2, 3, or 4 inches."*

HISTORY[1,2]

1733: First ever-arterial cannulation—Rev Stephen Hales.

1828: Poiseuille cannulation of small arteries, use of a mercury manometer for the measurement of arterial blood pressure. Also Ca^{++} for anticoagulation.

1856: Arterial cannulation of an artery in an amputee —Faivre.

1855: Vierordt suggested that arterial pressure can be measured by measuring the pressure required to stop the pulsations in the artery.

1881: The first sphygmomanometer was invented—Samuel Siegfried Karl Ritter von Basch.

1896: Improvement in the sphygmomanometer by Scipione Riva-Rocci.

1947: Direct measurement of the arterial pressure using strain gauge—Lambert and Wood.

1949: Continuous recording of arterial blood pressure in brachial artery—Peterson.

1961: Catheter over needle cannulation of artery—Barr.

INTRODUCTION

One of the most common parameters used to assess hemodynamic status of the critically ill patients is blood pressure. "Blood pressure may be the vital sign, we measure the most and understand the least." Blood pressure measurement techniques have evolved over last 3 centuries to improve its accuracy. There has been a technological evolution for increasing the accuracy in monitoring patient's blood pressure. This has involved measurement of manual blood pressure using a mercury sphygmomanometer to invasive arterial blood pressure (ABP) measurement. It has further evolved to include the oscillometry, applanation tonometry, and the volume clamp methods. Sir Otto Frank published his work on the analysis of arterial pressure pulse in 1899, which led to dynamic response monitoring.[3,4] Invasive blood pressure measurement has since become the gold standard for monitoring blood pressure. Since there are multiple components in the monitoring system and a human interface, multiple sources of errors exist. In this chapter, we describe these sources of error and ways to avoid these errors, to obtain accurate measurements.

CONVENTIONS TO REMEMBER WHILE MEASURING CARDIOVASCULAR PRESSURES

- All pressures are expressed as millimeters of mercury, except central venous pressure (CVP), which may be expressed as cmH_2O. 1 mm Hg = 1.36 cmH_2O.

Ideally, however, even CVP measurement should be done using a transducer because:

- Use of an open tubing, and improper handling of the tube, can cause infections.
- The frequency response of this system is slow, which is liable to cause inaccuracies in the measurement.

- All cardiovascular pressures are referenced to the heart, in what is known as the phlebostatic axis or plane **(Fig. 1)**. "Phlebostatic axis" was established by Winsor and Burch; as the external landmark for the right atrium and pulmonary catheter tip. It is located by identifying the patient's fourth intercostal space, and drawing an imaginary line that extends down the lateral aspect of the thorax.[5] The midaxillary line lies in the middle of anterior and posterior chest borders. Phlebostatic point is the point where these two lines converge. A line or plane passing through the phlebostatic point is termed as phlebostatic axis, or plane. There is an argument that the phlebostatic axis may not be located at exactly the same point in all patients. However, it does not matter in routine clinical practice, if the clinician marks the point on the chest with a marker pen while taking the first reading and levels the transducer at this point, and takes all subsequent readings with the transducer leveled consistently there, then it is accurate enough for clinical use. It is important to remember that it is the trend of change in the (monitored) variable, and not each single value observed, that is important for monitoring and therapy. The air-fluid zero point must be "leveled" or "referenced" horizontal to the precise point where the end of the pressure-monitoring catheter is located inside a vessel. This is necessary because pressure is being measured through a fluid-filled catheter and a certain length of connecting tubing. The weight of fluid within the tubing exerts "hydrostatic pressure" and is proportional to the height of the fluid column. Every 1 cm air-fluid interface difference from this leveling point will lead to an increase or decrease of 0.74 mmHg in the measured pressure. To cite an example, if the transducer level is off by 10 cm, there will be a difference of 7.4 mm Hg in the measured pressure in the either direction. While this may not be significant in the measurement of large pressures (arterial pressure), it can make the therapy inappropriate when measuring pressures, which are of lower magnitude [such as CVP and pulmonary artery occlusion pressure (PAOP)].
- All pressures, because the transducer is zeroed to atmosphere before measurement, are pressures above the ambient atmospheric pressure. During zeroing the transducer, the clinician is establishing the fact that the monitor has to treat the ambient pressure (760 mm Hg) as zero, and therefore all pressures measured by us at the bedside are 760 + measured pressure in mm Hg.

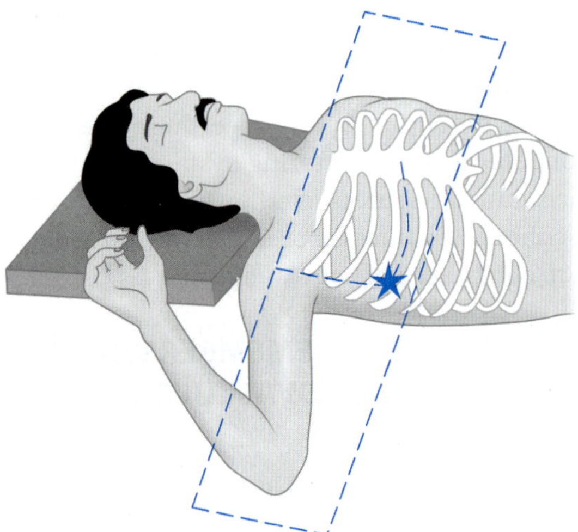

Fig. 1: Phlebostatic point, axis, and plane.

COMPONENTS OF THE MONITORING SYSTEM USED FOR INVASIVE PRESSURE MEASUREMENTS (FLOWCHART 1)

- An intravascular catheter to access/cannulate the patient's blood vessels.
- Connecting tubing (which is noncompliant) and stopcocks—to connect the intravascular catheter (in the patient's blood vessel) to the monitoring system.
- A pressure transducer to convert the mechanical impulse of a pressure wave into an electrical signal through movement of a displaceable sensing diaphragm. Modern transducers use a silicon wafer as the diaphragm, which is a stiff, low compliance pressure sensing device, capable of bending and creating a small volume change in response to applied pressure. The transducers function on the principle of the Wheatstone bridge (see later in the following test).
- A continuous flush device fills the pressure tubing with normal saline (in pediatric patients Ringer's lactate should be used, unless contraindicated) and helps prevent blood from clotting in the catheter by continuously flushing fluid through the system at a rate of 1–3 mL/hour.

Flowchart 1: Components of the monitoring system used for invasive pressure measurements, showing window for sources of errors and their rectification.

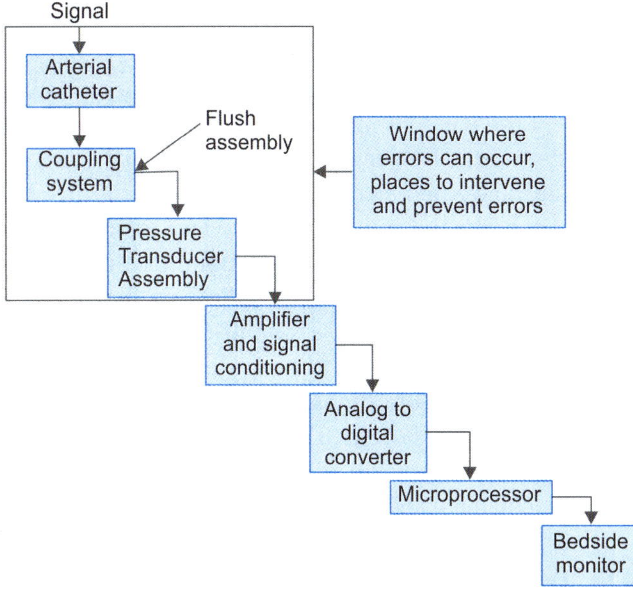

- An amplifier increases the low voltage signal from the pressure transducer (usually measured in microvolts) to a signal that can be displayed on an oscilloscope or other display device. Most amplifiers include electronic filters to filter out unwanted physiologic "noise."
- A monitor to display waveforms along with digital fields (to display numerical data).
- A processor or microcomputer, to calculate hemodynamic parameters from the measured variables.
- A recorder and a printer, for printing the patient data for the hospital records. Modern monitors are now equipped with interface, which allows direct storage of data in the electronic medical record (EMR).

ARTERIAL PRESSURE WAVEFORM: A FOURIER SERIES[6]

Fourier, a 19th century French mathematician, showed that complex repetitive waveforms could be analyzed as being the sum of a series of much simpler waveforms called sinusoids **(Fig. 2)**. A complex waveform thus can be broken down into a series of sinusoids in the same phase (same direction and passing through the zero amplitude) but of decreasing amplitudes (and having increasing frequency). Of these sinusoids, the first 6–10 sinusoids contribute the maximum information about the final waveform. The first sinusoid in this series, with the lowest frequency, is called fundamental frequency (or the first harmonic). For cardiovascular pressures, this equates to the heart rate. The second harmonic is a sinusoidal waveform that has twice the frequency and the third harmonic three times the frequency of the first harmonic, and so on. Arterial waveform, which is a complex waveform, can have as many as 30 harmonics. Therefore, reproducing the first 10 harmonics can produce a close approximation of the final arterial waveform.

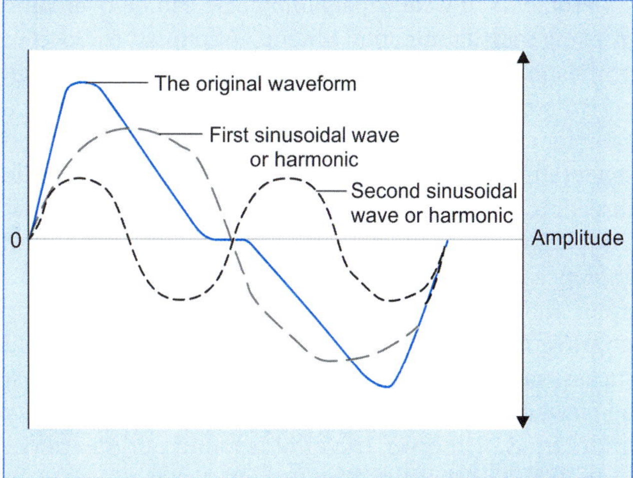

Fig. 2: Fourier series (multiple sinusoids or wavelets) forms the final complex waveform (see text for detailed explanation).

If the heart rate of patient is 60 beats/minute, then it has the frequency of 1 Hz, this is called the fundamental frequency. Since the arterial waveform can have as many as 30 harmonics, the monitoring recording system would require a frequency response that is undistorted up to 30 Hz to accurately reproduce the original waveform. The natural frequency of the arterial pulse (brachial and radial) ranges between 16 and 24 Hz. Thus, it follows that for faithfully reproduction of the original arterial waveform, the monitoring system should therefore have the natural frequency greater than this.

SITES OF CANNULATION, ARTERIAL CATHETER, AND END-HOLE ARTIFACT

The discussion about catheter types, techniques of insertion are beyond the scope of this write-up. Most clinicians perform arterial cannulation using the "catheter over needle" technique described by Barr in 1961. Nowadays commercial kits with Seldinger technique of different sizes are also available for cannulating arteries at various anatomical sites.

Problems of weakly palpable pulse can be overcome by using transillumination (infants) or miniature Doppler probes in adults. Difficulties in threading catheters can be overcome by using appropriately sized catheters, a catheter over guidewire (Seldinger technique) or a liquid stylet (after obtaining free-flow flushing with saline while threading the catheter), etc. A meta-analysis showed that first attempt success rate was higher when ultrasound guidance was used to cannulate the radial artery.[5] A recent meta-analysis suggested that though ultrasound may improve first success rate, it did not change the overall success rates, while cautioning that this conclusion must be viewed with caution due to significant heterogeneity in the trials.[6] However, use of ultrasound during arterial cannulation has become a routine practice now.

It is important to use a catheter of appropriate size (i.e., largest possible diameter but smallest length, see the formula for natural frequency in the following text). This is important because the arterial catheter tip points toward the heart. The blood flowing toward the catheter has kinetic energy. When the tip of catheter meets the blood having kinetic energy, some of this energy is converted into pressure, leading to a false increase (by 2–10 mm Hg) in the measured systolic blood pressure (SBP). This augmentation of systolic pressure due to addition of converted kinetic energy is known as the end-pressure product or the end-hole artifact.[7]

CONNECTING THE ARTERIAL CATHETER TO THE TRANSDUCER: THE COUPLING SYSTEM[8]

The typical catheter-transducer system used in the intensive care unit (ICU) setting is considered to be an "underdamped, second-order dynamic system." A second-order system is characterized by three mechanical parameters:

1. *Elasticity:* The stiffness of the system.
2. *Mass:* The weight of the material moving through the system.
3. *Friction:* The resistance encountered as the mass oscillates.

In the ICU, "elasticity" reflects the flexibility of the pressure transducer diaphragm and the compliance of the pressure tubing. "Mass" reflects the fluid or blood traveling through the catheter and tubing. "Friction" refers to both the resistance of the fluid, as it moves with each pulsatile change in blood pressure, as well as the viscosity of the fluid itself.

Each system has a characteristic natural frequency (the number of "oscillations" per unit time, natural frequency being the frequency at which it will oscillate freely, and in the absence of sustained stimulus). The arterial pressure waveform is propagated through the systemic circulation at a given frequency. The resulting sine wave, occurring at the rate of the patient's pulse, is called the first harmonic or fundamental frequency (see in the earlier text). If the natural frequency of the monitoring system is the same as the arterial pulse-pressure wave, or the pulse pressure wave reflects off a large catheter or obstruction in the system, then, a wave reflection or "harmonic" is generated which may be a sum of two waves, falsely augmenting the systolic blood pressure and reducing the diastolic blood pressure, though the mean arterial pressure will remain the same **(Fig. 3)**. The natural frequency at which a catheter-extension tubing system tends to oscillate can be calculated using the following formula:

$$f_n = \frac{1}{2\pi}\sqrt{\frac{\pi D^2}{4\rho L}\cdot\frac{\Delta V}{\Delta P}}$$

where, volume/change in pressure = compliance; D: diameter, L: length of the tubing, and ρ is density of the solution.

It is evident from the formula above that longer the length of the system, lower the natural frequency of the system, and the more likely it is to resonate with the pulse-pressure waves. In order to keep the natural frequency of the monitoring system higher than the frequencies in the pulse pressure wave (normally likely to be up to 20–30 Hz),

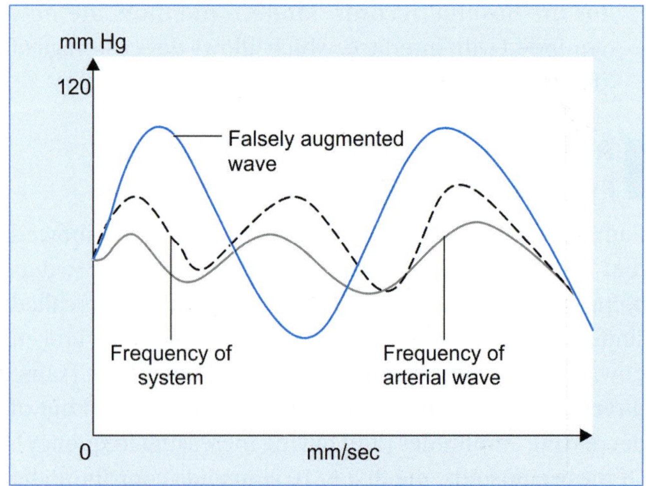

Fig. 3: Augmented systolic pressure due to summation of natural frequency of the monitoring system and of the waveform.

it is desirable to maximize the diameter of the catheter and tubing. The length of the catheter and the tubing should also be kept to the minimum (in the ideal world, the catheter would be directly connected to the transducer). This is because, if the length is increased to 6–8 feet, the resultant overshoot in SBP can vary from 2 to 31.3%. Small air bubbles in the tubing can cause hyperresonance due to summation, while large air bubbles in the tubing cause damping of the displayed waveform.

RESONANCE AND DAMPING IN THE MONITORING SYSTEM AND THEIR EFFECT ON THE WAVEFORM[9]

To prevent resonance (ringing) in the system, some degree of damping is essential in the system. There are frictional forces within the monitoring system or "damping factors" which include size and interval of the pressure wave, which affect the time it takes for the wave to dissipate and disappear. Without some extent of damping within the system (an "underdamped" system), the pressure waves would tend to reverberate, i.e., resonate (as discussed earlier) within the catheter and tubing, overestimation of systolic blood pressure. The damping coefficient can be calculated by the formula:

$$\beta = 1/r^3$$

A narrow, peaked waveform is characteristic of an underdamped pressure waveform **(Fig. 4 and Table 1)**. This waveform tends to overestimate SBP while underestimating diastolic blood pressure (DBP). At the opposite end of the spectrum is the overdamped system, which underestimates the SBP while overestimating DBP, this is seen at the bedside as a widened slurred tracing, a common phenomenon in the ICU **(Fig. 5 and Table 2)**.

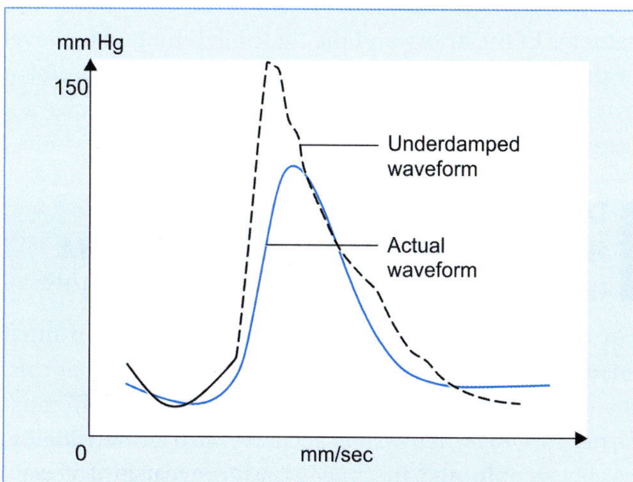

Fig. 4: Underdamped waveform.

TABLE 1: Characteristics and causes of underdamped waveforms.

Nature of waveform	*Effect on measurements*	*Causes*
Narrow, peaked tracing	Overestimates SBP	Long tubing increased vascular resistance
	Underestimates DBP	
	MAP remains unchanged	

(DBP: diastolic blood pressure; MAP: mean atrial pressure; SBP: systolic blood pressure)

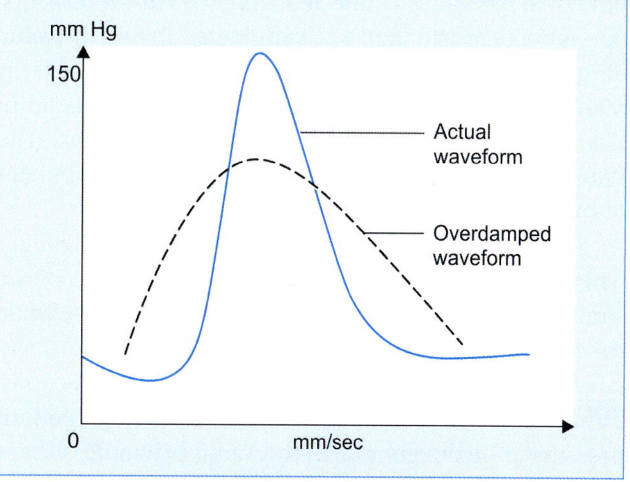

Fig. 5: Overdamped waveform.

TABLE 2: Characteristics and causes of overdamped waveforms.

Nature of waveform	*Effect on measurements*	*Causes*
Widened and slurred pressure tracing	Underestimates SBP	• Air bubbles • Overly compliant tubing • Blood clots/fibrin • Catheter kinks • Stopcocks/injection ports • No fluid in flush bag/low flush bag pressure
	Overestimates DBP	
	MAP remains unchanged	

(DBP: diastolic blood pressure; MAP: mean arterial pressure; SBP: systolic blood pressure)

Although damping seems to be a solely a theoretical issue, underdamped and overdamped waveforms are encountered on a daily basis in the ICU. The ability to recognize when these potential sources of error, or "dynamic response artifacts," are present is essential to being able to effectively analyze and apply hemodynamic measurements in the care of the critically ill and avoid potentially detrimental therapy.

THE WHEATSTONE BRIDGE PRINCIPLE (HOW THE TRANSDUCER FUNCTIONS)[8]

In 1833, Samuel Hunter Christie invented the Wheatstone bridge, which was improved and popularized by Sir Charles Wheatstone in 1843. The Wheatstone bridge is the *interconnection of four resistances* forming a bridge. The four resistances in circuit are referred to as arms of the bridge. The bridge is used for finding the value of an unknown resistance connected with two known resistors, one variable resistor and a galvanometer. To find the value of unknown resistance the deflection on galvanometer is made zero by adjusting the variable resistor. This point is known as balance point of Wheatstone bridge. The Wheatstone bridge can also be used for the measurement of small changes of resistance **(Fig. 6)**.

The pressure transducers contain four strain gauges which are designed so that the resistances of two of the strain gauges at opposite sides of the bridge increase while the resistances of the other two decrease. This results in a larger potential change at the galvanometer connections. The potential is then amplified before display. Modern pressure transducers utilize the same principle, except that they employ the semiconductor technology instead of wires. Silicon crystals also change resistance in linear proportion when pressure is applied. Using integrated circuit technology, a Wheatstone bridge is etched into the undersurface of the silicon pressure-sensing diaphragm. An epoxy coat is given over the entire structure to produce bonded strain gauge. As pressure is applied to the strain gauge, the wires increase in length and decrease in diameter, increasing the resistance to flow of current through the wires of the Wheatstone bridge. This change in the wire's electrical resistance causes a voltage change that can be quantified to reflect the amount of pressure that changed the wires length and diameter. The electrical signal can be amplified and measured; when calibrated, it is proportional to the pressure change. Thus, changes in resistance and current are measured, then electronically converted and displayed as systolic, diastolic, and mean arterial pressures. The preamplifier provides energizing current to the circuit and receives the output current from the transducer. It also contains the controls for calibration to preset pressure (by altering the resistance so that the output is equal to preset pressure) and zero it relative to atmosphere (by changing resistance so that the net output, i.e., output current to preamplifier is zero). After passing through the preamplifier, the electrical analog of the pulse-pressure wave passes through the amplifier section of the monitor, where the signal is boosted up to drive the readout device with sufficient voltage that is proportionate to the pressure change.

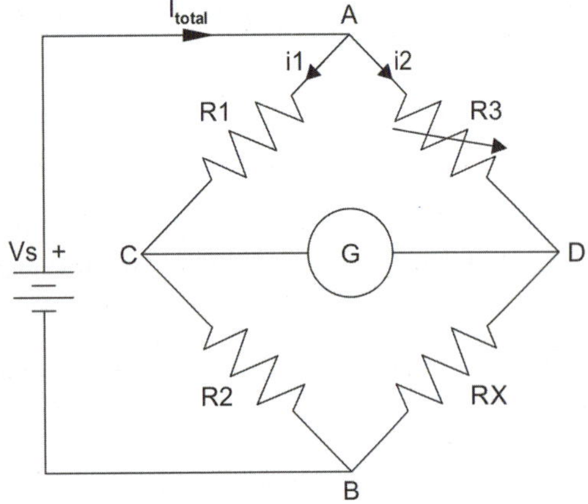

Fig. 6: Wheatstone bridge circuit diagram.

The clinician will have little control over actual electronic components. The system can be calibrated by connecting it to a manometer and raising the pressure to sequentially to 50 mm Hg, 100 mm Hg, and 200 mm Hg. We have a little more control than this, over the next components of the pressure monitoring system: the catheter in the artery and the fluid-filled tubing, the level of the transducer relative to heart, and we can perform dynamic response testing (DRT) for the system that we are using.

DYNAMIC RESPONSE TESTING OF A HEMODYNAMIC MONITORING SYSTEM (FAST FLUSH OR SQUARE WAVE TEST)[7,10]

For accurate capture of basic data, the clinician must ensure that the system is performing optimally. For this, the dynamic response characteristics of the system must be tested. Only when system accuracy, also termed fidelity, has been confirmed, the analog waveform can be accepted as an accurate reflection of a patient's status. The dynamic

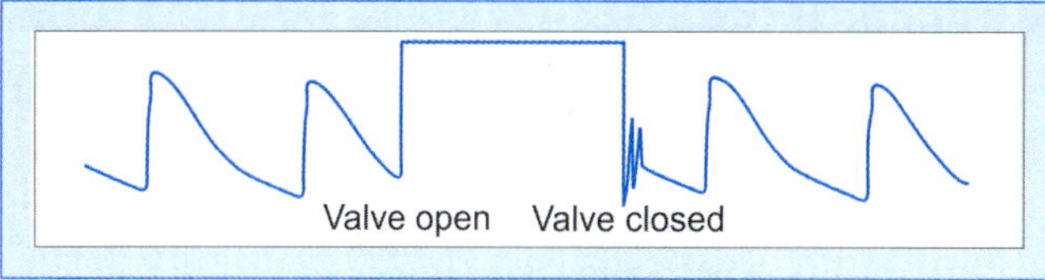

Fig. 7: Dynamic response testing using the square wave or fast flush test.

response of a hemodynamic monitoring system is defined by its natural frequency and the damping coefficient. Though performing DRT seems complicated at first, it can be performed quite easily using the fast flush test or square wave test.

Fast flush test (Square wave test): Open the valve of the continuous flush device to perform a "fast flush test;" this increases the flow through the catheter-tubing system is transiently to 30 mL/hour from the usual 1-3 mL/hour. This generates an acute rise in pressure within the system such that a square wave is generated on the bedside monitor. With closure of the valve, sinusoidal pressure waves (oscillations or wavelets) of progressively decreasing amplitude are generated. A system with appropriate dynamic response characteristics will return to the baseline pressure waveform within 1–2 oscillations. For actual calculation a strip chart recorder connected to the monitor is required. The rule of the thumb is, if there are more than two wavelets, the system is underdamped and if there are none, it is overdamped. After performing the fast flush test, record and print the resulting square waveform and subsequent oscillations on calibrated strip chart paper **(Fig. 7)**.

When and how Often the Dynamic Response Testing Should be Performed?[7,10]

The DRT should be performed as follows:

- After opening the system for the first time.
- When the accuracy of measurement is doubtful or when patient's clinical condition does not match the monitored parameters.
- When we suspect an overdamped or underdamped waveform.
- Before implementing interventions or making changes to ongoing interventions.
- Physiological changes place higher demands on the monitoring system.
- At least every 8–12 hours or at the time of each change of shift.

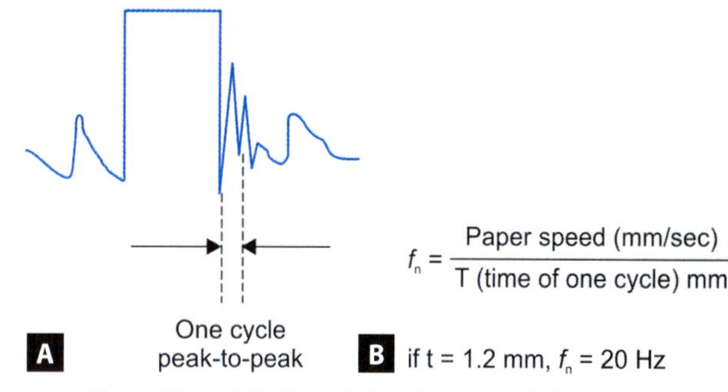

Figs. 8A and B: Calculating the natural frequency.

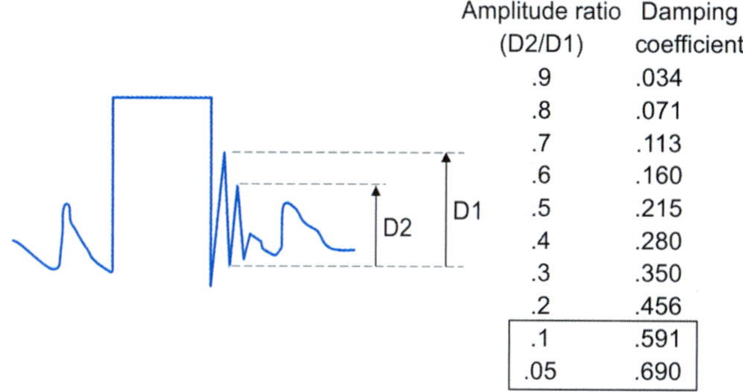

Amplitude ratio (D2/D1)	Damping coefficient
.9	.034
.8	.071
.7	.113
.6	.160
.5	.215
.4	.280
.3	.350
.2	.456
.1	.591
.05	.690

Fig. 9: Calculating damping coefficient and amplitude ratio.

- *Determining natural frequency (f_n):*[10]
  - Measure the distance [period (t) of one cycle] in millimeters between two oscillations (one small box on the calibrated strip chart paper equals 1 mm) **(Fig. 8A)**.
  - Calculate f_n by using the formula f_n = paper speed (mm/s)/t of one cycle (mm) (The standard paper speed is 25 mm/s) **(Fig. 8B)**.
- *Determining the amplitude ratio and damping coefficient:*[10]
  - Measure the amplitude (D) in millimeters of two successive oscillations (D1 and D2) **(Fig. 9)**.
  - *Calculate the amplitude ratio:* Divide D2 by D1 (D2/D1).
- *Determining the dynamic response characteristics of a monitoring system:*[10]
  - Plot fn along the x-axis.
  - Plot the amplitude ratio along the y-axis on the right.
  - Find the intersection of the two lines **(Fig. 10)**. Where the two lines intersect on the f_n-versus-amplitude ratio graph, determines if the system is able to correctly reproduce the hemodynamic waveform (adequate, optimal) or if the system is not functioning at a desirable level (overdamped, underdamped, and unacceptable).

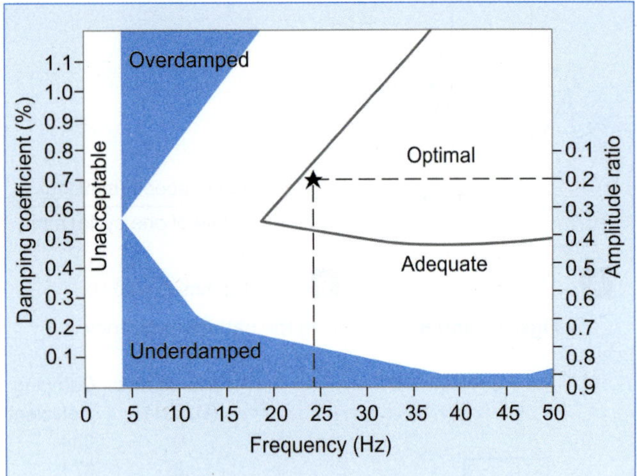

Fig. 10: Plotting the dynamic response characteristics of a monitoring system.[10]

CONCLUSION

It is important for every clinician to understand the physical principles behind pressure transduction in clinical medicine and understand where errors are likely to occur due to equipment related problems. Once optimal functioning of the monitoring is ensured, it is necessary that zeroing at the correct reference point, periodic calibration of the monitoring systems, and maintenance of the monitoring system such as removing blood from the catheter/tubing, ensuring that the flush bag is not empty, or ensuring adequate pressure in the flush bag will allow accurate acquisition of hemodynamic data.

REFERENCES

1. Booth J. A short history of blood pressure measurement. Proc R Soc Med. 1977;70:793-9.
2. Kapse CD, Patil BR. Auscultatory and Oscillometric methods of Blood pressure measurement: a survey. Int J Eng Res Appl. 2013;3:528-33.
3. Winsor T, Burch GE. Phlebostatic axis and phlebostatic level: reference levels for venous pressure measurements in man. Proc Soc Exp Biol Med. 1945;58:165-9.
4. FRCA. (2009). Physical principles of invasive blood pressure monitoring. [online] Available from https://www.frca.co.uk/Documents/137%20Physical%20 principles %20of%20intra-arterial%20blood%20pressure%20 measurement.pdf/ [Last accessed September, 2024].
5. Gao YB, Yan JH, Gao FQ, Pan L, Wang XZ, Lv CJ. Effects of ultrasound-guided radial artery catheterization: an updated meta-analysis. Am J Emerg Med. 2015;33(1):50-5.
6. Bhattacharjee S, Maitra S, Baidya DK. Comparison between ultrasound guided technique and digital palpation technique for radial artery cannulation in adult patients: An updated meta-analysis of randomized controlled trials. J Clin Anesth. 2018;47:54-9.
7. McGhee BH, Bridges EJ. Monitoring arterial blood pressure: what you may not know. Crit Care Nurse. 2002;22(2):60-4, 66-70.
8. CircuitDigest. (2017). What is Wheatstone bridge? [online] Available from https://circuitdigest.com/article/what-is-wheatstone-bridge/ [Last accessed September, 2024].
9. Derangedphysiology.com. (2017). Resonance, damping and frequency response. [online] Available from https://derangedphysiology.com/main/cicm-primary-exam/required-reading/cardiovascular-system/Chapter%20 734/resonance-damping-and-frequency-response/ [Last accessed September, 2024].
10. Gardner RM. Direct blood pressure measurement—dynamic response requirements. Anesthesiology. 1981; 54(3):227-36.

CHAPTER

Physiology of Arterial Pressure Monitoring

Vijaya Prakash Patil

INTRODUCTION

Blood pressure (BP) a commonly used terminology denotes the lateral pressure exerted by circulating blood against the walls of the arteries. Overall, BP is maintained by the interaction of the blood volume with the walls of the arteries and arterioles, and the force of the contraction of the heart. Arterial blood pressure (ABP) is the sum of kinetic and hydrostatic pressures. Kinetic pressure reflects energy associated with motion, which is imparted to the blood by contraction of the left ventricle (LV). When BP is measured in a direction perpendicular to the flow as in noninvasive BP measurement, it measures the lateral pressure exerted radially on the vessel wall. During invasive BP measurement, the catheter is pointed in a direction against blood flow and the final pressure measurement may have added a component of pressure wave artifact called end hole artifact which may falsely elevate BP though most often this rise is small. Hydrostatic pressure reflects fluid density and gravity contribution which is the pressure a column of fluids exerts on a container wall. This component affects BP reading if a transducer is not leveled properly.

Left ventricular contraction occurs due to ventricular depolarization and can be seen on the electrocardiograph (ECG) as an R wave. The interval between the R wave and the appearance of a pulse wave in the periphery reflects the time required for the spread of a depolarization wave, isovolumic left ventricular contraction, aortic valve opening, left ventricular ejection, the transmission of the aortic pressure wave to the radial artery, and of the pressure signal from a catheter to a transducer which is around 120–200 ms.[1]

The arterial tree starts with the aorta and the major branches. The aorta and its branches receive blood from the LV, distribute it to the whole body, and maintain arterial pressure. Arteries and arterioles control BP by manipulating systemic vascular resistance (SVR). Arterioles are the primary sites that contribute to SVR. During the compensatory state of shock, an increase in SVR and arteriovenous shunting help in mobilizing blood from peripheral circulation to central circulation and thus helps redirect blood flow to vital organs. This is the main reason why measurements of BP alone are not a good indicator of cardiac output (CO) and adequacy of peripheral perfusion.

WHAT IS A NORMAL BLOOD PRESSURE?

Normal or acceptable BP varies with age, state of health, and gestational age in the case of the fetus. In a full-term baby at birth (40 weeks), its BP is 80/50 mm Hg. It rises steadily throughout childhood and by the age of 15–17 years it becomes 120/80 mm Hg. It has been seen that systolic blood pressure (SBP) shows a continuous increase from the age of 30 years. However, diastolic blood pressure (DBP) shows an increase before 45 years of age and then slowly decreases afterward resulting in an increase in pulse pressure (PP) as age advances.[2] In late pregnancy and during sleep, BP is low as compared to other times.

COMPONENTS OF BLOOD PRESSURE

Systolic Blood Pressure

With each left ventricular contraction, blood is pumped into the aorta causing a rise in aortic pressure. Each ejection creates pressure and flow waves that propagate through an arterial tree. SBP is the highest pressure measured in the cardiovascular system. The main determinants of SBP are left ventricular stroke volume (SV), left ventricular ejection time, arterial wave reflection, and aortic compliance. As the site of BP measurement moves from center to periphery in a vascular tree, SBP increases due to the added component of the reflected wave.

Diastolic Blood Pressure

Diastolic blood pressure is the lowest BP measured in the central aorta and peripheral circulation during the cardiac cycle and corresponds with left ventricular diastole. Primary hemodynamic determinants of diastolic pressure include total peripheral resistance, heart rate (HR), arterial compliance, and SBP. As the site of BP measurement moves from the center to the periphery in a vascular tree, there is a slight drop in DBP.

Mean Arterial Blood Pressure

This is the average ABP throughout one cardiac cycle and not just the mathematical average of systolic and diastolic pressures. Mean arterial blood pressure (MAP) is determined exclusively by CO and total peripheral resistance. It is relatively steady and is generally closer to diastolic pressure because diastole represents about two-thirds of the cardiac cycle when the mean HR is 60 beats/min.

$$MAP = DP + 1/3(SP - DP) \text{ or } MAP = DP + 1/3(PP)$$

Most of the hemodynamic monitors measure MAP (during invasive BP measurement) from the ABP tracing by measuring the area under the pressure curve and dividing this area by the time interval involved **(Fig. 1)**. This is a more accurate way of measuring MAP than the aforementioned formula. For example, someone who has low SV, but high SVR may have the same MAP as someone with normal SV and normal SVR by using the aforementioned formula. Generally, MAP remains constant across the arterial tree, decreasing only slightly in the periphery. This component of BP is the most common therapeutic target for hemodynamically unstable patients since most organs autoregulate the blood flow around MAP.

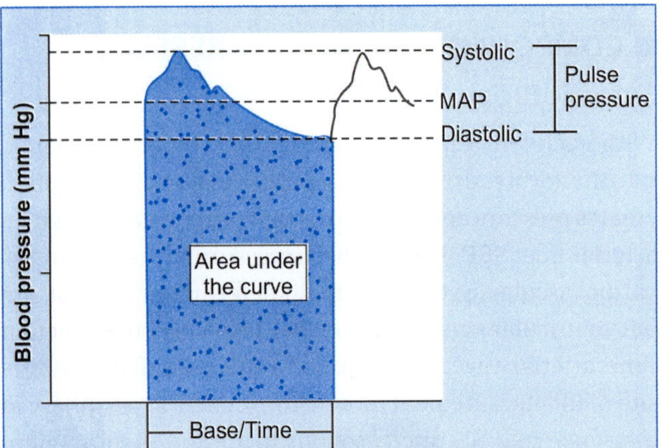

Fig. 1: Different components of blood pressure.

Pulse Pressure

Pulse pressure is the difference between the SBP and the DBP. The main factors influencing PP are SV and aortic compliance. PP is directly proportional to SV and inversely proportional to aortic compliance. An increased PP results from increased SV and peripheral vasodilatation as commonly seen during fever, exercise, anemia, and hyperthyroidism. Other causes of increased PP are bradycardia (increased SV), aortic regurgitation, and well-resuscitated vasodilatory states. Decreased PP is commonly seen in patients with decreased SV either due to hypovolemia or poor myocardial contractility.

Arterial PP varies depending on the site of measurement. As one moves away from the aorta to peripheral arteries, PP increases due to a rise in systolic pressure and a drop in diastolic pressure.

FACTORS REGULATING ARTERIAL BLOOD PRESSURE

Many organs autoregulate their blood flow to MAP. Autoregulation is the automatic variation of the radius of an arteriole in an organ to regulate local blood flow to meet the oxygen demand of that particular organ. This phenomenon is very prominent in renal, coronary, and cerebral circulation.

Mean arterial pressure is a product of CO and SVR. Factors, that affect either CO or SVR will affect the MAP. The force of ventricular contraction (inotropic state) and ventricular preload determines SV which in turn will affect CO. Ventricular preload is the force acting on ventricular muscles at the end of diastole. Preload is affected by many factors including ventricular compliance, venous return, venous compliance, intrapericardial and intrathoracic pressures, and blood volume. Kidneys are primarily responsible for the regulation of blood volume through its sodium- and water-handling mechanism. HR, inotropy, venous compliance, and renal function are all strongly influenced by neurohumoral mechanisms.

Systemic vascular resistance is determined by the anatomy of the vascular network and vascular diameter. Generally, vascular structure and density remain relatively unchanged over a period of time. Change in vascular diameter is the most common factor affecting SVR in acute settings. Neural factors such as the state of sympathetic nervous system activation; humoral factors such as endothelin, renin-angiotensin, and prostacyclin; and tissue factors such as adenosine, potassium ion, hydrogen ion, and histamine can significantly alter vessel diameter and thus SVR. SVR also gets affected by oxygen and carbon dioxide partial pressures through chemoreceptors.

UNDERSTANDING THE ARTERIAL PULSE WAVEFORM

Windkessel Effect[3,4]

Otto Frank in 1899 described the ascending thoracic aorta as being similar to the Windkessel (literal meaning air chamber or elastic reservoir) whose change in pressure is directly related to its change in volume (difference between LV ejection volume and outflow to peripheral vasculature) and, inversely, to its compliance (lower is the compliance of aorta higher will be the pressure change). The ascending and thoracic aortas are elastic structures that convert the phasic systolic inflow produced by ventricular ejection into a smoother, more continuous outflow to peripheral vessels. With each contraction of LV, blood is ejected into the ascending aorta, which in turn increases pressure. This gives rise to a pressure wave and a flow wave in the ascending aorta. This entire blood flow ejected by LV is not transmitted to the periphery with the BP wave but is partly absorbed by the distensible elastic aorta. As the blood flow ceases on the closure of the aortic valve, the walls of the ascending aorta and arch return back to initial dimensions due to their elastic properties (due to the presence of elastic fibers) maintaining forward flow. Thus, even though LV ejects intermittently, continuous forward flow is maintained. This also dampens large pressure swings and thus has a damping (or cushioning effect) on peripheral circulation. This reservoir property by which blood and potential energy are stored to be used in the later phase and maintain the forward flow of blood during diastole is termed as Windkessel effect **(Flowchart 1 and Fig. 2)**. This is the reason why it is only the ascending aortic pressure and not the peripheral arterial pressure, which ideally should be used to quantitate SV, left ventricular contractility, and SVR. The Windkessel effect diminishes with age as the aorta loses its compliance.

Reflected Wave Phenomenon[4]

Pressure and flow in a vascular tree are created by the periodic ejection of blood by LV in the ascending aorta. However, if one monitors the pressure wave and flow wave in the ascending thoracic aorta, one will realize that the two waveforms are distinctly different from each other. Pressure waves run forth and back toward the heart, with backward waves originating from the reflection of forward waves wherever there is a change in characteristic impedance such as branching sites, large atheromatous plaques, and any other sites of variation in arterial geometry. These reflected waves are similar to surface

Flowchart 1: Factors regulating arterial blood pressure.

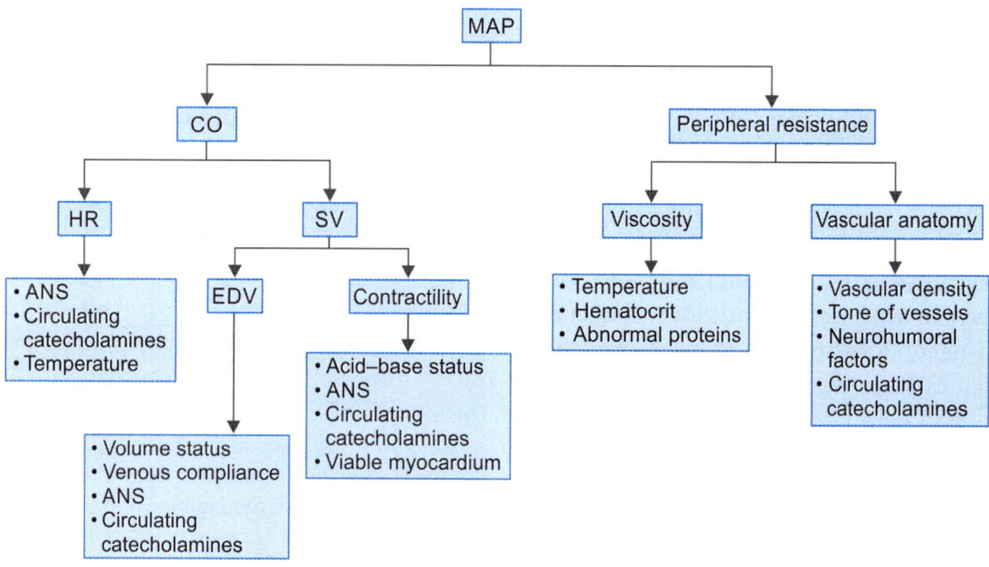

(ANS: autonomic nervous system; CO: cardiac output; EDV: end-diastolic volume; HR: heart rate; MAP: mean arterial pressure; SV: stroke volume)

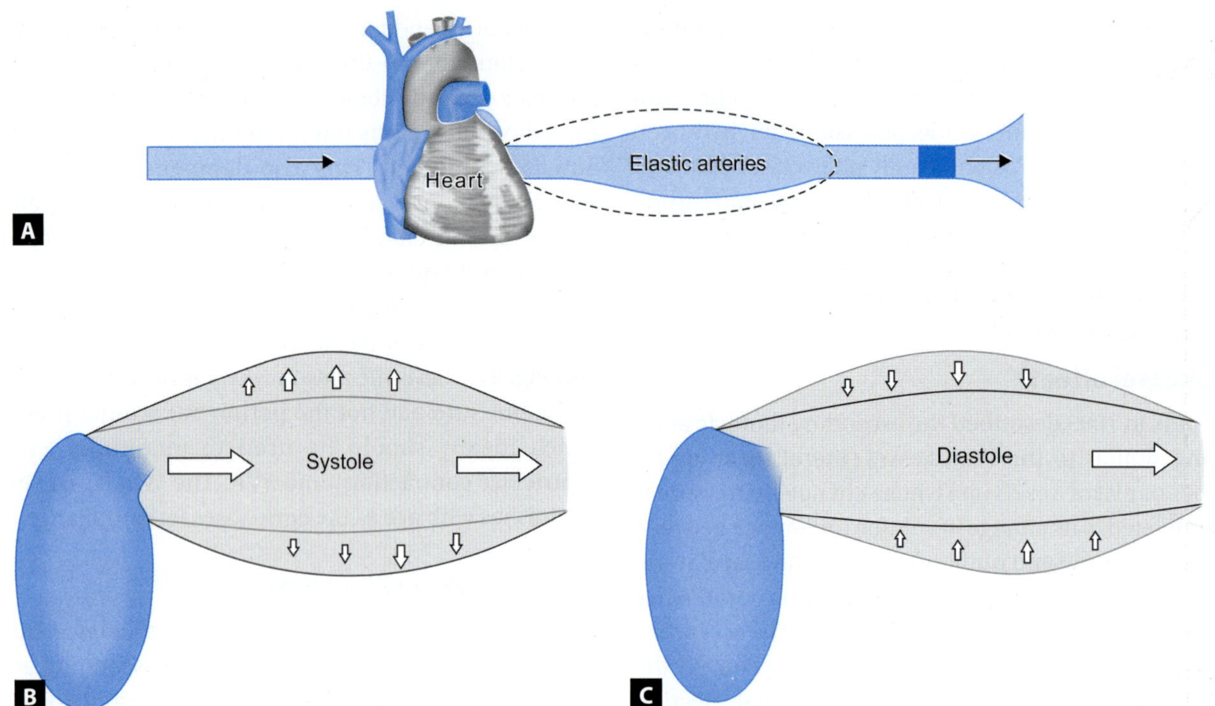

Figs. 2A to C: (A) The concept of Windkessel is applied to the cardiovascular system; (B) In the systolic phase, the aortic elastic fibers store the energy; and (C) In the diastole, this energy is imparted back to the blood in the aorta. This maintains the flow during the diastole in the absence of the left ventricular contractions.

Source: Wikimedia Commons. (2024). Category: CC-BY-SA-3.0. [Online] Available from https://commons. wikimedia.org/w/index. php?curid=31288770 [Last accessed September, 2024].

waves produced by dropping an object in a pool of water which on hitting the edge of the pool gets reflected back adding to the incident wave **(Fig. 3)**.

Murgo in 1980[5] measured input impedance reliably in the clinical cardiac catheterization laboratory and investigated the relationship of impedance to the aortic pressure waveform, with particular attention to reflection phenomena. He described three types of beats based on wave reflection patterns **(Fig. 4)**—the type A beats, related to an arterial system with large reflections, showing a secondary rise in pressure with a tendency toward a larger PP (classically seen in the elderly) and type C beats present in the system with little or more diffuse reflections, showing small secondary rises in pressure and have smaller PPs (mainly seen in young adults). Type B beats are in between type A and type C. In his study, most of the patients had wave reflection points 44–48 cm from the ascending aorta corresponding to the region of the terminal abdominal aorta and bifurcation into the iliac and femoral arteries. Though other investigators have shown that this reflection can occur at many points, probably the region

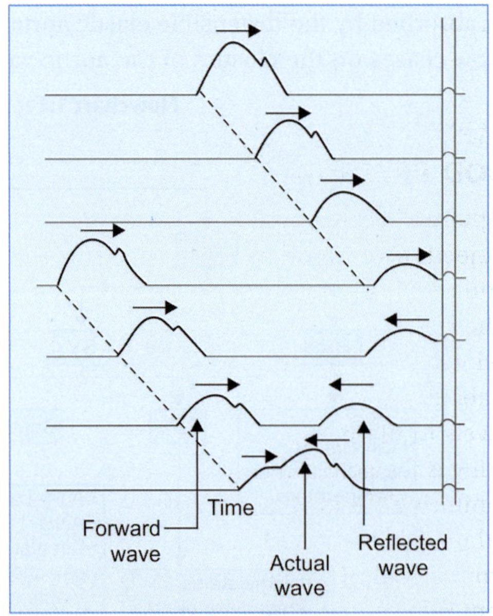

Fig. 3: The wave propagation and the phenomenon of wave reflection.

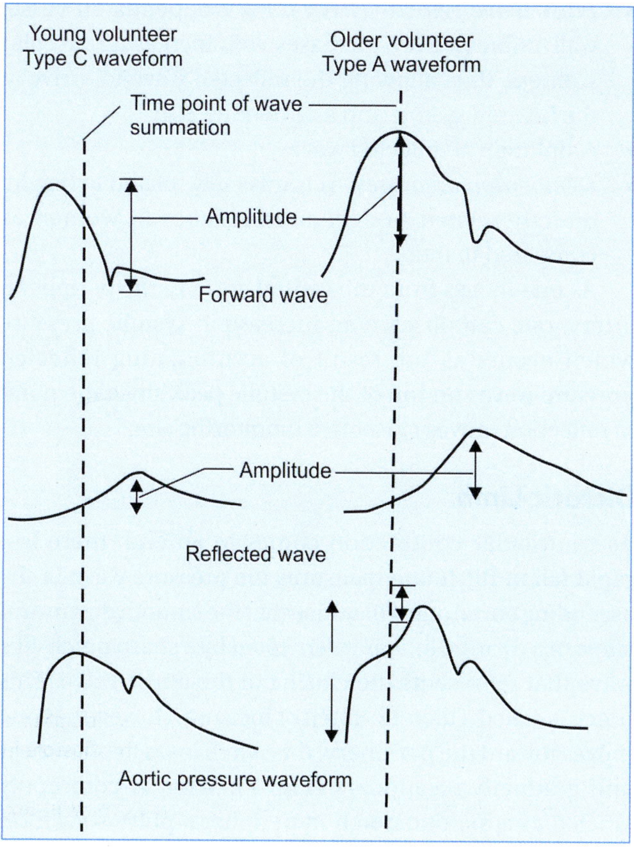

Fig. 4: Types of beats based on wave reflection patterns.

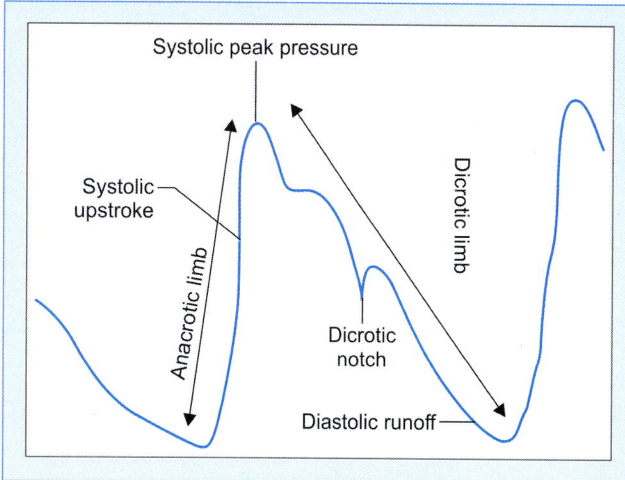

Fig. 5: Components of the normal arterial blood pressure (ABP) waveform.

of the terminal abdominal aorta generates reflections that dominate those arising from other locations in man.

COMPONENTS OF THE NORMAL ARTERIAL BLOOD PRESSURE WAVEFORM

Arterial pulse is created by a shock wave which is initiated by the ejection of blood by LV into the aorta and its interaction with elastic arterial walls. The speed with which these waves travel to the periphery is called pulse wave velocity (PWV) and is not the same everywhere. PWV is about 5 m/s in the ascending aorta and increases as it travels to the periphery. Invasive arterial pressure monitoring is the gold standard for accurately measuring and monitoring BP in real time. This plays a vital role during the assessment and management of shock state. Apart from actual BP values, analysis of waveform gives important information that can guide clinicians during treatment. For this reason, it is important to know the components of waveform and what factors contribute to the formation of waveform. Arterial pressure is the result of an interaction between the heart and the arterial system so the magnitude and shape of the pressure pulse will be affected by changes in the peripheral circulation or alterations in cardiac function.

Systolic Upstroke

This is created due to ventricular contraction and ejection of blood into the aorta. During early systole, LV acts predominantly as a pressure generator. When there is a strong contraction of LV, it will lead to a faster rise of systolic upstroke (pressure rises over time—dp/dt) and thus a steeper slope of the anacrotic limb, provided the aortic valve is normal. As against this, a weak contraction will give rise to a less steep upstroke. Studies have shown that dp/dt in radial artery waveform can be used to diagnose the systolic function of the heart.[6] Though changes in dp/dt can, and frequently do reflect changes in myocardial contractility, one needs to keep in mind that dp/dt is a complex function, subject not only to changes in contractility, but also to ventricular end-diastolic pressure, aortic diastolic pressure, the manner of ventricular activation, and intrinsic adjustments of contractility **(Fig. 5)**.[7]

Peak Systolic Pressure

This is the maximum pressure in the vascular system. The timing of the reflected wave has a strong influence on peak systolic pressure. For the same SV, peak systolic pressure will be lower in someone with compliant blood vessels, as the reflected waves will return back in diastole, augmenting DBP. As against this, with advancing age as vessels become stiffer, PWV increases and reflected waves

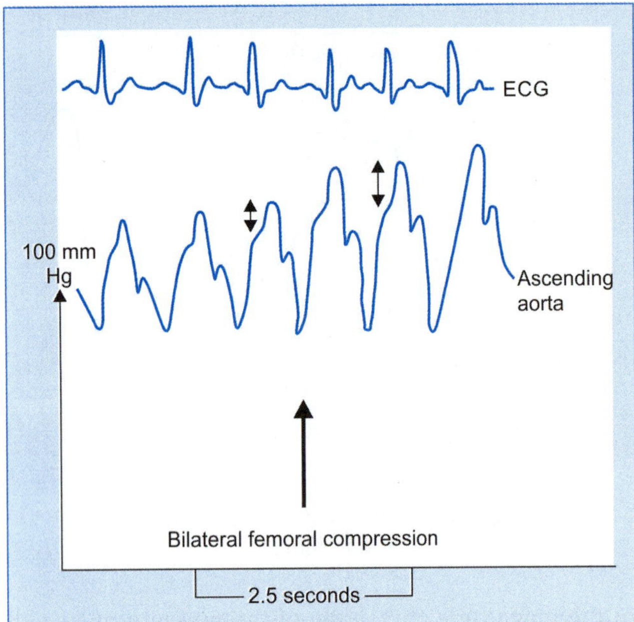

Fig. 6: Effect of vessel occlusion on systolic pressure augmentation.

return in systole, augmenting SBP (i.e., the afterload) and increasing the left ventricular workload. Augmentation index (AI) is defined as the ratio of the amplitude of the reflected wave to that of the forward ejection wave, and it signifies the cardiac load and arterial compliance (or noncompliance). The same augmentation effect can be seen when the major wave reflection point moves more proximally, as shown by Murgo[6] where he occluded both femoral arteries by external manual compression **(Fig. 6)**.

Augmentation Index

Augmentation index (AI) is a measure of systemic arterial stiffness derived from the ascending aortic pressure waveform. Wave reflection from the periphery to the central aorta augments the aortic pressure wave and imposes an excess workload on LV. AI is calculated as the height of the reflected wave as a percentage of the total height of the ascending aortic pressure wave. AI depends on:

- *Length of the cardiac cycle or HR:* This affects pulse wave augmentation by affecting the duration of systole. The slower the HR, the reflected wave is more likely to arrive in systole due to longer systolic time whereas an increase in HR will decrease the absolute duration of systole, effectively shifting the reflected wave into diastole.
- *Pulse wave velocity (PWV):* PWV depends on vessel wall stiffness. PWV increases with increasing vascular stiffness, thus allowing the reflected wave to arrive at the heart in systole and augmenting SBP.
- Amplitude of reflected wave
- *Demographic features:* AI is inversely related to height, directly related to age, and is higher in women as compared to men.

As one moves from the central aorta to the peripheral artery, one can observe an increase in systolic pressure which occurs as the result of accumulating reflected pressure waves on top of the systolic peak since the point of reflection moves closer to a monitoring site.

Dicrotic Limb

As ventricular contraction comes to an end, there is a rapid fall in BP. If one measures the pressure wave in the ascending aorta, one will notice that the smooth downward slope of a dicrotic limb is interrupted by a sharp notch-like wave that represents the closing of the aortic valve. This notch is called a dicrotic notch or incisura. However, as one moves toward the periphery, this notch loses its sharpness and gradually disappears **(Fig. 7)**. What is commonly labeled as a dicrotic notch in peripheral pulse waveform is a reflected wave and its position is related to SVR. One can see progressive delay in systolic upstroke in relation to R wave on ECG on moving further away from the root of the aorta, loss of sharpness and gradual disappearance of a dicrotic notch and change in morphology of arterial pressure waveform.

Area under the systolic portion of arterial pulse wave-systole is created due to ventricular ejection. Thus, a portion of waveform from the end-diastole to the end of the ejection phase (closure of the aortic valve) corresponds to left ventricular ejection. Many modern methods of measuring CO by minimally invasive methods using peripheral arterial waveforms use areas under the systolic portion to derive SV and CO.

Diastolic Run Off

Once the left ventricular contraction ceases, there is no more ejection of blood into the aorta and the BP starts decreasing, giving rise to a downstroke on the arterial waveform. The slope of this down stroke will depend on the resistance offered by peripheral vasculature. With constant SV, changes in peripheral vascular resistance will manifest as changes in the slope of the down stroke of an

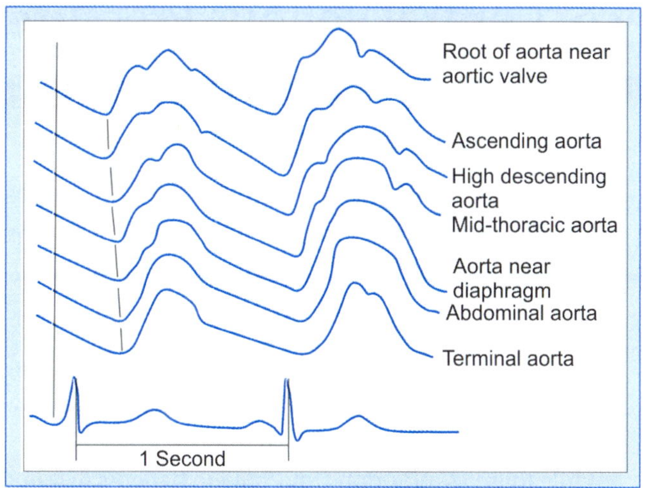

Fig. 7: Pressure waveforms as a function of location from the root of the aorta to the terminal aorta (iliac bifurcation).

arterial waveform. In vasodilatory states, this down stroke will be sharp as against in vasoconstricted states it will be shallow.

INDIRECT VERSUS DIRECT ARTERIAL BLOOD PRESSURE MONITORING

Arterial catheterization for direct measurement of BP is the gold standard. However, it is invasive and carries a risk of serious vascular complications. Factors such as under- or overdamping and end-hole artifact affect direct arterial pressure readings. On the other hand, noninvasive BP monitoring is safer and lacks all complications related to the invasive approach. However, in the present scenario, most noninvasive methods are intermittent. One can monitor noninvasive BP continuously using applanation tonometry but it is not widely available and clinical studies are lacking. In low-flow conditions where accurate beat-to-beat monitoring is crucial, noninvasive methods may yield lower and unreliable pressure readings, than invasive ABP monitoring. Though MAP is closely approximated when oscillometric and direct measurements are compared, more information can be gained from the shape of arterial pressure wave which is of much clinical use. This feature may be of clinical relevance when one wants to monitor CO or for functional hemodynamic monitoring to know volume responsiveness.

CONCLUSION

Arterial blood pressure gets affected by many factors and we can derive lots of information from morphology of arterial pressure wave.

ACKNOWLEDGMENT

We would like to acknowledge Ashwini Vitthalrao Wanjari for her help in drawing figures.

REFERENCES

1. Esper SA, Pinsky MR. Arterial waveform analysis. Best Pract Res Clin Anaesthesiol. 2014;28(4):363-80.
2. Lin JD, Chen YL, Wu CZ, Hsieh CH, Pei D, Liang YJ, et al. Identification of normal blood pressure in different age group. Medicine (Baltimore). 2016;95(14):e3188.
3. Davies JE, Hadjiloizou N, Leibovich D, Malaweera A, Alastruey-Arimon J, Whinnett ZI, et al. Importance of the aortic reservoir in determining the shape of the arterial pressure waveform–the forgotten lessons of Frank. Artery Res. 2007;1(2):40-5.
4. London GM, Pannier B. Arterial functions: how to interpret the complex physiology. Nephrol Dial Transplant. 2010;25(12):3815-23.
5. Murgo JP, Westerhof N, Giolma JP, Altobelli SA. Aortic input impedance in normal man: relationship to pressure wave forms. Circulation. 1980;62(1):105-16.
6. Tartiere JM, Logeart D, Beauvais F, Chavelas C, Kesri L, Tabet JY, et al. Non-invasive radial pulse wave assessment for the evaluation of left ventricular systolic performance in heart failure. Eur J Heart Fail. 2007;9(5):477-83.
7. Wallace AG, Skinner NS, Mitchell JH. Hemodynamic determinants of the maximal rate of rise of left ventricular pressure. Am J Physiol. 1963;205:30-6.

CHAPTER 3

Physiology of Central Venous Pressure and Pulmonary Artery Occlusion Pressure

Nishanth Baliga, Jigeeshu Vasistha Divatia

CENTRAL VENOUS PRESSURE

Central venous pressure (CVP) is the pressure in the thoracic veins near the right atrium and measured relative to atmospheric pressure. CVP is a major determinant of the filling pressure and, therefore, the preload of the right ventricle (RV).

Cardiac output is determined by preload, afterload, and contractility. Preload refers to volume of blood in the ventricle prior to contraction. This volume of blood leads to increase in muscle fiber length, which optimizes the overlapping of actin and myosin elements so that the contact of the cross-bridges are maximized which are the force-generating sites in both cardiac and skeletal muscle. Frank–Starling recognized that the benefit of filling the ventricle was not primarily related to the distending pressure, but rather to the increase in ventricular volume (or myocardial fiber length) during diastole. Hence, preload is the length of a muscle fiber prior to contraction, i.e., the end-diastolic volume of the chamber. Since end-diastolic volume is difficult to measure, pressure within the chamber is measured and equilibrated with volume based on a few assumptions:

- There is a linear relationship between ventricular volume and ventricular pressure during diastole
- This relationship is constant for a given patient (with varying degrees of illness/changes in pathology or physiology) and among different patients
- The left ventricular end-diastolic pressure (LVEDP) correlates well with atrial and CVP assuming there are no atrioventricular (A-V) valvular abnormalities.

Thus, CVP is assumed to closely resemble left atrial pressure (LAP), which in turn is thought to closely reflect left ventricular (LV) diastolic pressure, and is also assumed to correlate well with left ventricular end-diastolic (LVED) volume. Therefore, in healthy patients, CVP is generally considered to reflect LV preload.

While these assumptions may hold in patients without significant physiological abnormalities, they may not apply in critically ill patients.

Cardiac output and right atrial pressure (RAP) result from the interaction between the heart's function and the function of the circuit that returns blood to the heart. Cardiac function is typically represented by a "Starling Curve," which plots cardiac output against preload as estimated by RAP.[1] On the other hand, the venous return curve determines RV preload. The cardiac function curve is influenced by afterload, contractility, heart rate, and preload, while the venous return curve is influenced by stressed vascular volume (the portion of the total vascular volume that generates pressure in the vessels), vascular compliance, resistance to venous return, and RAP.[3] Therefore, RAP is a common factor in both cardiac and return functions, and it is determined by the interaction of these two functions **(Fig. 1)**.[3]

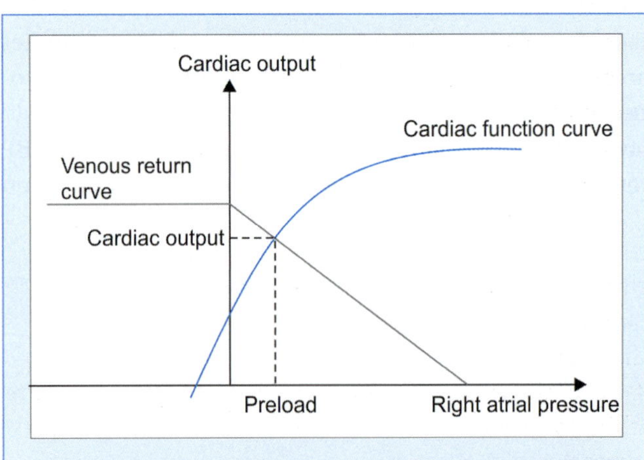

Fig. 1: Cardiac function curve and venous return curve.

MEASUREMENT OF CVP

Central venous pressure is traditionally measured using catheters placed in the large neck veins, such as the subclavian and internal jugular veins, and advanced into the superior vena cava (SVC). The ideal location for the catheter tip is at the junction where the SVC enters the right atrium. CVP can be measured using either a fluid-filled manometer or an electronic pressure transducer. Both methods require setting a reference level, which is defined as the right atrium, taken at the mid-axillary line in the fourth intercostal space, known as the phlebostatic axis.

The CVP waveform has three positive and two negative deflections.

- *"a" wave:* Represents atrial contraction.
- *"c" wave:* Corresponds to the closure of the tricuspid valve and its bowing into the atrium as the ventricle contracts.
- *"x descent":* Indicates atrial relaxation and a change in ventricular geometry.
- *"v" wave:* Represents venous return and atrial filling, occurring while the tricuspid valve is closed.
- *"y descent":* Marks the opening of the tricuspid valve and the subsequent emptying of the atrium.

Due to its location within the thorax, intrathoracic pressure influences central venous pressure and, consequently, CVP readings. In spontaneously breathing patients, intrathoracic pressure decreases during inspiration, resulting in lower CVP, while during expiration, intrathoracic pressure and CVP increase. Conversely, in patients receiving positive pressure ventilation, intrathoracic pressure and CVP increase during inspiration and decrease during expiration. Therefore, CVP measurements should be taken at the end of the expiration phase for both spontaneously breathing and mechanically ventilated patients, as intrathoracic pressure is more stable then, and pleural pressure is closer to atmospheric pressure.[4]

CVP is measured at the level of the "c" wave, which marks the protrusion of the tricuspid valve into the right atrium just before ventricular systole. This pressure corresponds to the right ventricular end-diastolic pressure and aligns with the R wave on an electrocardiogram (ECG). If the "c" waves are not clearly visible, the average pressure at the "a" wave can be used as the CVP value. In cases where the "a" wave is also not discernible, the z point—the pressure corresponding to the end of the QRS complex—should be recorded as the CVP **(Fig. 2)**.[3]

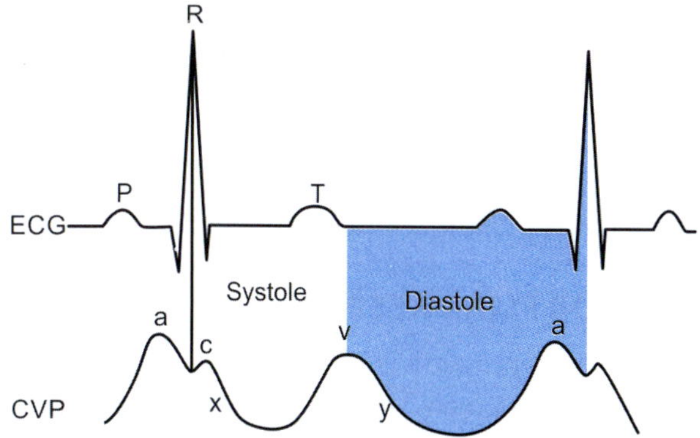

Fig. 2: Normal central venous tracing. (CVP: central venous pressure; ECG: electrocardiogram)

Problems with Measuring CVP

Preload refers to the end-diastolic volume in the ventricle before contraction, which represents the length of the muscle fiber at the end of diastole. The pressure that distends the ventricle is known as transmural pressure, defined as the difference between intraventricular pressure and intrathoracic pressure. Various factors can influence intrathoracic pressures, such as positive end-expiratory pressure (PEEP), increased intra-abdominal pressure, and pericardial or pleural effusions, all of which can affect transmural pressure. Determining the extent of these effects is challenging, making it difficult to accurately assess transmural pressure. It is important to note that CVP measures intravascular pressure, not transmural pressures.

The venous return to the right atrium depends on the pressure gradient between mean systemic filling pressure (MSFP) and intravascular pressure (CVP). MSFP represents the mean pressure that distends elastic vascular structures when the heart ceases to beat, primarily determined by stressed volume. Stressed volume refers to the portion of blood volume that stretches the vessel wall, while unstressed volume is the additional volume that fills the vessel but does not contribute to wall tension.

Research conducted on hypothermic patients in circulatory arrest found that approximately 30% of total blood volume constituted stressed volume, while the remaining 70% was classified as unstressed volume.[5] Unstressed volume can be recruited to sustain MSFP. As such, CVP does not provide information about MSFP or stressed volume. Patients may exhibit normal CVP, mean circulating filling volume, and cardiac output, even when total blood volume is reduced due to an increase in stressed volume and a decrease in unstressed volume. Additionally, a reduction in venous resistance can lead to higher CVP without changing stressed volume, as the venous return curve intersects the cardiac function curve at a higher RAP. Consequently, CVP is not considered an ideal predictor of right ventricular preload.[6]

CVP FOR FLUID RESPONSIVENESS

Central venous pressure is often used in fluid challenges based on the "2–5 rules." In this approach, the initial CVP is measured, and a fluid bolus is administered. If, after 10 minutes, there is no increase in CVP by more than 2 mm Hg, additional fluid boluses are given. However, if the increase in CVP is greater than 5 mm Hg, the fluid bolus is stopped. If the increase falls between 2 and 5 mm Hg, the infusion is halted, and CVP is remeasured after another 10 minutes. If this subsequent measurement indicates an increase of more than 5 mm Hg, the infusion is terminated.

A modified fluid challenge has been developed in which a fixed amount of crystalloid or colloid is infused over 30 minutes, targeting a predefined goal, such as an improvement in mean arterial pressure. CVP is then measured every 10 minutes and serves as a safety limit; the infusion is stopped once the predetermined safety limit is reached.[7]

Numerous studies suggest that CVP is a poor indicator of fluid responsiveness. One trial that investigated the use of CVP and pulmonary artery occlusion pressure (PAOP) as predictors of fluid responsiveness found that baseline CVP values were similar in both responders and non-responders. This indicated that using CVP and PAOP for predicting fluid responsiveness was ineffective.[8]

A systematic review and meta-analysis conducted by Marik et al. further revealed that CVP correlates poorly with intravascular volume, with an area under the receiver operating characteristic curve of only 0.56. The study showed that the CVP and change in CVP (delta CVP) were inadequate in predicting the hemodynamic response to fluid challenges. The authors concluded that CVP should not be used for making clinical decisions regarding fluid administration.[9-11]

Dynamic measures outperform static measures like CVP for prediction of fluid responsiveness and are now recommended in the Surviving Sepsis Campaign guidelines.[12,13]

PULMONARY ARTERY OCCLUSION PRESSURE

Pulmonary artery occlusion pressure is measured using a Swan–Ganz pulmonary artery catheter (PAC). This catheter is inserted into the distal pulmonary artery, with the balloon inflated to obtain a pressure reading. PAOP reflects LAP.

The Swan–Ganz PAC is typically placed in the intensive care unit using a technique called flow-directed balloon flotation, without the need for radiological assistance. The catheter is usually inserted via the internal jugular, subclavian, or femoral vein. The inflated balloon acts like a "sail" that steers the catheter in the direction of blood flow. Continuous monitoring of the pressures at the catheter tip helps guide its positioning within the various cardiac chambers and ensures proper placement in the pulmonary artery **(Fig. 3)**.

As the catheter is advanced from the right atrium and ventricle into the pulmonary artery and its branches, it may occlude a branch of the artery, halting blood flow in the vessel bed that lies between the occluded arterial branch and the venous radicles supplied by that branch. This creates a static column of blood that allows for pressure measurement in the adjacent venous bed where blood flow continues. Since the pulmonary veins do not offer resistance to flow, this pressure can be considered a reasonable estimate of the LAP. If the mitral valve apparatus is functioning normally, it also correlates with left ventricular (LV) diastolic pressures.

Pulmonary artery pressure (PAP) is determined by the flow generated by RV contraction, the resistance

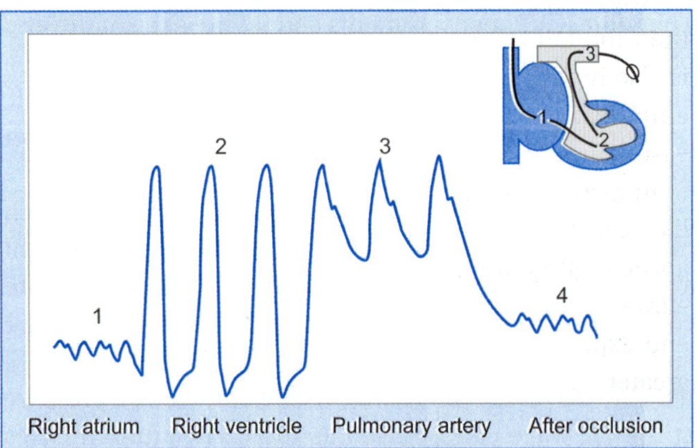

Fig. 3: Pressure tracings during placement of a pulmonary artery catheter.

within the pulmonary vascular bed, and the downstream pulmonary venous pressure. Typically, the pulmonary vasculature operates as a low-resistance, high-volume circuit, which means that the normal pulmonary artery diastolic pressure (PADP) only slightly exceeds PAOP and LAP. Therefore, under normal conditions, PADP serves as a continuous surrogate for left ventricular end-diastolic pressure (LVEDP). However, this relationship may not hold if pulmonary vascular resistance is elevated, in which case the PADP will be significantly higher than the LVEDP. Several assumptions are made during the measurement of PAOP.

PAOP Waveform

The pulmonary artery (PA) occlusion tracing resembles the CVP tracing, but it exhibits a slight delay, with the "a" and "v" waves being more distinguishable than the "c" wave. Due to the dampened nature of the pressure wave, the "c" wave is usually absent. Typically, the "v" wave surpasses the "a" wave in the PA occlusion pressure (PAOP) tracing. When comparing this to the ECG, the onset of the corresponding pressure wave is significantly delayed. The peak of the "a" wave usually occurs after the P wave on the ECG, about 240 ms later, compared to 80 ms in the right atrial tracing. This delay is due to the time it takes for the LAP waveform to travel through the pulmonary veins, capillaries, arterioles, and arteries. Likewise, the peak of the "v" wave follows the T wave on the ECG.

Normally, PAOP equals LAP, which in turn equals LVEDP. However, there are certain conditions in which PAOP may not accurately reflect LVEDP. For example, in instances of mitral stenosis, left atrial obstruction from a myxoma, or mitral regurgitation, the LAP can be higher than the LVEDP, resulting in a PAOP measurement that is also higher. Conversely, conditions such as pulmonary embolism and hypoxemia, which lead to pulmonary vasoconstriction, can cause pulmonary venous pressure to increase, making PAOP greater than LVEDP.[15] In cases like diastolic dysfunction, myocardial infarction, or aortic regurgitation, LVEDP may exceed PAOP. Similarly, elevated intrathoracic pressure, such as with high positive end-expiratory pressure (PEEP), can result in LVEDP being greater than PAOP.[16]

CHALLENGES IN MEASURING PAOP

Despite its usage as an indicator of left ventricular preload, PAOP may not accurately reflect this preload due to various influencing factors. The lung is divided into three physiological zones based on the relationship between the alveolar, pulmonary arterial, and pulmonary venous pressures, known as West's zones.

- Zone 1, located at the lung apex, has alveolar pressure that is higher than both arterial and venous pressures.
- Zone 2, found in the mid-zones of the lung, is characterized by arterial pressure exceeding alveolar pressure, which is greater than pulmonary venous pressure.

Neither Zone 1 nor Zone 2 is ideal for placing a pulmonary artery catheter (PAC) because capillary collapse occurs and there is no static column of blood between the left atrium and the wedged catheter tip. In contrast, Zone 3, typically at the base of the lung, is characterized by alveolar pressure that is lower than both pulmonary arterial and pulmonary venous pressures, allowing for direct pressure transmission from the left atrium to the wedged catheter tip. Zone 3 is the optimal position for measuring PAOP, which is generally achieved when the pulmonary catheter is placed in a supine position.[17]

In situations where alveolar pressure exceeds LAP, PAOP may reflect the alveolar pressure instead of LVEDP. Clinicians can identify these conditions at the bedside if the increase in wedge pressure during respiration exceeds the swings in PADP, as wedge pressure senses airway pressures rather than pleural pressure (Ppl).

Significant changes in Ppl, which occur in both spontaneous and mechanical ventilation, can affect PAOP measurement. Therefore, PAOP should ideally be measured at the end of expiration when physiological changes are minimal. This point is represented by the highest pressure in the tracing during spontaneous breathing and the lowest during positive pressure ventilation. PEEP can also influence Ppl, either through externally applied PEEP or intrinsic PEEP that develops from dynamic hyperinflation. PEEP increases alveolar pressure, which can hinder the static column of blood necessary for PAOP to accurately reflect LAP, or it can elevate transmural pressure, leading to an overestimation of LVEDP. As PEEP rises, PAOP and LVEDP may diverge, resulting in a scenario where PAOP is not a reliable measure of preload.

Direct measurement through the transient interruption of PEEP has been suggested, as the lowest vascular pressures have correlated with true distending pressures. However, temporarily discontinuing PEEP may create hemodynamic artifacts and pose risks to patients.[18] An empirical method aims to adjust for variability in pressure transmission without subjecting patients to the risks associated with the transient loss of PEEP. By measuring the change in airway pressure during ventilation and the fluctuations in vascular pressures within each respiratory cycle, it is possible to calculate the proportion of airway pressure transmitted to vascular structures. This is defined as the Index of Transmission (It), calculated as follows:

Index of transmission (It)

$$= \frac{(\text{End-inspiratory PAOP} - \text{End expiratory PAOP})}{(\text{Plateau pressure} - \text{total PEEP})}$$

The effect of PEEP on end-expiratory vascular pressures would be proportional to this index. Therefore, the Corrected PAOP can be calculated as:

$$\text{Corrected PAOP} = \text{End expiratory PAOP} - (\text{It} \times \text{PEEP})$$

This calculated pressure has shown a strong correlation with the "nadir" PAOP in ventilated patients without intrinsic PEEP, and it is believed to be an adequate measurement even in patients exhibiting intrinsic PEEP.[19]

PAOP for Fluid Responsiveness

Research examining the use of PAOP as a predictor for fluid responsiveness has revealed that PAOP measured before a volume challenge does not significantly differ between responders and nonresponders. Additionally, it does not correlate with the changes in cardiac index induced by volume expansion. The studies concluded that no specific value of RAP or PAOP could reliably predict whether a patient would experience an increase in stroke volume.

Moreover, studies comparing dynamic measures—such as stroke volume variation, pulse pressure variation, and respiratory variations in aortic blood velocity—with static measures like CVP, PAOP, Right Ventricular End-Diastolic Volume (RVEDV), and Left Ventricular End-Diastolic Area (LVEDA) found that the dynamic parameters were more effective at predicting fluid responsiveness than the static measures. Therefore, PAOP has limited utility in predicting fluid responsiveness in critically ill patients.[20]

PULMONARY CAPILLARY PRESSURE

It is important to note that PAOP is not the same as pulmonary capillary pressure. Pulmonary capillary pressure can be estimated from the pulmonary artery (PA) tracing at the moment of occlusion. Flow through the pulmonary vasculature consists of two dynamic components: first, flow from a proximal pulmonary arterial capacitance system into a pulmonary capillary capacitance system across an arterial resistance; second, flow through a pulmonary venous resistance into the pulmonary venous capacitance system. The pressure in the venous system is reflected as PAOP. This measurement often displays an inflection point that indicates pulmonary capillary pressure, typically occurring two-thirds of the way between pulmonary diastolic pressure and PAOP, as approximately two-thirds of the pulmonary vascular resistance occurs in the arteries.[21]

Estimating Pulmonary Capillary Pressure at the Bedside

Pulmonary capillary pressure can be visually observed while monitoring the PAP tracing with the balloon inflated. To mitigate the effects of intrathoracic pressures and volumes in patients who are mechanically ventilated, it is advisable to perform an expiratory hold maneuver. During balloon inflation, one may notice an initial rapid decline in pressure that subsequently slows as it approaches PAOP. Drawing a tangent at the point where this change occurs—from a rapid to a slower decrease—will help denote the likely pulmonary capillary pressure.

The pulmonary capillary pressure can be calculated as: Pcap = PAOP + 0.4 (PAP – PAOP) where Pcap is pulmonary capillary pressure, PAP is the mean pulmonary artery pressure, and PAOP is the pulmonary artery occlusion pressure.

Physiological Relevance of Pulmonary Capillary Pressure

Pulmonary capillary pressure plays a crucial role in determining fluid movement across the capillary wall and the formation of lung edema. Under normal conditions, some fluid and protein are filtered through the capillary into the pulmonary interstitium and subsequently drained into the systemic circulation by the lung lymphatics. When the capacity of the lung lymphatics is surpassed, interstitial and, eventually, alveolar edema can occur. The rate of fluid filtration from the capillary to the interstitium can be estimated by the Starling equation:

$$\text{Fluid efflux} = \text{Kfc} \times [(P_{\text{capillary}} - P_{\text{interstitium}})] - \text{Kd}\,[(\pi_{\text{capillary}} - \pi_{\text{interstitium}})]/[(\pi_{\text{capillary}} - \pi_{\text{interstitium}})]$$

Where P = hydrostatic pressure, π = oncotic pressure, Kfc = capillary filtration coefficient (product of capillary wall hydraulic conductivity and capillary surface area), and

Kd = reflection coefficient (values from 0–1; 0 = capillary freely permeable to proteins, 1 = capillary impermeability to proteins). Whenever there is an increase in the fluid efflux, the lymph flow simultaneously increases leading to washing out of proteins in the interstitium causing a decrease in oncotic pressure in the compartment. This leads to an increase in the oncotic gradient making interstitial fluid flow back into the blood and preventing edema formation. With an increase in permeability of the capillary endothelium to protein, there is decreased Kd (π capillary – π interstitium) leading to loss of protein.

It is essential to remember that any increase in pulmonary capillary pressure will cause fluid to move into the interstitium, regardless of the oncotic pressure gradient. Under normal capillary permeability, a higher capillary pressure will be necessary for tissue edema to form. Conversely, when permeability increases, edema may develop at lower pulmonary capillary pressures.[22,23]

CLINICAL UTILITY OF PAOP

Pulmonary artery occlusion pressure values lower than 18–20 mm Hg suggest a nonhydrostatic cause for interstitial edema. PAOP may be lower than 18–20 mm Hg in a patient with hydrostatic edema if either the PAOP increase had been transient, or if pulmonary capillary pressure significantly exceeds PAOP. In acute respiratory distress syndrome, (ARDS), once pulmonary vascular obliteration occurs, pulmonary capillary pressure often exceeds PAOP by a considerable amount because pulmonary venous resistance increases. Thus, some "low pressure" pulmonary edema characterized by low PAOP values in a hyperdynamic state may actually reflect hydrostatic pulmonary edema.

Conversely, PAOP may exceed 18–20 mm Hg in the absence of hydrostatic pulmonary edema, as any increase in pulmonary pressure (Ppl) raises the measured PAOP, potentially due to either intrinsic or extrinsic PEEP or active expiratory muscle contraction.

REFERENCES

1. Braunwald, E, Frahm C, Ross J. Studies on Starling's law of the heart. V. Left ventricular function in man. J Clin Invest. 1961;40(10):1882-90.
2. Beard DA, Feigl EO. Understanding Guyton's venous return curves. Am J Physiol Heart Circ Physiol. 2011;301(3):H629-33.
3. Magder S. Central venous pressure: A useful but not so simple measurement. Crit Care Med. 2006;34(8):2224-7.
4. Izakovic M. Central venous pressure-evaluation, interpretation, clinical implications. Bratisl Lek Listy. 2008:109(4):185-7.
5. Magder S, De Varennes B. Clinical death and the measurement of stressed vascular volume. Crit Care Med. 1998;26(6):1061-4.
6. Michard F, Alaya S, Zarka V, Bahloul M, Richard C, Teboul JL. Global end-diastolic volume as an indicator of cardiac preload in patients with septic shock. Chest. 2003;124(5):1900-8.
7. Vincent JL, Weil MH. Fluid challenge revisited. Crit Care Med. 2006;34(5):1333-7.
8. Osman D, Ridel C, Ray P, Monnet X, Anguel N, Richard C, et al. Cardiac filling pressures are not appropriate to predict hemodynamic response to volume challenge. Crit Care Med. 2007;35(1):64-8.
9. Marik PE, Baram M, Vahid B. Does central venous pressure predict fluid responsiveness? A systematic review of the literature and the tale of seven mares. Chest. 2008;134(1):172-8.
10. Marik PE, Cavallazzi R. Does the central venous pressure predict fluid responsiveness? An updated meta-analysis and a plea for some common sense. Crit Care Med. 2013;41(7):1774-81.
11. De Backer D, Vincent JL. Should we measure the central venous pressure to guide fluid management? Ten answers to 10 questions. Crit Care. 2018;22(1):43.
12. Rhodes A, Evans LE, Alhazzani W, Levy MM, Antonelli M, Ferrer R, et al. Surviving sepsis campaign: International Guidelines for Management of Sepsis and Septic Shock: 2016. Intensive Care Med. 2017;43(3):304-77.
13. Marik PE, Cavallazzi R, Vasu T, Hirani A. Dynamic changes in arterial waveform derived variables and fluid responsiveness in mechanically ventilated patients. A systematic review of the literature. Crit Care Med. 2009;37(9):2642-7.
14. O'Quin R, Marini JJ. Pulmonary artery occlusion pressure: clinical physiology, measurement, and interpretation. Am Rev Respir Dis. 1983;128(8):319-26.
15. Robin E, Costecalde M, Lebuffe G, Vallet B. Clinical relevance of data from the pulmonary artery catheter. Crit Care. 2006;10(Suppl 3):S3.
16. Pinsky MR. Pulmonary artery occlusion pressure. Intensive Care Med. 2003;29(1):19-22.
17. Silverman HJ, Eppler HJ, Pitman AP, Patz D. Pulmonary capillary wedge pressure measurements in patients on assisted ventilation. J Crit Care. 1987;2:115-20.
18. Pinsky M, Vincent JL, De Smet JM. Estimating left ventricular filling pressure during positive end-expiratory pressure in humans. Am Rev Respir Dis. 1991;143(1):25-31.

19. Teboul JL, PinskyMR, Mercat A, Anguel N, Bernardin G, Achard JM, et al. Estimating cardiac filling pressure in mechanically ventilated patients with hyperinflation. Crit Care Med. 2000;28(11):3631-6.
20. Michard F, Boussat S, Chemla D, Anguel N, Mercat A, Lecarpentier Y, et al. Relation between respiratory changes in arterial pulse pressure and fluid responsiveness in septic patients with acute circulatory failure. Am J Respir Crit Care Med. 2000;162(1):134-8.
21. Cope DK, Allison RC, Parmentier JL, Miller JN, Taylor AE. Measurement of effective pulmonary capillary pressure using the pressure profile after pulmonary artery occlusion. Crit Care Med. 1986;14(1):16-22.
22. Cope DK, Grimbert F, Downey JM, Taylor AE. Pulmonary capillary pressure: a review. Crit Care Med. 1992;20(7):1043-56.
23. Takala J. Pulmonary capillary pressure. In: Pinsky MR, Brochard L, Mancebo J (Eds). Applied Physiology in Intensive Care Medicine, 1st edition. Berlin, Heidelberg: Springer; 2006.

CHAPTER

Heart–Lung Interactions in the Critically Ill

Jacob George Pulinilkunnathil, Amol Trimbakrao Kothekar, Atul Prabhakar Kulkarni

INTRODUCTION

Both the respiratory and circulatory systems work in tandem to achieve optimal tissue oxygenation through the processes of ventilation and blood circulation to and from the heart and peripheral tissues. The physiology of the heart and lungs is interdependent due to their shared location in the thorax. The functions of both systems influence each other and are also affected by the changes in the intrathoracic pressure (ITP) and volume, a phenomenon known as heart–lung interactions. These interactions can be further altered or magnified by positive-pressure ventilation in the critically ill.

GLOSSARY OF TERMS

Preload: The passive stress at the end of diastole in the left ventricle (LV) is known as preload. This is influenced by the end-diastolic filling pressure and the net end-diastolic volume as described by the Laplace–Young formula: σ = Pressure × Radius/2 × Thickness of left ventricle.[1]

Afterload: Afterload is the total myocardial stress experienced during the ejection of stroke volume. Similar to preload, the afterload is determined to by the left ventricular systolic pressure, the left ventricular systolic radius, and wall thickness. It is distinct from systemic vascular resistance which reflects the vasomotor tone of the circulation.

Heart–lung interaction: This refers to the complex interactions between cardiovascular and respiratory physiology resulting from phasic changes in intrathoracic pressure (ITP) during respiration.

Transmural pressure: The distending pressure of a chamber is called transmural pressure. It is calculated as the difference between internal expanding forces and the external collapsing forces. For example, in the LV, the pressure around the heart (pericardial pressure) is generally considered equivalent to the pleural pressure, except in cases of pericardial diseases, where there is a significant difference between the pleural and pericardial pressure. The transmural pressure of the LV is calculated as left ventricular intracavitary pressure minus pericardial pressure. Similarly, the transmural pressure of the alveoli is known as transpulmonary pressure.

Mean systemic filling pressure (MSFP): MSFP is the mean pressure in the central circulation when there is no blood flow. It is related to the effective blood volume, compliance of blood vessels, and the pressure exerted by the blood volume on the vasculature. The normal mean systemic pressure is around 7 mm Hg and is highly sensitive to changes in blood volume.[2-4] Within physiological limits, the MSFP-blood volume relationship can be depicted as a linear curve.

Ventricular interdependence: Ventricular interdependence refers to the physiological state where the function of one ventricle is affected by the dynamic changes in the other ventricle due to sharing of interventricular septum, and pericardium (ventricular interdependence in parallel), and by the variations in the preload and afterload (ventricular interdependence in series).

Stressed circulatory volume: The circulatory system behaves more like a water-filled balloon than a water-filled pot. Blood in the circulatory system exerts some pressure on vessel walls as its volume of the blood exceeds the capacity of the circulatory system to accommodate the blood without stretching. Approximately 60% of the blood volume can be easily accommodated in the circulatory system without causing vessel stretch; this is called the *unstressed* volume. Once this volume is exceeded, any further increase in volume begins to stretch the vessel walls, resulting in what is known as the stressed volume. Approximately 40% of blood volume constitutes the

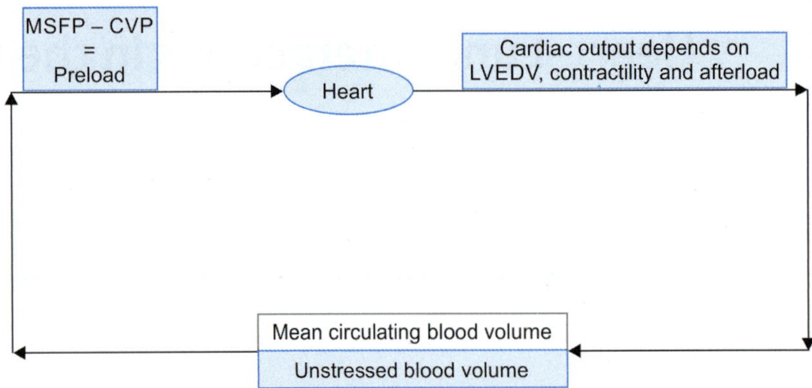

Fig. 1: Simplified overview of the circulatory system. (CVP: central venous pressure; LVEDV: end diastolic volume of left ventricle; MSFP: mean systemic filling pressure)

stressed volume. This portion of the blood volume is hemodynamically active, contributing to the pressure generated on the vessel walls. If pressure is measured throughout the circulatory system in a steady state (no-flow state), the resulting pressure is called MSFP (P_{MSFP}). Because most of the blood volume is occupied in the low-pressure venous system, P_{MSFP} is much closer to central venous pressure than to arterial pressure.

OVERVIEW OF THE CIRCULATORY SYSTEM

The primary function of the heart is to receive venous blood flow on the atrial side and eject as stroke volume from the ventricular side. Therefore, the cardiovascular system can thus be viewed as a simple conduit through which blood circulates throughout the body **(Fig. 1)**.

Physiology of Venous Return

The gradient between the mean systemic filling pressure (P_{MSFP}) and the central venous pressure (CVP) [right atrial pressure (RAP)] creates the driving pressure for return of blood from the venous part of circulation to the right heart, a process known as the venous return.

Physiology of Ejection of Stroke Volume

The amount of blood pumped from the left ventricle (LV) depends on three key factors: (1) The stretch on the resting LV, i.e., the end diastolic volume of left ventricle (LVEDV), known as preload; (2) the intrinsic ability of the cardiac muscles to contract, known as contractility of the heart; and (3) the resistance against which the heart must pump blood into the circulatory system, known as afterload.

A more complex model of circulation is shown in **Figure 2**. It depicts both ventricles encased by the pericardium and sharing the pleural cavity along with the lungs. The pulmonary circulation is further divided into intra-alveolar and extra-alveolar vessels, which respond in opposite ways to alveolar distension **(Fig. 3)**, resulting in changes in the pulmonary vascular resistance (PVR). The systemic circulation comprises two components: the vessels in the abdomen, which are influenced by the abdominal pressure (P_{ab}), and vessels outside the abdomen. The resistance to venous return is the sum of the individual venous resistances offered by these two vascular beds. The autonomic nervous system, which controls the systemic vascular resistance, arterial compliance, and cardiac contractility, has the overall control over the entire circulatory system.

Physiology of Heart–Lung Interaction

During respiration, cyclic changes in ITP are transmitted to the heart and the circulating blood volume. The movement of the diaphragm further alters intra-abdominal venous capacitance, influencing venous return. These physiological changes occur during both spontaneous and controlled ventilation.

DETERMINANTS OF HEART–LUNG INTERACTION

The magnitude of heart–lung interactions depends primarily on four simultaneous factors:

1. The effect of phasic variations in ITP on the larger vessels and cardiac chambers.
2. The impact of changes in lung volume on pulmonary circulation.

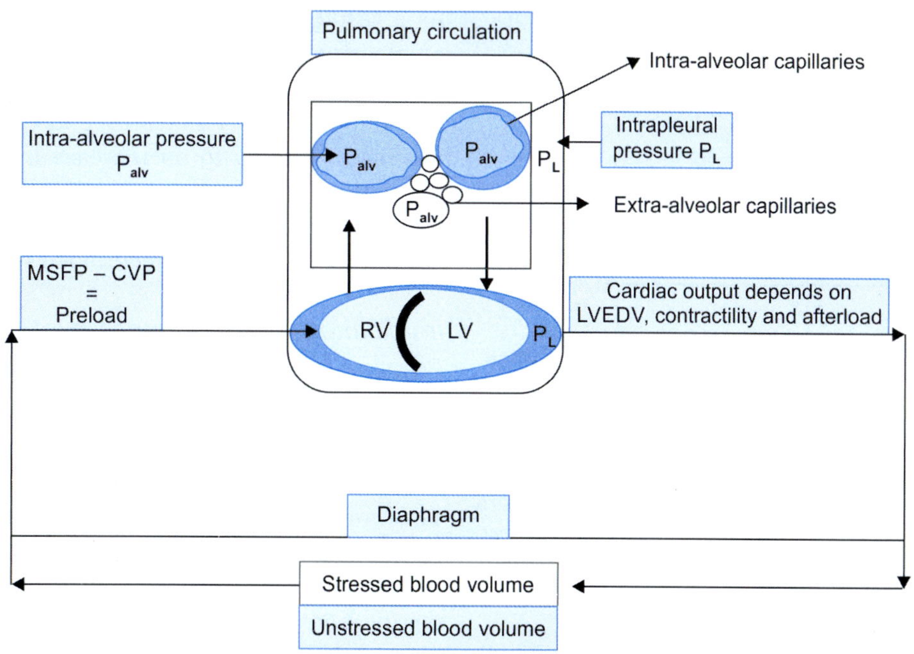

Fig. 2: A complex view of circulation. (CVP: central venous pressure; LV: left ventricle; LVEDV: end diastolic volume of left ventricle; MSFP: mean systemic filling pressure; RV: right ventricle)

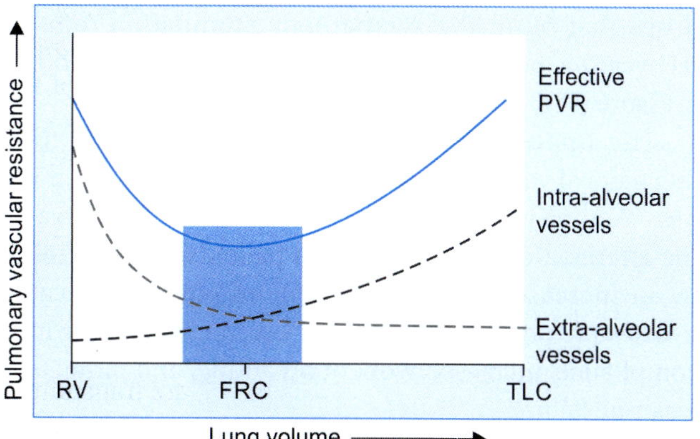

Fig. 3: Effect of lung volumes on extra-alveolar, intra-alveolar blood vessels, and the net PVR. (FRC: functional residual capacity; PVR: pulmonary vascular resistance; RV: right ventricle; TLC: total lung capacity)

3. Alterations due to ventricular interdependence, both in series and in parallel.
4. The effect of changes in intra-abdominal pressure, caused by diaphragm displacement, on the abdominal vessels.

The overall impact of heart–lung interactions is influenced by several factors, including intravascular blood volume, the intrinsic ability of the cardiac muscles to generate contraction in response to the changing preload, heart contractility, end-expiratory lung volume, lung compliance, and sympathetic stimulation. Each of these factors is explained in detail here.

Effects of Changes in Intrathoracic Pressure on Venous Return and Ventricular Function

Effect of Intrathoracic Pressure on Venous Return and Preload of the Ventricles

As explained by the Guytonian principle of venous return, venous return is considered a passive process that depends on the pressure gradient between P_{MSFP} and the CVP or RAP. Under normal physiological conditions, spontaneous respiration causes a reduction in ITP, leading to an increase in the MSFP–CVP gradient. This results in an increase in both venous return and right ventricle (RV) preload, subsequently enhancing RV output. Venous return continues to increase as ITP decreases until it falls below atmospheric pressure. However, at further subatmospheric pressures, there is no further significant increase in venous return due to the collapse of the great veins at their entry point into the thorax. The opposite occurs with positive-pressure ventilation. Any increase in ITP is transmitted to the right atrium, raising the RAP. This

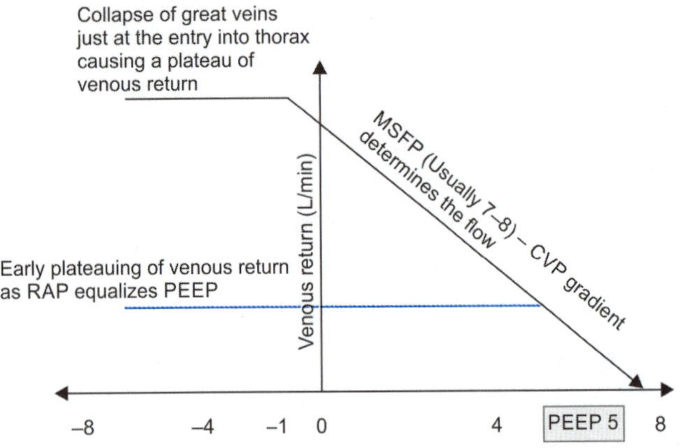

Fig. 4: The relationship between RAP, P_{MSFP}–RAP gradient, venous return, and expected graph of reduced venous return with addition of PEEP. (CVP: central venous pressure; MSFP: mean systemic filling pressure; PEEP: positive end-expiratory pressure; RAP: right atrial pressure)

reduces the gradient between the P_{MSFP} and the CVP or RAP, reduces resulting in a decreased venous return and a reduced right-sided cardiac output **(Fig. 4)**.

Effect of Intrathoracic Pressure on Ventricular Afterload

The transmural pressure (P_{tm}), which is the distending force of a cardiac chamber, is the difference between the pressure inside the cardiac chamber (intramural pressure: $P_{intramural}$) and the surrounding pressure [pericardial pressure (P_{pc}) and pleural pressure (P_{pl})]. Since measuring P_{pc} is challenging in clinical practice, intrapleural pressure is typically used as its surrogate in the absence of pericardial disease.

The P_{tm} is a key determinant of the afterload and, consequently, of ventricular function. In spontaneously breathing patients, as the intrapleural pressure becomes negative, the P_{tm} is calculated as:

$$P_{tm} = P_{intramural} - (-P_{pleural}), \text{ thus, } P_{tm} = P_{intramural} + P_{pleural}$$

Therefore, in spontaneously breathing patients, the P_{tm} increases, resulting in an increase in the LV afterload and decrease in ventricular function.

In contrast, positive-pressure ventilation increases the P_{pl} and application of positive pressure reduces the P_{tm} and the afterload for LV.

$$P_{tm} = P_{intramural} - P_{pleural}$$

As a result, positive-pressure ventilation reduces the afterload of LV and facilitates the function of LV.

To sum up, during spontaneous breathing, the venous return to right heart increases, and the LV afterload also increases, leading to an increase in blood volume in the thorax. Conversely, application of positive pressure reduces the venous return and augments the LV outflow, thereby reducing intrathoracic blood volume.

Implications of the Changes in Intrathoracic Pressure on Heart–Lung Interactions

Initiating positive-pressure ventilation causes a decrease in venous return due to an increase in ITP, leading to hypotension and reduced cardiac output. The normal compensatory response to hypotension involves increased sympathetic stimulation, resulting in tachycardia and vasoconstriction. Vasoconstriction helps recruit more blood from the unstressed volume into the hemodynamically active pool of stressed circulating blood volume, while tachycardia helps maintain the cardiac output. However, if the patient is hypovolemic, the additional blood recruited will be minimal, leading to a further drop in cardiac output. Similarly, administering drugs that blunt the sympathetic stimulation reduces tachycardia, potentially causing a precipitous fall in blood pressure **(Fig. 5)**.

The opposite effects occur during weaning from mechanical ventilation. During weaning, the reduced ITP increases the venous return to the heart and also increases the afterload of LV. In vulnerable patients, this can result in an increased intrathoracic blood volume, elevated hydrostatic pressure, pulmonary edema, worsening lung compliance, increased work of breathing, and ultimately, weaning failure.

Hemodynamic Effects Due to Changes in Lung Volume

Changes Due to a Change in Autonomic Tone

Lung inflation with normal tidal volumes exerts a vagolytic effect, resulting in tachycardia (sinus arrhythmia). However, if the lungs are inflated with a volume exceeding 10 mL/kg, it can lead to bradycardia and vasodilation. Positive-pressure ventilation can also increase prostaglandin synthesis while reducing atrial natriuretic peptide (ANP) synthesis, leading to weight gain due to salt and water retention.[5]

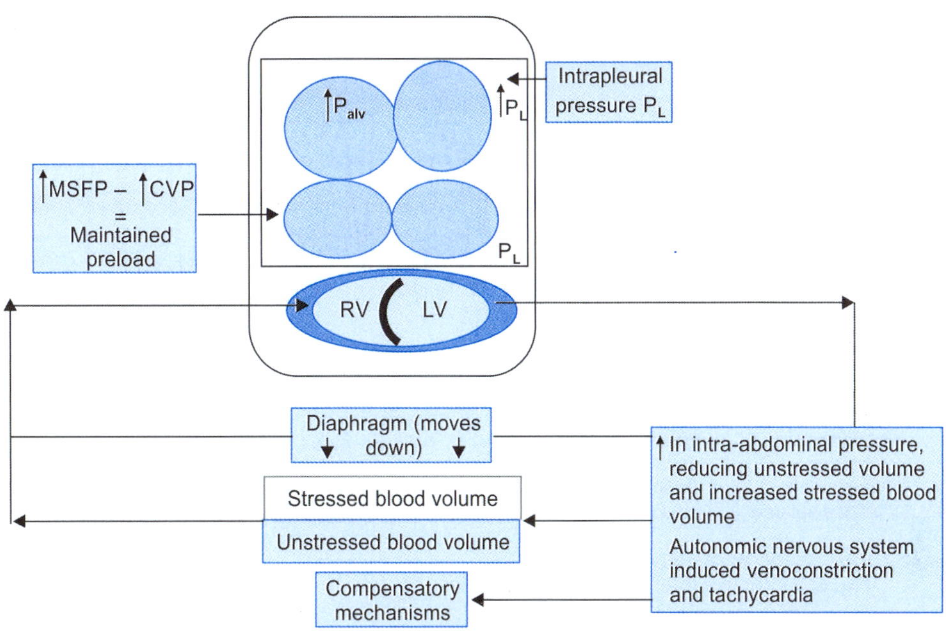

Fig. 5: Compensatory mechanisms to prevent hypotension during initiation of positive-pressure ventilation. (CVP: central venous pressure; LV: left ventricle; MSFP: mean systemic filling pressure; RV: right ventricle)

Effects of Changes in Lung Volume on Cardiovascular System

During positive-pressure ventilation, as the lungs expand, the pulmonary vessels are compressed, leading to a transient increase in blood volume entering the left atrium. However, this effect on preload is short-lived and is overshadowed by the impact of positive ITP on venous return, which results in a reduced preload to both atria.

Another clinically significant effect of lung inflation is the compression of the heart in the cardiac fossa, which reduces the diastolic compliance of the heart. This effect is proportional to the increase in the mean airway pressure and is significantly enhanced during ventilation with high positive end-expiratory pressure (PEEP) and recruitment maneuvers.[6]

Effects of Changes in Lung Volume on Pulmonary Vascular Resistance

The RV afterload is primarily determined by pulmonary vascular resistance (PVR). Increases in PVR can occur due to hyperinflation alveolar collapse. Therefore, it is essential to avoid high airway pressures and prevent alveolar collapse by using optimal PEEP **(Fig. 3)**.

In summary, during positive-pressure ventilation, the changes in lung volume can lead to sinus tachycardia, atrial natriuretic peptide (ANP) secretion (resulting in salt and water retention), and a reduction in end-diastolic compliance. Depending on the functional residual capacity, the RV function may either improve or deteriorate. Recognizing the causes of edema and weight gain in mechanically ventilated patients is crucial, as is selecting optimal PEEP to facilitate optimal biventricular function.

Hemodynamic Effects Due to Ventricular Interdependence

Both ventricles are connected in series through the pulmonary circulation in series and are also enclosed together within a thick fibrous pericardium. As a result, they exhibit interdependence through both series and parallel mechanisms.

Ventricular Interdependence Due to the Series Effect

During positive-pressure ventilation, inspiration leads to a reduction in RV preload and RV stroke volume, which is reflected as a reduced LV preload after a delay of three heartbeats (due to transit time through the pulmonary circulation). Simultaneously, LV experiences a transient increase in preload due to squeezing of the intra-alveolar vessels, and a reduction in afterload resulting in an increased stroke volume. After three to four heartbeats as the decreased RV stroke volume reaches the LV, the LV

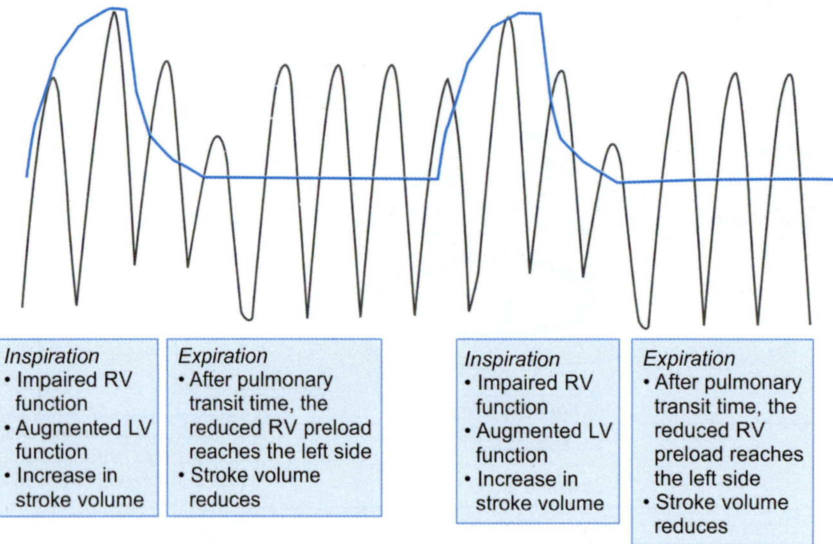

Fig. 6: Ventricular interdependence (in series). (LV: left ventricle; RV: right ventricle)

output transiently reduces.[7] These phasic variations in LV stroke volume, in the absence of RV failure, signify that LV is operating on the steep portion of Frank–Starling curve. These variations can be directly measured as stroke volume variation (SVV) or through its surrogates such as systolic pressure variation (SPV) and pulse pressure variation (PPV). These parameters help to identify patients who are preload dependent **(Fig. 6)**. It is important to recognize that these phasic variations in the LV stroke volume can also occur in presence of right ventricular failure, and even in volume overload, where fluid expansion may be detrimental in both these conditions.

Ventricular Interdependence (in Parallel)

The left heart operates as a high-pressure system as compared to the right heart, with the septum typically bulging toward the RV. In cases of a rapid increase in volume or pressure within the right-sided circulation, the RV dilates to accommodate these changes. However, the outward dilatation is limited by the pericardium and further dilatation causes the septum to shift toward the LV, reducing its filling volume resulting in decreased LV preload and stroke volume **(Fig. 7)**.

In summary, both ventricles are interconnected in series and in parallel. Therefore, a reduction in the preload on the right side will eventually affect the preload on the left side. Due to this parallel interdependence, acute RV failure or a noncompliant pericardium can impair LV function and potentially precipitate LV failure.

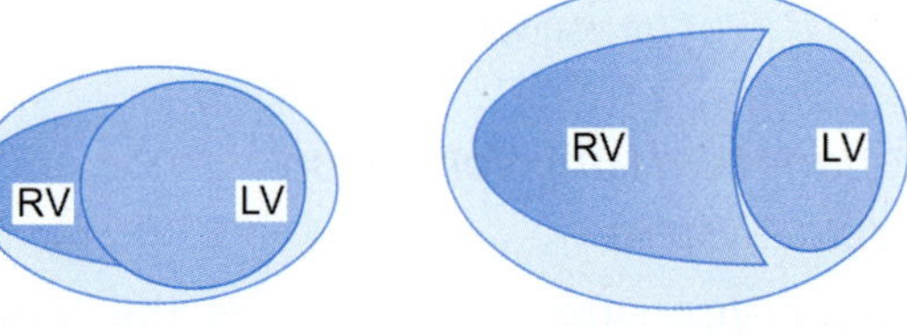

Fig. 7: Ventricular interdependence (in parallel). (LV: left ventricle; RV: right ventricle)

Hemodynamic Changes Due to Diaphragmatic Displacement

As mentioned earlier, positive-pressure ventilation results in a reduction in venous return. The effect of reduced venous return is mitigated by the simultaneous downward movement of the diaphragm and compensatory sympathetic stimulation. Due to the caudal displacement of the diaphragm, the intra-abdominal pressure increases, resulting in compression of the splanchnic circulation. If intravascular pressure exceeds intra-abdominal pressure, the venous return will increase, maintaining the mean circulating volume. If the intra-abdominal pressure exceeds intravascular pressure (as in cases of severe hypovolemia), the veins will collapse, causing a reduction in venous return and effective circulating volume.[8]

UNDERSTANDING THE PHYSIOLOGICAL ASPECTS OF HEART–LUNG INTERACTION

Pulsus Paradoxus and Reverse Pulsus Paradoxus

Pulsus paradoxus is a normal physiological phenomenon that occurs due to ventricular interdependence. In normal subjects during quiet breathing, inspiration causes an increase in venous return to the right side of heart. On the left side, the preload decreases due to the combined effect of pooling of blood in the pulmonary vasculature, which reduces LV preload, reduction in diastole due to sinus tachycardia, and due to the phenomenon of ventricular interdependence in parallel. Simultaneously, the afterload of the LV also increases and the net effect is a drop in stroke volume, which is manifested as a drop in systolic blood pressure. Among all the factors mentioned in the earlier text, in normal subjects, the effect of ventricular interdependence in parallel is least likely to contribute to the drop in stroke volume, in the absence of any restrictive pericardial disease. The mechanism of pulsus paradoxus varies according to the underlying conditions, such as status asthmaticus or pericardial diseases **(Table 1)**.[9]

The converse of pulsus paradoxus occurs with positive-pressure ventilation in patients with relative hypervolemia or LV failure. The reduction in left ventricular afterload results in an augmentation of the left ventricular function, which is manifested as an increase in systolic pressure during inspiration, followed by a decrease in systolic pressure during expiration. This is called reverse pulsus paradoxus or respirator paradox.[10]

Kussmaul Sign

As mentioned earlier, during spontaneous breathing, inspiration is associated with an increase in venous return due to a drop in the ITP. The right ventricular outflow need to match the increase in the venous inflow to maintain normal CVP and RAP. In conditions of poor RV compliance (RV failure/RV infarction) or in conditions of increased RV afterload (pulmonary embolism), the RV outflow will be impaired and the increase in venous return will be transmitted to the great veins as an increase in CVP. This paradoxical increase in CVP during inspiration is called Kussmaul sign.[11]

Negative Pressure Pulmonary Edema

A sustained negative ITP, as seen during inspiration against a closed glottis (Müller maneuver), results in a significant rise in the venous return to the right side of the heart. Simultaneously, as the P_{tm} and afterload of LV increases, left ventricular stroke volume decreases. This combination of increased venous pooling in the thorax combined with reduced left ventricular stroke volume raises the hydrostatic pressure in the pulmonary capillaries, leading to increased transudation into the lungs. If the outward hydrostatic forces are not matched by lymphatic resorption, fluid leaks into the lungs, resulting in negative pressure pulmonary edema.[12]

Measuring Central Venous Pressure during Positive-pressure Ventilation

It is recommended to measure CVP at the end of expiration when the influence of ITPs is minimal, and intrapericardial/intrapleural pressures are closest to the atmospheric pressure. During positive-pressure ventilation, the ITP increases, and a portion of this pressure is transmitted to the right atrium and the great veins. Consequently, after initiating positive-pressure ventilation, the measured values of CVP and pulmonary artery

TABLE 1: Mechanisms attributed to the development of pulsus paradoxus in various conditions.[9]

Pathophysiology	*Normal subjects*	*Cardiac tamponade*	*Acute asthma*
Reduction in intrathoracic pressure during inspiration causing an increased venous return to right side	Possible	Possible	One of the major determinants
Stagnation of blood in pulmonary circulation	Possible	Possible	Possible
Ventricular interdependence in series	Possible	Equal determinants	Possible
Ventricular interdependence in parallel	No effect	Equal determinants	Dominant mechanism due to increased PVR and acute cor pulmonale
Increased left ventricular afterload with deep inspiration	No effect	Possible	Possible

(PVR: pulmonary vascular resistance)

occlusion pressure (PAOP) will be spuriously elevated. The magnitude of these changes is difficult to calculate, as it depends upon the transmission of airway pressure to the right heart, which in turn is influenced by the compliance of the underlying lung. Although complex formulas have been proposed to compute the transmission index based on pulmonary compliance, their utility at the bedside remains limited.[13] As long as the pulmonary compliance does not vary drastically, the transmitted pressure will remain similar meaning that, tracking changes in the measured CVP over time should also provide the same clinical information. Therefore, disconnecting the ventilator or transiently reducing applied PEEP to zero for the purpose of measuring CVP is not advisable and is considered potentially harmful.

CLINICAL USE OF HEART–LUNG INTERACTIONS

Prediction of Fluid Responsiveness

Predicting Fluid Responsiveness Based on Ventricular Interdependence

Due to the heart–lung interactions, the phases of respiration are associated with phasic reductions in the LV preload and LV afterload. In a hypovolemic patient, these effects are accentuated and can be observed at the bedside as wide swings in the pulse pressure, systolic pressure or stroke volume (PPV, SVV, or SPV). These wide swings result from the combined effects of an augmented left ventricular function due to reduction in LV afterload causing an increase in stroke volume from baseline (Δ up) which alternates with a decrease in stroke volume due to reduction in LV preload (Δ down).[14] In euvolemic patients with normal biventricular function, both delta up and delta down contribute equally to this variation, whereas in hypovolemic patients, Δ down predominates.

The dynamic variables such as PPV and SVV are indicators of the biventricular function and can be easily obtained at the bedside to identify fluid responsiveness in patients on controlled ventilation. However, these variables should be interpreted in the appropriate context and not used as direct markers of hypovolemia, or as automatic indications for fluid administration. Fluid administration should be considered only in patients with signs of circulatory insufficiency. Further details on the assessment of fluid responsiveness can be found in Chapter 5 of this textbook. If PPV or SVV values remain elevated despite fluid therapy, the possibility of underlying ventricular dysfunction or a relative hypervolemia should be considered as potential causes.

Identifying Preload Responders Based upon Dynamic Changes in Central Venous Pressure in Spontaneously Breathing Patients

Magder et al. suggested that in patients who are spontaneously breathing, preload responsiveness can be identified by measuring the inspiratory decrease of CVP. A decrease of CVP of >1 mm Hg during spontaneous breathing was proposed as a marker of preload responsiveness; however, this method has not been rigorously validated. Accurate identification of the decrease in the "a" wave of the CVP tracing and assessment of the adequacy of inspiratory effort are required for this test.[15] While this method does not indicate how close the heart is to the plateau of the Frank–Starling curve, the absence of an inspiratory fall in CVP suggests that the heart is already functioning on the flat part of the Frank–Starling curve, indicating that further fluid administration may be ineffective.

Therefore, this test can be used to rule out fluid responsiveness in appropriate patients.

Management of Pulmonary Edema

Cardiogenic pulmonary edema develops due to relative or absolute fluid overload in the presence of impaired left ventricular function. The resulting low cardiac output leads to circulatory insufficiency, increased oxygen extraction tissues, and both venous and arterial hypoxemia, which further increases myocardial stress and can precipitate myocardial ischemia. Hypoxia and tachypnea cause wide pressure swings in the thorax, leading to increased venous pooling and decreased left ventricular output. Therefore, the management of pulmonary edema requires a reduction in venous return, augmentation of left ventricular output by a reducing afterload, correction of hypoxia, and rest for the fatigued respiratory muscles.

With positive-pressure ventilation, intrathoracic positive pressure rises, leading to a reduction in venous return. Hypoxia is also corrected with oxygen supplementation. Optimal PEEP maintains the functional residual capacity (FRC) and reduces PVR, thereby improving RV function. This transiently improves left ventricular preload. Positive airway pressure increases P_{pc}, which reduces the P_{tm} of the LV. This leads to improved left ventricular ejection and improved cardiac output. Thus, positive-pressure ventilation unloads the respiratory muscles, reduces the intrathoracic blood volume, decreases the RV preload, improves PVR and RV function, and enhances LV preload and LV afterload, thereby simulating a multi-model approach to heart failure.

Management of Weaning-induced Pulmonary Edema

Weaning trials significantly increase the mechanical load on the respiratory muscles, raising the oxygen consumption and oxygen demand by as much as 15%. Failure to meet this increased oxygen demand results in blood flow redistribution, tissue hypoxia, and lactic acidosis, which can lead to weaning failure.[16] During weaning, as positive pressure is reduced or abolished, the venous return increases, and the left ventricular afterload rises. This leads to an increased intrathoracic blood volume, which places additional stress on a failing LV, worsening the demand supply balance and causing myocardial ischemia. These patients should be aggressively managed with measures to reduce preload and afterload, including vasodilators, diuretics, or noninvasive ventilatory support after extubation.

CONCLUSION

Heart–lung interactions are physiological relationships that can be altered or magnified in the intensive care unit (ICU) due to the application of positive-pressure ventilation. In daily practice, these interactions can be easily evaluated and monitored using tools such as echocardiography, PPV, and SVV. Monitoring heart-lung interactions can serve as both a therapeutic and diagnostic strategy in the ICU for managing common situations, such as predicting fluid responsiveness, identifying occult hypervolemia, diagnosing right heart failure, recognizing weaning-induced pulmonary edema, managing pulmonary edema, and predicting the severity of acute asthma or pericardial effusion. Therefore, a thorough physiological understanding of heart-lung interactions and their application at the bedside is of paramount importance for the intensive care physician.

REFERENCES

1. Norton JM. Toward consistent definitions for preload and afterload. Adv Physiol Educ. 2001;25(1-4):53-61.
2. Guyton AC, Armstrong GG, Chipley PL. Pressure-volume curves of the arterial and venous systems in live dogs. Am J Physiol. 1956;184(2):253-8.
3. Henderson WR, Griesdale DE, Walley KR, Sheel AW. Clinical review: Guyton—the role of mean circulatory filling pressure and right atrial pressure in controlling cardiac output. Crit Care. 2010;14(6):243.
4. Guyton AC, Polizo D, Armstron GG. Mean circulatory filling pressure measured immediately after cessation of heart pumping. Am J Physiol. 1954;179(2):261-7.
5. Pinsky MR. Heart-lung interactions. Curr Opin Crit Care. 2007;13(5):528-31.
6. Gomez H, Pinsky M. Effects of mechanical ventilation on heart-lung interactions. In: Tobin MJ (Ed). Principles and Practice of Mechanical Ventilation, 3rd edition. Columbus: McGraw-Hill Education; 2012.
7. Michard F, Teboul JL. Using heart-lung interactions to assess fluid responsiveness during mechanical ventilation. Crit Care. 2000;4(5):282-9.
8. Fessler HE. Heart-lung interactions: applications in the critically ill. Eur Respir J. 1997;10(1):226-37.
9. Hamzaoui O, Monnet X, Teboul JL. Pulsus paradoxus. Eur Respir J. 2013;42(6):1696-705.
10. Rick JJ, Burke SS. Respirator paradox. South Med J. 1978;71(11):1376-82.
11. Mansoor AM, Karlapudi SP. Images in clinical medicine. Kussmaul's sign. N Engl J Med. 2015;372(2):e3.
12. Bhattacharya M, Kallet RH, Ware LB, Matthay MA. Negative-pressure pulmonary edema. Chest. 2016;150(4):927-33.
13. Teboul JL, Pinsky MR, Mercat A, Anguel N, Bernardin G, Achard JM, et al. Estimating cardiac filling pressure in mechanically ventilated patients with hyperinflation. Crit Care Med. 2000;28(11):3631-6.
14. Cannesson M, Aboy M, Hofer CK, Rehman M. Pulse pressure variation: where are we today? J Clin Monit Comput. 2011;25(1):45-56.
15. Magder S. Hemodynamic monitoring in the mechanically ventilated patient. Curr Opin Crit Care. 2011;17(1):36-42.
16. Mohsenifar Z, Hay A, Hay J, Lewis MI, Koerner SK. Gastric intramucosal mechanical, pH as a predictor of success or failure in weaning patients from ventilation. Ann Intern Med. 1997;119(8):794-8.

CHAPTER

Preload Responsiveness

Sheila Nainan Myatra

INTRODUCTION

Fluid administration is usually the first step in the management of a patient with acute circulatory failure. Fluids are given with the goal of increasing cardiac output (CO) and thus oxygen delivery. Therefore, if the CO does not increase, giving fluid is not beneficial. The ability of the left ventricle to increase its stroke volume in response to fluid administration is called "fluid responsiveness."[1] According to the Frank–Starling principle, increasing preload increases the left ventricular (LV) stroke volume, when the ventricle is functioning on the steep part of the Frank–Starling curve. However, when the ventricle is functioning on the flat portion of the curve, giving more fluid will not increase the stroke volume much. In a normal heart, both ventricles usually operate on the steep portion of the Frank–Starling curve and the patient is usually fluid responsive, provided a large amount of fluid has not been already administered. A failing heart usually operates on the flat part of the curve; the exception is when the preload is very low. Thus, the same increase in preload by giving fluids as in a normal heart may result in only a minimal increase in stroke volume **(Fig. 1)**. A meta-analysis has shown that only about 50% of the patients presenting to the intensive care unit (ICU) in shock will respond positively to a fluid challenge. If a patient remains hypovolemic, tissue oxygenation may get affected, while on the other hand, increased fluid loading also leads to increased morbidity and mortality.[2-4] Thus, it is necessary to detect fluid responders before giving the patient fluid when the patient remains in shock despite initial resuscitation. However, identifying which patients will respond positively to fluid administration is a challenge in the ICU patients.

METHODS OF ASSESSING FLUID RESPONSIVENESS (TABLE 1)

Patient who can increase his stroke volume/CO by >10–15% after a fluid bolus is called a fluid responder.

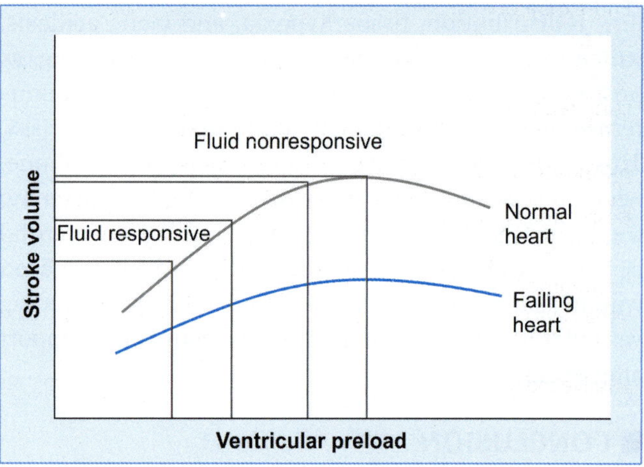

Fig. 1: Frank–Starling curves of a normal and a failing heart. The same increase in cardiac preload by fluid administration may result in a significant increase in stroke volume in a normal heart or a negligible increase in a failing heart, depending upon the shape of the curve.

A fluid challenge is when a small amount of fluid is given intravenously over a short time.[5] Fluid responsiveness can be assessed either by giving a fluid challenge and observing the changes in CO or it can be predicted by using various static and dynamic indices. The former requires fluid to be administered, which may be harmful in a fluid nonresponder, while the latter can be used without administering fluids.

Fluid Challenge to Assess Fluid Responsiveness

The gold standard of assessing fluid responsiveness is to give a fluid bolus and observe the response to the CO. Conventionally, a bolus of 500 mL of fluid was given over 30 minutes.[6] There are two problems with this approach. The first being that you can know if the patient is a fluid responder or not, only after giving fluids, hence this may run the risk of fluid overload in fluid nonresponders. The

TABLE 1: Methods for assessing fluid responsiveness.

Methods used	***Variable assessed***	***Limitations***
Conventional fluid challenge	Cardiac output	Requires a direct measurement of cardiac output to be reliable. Fluid overload in nonresponders
Mini-fluid challenge (MFC)	Cardiac output	Requires a precise technique for measuring cardiac output. Repeated challenges can also result in fluid overload in nonresponders
Pulse pressure variation (PPV) Stroke volume variation (SVV)	Pulse pressure/stroke volume	Cannot be used in case of spontaneous breathing, low tidal volume/lung compliance
Tidal volume challenge (TVC)	PPV/SVV	Cannot be used during spontaneous breathing and low lung compliance
End-expiratory-occlusion test (EEOT)	Cardiac output	Cannot be used in nonintubated patients Cannot be used in patients in whom a 15-second respiratory hold is not feasible
Lung recruitment maneuver	Cardiac output	Risk of adverse hemodynamic effects and overdistension of alveoli leading to ventilator induces lung injury
Positive end-expiratory pressure test	Cardiac output	Risk of decruitment and hypoxemia
Respiratory variations in inferior vena cava (IVC)	IVC diameter	Cannot be used in case of spontaneous breathing, low tidal volume/lung compliance diameter
Respiratory variations in superior vena cava (SVC) diameter	SVC diameter	Cannot be used in case of spontaneous breathing, low tidal volume/lung compliance Needs expertize
Passive leg raising (PLR)	Cardiac output	Requires a direct measurement of cardiac output

second issue is in order to assess the response to the fluid challenge reliably, you need a real time measurement of CO, since changes in mean arterial pressure (MAP) do not reliably track changes in CO.[7]

To overcome the problem of large volume, a "mini-fluid challenge" (MFC) was proposed, using a volume of 100 mL of hydroxyethyl starch and then observing a change in velocity time integral (VTI) of the LV outflow tract (ΔVTI 100) by echocardiography. The authors found that a ΔVTI 100 ≥10% predicted fluid responsiveness with a 95% and 78%, sensitivity and specificity, respectively.[8]

The main limitation of this test is that since the volume used for the challenge is less, it induces only small changes in CO; hence, very precise measurements are required, which require an expert echocardiographer. A minimum volume of 4 mL/kg of fluid is shown to be required to produce a significant hemodynamic effect.[9] This may suggest that the volume used in the MFC may not be adequate. One also needs to keep in mind that repeated testing, even with small volumes, might still result in a large volume being administered to the patient. In addition to the volume, the time taken for administering the bolus is important. It has been recently shown that the longer the duration of administering the fluid challenge, the lesser the proportion of fluid responders. A fluid challenge given in ≥30 minutes showed less fluid responders than when a fluid challenge was given in <15 minutes ($p = 0.045$).[10] Considering the limitations above an accurate way of predicting preload responsiveness without actually giving fluids is desired. Some of these indices are described in the following text.

Use of Static and Dynamic Indices to Assess Preload Responsiveness

The most commonly used static indices are the central venous pressure (CVP) and pulmonary artery occlusion pressure (PAOP); which commonly used markers of right and left cardiac ventricular preload, respectively. Other static markers of cardiac preload are the global end-diastolic volume, the left end-diastolic area/volume or aortic blood flow measured by transpulmonary thermodilution, echocardiography and esophageal Doppler, respectively. However, it has been well-demonstrated that all these indices are not reliable in predicting fluid responsiveness.[11,12] The reason for this being that the same value of these static indices could correspond to a preload responsive or unresponsive state depending on the kind of slope of the Frank–Starling curve, which may be variable depending on the systolic function of the heart. In addition, the values of these static indices may depend on the transmission of the pleural pressure on the heart, during mechanical ventilation, use of positive end-expiratory pressure (PEEP), conditions when the intrathoracic or abdominal pressures are raised, etc. Despite the unreliability of these indices to predict fluid responsiveness, the FENICE study showed that CVP is still the most commonly used variable for this purpose.[13] Dynamic indices such as stroke volume variation (SVV), pulse pressure variation (PPV), etc., have been shown to be superior to traditionally used static indices, such as CVP and PAOP, to predict fluid responsiveness.[1,14-16] The recent Surviving Sepsis guidelines have recommended the use of dynamic over static variables to predict fluid responsiveness.[17]

Most of the dynamic indices to predict preload responsiveness are based on heart–lung interaction during mechanical ventilation, except the passive leg raising (PLR) test, which does not depend on this and hence can overcome most of the limitations related to methods using heart–lung interactions.

Dynamic Indices Using Heart–Lung Interactions to Assess Fluid Responsiveness

The changes in preload produced by intrathoracic pressure changes during the respiratory cycle, during mechanically ventilation in a patient, and have been used to develop dynamic tests to assess fluid responsiveness. The principal mechanisms underlying these tests are based on heart–lung interactions during mechanical ventilation described earlier. These include PPV, SVV, tidal volume challenge (TVC), end-expiratory-occlusion test (EEOT), plethysmography variability index (PVI), and echocardiographic variables.

Heart–Lung Interaction During Mechanical Ventilation

During mechanical ventilation, the intrathoracic and transpulmonary pressures increase during inspiration, resulting in variable changes in the loading conditions of both the ventricles. Due to this increase, there is a decrease in venous return and therefore a drop in the right ventricular (RV) preload, while an increase in transpulmonary pressure increases RV afterload causing a decrease in the RV stroke volume (lowest at the end of inspiration). At the same time, this increase in the intrathoracic and transpulmonary pressures results in decreased LV afterload and an increase in LV preload, due to the blood that is squeezed out of alveolar. This leads to an increase in LV stroke volume, which will be maximum at the end of inspiration. The reduction in RV stroke volume during inspiration leads to decreased LV preload which causes decreased LV stroke volume (lowest during expiration). During mechanical ventilation, there are cyclical changes in the LV stroke volume, which are maximum during inspiration and minimum during expiration. The magnitude of this change in LV stroke volume, or its surrogates, like pulse pressure, is magnified when the patient is preload-dependent (See Chapter 4: Heart–Lung Interaction in the Critically Ill for details).[18]

Hemodynamic Variables Based on Heart–Lung Interactions to Predict Fluid Responsiveness

Pulse Pressure Variation and Stroke Volume Variation

These indices are derived from the arterial waveform analysis and are the most commonly used indices in the ICU. The PPV is the difference between the maximum and minimum pulse pressure value over one ventilatory cycle, divided by the average value of the two values.[14] Several hemodynamic monitors can automatically calculate and display the PPV values. The SVV is derived from the analysis of the arterial pressure waveform. The CO monitors using calibrated and uncalibrated pulse contour analysis automatically calculate these parameters.[14] In a preload responsive patient, the PPV and SVV values are high, while low values are associated with preload unresponsiveness. Three systematic reviews have shown good predictive value of these variables to predict fluid responsiveness. In patients ventilated with a tidal volume is >8 mL/kg predicated body weight (PBW), the threshold value for PPV is >12–13% and for SVV it is 10%.[15,19,20] These tests have some limitations. These include arrhythmias, spontaneous breathing activity, low tidal volume (V_t) ventilation, low lung compliance, increased intra-abdominal pressure, open thorax, and a heart rate to respiratory rate ratio <3.6.[21]

Tidal Volume Challenge

The dynamic indices, PPV and SVV, are not reliable in predicting fluid responsiveness during low V_t ventilation (V_t ≤6 mL/kg PBW).[22,23] It has been shown that PPV is a reliable predictor of fluid responsiveness only when the tidal volume was at least 8 mL/kg PBW.[22] A low V_t might not be sufficient to produce significant change in the intrathoracic pressure, making these indices indicate a nonresponsive state even in a responder.[24,25] This may limit the use of PPV and SVV during low V_t ventilation. To overcome this limitation, the "TVC" has been proposed. This is a novel test to improve the reliability of PPV and SVV during low V_t ventilation.[26] The test involves transiently increasing tidal volume from 6–8 mL/kg PBW for 1 minute in a paralyzed patient and observing the change in PPV (ΔPPV_{6-8}) and SVV (ΔSVV_{6-8}) from baseline to that at 8 mL/kg PBW. A change in PPV of 3.5% or SVV of 2.5%, after performing the TVC, reliably predicted fluid responsiveness. This test is very simple and can be performed at the bedside. If the PPV can be obtained from a simple bedside hemodynamic monitor, then this test does not require a CO monitor, making this useful even in resource-limited settings. A recent study showed that TVC is able to reliably predict fluid responsiveness in neurosurgical patients.[27]

Recruitment Maneuvers

The hemodynamic effects of using recruitment maneuvers to predict preload responsiveness has been recently tested. A recruitment maneuver produces a transient increase in intrathoracic pressure, thus reducing the venous return and the cardiac preload. The resultant drop in stroke volume as shown in two studies could reliably distinguish responders from nonresponders.[28,29] The drop in stroke volume was to a lesser extent in some patients than in other among nonresponder, which may suggest that increase in afterload may also contribute to this effect. More studies are needed to better understand the mechanisms involved in this test and to validate these tests before incorporating them into clinical practice.

Indices Using Plethysmographic Waveform

The PPV and SVV both require invasive arterial pressure measurements. The pulse oximetry plethysmographic (POP) waveform can be captured noninvasively. This depends on the arterial pulsatility and the stroke volume. Canneson et al. showed a good correlation and agreement between respiratory variation in POP waveform amplitude and respiratory variation in arterial pulse pressure.[30] Other studies have also shown the respiratory changes in the amplitude of the POP pulse wave to reliably predict fluid responsiveness in ventilated patients, with a cutoff of around 14–17%.[30,31] Currently commercial monitors automatically calculate the respiratory variation of the POP and this is called PVI. The PVI reliably predicts fluid responsiveness in perioperative settings.[32,33] The reliability of this index depends on good signal capture, which may not be always possible in patients who are hypothermic. In addition, it has been shown to be unreliable in patients on vasopressors.[34] Thus, the applicability of these indices may be limited in the ICU patients, and this variable may be more useful for hemodynamic monitoring in the operating room.

End-expiratory-occlusion Test

The EEOT is based on the heart–lung interactions. This test is performed by giving a 15-second hold at the end of expiration in a mechanically ventilated patient.[35] During this, inspiration is prevented when the hold is given, thereby preventing an increase in the intrathoracic pressure. In addition, the increase in transpulmonary pressure during inspiration will also not occur. The resultant effect is an increase in the venous return, increasing ventricular preload, which results in an increased RV stroke volume in a fluid responsive patient. An increase in CO of >5% after an EEOT reliably predicts fluid responsiveness. This test is like giving a mini auto fluid challenge. This test has been shown to be more reliable when used with a continuous CO monitor (See Chapter 6: End-expiratory Occlusion and Passive Leg Raising Tests).

Lung Recruitment Maneuver and Positive End-expiratory Pressure Test

Hemodynamic alterations caused by lung recruitment maneuvers (LRM) using continuous positive airway pressure have been shown to identify fluid responders.[1,2] Biais et al. demonstrated that a 30% decrease in stroke volume during an LRM (a continuous positive airway pressure of 30 cmH_2O for 30 seconds) predicted fluid responsiveness (sensitivity of 88% and specificity of 92%).[2] However, the adverse hemodynamic effects and risks of overstretching the alveoli which may lead to ventilator-induced lung injury, have always been a concern.[3] More recently authors have demonstrated the ability of a stepwise LRM, given by increasing PEEP with a constant driving pressure for predicting fluid responsiveness in patients under protective lung ventilation.[4,5]

In mechanically ventilated patients, the use of PEEP can decrease the CO by decreasing the preload and/or increasing the RV afterload. In a recent study including 64 mechanically ventilated patients with PEEP ≥10 cmH_2O, a transient decrease in PEEP level to 5 cmH_2O for 1 minute (PEEP-test), was used to detect fluid responsiveness. An increase in cardiac index (CI) > 8.6% during the PEEP-test had area under the receiver operating characteristic curve of 0.94 for detecting volume responsiveness (sensitivity of 96.8% and a specificity of 84.9%).[6]

Further studies are required to standardize and validate LRM and the PEEP test before using them in clinical practice.

Echocardiographic Variables

Echocardiography is used to directly visualize the heart and major vessels and assess cardiac function. The changes in the diameter of the superior vena cava (SVC) or inferior vena cava (IVC) with respiration, or changes in aortic flow velocity can be measured.[36] During controlled mechanical ventilation, the IVC diameter is maximum during inspiration. The respiratory variations in the diameter of the IVC are used to calculate the IVC distensibility index (calculated as maximum minus minimum diameter, divided by the minimum diameter). A cutoff value of ≥18% has been shown to reliably predict fluid responsiveness.[37] Transesophageal echocardiography can be used to measure changes in the diameter of the SVC. A change in SVC diameter >36% during controlled ventilation has been shown to be reliability predictive of fluid responsiveness.[38] These echocardiographic variables have the same limitations as PPV and SVV to predict fluid responsiveness, however, they are reliable in patients with arrhythmias. A recent study showed this parameter to have moderate to poor reliability to predict fluid responsiveness (See Chapter 40: TTE for ICU and Chapter 41: TEE for ICU).[36]

PASSIVE LEG RAISING

These tests, described in the earlier text, use the heart-lung interaction during mechanical ventilation to assess fluid responsiveness. However, these tests are not without limitations, their applicability in certain situations such as presence of spontaneous breathing activity, arrhythmias, low tidal volume ventilation, low lung compliance, open thorax, etc., is limited. The PLR can reliably predict fluid responsiveness in these situations, since it does not depend on heart-lung interactions.[39] This test involves transiently raising the legs to 45° with the horizontal. This results in an auto-fluid challenge, mimicking the effects of volume expansion and with the advantage of being completely reversible. A PLR-induced change in CO >10% reliably predicts fluid responsiveness in patients with acute circulatory failure. However, this test requires the use of continuous CO monitoring and is contraindicated in neurotrauma patients and those requiring immobilization of the lower limbs (See Chapter 6: End-expiratory Occlusion and Passive Leg Raising Tests).[40]

The various tests described earlier can help to predict fluid responsiveness with reasonable reliability. However, it is important to remember that all patients who are fluid responsive may not require fluids, if they are not in acute circulatory failure. Some patients are at an increased risk of receiving fluid. Even though a patient may be fluid responsive, if there is a risk of giving fluids, fluid administration should be avoided and alternative therapies like vasopressors should be considered (See Chapter 31: Fluid Therapy in Shock and Chapter 32: Vasopressors in the Critically Ill).

CONCLUSION

Assessing preload responsiveness before giving fluid is essential, especially following the initial resuscitation phase. Dynamic rather than static indices, such as PPV, SVV, TVC, EEOT, echocardiographic variables, PLR, etc., are more reliable and should be used to predict fluid responsiveness. However, these tests have their limitations, thus an integration of various dynamic indices and clinical assessment is essential. It is important to remember that even if a patient is preload responsive, fluid should only be given only if there are signs of acute circulatory shock and reduced tissue perfusion and if there is no risk of giving fluids.

REFERENCES

1. Michard F, Teboul JL. Predicting fluid responsiveness in ICU patients: a critical analysis of the evidence. Chest. 2002;121(6):2000-8.
2. Pinsky MR, Brophy P, Padilla J, Paganini E, Pannu N. Fluid and volume monitoring. Int J Artif Organs. 2008;31(2):111-26.
3. National Heart, Lung, and Blood Institute Acute Respiratory Distress Syndrome (ARDS) Clinical Trials Network;

Wiedemann HP, Wheeler AP, Bernard GR, Thompson BT, Hayden D, deBoisblanc B, et al. Comparison of two fluid-management strategies in acute lung injury. N Engl J Med. 2006;354(24):2564-75.
4. Acheampong A, Vincent JL. A positive fluid balance is an independent prognostic factor in patients with sepsis. Crit Care. 2015;19(1):251.
5. Cecconi M, Parsons AK, Rhodes A. What is a fluid challenge? Curr Opin Crit Care. 2011;17(3):290-5.
6. Vincent JL, Weil MH. Fluid challenge revisited. Crit Care Med. 2006;34(5):1333-7.
7. Pierrakos C, Velissaris D, Scolletta S, Heenen S, De Backer D, Vincent JL. Can changes in arterial pressure be used to detect changes in cardiac index during fluid challenge in patients with septic shock? Intensive Care Med. 2012;38(3):422-8.
8. Muller L, Toumi M, Bousquet PJ, Riu-Poulenc B, Louart G, Candela D, et al. An increase in aortic blood flow after an infusion of 100 mL colloid over 1 min can predict fluid responsiveness: the mini-fluid challenge study. Anesthesiology. 2011;115(3):541-7.
9. Toscani L, Aya HD, Antonakaki D, Bastoni D, Watson X, Arulkumaran N, et al. What is the impact of the fluid challenge technique on diagnosis of fluid responsiveness? A systematic review and meta-analysis. Crit Care. 2017;21(1):207.
10. Aya HD, Rhodes A, Chis Ster I, Fletcher N, Grounds RM, Cecconi M. Hemodynamic effect of different doses of fluids for a fluid challenge: a quasi-randomized controlled study. Crit Care Med. 2017;45(2):e161-8.
11. Monnet X, Marik P, Teboul JL. Prediction of fluid responsiveness: an update. Ann Intensive Care. 2016;6(1): 111.
12. Marik PE, Cavallazzi R. Does the central venous pressure predict fluid responsiveness? An updated meta-analysis and a plea for some common sense. Crit Care Med. 2013;41(7):1774-81.
13. Cecconi M, Hofer C, Teboul JL, Pettila V, Wilkman E, Molnar Z, et al. Fluid challenges in intensive care: the FENICE study: A global inception cohort study. Intensive Care Med. 2015;41(9):1529-37.
14. Michard F, Boussat S, Chemla D, Anguel N, Mercat A, Lecarpentier Y, et al. Relation between respiratory changes in arterial pulse pressure and fluid responsiveness in septic patients with acute circulatory failure. Am J Respir Crit Care Med. 2000;162(1):134-8.
15. Marik PE, Cavallazzi R, Vasu T, Hirani A. Dynamic changes in arterial waveform derived variables and fluid responsiveness in mechanically ventilated patients. A systematic review of the literature. Crit Care Med. 2009;37(9):2642-7.
16. Perel A, Pizov R, Cotev S. Respiratory variations in the arterial pressure during mechanical ventilation reflects volume status and fluid responsiveness. Intensive Care Med. 2014;40(6):798-807.
17. Rhodes A, Evans LE, Alhazzani W, Levy MM, Antonelli M, Ferrer R, et al. Surviving sepsis campaign: International guidelines for management of sepsis and septic shock: 2016. Intensive Care Med. 2017;43(3):304-77.
18. Michard F, Teboul JL. Using heart lung interactions to assess fluid responsiveness during mechanical ventilation. Crit Care. 2000;4(5):282-9.
19. Hong JQ, He HF, Chen ZY, Du ZS, Liu WF, Weng PQ, et al. Comparison of stroke volume variation with pulse pressure variation as a diagnostic indicator of fluid responsiveness in mechanically ventilated critically ill patients. Saudi Med J. 2014;35(3):261-8.
20. Yang X, Du B. Does pulse pressure variation predict fluid responsiveness in critically ill patients: A critical review and meta-analysis. Crit Care. 2014;18(6):650.
21. Myatra SN, Monnet X, Teboul JL. Use of "tidal volume challenge" to improve the reliability of pulse pressure variation. Crit Care. 2017;21(1):60.
22. De Backer D, Heenen S, Piagnerelli M, Koch M, Vincent JL. Pulse pressure variations to predict fluid responsiveness: Influence of tidal volume. Intensive Care Med. 2005;31(4):517-23.
23. Lansdorp B, Lemson J, van Putten MJ, de Keijzer A, van der Hoeven JG, Pickkers P. Dynamic indices do not predict volume responsiveness in routine clinical practice. Br J Anaesth. 2012;108(3):395-401.
24. Teboul JL, Monnet X. Pulse pressure variation and ARDS. Minerva Anestesiol. 2013;79(4):398-407.
25. Pinsky MR. Using ventilation-induced aortic pressure and flow variation to diagnose preload responsiveness. Intensive Care Med. 2004;30(6):1008-10.
26. Myatra SN, Prabu NR, Divatia JV, Monnet X, Kulkarni AP, Teboul JL. The changes in pulse pressure variation or stroke volume variation after a "Tidal Volume Challenge" reliably predict fluid responsiveness during low tidal volume ventilation. Crit Care Med. 2017;45(3):415-21.
27. Messina A, Montagnini C, Cammarota G, De Rosa S, Giuliani F, Muratore L, et al. Tidal volume challenge to predict fluid responsiveness in the operating room: An observational study. Eur J Anaesthesiol. 2019;36(8):583-91.
28. De Broca B, Garnier J, Fischer MO, Archange T, Marc J, Abou-Arab O, et al. Stroke volume changes induced by a recruitment maneuver predicts fluid responsiveness in patients with protective ventilation in the operating theater. Medicine (Baltimore). 2016;95(28):e4259.
29. Biais M, Lanchon R, Sesay M, Le Gall L, Pereira B, Futier E, et al. Changes in stroke volume induced by lung recruitment maneuver predicts fluid responsiveness in mechanically ventilated patients in the operating room. Anesthesiology. 2017;126(2):260-7.
30. Feissel M, Teboul JL, Merlani P, Badie J, Faller JP, Bendjelid K. Plethysmographic dynamic indices predict fluid responsiveness in septic ventilated patients. Intensive Care Med. 2007;33(6):993-9.

31. Cannesson M, Attof Y, Rosamel P, Desebbe O, Joseph P, Metton O, et al. Respiratory variations in pulse oximetry plethysmographic waveform amplitude to predict fluid responsiveness in the operating room. Anesthesiology. 2007;106(6):1105-11.
32. Hood JA, Wilson RJ. Pleth variability index to predict fluid responsiveness in colorectal surgery. Anesth Analg. 2011;113(5):1058-63.
33. Zimmermann M, Feibicke T, Keyl C, Prasser C, Moritz S, Graf BM, et al. Accuracy of stroke volume variation compared with pleth variability index to predict fluid responsiveness in mechanically ventilated patients undergoing major surgery. Eur J Anaesthesiol. 2010;27(6):555-61.
34. Monnet X, Guérin L, Jozwiak M, Bataille A, Julien F, Richard C, et al. Pleth variability index is a weak predictor of fluid responsiveness in patients receiving norepinephrine. Br J Anaesth. 2013;110(2):207-13.
35. Monnet X, Osman D, Ridel C, Lamia B, Richard C, Teboul JL. Predicting volume responsiveness by using the end-expiratory occlusion in mechanically ventilated intensive care unit patients. Crit Care Med. 2009;37(3):951-6.
36. Vignon P, Repessé X, Begot E, Léger J, Jacob C, Bouferrache K, et al. Comparison of echocardiographic indices used to predict fluid responsiveness in ventilated patients. Am J Respir Crit Care Med. 2017;195(8):1022-32.
37. Barbier C, Loubières Y, Schmit C, Hayon J, Ricôme JL, Jardin F, et al. Respiratory changes in inferior vena cava diameter are helpful in predicting fluid responsiveness in ventilated septic patients. Intensive Care Med. 2004;30(9):1740-6.
38. Vieillard-Baron A, Chergui K, Rabiller A, Peyrouset O, Page B, Beauchet A, et al. Superior vena caval collapsibility as a gauge of volume status in ventilated septic patients. Intensive Care Med. 2004;30(9):1734-9.
39. Monnet X, Marik P, Teboul JL. Passive leg raising for predicting fluid responsiveness: a systematic review and meta-analysis. Intensive Care Med. 2016;42(12):1935-47.
40. Monnet X, Teboul JL. Passive leg raising. Intensive Care Med. 2008;34(4):659-63.

CHAPTER 6 End-expiratory Occlusion and Passive Leg Raising Tests

Rui Shi, Xavier Monnet, Jean-Louis Teboul

INTRODUCTION

Hypovolemia is present in almost all patients with acute circulatory failure so fluid should be infused urgently in such patients without using any predictor of fluid responsiveness. If the initial fluid bolus is insufficient to completely correct tissue hypoxia, continuing fluid resuscitation can be a therapeutic dilemma. On the one hand, hemodynamic benefits can still be expected. On the other hand, not all patients are fluid responsive at this stage,[1] and it is now widely recognized that fluid overload results in lung and tissue edema, delays weaning from mechanical ventilation, and is an independent predictor of mortality in acutely ill patients, in particular in septic patients[2,3] and those with acute respiratory distress syndrome (ARDS).[4] Thus, at this stage, prediction of fluid responsiveness is essential to deciding to continue fluid administration.[5] Historically, static markers of cardiac preload, such as the central venous pressure (CVP) have been used to guide fluid administration but clinical studies showed that CVP was a poor indicator of fluid responsiveness.[6] In this regard, the current Surviving Sepsis Campaign guidelines no longer recommend the use of CVP to guide fluid resuscitation in septic patients.[7] More recently, dynamic tests have been developed to predict fluid responsiveness.[8] Most of them, such as pulse pressure variation (PPV) or stroke volume variation (SVV),[9] end-expiratory occlusion (EEO) test,[10] and tidal volume challenge[11] are based on heart–lung interactions during mechanical ventilation. Another test, called *passive leg raising (PLR)*, is feasible in patients receiving mechanical ventilation as well as in nonintubated patients.

In this chapter, we describe the EEO and the PLR tests and their place in the strategy of fluid management.

THE END-EXPIRATORY OCCLUSION TEST

This test can be performed only in patients who receive mechanical ventilation.

What is the underlying hypothesis?

Each mechanical insufflation increases the intrathoracic pressure. This increases the right atrial pressure, which is the downstream pressure for venous return, and thus impedes the venous return as the mean systemic filling pressure, which is the upstream pressure for venous return, does not increase in the same degree. Therefore, interrupting mechanical ventilation at end-expiration (i.e., just before the next insufflation) for a few seconds should prevent the cyclic decrease in venous return and cardiac preload, which increases transiently. This "preload challenge" will result in an increase in cardiac output if the patient's heart is preload responsive **(Fig. 1)**. Thus, as a preload challenge, the EEO maneuver can serve as a preload responsiveness test provided that cardiac output measurements are obtained before and during the test. As the test lasts a few seconds (15 seconds), real-time cardiac output monitoring is required.

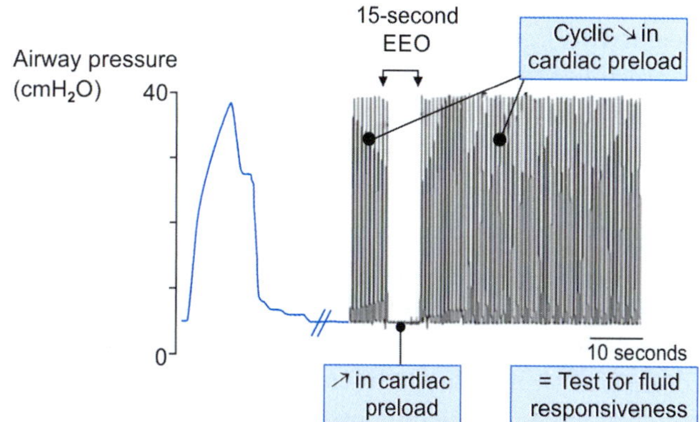

Fig. 1: End-expiratory occlusion (EEO) test. The EEO test in mechanically ventilated patients, performing by interrupting mechanical ventilation at end-expiration for 15 seconds, is expected to increase venous return and cardiac output transiently. An increase in cardiac output ≥5% during the test could be used to predict fluid responsiveness in critically ill patients.

Clinical Validation

The EEO test was proposed 10 years ago in a clinical study where 34 critically ill patients ventilated with a tidal volume of 6.8 mL/kg on average were included.[10] 11 patients had arrhythmias; the 23 remaining patients had spontaneous breathing activity. Fluid responsiveness was defined as an increase in cardiac output by >15% after a fluid challenge (500 mL over 10 minutes). The pulse contour cardiac output method was used to assess the hemodynamic effects of the 15-second EEO.[10] An increase in cardiac output ≥5% during an EEO predicted fluid responsiveness with excellent accuracy: Area under the receiver operating characteristics (AUROC) of 0.97, sensitivity of 91%, and specificity of 100%. In the subgroup of patients with spontaneous breathing activity, the prediction of fluid responsiveness using EEO was also excellent (AUROC: 0.97) and significantly better than that using PPV (AUROC: 0.68) and SVV (AUROC: 0.57).[10] Another study showed that EEO was accurate in predicting fluid responsiveness in patients with compliance of the respiratory system (Crs) >30 mL/cmH_2O as well as in those with Crs <30 mL/cmH_2O (AUROC: 0.97 vs. 0.93, respectively).[12] In the latter subgroup, the AUROC for EEO was far larger than that for PPV (0.93 vs. 0.64, respectively).[12] A study performed in patients with ARDS showed that the good predictive value of the EEO test was not modified when the level of positive end-expiratory pressure (PEEP) changed from 5 to 15 cmH_2O.[13] Other more recently published studies reported an accurate prediction of fluid responsiveness by the EEO test.[14-18]

Two studies reported a relatively poor predictive value of the EEO test with a tidal volume of 6 mL/kg of ideal body weight (IBW), compared with 8 mL/kg (IBW).[11,19] However, as previous studies have already shown robust results in patients receiving protective ventilation with a tidal volume <8 mL/kg (IBW),[10,12,13,15-18] further validation in larger and more heterogeneous patients is expected. One study failed to confirm the accuracy of the EEO test in severe ARDS patients during a prone position.[20] It cannot be excluded that this finding was due to the low tidal volume used in these patients. Another study conducted in the operating room also showed negative results.[21] Nevertheless, its conclusion should be interpreted with caution since the effect of the EEO test on cardiac output was assessed by an esophageal Doppler device, which does not measure the aortic diameter but only the aortic blood velocity.[22]

How to perform the EEO test?

The EEO test is an easy-to-use maneuver. As mentioned before, it has the advantage of remaining reliable in various clinical settings, including arrhythmias, moderate spontaneous breathing activity (but not sufficient to interrupt the occlusion), low tidal volume low compliance, and is independent on PEEP level.[10-13,15-18]

The method of performing the EEO test is similar to the way to measure the intrinsic PEEP in mechanically ventilated patients. It consists in interrupting the ventilator at the end of expiration for 15 seconds. The effect of the EEO test should be assessed by the changes in cardiac output. The maximal changes should be taken into consideration. In general, they occur at the end of the 15-second test. The test is considered positive (i.e., the patient to be preload responsive) when cardiac output increases by ≥5%.[10,12,16] Due to the low threshold value (5%), the use of a precise cardiac output monitoring device is mandatory. In this regard, in several studies, the response to the EEO test was assessed by using a pulse contour analysis-derived cardiac output monitor, which most often requires an invasive hemodynamic approach.[10,12-16] The precision of this technique is sufficiently acceptable to detect changes in cardiac output by <5%.[23]

Interestingly, our group and others have recently demonstrated that the EEO test could be used with echocardiography to estimate cardiac output.[15,17] An increase ≥5% or ≥9% in the velocity-time integral (VTI) of the left ventricular outflow tract induced by a 15-second or a 12-second[17] expiratory hold could reliably predict fluid responsiveness.[15,17] Nevertheless, these threshold values found in these studies were lower than the least significant changes found for VTI (11%) in a series of measurements performed on 100 critically ill patients.[24] In other words, the prediction of fluid responsiveness from the changes in VTI during EEO might be limited by the precision of echocardiography. In this regard, our group has proposed to combine EEO with end-inspiratory occlusion (EIO) sequentially performed, to predict fluid responsiveness in order to circumvent limits of interpretation due to the lack of precision of echocardiography. Adding the absolute changes in VTI induced by EEO and EIO, predicted accuracy fluid responsiveness with a threshold value of 13%, which is a value compatible with the precision of echocardiography.[15,24] Similar results were found when esophageal Doppler was used.[18]

What are the limitations of the EEO test?

The patients should not interrupt the EEO test by triggering the ventilator due to marked inspiratory efforts. This can occur in 22% of the cases.[10] As detailed above; the technique used to assess the changes in cardiac output should be precise. If a less precise method is used, for instance, echocardiography or esophageal Doppler, it is better to combine the results of the EEO test and EIO in order to increase the reliability of the test.[15,18]

THE PASSIVE LEG-RAISING TEST

What is the underlying hypothesis?

The PLR test is considered an "internal preload challenge."[8] Boulain et al. showed that this postural maneuver resulted in an increase in both the right and the left ventricular preload.[25] Interestingly, the changes in stroke volume induced by PLR and by a fluid challenge are strongly correlated suggesting that PLR might mimic the hemodynamic effects of a fluid challenge of about 300 mL.[25,26] Furthermore, in fluid-responsive patients, PLR increases cardiac output by increasing the mean systemic pressure to a larger extent than CVP.[27] Conversely, in fluid nonresponsive patients, PLR does not increase cardiac output as the mean systemic pressure and the CVP increase to a similar extent, thus resulting in an unchanged venous return pressure gradient.[27]

Clinical Validation

The first study that demonstrated that a PLR test can predict fluid responsiveness in critically ill patients used the esophageal Doppler to assess the hemodynamic effect of PLR.[28] Other studies using different devices confirmed the excellent accuracy of PLR in predicting fluid responsiveness.[8] The two most recent meta-analyses pooling respectively 21 studies involving 991 patients and 23 studies involving 1,013 patients found a pooled sensitivity of ≥85% and a pooled specificity of >90%, a pooled AUROC of 0.95, and a threshold value of 10%.[29,30] Thus, the PLR test is now recommended to assess fluid responsiveness in the consensus on circulatory shock and hemodynamic monitoring of the European Society of Intensive Care Medicine, as well as in the most recent Surviving Sepsis Campaign guidelines.[7,31]

How to perform the PLR test?

Conversely to most of the other dynamic tests, the PLR test can be used in almost all patients, including those with partial or total spontaneous breathing, atrial fibrillation, or low lung compliance, as long as the effects of PLR are assessed by direct measurement of cardiac output.[12,29,30,32-33]

Importantly, the use of PLR to reliably assess fluid responsiveness needs to respect strict rules **(Fig. 2)**.[34] Firstly, PLR should start from the semirecumbent and not the supine position to make the test more sensitive.[26] Secondly, the effects of PLR must be assessed using a real-time measurement of cardiac output with a technique sensitive enough to track short-term and transient changes in cardiac output. Several invasive or noninvasive techniques can be used for this purpose. It has been shown that the pulse contour analysis method, the esophageal Doppler, and the transthoracic echocardiography had

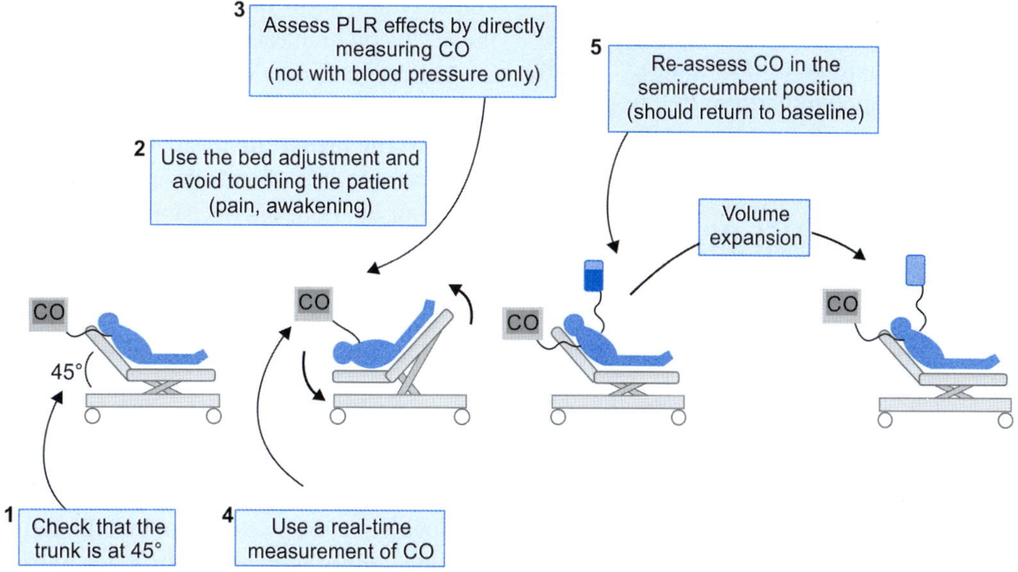

Fig. 2: Procedures to perform a PLR test. (CO: cardiac output; PLR: passive leg raising).

similar diagnostic performance.[30] The use of PLR-induced changes in cardiac output measured by bioreactance to assess fluid responsiveness is a matter of debate. One study showed an excellent accuracy, another reported poor results, while a more recent one concluded to a reasonable but not perfect accuracy.[35-37] PLR-induced changes in the peak velocity of the carotid and the femoral arteries, in end-tidal carbon dioxide, in transcutaneous partial pressure of oxygen, and in perfusion index (using a pulse oximeter) have also been proposed to assess the effects of PLR.[32,35,38-42] Finally, some precautions must be taken. Confounding factors such as pain, cough, and other discomfort, which might induce adrenergic stimulation leading to erroneous interpretation, should be avoided.[34] Accordingly, some practical tips such as using the automatic pivotal motion of the patient's bed and ensuring that the heart rate remains stable during the PLR test have been suggested.[43]

What are the limitations of the PLR test?

Some limitations and contraindications of the PLR test must be acknowledged. Firstly, as mentioned before, a real-time and precise hemodynamic monitoring device, which is able to track the changes in cardiac output during 1 minute is indispensable.[34] It is important to keep in mind that the effects of PLR cannot be reliably assessed by the changes in arterial pulse pressure due to a decreased sensitivity and that procedures that induce adrenergic stimulation should be avoided.[29,30,43] Secondly, some cases of false negatives have been reported in patients with intra-abdominal hypertension.[44,45] The increased abdominal volume during PLR might squeeze the inferior vena cava.[46] Thirdly, some data suggested that the effects of the PLR test might be compromised by using compression stockings because of inadequate venous return.[47] Finally, it is obviously contraindicated to perform PLR in patients with head trauma due to the risk of increasing intracerebral pressure.[43]

WHAT IS THE CLINICAL USE OF FLUID RESPONSIVENESS TESTS SUCH AS EEO AND PLR?

The interest of testing fluid responsiveness at the bedside is twofold. On the one hand, testing fluid responsiveness may help physicians to know when to start when to continue, and when to stop fluid administration **(Flowchart 1)**. On the other hand, testing fluid responsiveness may help physicians to manage fluid removal and predict weaning failure from mechanical ventilation.

Fluid Responsiveness to Guide Fluid Administration

Some important points must be kept in mind.

Firstly, it is important to highlight that preload responsiveness is a physiological phenomenon. In other words, a positive predictive test of fluid responsiveness must not necessarily prompt fluid administration. Indeed, as previously discussed, the main goal of fluid administration is to increase cardiac output, oxygen delivery, and ultimately oxygen consumption. Thus, the question of fluid administration makes sense only in patients with preload responsiveness and signs of tissue hypoxia.[48]

Secondly, even if it is recommended to predict fluid responsiveness in patients with acute circulatory failure, there are some cases where testing fluid responsiveness is not recommended and could even be deleterious by delaying fluid administration.[31] In particular, at the initial phase of hypovolemic or septic shock, hypovolemia is constant and most of the patients should be responsive to initial fluid resuscitation.[49] In this regard, our group recently proposed a more individualized approach to fluid administration in septic shock patients.[5] Within the first hour of resuscitation, fluids should be infused urgently without using any predictor of fluid responsiveness. A rate of around 10 mL/kg within the first hour (e.g., from 30 to 60 minutes) of resuscitation should be reasonable. A higher rate should be considered in cases of evident fluid losses, evident signs of hypovolemia, or abdominal origin of infection, and a lower rate of infusion should be considered if signs of pulmonary edema appear during fluid infusion or in cases of severe lung injury.[5]

Thirdly, it is now well established that positive fluid balance is associated with a poor outcome in critically ill patients: the higher the positive fluid balance, the poorer the outcome.[2-4,50,51] That is the reason why after the initial fluid resuscitation, the decision on further fluid infusion, if signs of shock persists, should be made, after assessing the benefits/risks ratio based on individual management. Using dynamic tests of fluid responsiveness such as EEO and PLR is suggested in order to prevent fluid overload in fluid-unresponsive patients, who represent 50% of the critically ill patients.[1]

If the risks are judged to be greater than the benefits, especially in patients with ARDS, other therapies such as cardiovascular drugs, should be considered even if preload responsiveness is present. In such patients, objective

Flowchart 1: An algorithmic approach to the use of the concept of fluid responsiveness at the bedside.

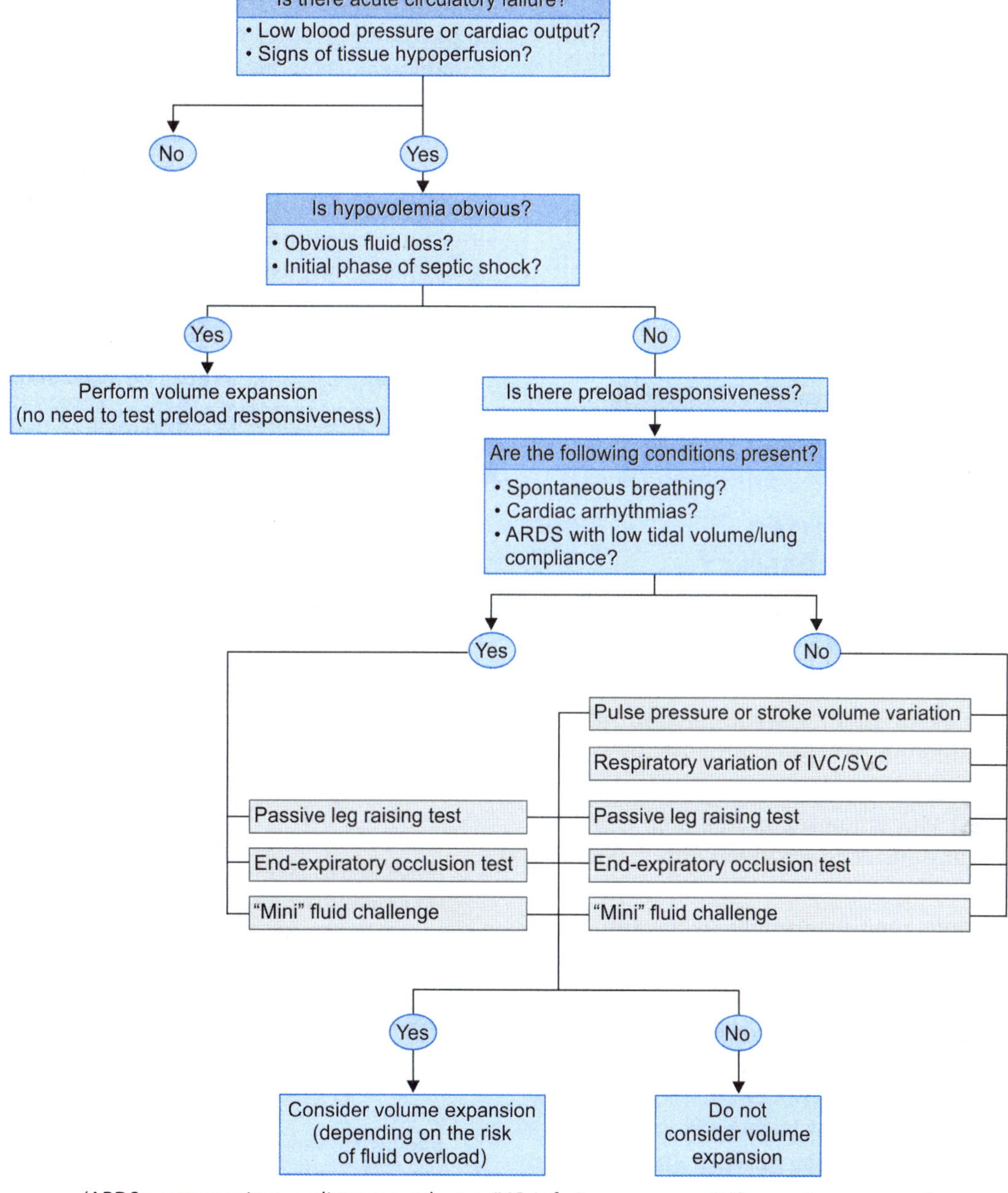

(ARDS: acute respiratory distress syndrome; IVC: inferior vena cava; SVC: superior vena cava)

markers evaluating the risk of fluid loading are mandatory. The transpulmonary thermodilution technique could be interesting to help guide fluid management since it allows us to measure the extravascular lung water and the pulmonary vascular permeability index.[52] Both of them are independent predictors of mortality and could be used as safety parameters of fluid administration in patients with ARDS.[4,52]

Fluid Responsiveness to Guide Fluid Removal During Renal Replacement Therapy

Fluid removal through diuretics or ultrafiltration is common in patients with acute circulatory failure or/and ARDS, especially at the late phase of shock management, since positive fluid balance is an independent risk factor of mortality.[2,48-53] However, the risk of fluid removal is dehydration and can impair the hemodynamic condition.[54]

Our group reported that hemodynamic intolerance during intermittent renal replacement therapy (RRT) is related to the presence of preload responsiveness, and a positive PLR test before starting ultrafiltration could reliably predict intradialytic hypotension (AUROC: 0.89).[55] One recent study showed that preload dependence-associated hypotension during intermittent hemodialysis was observed in 19% of the cases.[56] High values of the pulmonary vascular permeability index and use of mechanical ventilation were found to be risk factors for preload dependence-related hypotension during hemodialysis. It is thus reasonable to prompt a reduction of planned fluid removal therapy in these patients.[56] Further studies are needed to validate the hypothesis that protocolized RRT should include fluid responsiveness tests such as the PLR test.

ASSESSMENT OF PRELOAD RESPONSIVENESS TO PREDICT WEANING FAILURE FROM MECHANICAL VENTILATION

Another clinical application of testing preload responsiveness is to predict weaning failure from mechanical ventilation. Weaning-induced pulmonary edema (WiPO) is one of the most common causes of weaning failure.[57] Our group reported a high incidence of WiPO (58%) in difficult-to-wean patients.[58] Potential mechanisms including decreased intrathoracic pressure, activated adrenergic tone, hypoxemia, hypercapnia, and increased work of breathing result in increased right and left ventricular preload and afterload, and ultimately in WiPO.[57] One study showed that the occurrence of WiPO was associated with preload unresponsiveness before an spontaneous breathing trial (SBT).[59] In this study, preload unresponsiveness assessed by a negative PLR test before a SBT predicted weaning failure due to WiPO with an AUROC of 0.88.[59] A further study confirmed previous results and reported that a fluid removal therapy, changing preload unresponsiveness to preload responsiveness, facilitates the following SBT.[58] Conversely, patients with a sustained negative PLR test were more likely to have another failed SBT.[58] Hence, the presence of preload unresponsiveness assessed by a negative PLR test before SBT could be useful to predict weaning failure due to WiPO, while a positive PLR test could exclude a WiPO as the cause of weaning failure so that a diuretic therapy should not be recommended in this context.[58]

CONCLUSION

Since fluid overload has deleterious effects in critically ill patients, prediction of fluid responsiveness is fundamental. Dynamic tests are better predictors of fluid responsiveness than static markers of cardiac preload. Dynamic indices such as PPV and SVV are based on the heart–lung interactions and share important limitations. The EEO and PLR tests are reliable and usable in many situations encountered in the intensive care unit. Nevertheless, it must be kept in mind that the decision of fluid administration must not only be based on the presence of fluid responsiveness but also on the presence of signs of tissue hypoxia and on the individual assessment of its benefits/risks ratio.

REFERENCES

1. Michard F, Teboul JL. Predicting fluid responsiveness in ICU patients: a critical analysis of the evidence. Chest. 2002;121(6):2000-8.
2. Vincent JL, Sakr Y, Sprung CL, Ranieri VM, Reinhart K, Gerlach H, et al. Sepsis in European intensive care units: results of the SOAP study. Crit Care Med. 2006;34(2):344-53.
3. Sakr Y, Rubatto Birri PN, Kotfis K, Nanchal R, Shah B, Kluge S, et al. Higher fluid balance increases the risk of death from sepsis: results from a large international audit. Crit Care Med. 2017;45(3):386-94.
4. Jozwiak M, Silva S, Persichini R, Anguel N, Osman D, Richard C, et al. Extravascular lung water is an independent prognostic factor in patients with acute respiratory distress syndrome. Crit Care Med. 2013;41(2):472-80.
5. Jozwiak M, Hamzaoui O, Monnet X, Teboul JL. Fluid resuscitation during early sepsis: a need for individualization. Minerva Anestesiol. 2018;84(8):987-92.
6. Marik PE, Cavallazzi R. Does the central venous pressure predict fluid responsiveness? An updated meta-analysis and a plea for some common sense. Crit Care Med. 2013;41(7):1774-81.
7. Rhodes A, Evans LE, Alhazzani W, Levy MM, Antonelli M, Ferrer R, et al. Surviving Sepsis Campaign: International Guidelines for Management of Sepsis and Septic Shock: 2016. Intensive Care Med. 2017;43(3):304-77.
8. Monnet X, Marik P, Teboul JL. Prediction of fluid responsiveness: an update. Ann Intensive Care. 2016;6(1):111.
9. Teboul JL, Monnet X, Chemla D, Michard F. Arterial Pulse Pressure Variation with Mechanical Ventilation. Am J Respir Crit Care Med. 2019;199(1):22-31.
10. Monnet X, Osman D, Ridel C, Lamia B, Richard C, Teboul JL. Predicting volume responsiveness by using the end-expiratory occlusion in mechanically ventilated intensive care unit patients. Crit Care Med. 2009;37(3):951-6.

11. Myatra SN, Prabu NR, Divatia JV, Monnet X, Kulkarni AP, Teboul JL. The changes in pulse pressure variation or stroke volume variation after a "tidal volume challenge" reliably predict fluid responsiveness during low tidal volume ventilation. Crit Care Med. 2017;45(3):415-21.
12. Monnet X, Bleibtreu A, Ferré A, Dres M, Gharbi R, Richard C, et al. Passive leg-raising and end-expiratory occlusion tests perform better than pulse pressure variation in patients with low respiratory system compliance. Crit Care Med. 2012;40(1):152-7.
13. Silva S, Jozwiak M, Teboul JL, Persichini R, Richard C, Monnet X. End-expiratory occlusion test predicts preload responsiveness independently of positive end-expiratory pressure during acute respiratory distress syndrome. Crit Care Med. 2013;41(7):1692-701.
14. Monnet X, Dres M, Ferré A,Jozwiak M, Bleibtreu A, Le Deley MC, et al. Prediction of fluid responsiveness by a continuous non-invasive assessment of arterial pressure in critically ill patients: comparison with four other dynamic indices. Br J Anaesth. 2012;109(3):330-8.
15. Jozwiak M, Depret F, Teboul JL, Alphonsine JE, Lai C, Richard C, et al. Predicting fluid responsiveness in critically ill patients by using combined end-expiratory and end-inspiratory occlusions with echocardiography. Crit Care Med. 2017;45(11):e1131-e8.
16. Biais M, Larghi M, Henriot J, de Courson H, Sesay M, Nouette-Gaulain K. End-expiratory occlusion test predicts fluid responsiveness in patients with protective ventilation in the operating room. Anesth Analg. 2017;125(6):1889-95.
17. Georges D, de Courson H, Lanchon R, Sesay M, Nouette-Gaulain K, Biais M. End-expiratory occlusion maneuver to predict fluid responsiveness in the intensive care unit: an echocardiographic study. Crit Care. 2018;22:32.
18. Dépret F, Jozwiak M, Teboul JL, Alphonsine JE, Richard C, Monnet X. Esophageal Doppler can predict fluid responsiveness through end-expiratory and end-inspiratory occlusion tests. Crit Care Med. 2019;47(2):e96-e102.
19. Messina A, Montagnini C, Cammarota G, De Rosa S, Giuliani F, Muratore L, et al. Tidal volume challenge to predict fluid responsiveness in the operating room: An observational study. Eur J Anaesthesiol. 2019;36(8):583-91.
20. Yonis H, Bitker L, Aublanc M, Perinel Ragey S, Riad Z, Lissonde F, et al. Change in cardiac output during the Trendelenburg maneuver is a reliable predictor of fluid responsiveness in patients with acute respiratory distress syndrome in the prone position under protective ventilation. Crit Care. 2017;21(1):295.
21. Guinot PG, Godart J, de Broca B, Bernard E, Lorne E, Dupont H. End-expiratory occlusion manoeuvre does not accurately predict fluid responsiveness in the operating theatre. Br J Anaesth. 2014;112(6):1050-4.
22. Monnet X, Teboul JL. End-expiratory occlusion test: please use the appropriate tools! Br J Anaesth. 2015;114(1):166-7.
23. Hamzaoui O, Monnet X, Richard C, Osman D, Chemla D, Teboul JL. Effects of changes in vascular tone on the agreement between pulse contour and transpulmonary thermodilution cardiac output measurements within an up to 6-hour calibration-free period. Crit Care Med. 2008;36(2):434-40.
24. Jozwiak M, Mercado P, Teboul JL, Benmalek A, Gimenez J, Dépret F, et al. What is the lowest change in cardiac output that transthoracic echocardiography can detect? Crit Care. 2019;23:116.
25. Boulain T, Achard JM, Teboul JL, Richard C, Perrotin D, Ginies G. Changes in BP induced by passive leg raising predict response to fluid loading in critically ill patients. Chest. 2002;121(4):1245-52.
26. Jabot J, Teboul JL, Richard C, Monnet X. Passive leg raising for predicting fluid responsiveness: importance of the postural change. Intensive Care Med. 2009;35(1):85-90.
27. Guerin L, Teboul JL, Persichini R, Dres M, Richard C, Monnet X. Effects of passive leg raising and volume expansion on mean systemic pressure and venous return in shock in humans. Crit Care. 2015;19:411.
28. Monnet X, Rienzo M, Osman D, et al. Passive leg raising predicts fluid responsiveness in the critically ill. Critical Care Medicine. 2006;34(5):1402-7.
29. Monnet X, Marik P, Teboul JL. Passive leg raising for predicting fluid responsiveness: a systematic review and meta-analysis. Intensive Care Med. 2016;42(12):1935-47.
30. Cherpanath TG, Hirsch A, Geerts BF, Lagrand WK, Leeflang MM, Schultz MJ, et al. Predicting fluid responsiveness by passive leg raising: a systematic review and meta-analysis of 23 clinical trials. Crit Care Med. 2016;44(5):981-91.
31. Cecconi M, De Backer D, Antonelli M, Beale R, Bakker J, Hofer C, et al. Consensus on circulatory shock and hemodynamic monitoring. Task force of the European Society of Intensive Care Medicine. Intensive Care Med. 2014;40(12):1795-815.
32. Préau S, Saulnier F, Dewavrin F, Durocher A, Chagnon JL. Passive leg raising is predictive of fluid responsiveness in spontaneously breathing patients with severe sepsis or acute pancreatitis. Crit Care Med. 2010;38(3):819-25.
33. Kim N, Shim JK, Choi HG, Kim MK, Kim JY, Kwak YL. Comparison of positive end-expiratory pressure-induced increase in central venous pressure and passive leg raising to predict fluid responsiveness in patients with atrial fibrillation. Br J Anaesth. 2016;116(3):350-6.
34. Monnet X, Teboul JL. Passive leg raising: five rules, not a drop of fluid! Crit Care. 2015;19(1):18.
35. Marik PE, Levitov A, Young A, Andrews L. The use of bioreactance and carotid Doppler to determine volume responsiveness and blood flow redistribution following passive leg raising in hemodynamically unstable patients. Chest. 2013;143(2):364-70.
36. Kupersztych-Hagege E, Teboul JL, Artigas A, Talbot A, Sabatier C, Richard C, et al. Bioreactance is not reliable for estimating cardiac output and the effects of passive leg raising in critically ill patients. Br J Anaesth. 2013;111(6):961-6.

37. Galarza L, Mercado P, Teboul JL, Girotto V, Beurton A, Richard C, et al. Estimating the rapid haemodynamic effects of passive leg raising in critically ill patients using bioreactance. Br J Anaesth. 2018;121(3):567-73.
38. Monge García MI, Gil Cano A, Gracia Romero M, Monterroso Pintado R, Pérez Madueño V, et al. Non-invasive assessment of fluid responsiveness by changes in partial end-tidal CO_2 pressure during a passive leg-raising maneuver. Ann Intensive Care. 2012;2:9.
39. Monnet X, Bataille A, Magalhaes E, Barrois J, Le Corre M, Gosset C, et al. End-tidal carbon dioxide is better than arterial pressure for predicting volume responsiveness by the passive leg raising test. Intensive Care Med. 2013;39(1):93-100.
40. Xiao-ting W, Hua Z, Da-wei L, Hong-min Z, Huai-wu H, Yun L, et al. Changes in end-tidal CO_2 could predict fluid responsiveness in the passive leg raising test but not in the mini-fluid challenge test: A prospective and observational study. J Crit Care. 2015;30(5):1061-6.
41. Xu J, Peng X, Pan C, Cai S, Zhang X, Xue M, et al. Fluid responsiveness predicted by transcutaneous partial pressure of oxygen in patients with circulatory failure: a prospective study. Ann Intensive Care. 2017;7:56.
42. Beurton A, Teboul JL, Gavelli F, Gonzalez FA, Girotto V, Galarza L, et al. The effects of passive leg raising may be detected by the plethysmographic oxygen saturation signal in critically ill patients. Crit Care. 2019;23(1):19.
43. Monnet X, Teboul JL. Passive leg raising. Intensive Care Med. 2008;34(4):659-63.
44. Mahjoub Y, Touzeau J, Airapetian N, Lorne E, Hijazi M, Zogheib E, et al. The passive leg-raising maneuver cannot accurately predict fluid responsiveness in patients with intra-abdominal hypertension. Crit Care Med. 2010;38(9):1824-9.
45. Beurton A, Teboul JL, Girotto V, Galarza L, Anguel N, Richard C, et al. Intra-abdominal hypertension is responsible for false negatives to the passive leg raising test. Crit Care Med. 2019;47(8):e639-47.
46. Malbrain ML, Reuter DA. Assessing fluid responsiveness with the passive leg raising maneuver in patients with increased intra-abdominal pressure: be aware that not all blood returns! Crit Care Med. 2010;38(9):1912-5.
47. Chacko CJ, Wise MP, Frost PJ. Passive leg raising and compression stockings: a note of caution. Crit Care. 2015;19(1):237.
48. Lira A, Pinsky MR. Choices in fluid type and volume during resuscitation: impact on patient outcomes. Ann Intensive Care. 2014;4:38.
49. Leisman DE, Doerfler ME, Schneider SM, Masick KD, D'Amore JA, D'Angelo JK. Predictors, prevalence, and outcomes of early crystalloid responsiveness among initially hypotensive patients with sepsis and septic shock. Crit Care Med. 2018;4(2)6:189-98.
50. Li DK, Wang XT, Liu DW. Association between elevated central venous pressure and outcomes in critically ill patients. Ann Intensive Care. 2017;7(1):83.
51. Acheampong A, Vincent JL. A positive fluid balance is an independent prognostic factor in patients with sepsis. Crit Care. 2015;19(1):251.
52. Jozwiak M, Teboul JL, Monnet X. Extravascular lung water in critical care: recent advances and clinical applications. Ann Intensive Care. 2015;5(1):38.
53. Vincent JL, De Backer D. Circulatory shock. N Engl J Med. 2013;369(18):1726-34.
54. Schortgen F. Hypotension during intermittent hemodialysis: new insights into an old problem. Intensive Care Med. 2003;29(10):1645-9.
55. Monnet X, Cipriani F, Camous L, Sentenac P, Dres M, Krastinova E, et al. The passive leg raising test to guide fluid removal in critically ill patients. Ann Intensive Care. 2016;6:46.
56. Bitker L, Bayle F, Yonis H, Gobert F, Leray V, Taponnier R, et al. Prevalence and risk factors of hypotension associated with preload-dependence during intermittent hemodialysis in critically ill patients. Crit Care. 2016;20:44.
57. Teboul JL. Weaning-induced cardiac dysfunction: where are we today? Intensive Care Med. 2014;40(8):1069-79.
58. Liu J, Shen F, Teboul JL, Anguel N, Beurton A, Bezaz N, et al. Cardiac dysfunction induced by weaning from mechanical ventilation: incidence, risk factors, and effects of fluid removal. Crit Care. 2016;20(1):369.
59. Dres M, Teboul JL, Anguel N, Guerin L, Richard C, Monnet X. Passive leg raising performed before a spontaneous breathing trial predicts weaning-induced cardiac dysfunction. Intensive Care Med. 2015;41(3):487-94.

CHAPTER

Is it High Time to Start Checking Fluid Tolerance?

Sumalatha A, Atul Prabhakar Kulkarni

INTRODUCTION

The main goal of fluid resuscitation is to increase cardiac output (CO) in a preload-responsive patient to increase tissue perfusion. However, this may also result in increased venous pressure in various organs such as the kidney, lungs, liver, and gut, especially in the presence of damaged endothelial glycocalyx. There is now widespread evidence that overzealous administration of intravenous (IV) fluids is detrimental. It leads to worsening respiratory function, increased risk of infections, increased risk of acute kidney injury (AKI), increased length of intensive care unit (ICU) stays, and increased mortality. Hence, despite the patient being fluid-responsive, it is important to assess the ability of end organs to handle the "venous congestion."

WHAT IS FLUID TOLERANCE?

Fluid tolerance (FT) is the ability of the body to receive an infusion of fluids without progressing to organ dysfunction. Fluid intolerance may be caused by a variety of mechanisms, such as:

- Tissue damage in the microcirculation from increased oxygen diffusion distance to the cells and hemodilution leading to a decrease in oxygenated red blood cells.[1]
- Changes in the endothelial glycocalyx with altered vascular permeability and increased tissue edema.[2]
- Increased intraparenchymal pressure in encapsulated organs, such as the liver and kidneys, which causes lower tissue blood flow and lower perfusion pressure.[3]

Fluid Responsiveness versus Fluid Tolerance

Fluid responsiveness is a state wherein the focus is on the ability of a biventricular system to increase CO to >10–15% of baseline after a fluid bolus.[4] It does not describe or assess the state of downstream organs such as the renal and respiratory systems which receive this additional CO. Here lies the inherent fallacy of fluid responsiveness. The assumption that increases in CO will lead to increased tissue perfusion in end organs may not hold ground as organ perfusion is also dependent on the venous pressure of individual organs.

For example, the renal perfusion pressure = Mean arterial pressure – renal venous pressure.

Whereas during an assessment of fluid tolerance, the focus is on the end organ receiving the increased perfusion. Fluid tolerance therefore describes the ability of organs to undergo fluid expansion without experiencing the harmful effects of fluid overload. It may be plausible that a patient might be fluid-responsive but fluid-intolerant. Studies by Muñoz et al.[5] and Osman et al.[6] have shown that the prevalence of venous congestion is almost equal in both fluid-responsive and volume-overloaded patients. Therefore, the intensivist should be aware of the possibility that despite being in shock and fluid responsive, the patient may be harmed by fluid therapy if their end organs are fluid intolerant. This concept raises questions about a traditionally accepted universal strategy of administering IV fluid to patients who are fluid-responsive. Intensivists need to be now aware of the possibility of venous congestion in such patients and understand the limits of fluid therapy.

Assessment of Fluid Tolerance

The assessment of fluid tolerance necessitates the utilization of various indices, pressures, and ultrasound (USG)-based markers. These markers can be broadly categorized into three groups:

1. Those indicating fluid tolerance on the right side of the circulation
2. Those indicating fluid tolerance on the left side of the circulation
3. Organ-specific markers

Indicators of Fluid Tolerance on the Right Side of Circulation

Mean central venous pressure (CVP): CVP is recognized as neither a measure of volume status nor fluid responsiveness, yet it remains a critical determinant of venous return since venous return is the difference between mean systemic filling pressure (MSFP) and CVP. With the increasing importance of dynamic markers of fluid responsiveness, the relevance of measuring CVP has diminished. Nonetheless, CVP is a significant marker of downstream pressure influencing venous return and organ function.

Typically, CVP is low, ranging from 4 to 8 cmH_2O, and elevated CVP values are associated with poorer outcomes in ICU settings. Some studies have reported higher mortality rates in patients with CVP exceeding 8 cmH_2O compared to those with lower values, although this association is not causal.[7,8] An increase of 1 cmH_2O in CVP is associated with an increased risk of AKI by an odds ratio of 1.02.[9] The risk of AKI is higher in patients with acute decompensated heart failure (ADHF) who have a CVP >8 cmH_2O compared to those with lower CVP levels.[10] Thus, a high CVP serves as a surrogate marker for venous congestion and can be used to assess fluid tolerance.

Despite the reliability of CVP as a marker of fluid tolerance, there is no defined optimal threshold to classify patients as fluid intolerant. Various studies have used a threshold of 12 cm of water,[5,7] but this cut-off was not sensitive and identified only 25% of patients as fluid intolerant.[11] When a threshold of 8 cm of water was used, sensitivity improved.[11] However, further studies in different subpopulations are necessary to determine an optimal cutoff. Beyond its threshold, a significant limitation of CVP in evaluating venous congestion is its inability to provide direct information on organ perfusion. Ideally, venous congestion should be measured in individual organs such as the kidney, gut, brain, and liver. Additionally, CVP cannot assess congestion in the lungs. Given these limitations, along with potential pitfalls and errors during CVP measurement, intensivists must exercise caution when using CVP alone to determine fluid tolerance.

VExUS score: Based on an original concept by Andre Y Denault and Philippe Role, a venous excess ultrasound score (VExUS) was developed in patients who underwent cardiac surgery to predict the incidence of acute kidney injury based on venous congestion.[12] It involves ultrasound

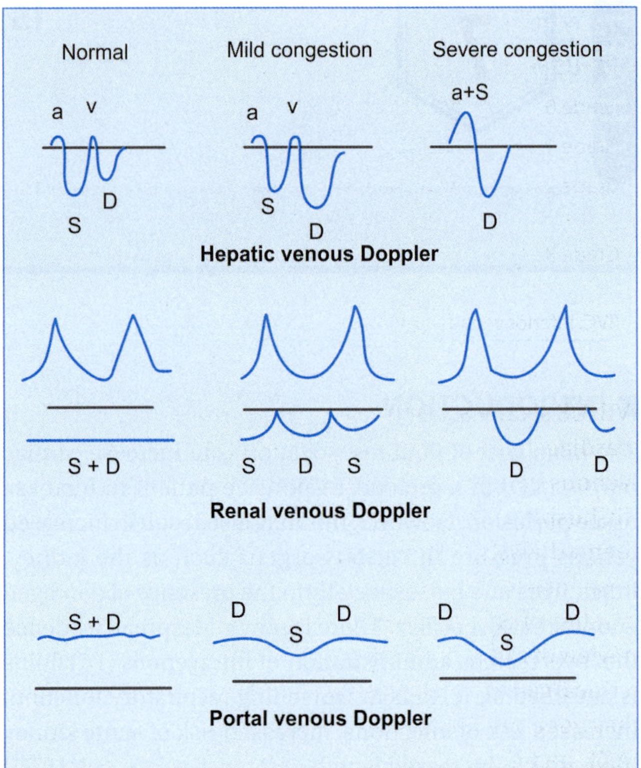

Fig. 1: Grading of venous Doppler of the hepatic, portal, and intrarenal veins.
Source: Modified from Karki et al.[13]

assessment of hepatic, portal, and renal vein Doppler along with inferior vena cava (IVC). The physiological basis while developing the VExUS score was that flow patterns in the hepatic, portal, and renal veins describe the congestion in the liver, gut, and kidneys respectively **(Fig. 1)**.[13] The extra volume brought on by congestive causes in any venous vascular system will eventually exceed the maximum limitations creating a sharp increase in venous pressure due to the systemic venous capacitance. Dilated large veins (vena cava and internal jugular) and abnormal venous waveforms of organ-specific major veins (portal, hepatic, and renal veins) suggest the limit of systemic venous compliance.

Based on the venous Doppler of the aforementioned three veins and IVC diameter, the VExUS grade is given in **Table 1**.

Evidence for VExUS score—After the seminal publication of the VExUS score by Beaubien-Souligny W et al.,[12] multiple observational studies and case series have shown positive effects of the VExUS score in fluid management.[14-21]

TABLE 1: Grading of VExUS score.

VExUS grade	*Findings*
Grade 0	IVC <2 cm
Grade 1	IVC ≥2 cm with normal/mild abnormalities
Grade 2	IVC ≥2 cm with severe abnormality in at least one of the veins
Grade 3	IVC ≥2 cm with severe abnormalities in multiple veins

(IVC: inferior vena cava; VExUS: venous excess ultrasound score)

VExUS score has been shown to predict AKI in congestive cardiac failure,[14] and cardiorenal syndrome,[18] assess venous congestion in acute heart failure and predicted in-hospital mortality,[16] and to guide ultrafiltration in hemodialysis.[17] However, it could not reliably predict response to diuretic therapy when compared to Doppler studies of the portal and intrarenal veins.[19] A systematic review of 15 publications on the VExUS score in emergency, critical care, and perioperative settings showed that VExUS has good reliability in predicting venous congestion and AKI, had good correlation with CVP measurements but questionable specificity for predicting outcomes in acute heart failure patients.[21] High-quality studies are needed to further confirm these findings.

Venous reflux status (VRS): Zhao et al.[22] hypothesized that venous compliance is decreased in patients with right ventricular dysfunction due to various disorders in the ICU such as acute respiratory distress syndrome (ARDS), sepsis, inappropriate mechanical ventilation, poisoning, postcardiac surgery, and congestive cardiac failure. Any altered venous compliance leads to altered venous flow and they labeled it as "venous reflux status." Evaluation of VRS and normalization of venous reflux may mitigate acute kidney injury. They proposed evaluation of VRS using bedside Doppler ultrasound of hepatic, portal, renal and intrarenal, common femoral, and pulmonary veins **(Fig. 2)**.

They propose a sequential examination of VRS in a particular order based on the distance of various venous systems from the heart **(Fig. 3)**. They argue that any rise in distal venous pressure without elevation of pressures in more proximal veins (for example, common femoral venous reflux seen without reflux in hepatic vein suggests local pathologies than systemic venous congestion). Pulmonary VRS evaluates tolerance to fluid therapy in the pulmonary circulation.

Studies comparing VRS over VExUS scores are needed to confirm their predictive ability for fluid tolerance.

IVC diameter: IVC alone can be used to measure fluid tolerance.[23,24] A dilated noncollapsible IVC indicates fluid intolerance and venous congestion. The risk of AKI is less in patients with normal IVC.[24] There are no studies so far comparing VExUS score and IVC diameter for predicting fluid tolerance.

Indicators of Fluid Tolerance on the Left Side of Circulation (Cardiopulmonary System)

- Pulmonary artery occlusion pressure (PAOP)
- Diastolic indices by echocardiography (E/E' and E/A)
- B lines on lung ultrasound
- Extravascular lung water (EVLW) and pulmonary vascular permeability index (PVPI)

Organ-specific Measures of Fluid Tolerance

It is also plausible that a patient may be fluid responsive and fluid tolerant for some organs (kidneys, liver) but fluid nontolerant for others (respiratory system). Hence, it is important to assess the fluid tolerance of individual internal organs, especially in patients with multiorgan dysfunction. **Table 2** summarizes the organ-specific measures of fluid tolerance.

Based on these hemodynamic profiles, Melo HR et al.[25] proposed the following classification and management of patients based on fluid status **(Table 3)**.

Incorporating the concept of fluid tolerance into daily practice

It is evident from the currently available evidence that fluid responsiveness and fluid intolerance are two distinct entities and can coexist in the same patient and hence not mutually exclusive phenomena. Thus, in a hemodynamically unstable patient, an intensivist should assess both the fluid responsiveness and fluid tolerance status of the patient **(Flowchart 1)**. Also, organ-specific assessment of fluid tolerance should be performed tailoring to the patient's diagnosis before giving fluids despite the patient being fluid responsive; some examples are discussed in **Table 4**.

The concept of fluid tolerance represents a critical evolution in the management of critically ill patients, particularly in the context of fluid resuscitation. While fluid responsiveness has traditionally guided treatment, focusing solely on the ability to increase CO may lead

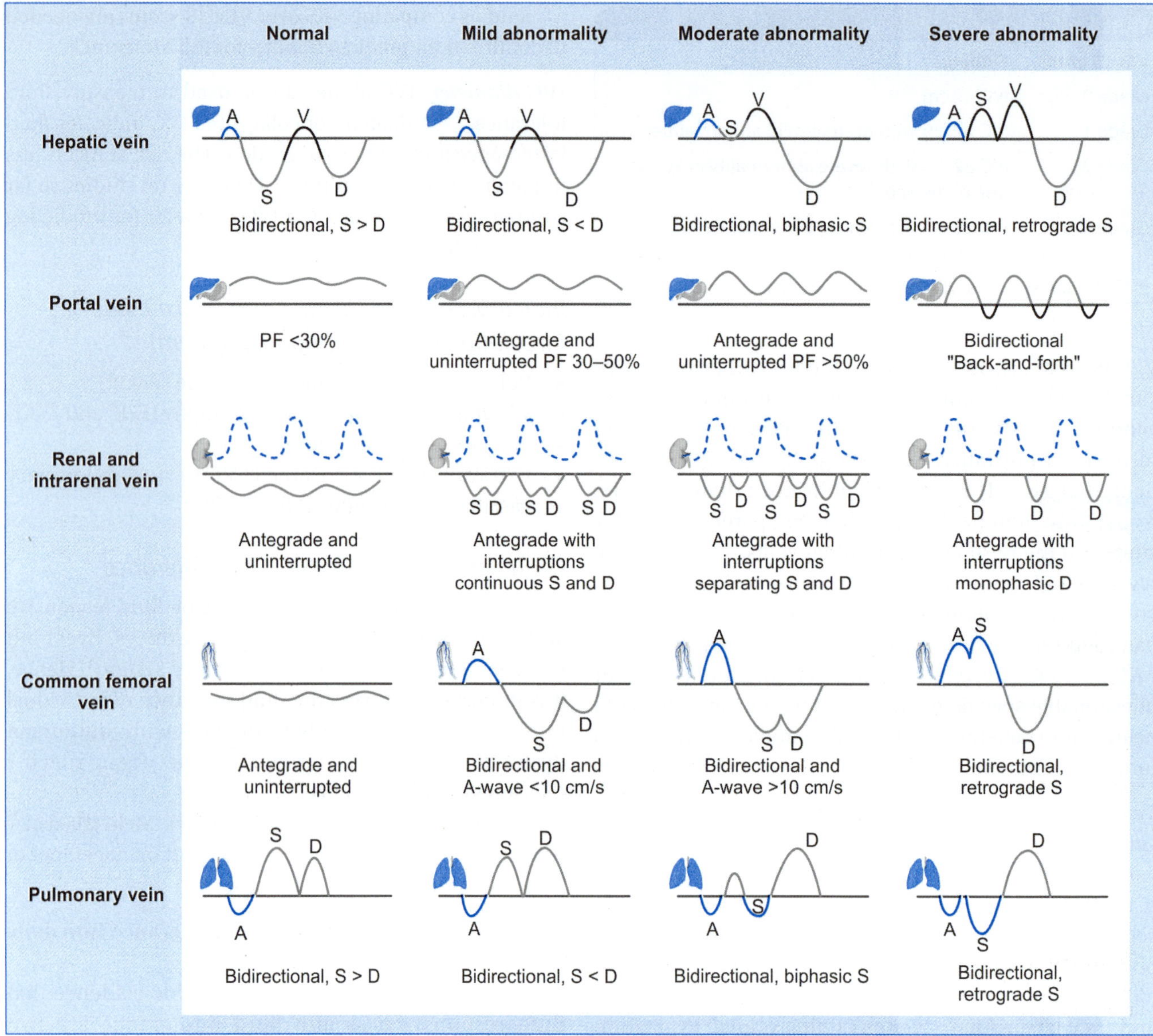

Fig. 2: Grading of VRS. (VRS: venous reflux status)
Source: Modified from Zhao et al.[22]

to significant harm if the end-organ capacity to tolerate increased venous pressure is overlooked. Fluid tolerance acknowledges the limitations of downstream organs in handling additional fluid load, emphasizing the need for a more nuanced approach to fluid therapy.

Incorporating assessments of fluid tolerance into clinical practice requires the utilization of advanced monitoring tools, such as the VExUS score, venous reflux status, and specific organ-focused assessments. By evaluating both fluid responsiveness and fluid tolerance, intensivists can make more informed decisions, avoiding the potential pitfalls of fluid overload that can exacerbate organ dysfunction.

As evidence continues to emerge, the integration of fluid tolerance assessments promises to refine fluid management strategies, ultimately improving patient outcomes by tailoring interventions to the unique hemodynamic and organ-specific needs of each patient.

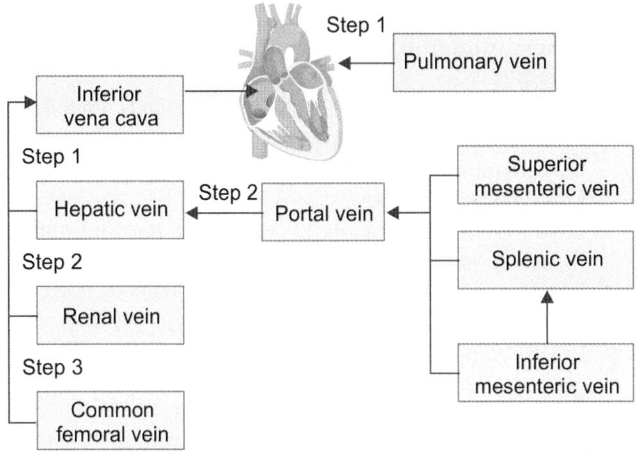

Fig. 3: Sequential evaluation of venous reflux status (VRS). *Source:* Modified from Zhoa et al.[22]

TABLE 2: Organ-specific measures of fluid tolerance.

Organs	*Measures of fluid tolerance*
Respiratory system	• B lines on USG • EVLW and PVPI
Abdominal compartment	• Dilated, noncollapsing IVC • VExUS score • Venous reflux status • Intra-abdominal pressure monitoring
Renal	• Dilated, noncollapsing IVC • VExUS score • Venous reflux status
Cardiac system	• Lack of fluid responsiveness • D-shaped septum • Systolic or diastolic dysfunction

(EVLW: extravascular lung water; IVC: inferior vena cava; PVPI: pulmonary vascular permeability index; VExUS: venous excess ultrasound score)

TABLE 3: Classification of patients into four hemodynamic profiles based on fluid status and their management.

Patient subgroup	*Fluid responsive*	*Fluid tolerance*	*Management*
A	Present	Present	Fluid resuscitation
B	Absent	Present	Fluid restriction
C	Absent	Absent	Diuretics, ultrafiltration
D	Present	Absent	Early use of vasopressors

Source: Modified from Melo et al.[25]

Flowchart 1: An approach to patients with hemodynamic instability incorporating tests of fluid responsiveness and fluid tolerance status.

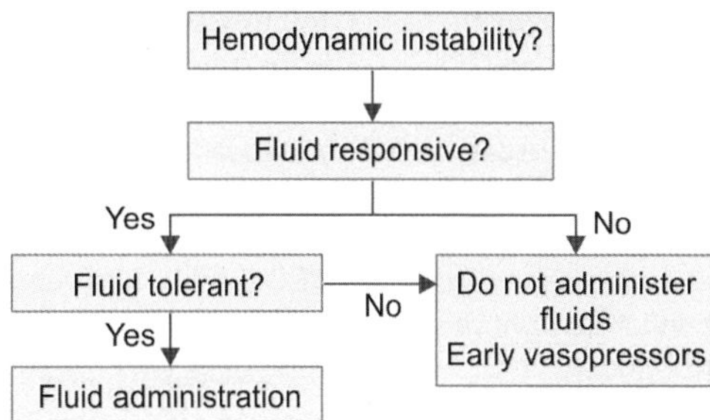

Source: Adapted and modified from Melo et al.[25]

TABLE 4: Incorporation of tests evaluating organ-specific measures of fluid tolerance in specific case scenarios.

Case scenario	*Assessment for fluid tolerance*
Acute severe pancreatitis with septic shock on invasive mechanical ventilation with ARDS	• Measure VExUS score and intra-abdominal pressure to assess fluid tolerance status of kidneys and gut • EVLW, PVPI, and B lines on USG for lungs • D-shaped ventricle, E/E', E/A, PAOP for the heart
Community-acquired pneumonia with morbid obesity and ARDS on prone ventilation with acute kidney injury	• Measure hepatic venous and renal venous flow (limited VExUS scoring excluding IVC) and intra-abdominal pressure to assess the fluid tolerance status of kidneys and gut • EVLW, PVPI, and B lines on USG for lungs • CVP is valuable in assessing the fluid tolerance status of the right heart
Postmitral valve replacement surgery for infective endocarditis with acute glomerulonephritis on invasive mechanical ventilation with septic and cardiogenic shock	• Dilated, noncollapsing IVC, VExUS score, and venous reflux status for the kidneys • D-shaped septum, PAOP, CVP, systolic or diastolic dysfunction for the heart
Acute exacerbation of bronchial asthma with cor pulmonale, obesity secondary to steroid dependency, and cardiorenal syndrome on invasive mechanical ventilation	• CVP, D-shaped ventricle, E/E', E/A, PAOP for the heart • Dilated, noncollapsing IVC, VExUS score, and venous reflux status for the kidneys

Contd...

Contd...

Case scenario	*Assessment for fluid tolerance*
Diffuse axonal injury with raised ICP due to road traffic injury, paralytic ileus secondary to psoas hematoma, cellulitis of right thigh, acute kidney injury due to myoglobinuria caused by crush injury to right thigh with septic shock	• IAP to assess the fluid tolerance status of the gut. Fluid intolerance is reflected by increased IAP which will also worsen ICP • Dilated, noncollapsing IVC, VExUS score, and venous reflux status for the kidneys

(EVLW: extravascular lung water; IAP: intra-abdominal pressure; ICP: intracranial pressure; PAOP: pulmonary artery occlusion pressure; PVPI: pulmonary vascular permeability index; USG: ultrasound; VExUS: venous excess ultrasound score)

CONCLUSION

Intensivists need to be aware of the possibility of venous congestion in patients who are fluid-responsive and are receiving intravenous fluids, and understand the limits of fluid therapy.

It is evident from the currently available evidence that fluid responsiveness and fluid intolerance are two distinct entities and can coexist in the same patient and hence not mutually exclusive phenomena. Thus, in a hemodynamically unstable patient, an intensivist should assess both the fluid responsiveness and fluid tolerance status of the patient. The assessment of fluid tolerance involves the utilization of various indices, pressures, and ultrasound (USG)-based markers. IVC diameter, VExUS score, E/E', and E/A should be routinely done in all patients who are receiving volume expansion.

REFERENCES

1. Wollborn J, Hassenzahl LO, Reker D, Staehle HF, Omlor AM, Baar W, et al. Diagnosing capillary leak in critically ill patients: development of an innovative scoring instrument for non-invasive detection. Ann Intensive Care. 2021;11(1):175.
2. Uchimido R, Schmidt EP, Shapiro NI. The glycocalyx: a novel diagnostic and therapeutic target in sepsis. Crit Care Lond Engl. 2019;23(1):16.
3. Rajendram R, Prowle JR. Venous congestion: are we adding insult to kidney injury in sepsis? Crit Care Lond Engl. 2014;18(1):104.
4. Monnet X, Shi R, Teboul JL. Prediction of fluid responsiveness. What's new? Ann Intensive Care. 2022;12(1):46.
5. Muñoz F, Born P, Bruna M, Ulloa R, González C, Philp V, et al. Coexistence of a fluid responsive state and venous congestion signals in critically ill patients: a multicenter observational proof-of-concept study. Crit Care. 2024;28(1):52.
6. Osman D, Ridel C, Ray P, Monnet X, Anguel N, Richard C, et al. Cardiac filling pressures are not appropriate to predict hemodynamic response to volume challenge. Crit Care Med. 2007;35(1):64-8.
7. Boyd JH, Forbes J, Nakada TA, Walley KR, Russell JA. Fluid resuscitation in septic shock: a positive fluid balance and elevated central venous pressure are associated with increased mortality. Crit Care Med. 2011;39(2):259-65.
8. Li DK, Wang XT, Liu DW. Association between elevated central venous pressure and outcomes in critically ill patients. Ann Intensive Care. 2017;7(1):83.
9. Chen KP, Cavender S, Lee J, Feng M, Mark RG, Celi LA, et al. Peripheral Edema, Central Venous Pressure, and Risk of AKI in Critical Illness. Clin J Am Soc Nephrol CJASN. 2016;11(4):602-8.
10. Mullens W, Abrahams Z, Francis GS, Sokos G, Taylor DO, Starling RC, et al. Importance of venous congestion for worsening of renal function in advanced decompensated heart failure. J Am Coll Cardiol. 2009;53(7):589-96.
11. Joseph A, Petit M, Vignon P, Vieillard-Baron A. Fluid responsiveness and venous congestion: unraveling the nuances of fluid status. Crit Care. 2024;28(1):140.
12. Beaubien-Souligny W, Rola P, Haycock K, Bouchard J, Lamarche Y, Spiegel R, et al. Quantifying systemic congestion with point-of-care ultrasound: development of the venous excess ultrasound grading system. Ultrasound J. 2020;12(1):16.
13. Karki B, Ghimire S, Vaddi B, Shrestha GS, Soliman-Aboumarie H. VExUS: The Holy Grail or Achilles Heel of fluid management? J Nepal Soc Crit Care Med. 2024;2:18-24.
14. Singh K, Carvalho R. Perioperative Venous Excess Ultrasound Score (VExUS) to Guide Decongestion in a Dilated Cardiomyopathy Patient Presenting for Urgent Surgery. Cureus. 2021;13(12):e20545.
15. Rola P, Miralles-Aguiar F, Argaiz E, et al. Clinical applications of the venous excess ultrasound (VExUS) score: conceptual review and case series. Ultrasound J. 2021;13(1):32.
16. Anastasiou V, Peteinidou E, Moysidis DV, Beaubien-Souligny W, Haycock K, Karimov T, et al. Multiorgan Congestion Assessment by Venous Excess Ultrasound Score in Acute Heart Failure. J Am Soc Echocardiogr Off Publ Am Soc Echocardiogr. 2024;S0894-7317(24)00234-7.
17. Koratala A, Ibrahim M, Gudlawar S. VExUS to Guide Ultrafiltration in Hemodialysis: Exploring a Novel Dimension of Point of Care Ultrasound. POCUS J. 2024;9(1):16-9.
18. Bhardwaj V, Vikneswaran G, Rola P, Raju S, Bhat RS, Jayakumar A, et al. Combination of Inferior Vena Cava Diameter, Hepatic Venous Flow, and Portal Vein Pulsatility Index: Venous Excess Ultrasound Score (VEXUS Score) in Predicting Acute Kidney Injury in Patients with Cardiorenal

Syndrome: A Prospective Cohort Study. Indian J Crit Care. 2020;24(9):783-9.
19. Guinot PG, Bahr PA, Andrei S, Popescu BA, Caruso V, Mertes PM, et al. Doppler study of the portal vein and renal venous velocity predict the appropriate fluid response to the diuretic in ICU: a prospective observational echocardiographic evaluation. Crit Care. 2022;26(1):305.
20. Menéndez-Suso JJ, Rodríguez-Álvarez D, Sánchez-Martín M. Feasibility and Utility of the Venous Excess Ultrasound Score to Detect and Grade Central Venous Pressure Elevation in Critically Ill Children. J Ultrasound Med Off J Am Inst Ultrasound Med. 2023;42(1):211-20.
21. Gupta B, Ahluwalia P, Gupta A, Ranjan N, Kakkar K, Aneja P. Utility of VExUS score in the perioperative care unit, intensive care unit, and emergency setting - A systematic review. Indian J Anaesth. 2023;67(Suppl 4):S218-26.
22. Zhao H, Gao B, Zhang H, Wang X; Critical Care Ultrasound Study Group. The Importance of Venous Reflux Status Evaluation in the Intensive Care Unit. Aging Dis. 2024;15(3):953-64.
23. Argaiz ER, Rola P, Haycock KH, Verbrugge FH. Fluid management in acute kidney injury: from evaluating fluid responsiveness towards assessment of fluid tolerance. Eur Heart J Acute Cardiovasc Care. 2022;11(10): 786-93.
24. Rola P, Haycock K, Spiegel R. What every intensivist should know about the IVC. J Crit Care. 2024;80:154455.
25. Melo RH, dos Santos MHC, Ramos FJ da S. Beyond fluid responsiveness: the concept of fluid tolerance and its potential implication in hemodynamic management. Crit Care 2023;35(2):226-9.

SECTION

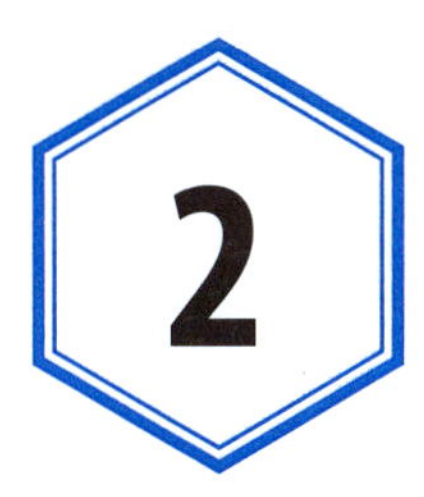

Cardiac Output Measurement

CHAPTER

Pulmonary Artery Catheterization

Nishanth Baliga, Atul Prabhakar Kulkarni, Jigeeshu Vasistha Divatia

INTRODUCTION

Pulmonary artery catheterization (PAC) was first done under fluoroscopic guidance in the mid-1940s. Balloon floatation pulmonary artery catheter was introduced in the 1970s by Dr HJC Jeremy Swan and Dr William Ganz for assessment of heart function at the bedside. Initially utilized in cardiac catheterization laboratories, PAC subsequently was being used in cardiac surgery, coronary care units, medical and surgical ICU for assessment of hemodynamics, measure cardiac output as well as to monitor response to treatment. For the next 30 years PAC was being extensively used until the advent of less invasive devices especially bedside echocadiography with which frequency of use declined.

INDICATIONS

The current indications for the insertion of PAC in the ICU are limited. It should be inserted in centers with nursing expertise in the management of catheters and sufficient physician experience in the interpretation of data in the following conditions:

1. *Cardiac surgery:* Patients undergoing complex cardiac surgeries such as complex valvular heart disease, congenital heart disease, left to right shunt, severe underlying cardiovascular disease who are undergoing corrective surgery.
2. *Right heart failure and pulmonary hypertension*: Bedside echocardiography is not very sensitive for determination or measurement of pulmonary artery pressures as well as right heart function. Hence, in patients with right heart failure and pulmonary hypertension, PAC gives direct measurement of pulmonary artery and right ventricular pressures which can be used to guide therapy.
3. *Unexplained or complicated shock:* In patients with complicated shock with combination of septic, obstructive, cardiogenic or hypovolemic shock, PAC helps in guiding therapy such as fluids, vasopressors, inotropes by direct measurements of pressures along with calculated variables.
4. *Severe heart failure*: Few subset of patients who have right as well as left heart failure, data obtained from insertion of PAC can help to determine severity of hemodynamic abnormalities to guide therapy as well as to assess prognosis.
5. As part of workup or bridge to cardiac transplantation or left ventricular assist device (LVAD).[1-3]

CONTRAINDICATIONS

Some of the contraindications for the placement of PAC are:

- Infection at the insertion site
- Coagulopathy
- Right sided cardiac mass
- Right ventricular assist device
- Prosthesis at the site of pulmonary or tricuspid valve
- Tricuspid or pulmonary valve endocarditis
- Severe tricuspid regurgitation
- Lack of consent[4]

PARTS OF THE PULMONARY ARTERY CATHETERIZATION

Pulmonary artery catheter is usually 7–9 Fr in size and length is 110 cm which is marked at 10 cm intervals. It usually has four or five ports.

1. The distal port usually yellow color is at the catheter tip which is used for monitoring of pulmonary artery pressure and to collect specimens for mixed venous oxygen saturation.

2. The second port blue in color opens 30 cm proximal from the tip is used for monitoring central venous pressure (CVP) as well as infusion of fluids and drugs.
3. The third port red in color leads to a balloon near the tip with a locking port is used for inflation and deflation of balloon during insertion.
4. The fourth port houses wires that lead to a temperature thermistor just proximal to the balloon. It is used to monitor pulmonary artery temperature during thermodilution for cardiac output monitoring.
5. The fifth port is the right ventricle infusion port which can be used for pacing.

Figure 1 shows a pulmonary artery catheter and its parts

Some catheters may have extra ports with additional capabilities like:

1. Continuous mixed venous oxygen saturation measurement
2. Continuous cardiac output measurement
3. Temporary venous pacing
4. Right ventricular end-diastolic volume and ejection fraction measurement.

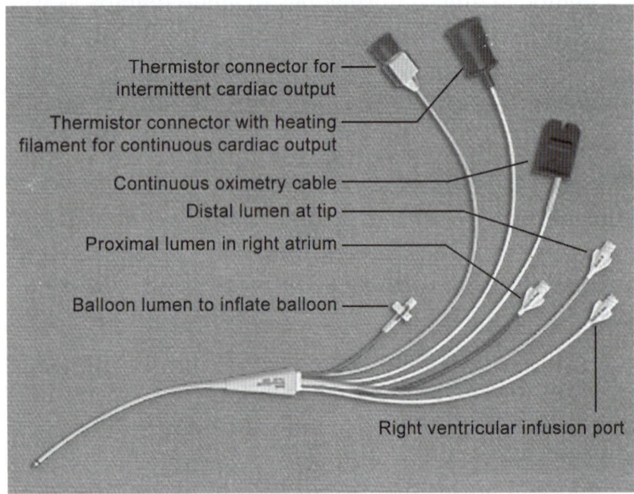

Fig. 1: Pulmonary artery catheter *(For color version, see Plate 1).*

INSERTION OF PULMONARY ARTERY CATHETERIZATION

After obtaining consent for the procedure, the placement site for the pulmonary artery catheter (PAC) insertion is selected, typically either the right internal jugular vein or the left subclavian vein. These locations are preferred because the natural curve of the catheter facilitates easier insertion into the pulmonary artery. Universal aseptic precautions are taken to prepare and drape the site.

A vein is located using either a landmark or ultrasound-guided technique. A large-bore introducer sheath is placed in the vessel using the Seldinger technique. The proximal tip of the sheath is connected to the transducer, the lumen is flushed, and the transducer is zeroed to atmospheric pressure. The other lumens of the catheter are also flushed.

The PAC is introduced with the catheter rotated so that its curvature is positioned at the 11 o'clock angle from the patient's head. The catheter is advanced through the introducer up to about 20 cm with the balloon deflated. As the catheter enters the right atrium, central venous pressure (CVP) is noted. The balloon is then gently inflated with 1.5 cc of air, and the inflation port is locked. The catheter is advanced slowly while monitoring for the right ventricle waveform, which is identified by an increase in systolic pressure (up to 25–35 mm Hg) and near-zero diastolic pressure. The catheter typically reaches the right ventricle at around 30–35 cm. **Figure 2** shows pressure recordings traced from PAC from right atrium, right ventricle, pulmonary artery catheter and on occlusion.

If it is difficult to enter the right ventricle or pulmonary artery, the patient may be asked to take a deep breath, the head of the bed can be raised, or the table can be tilted

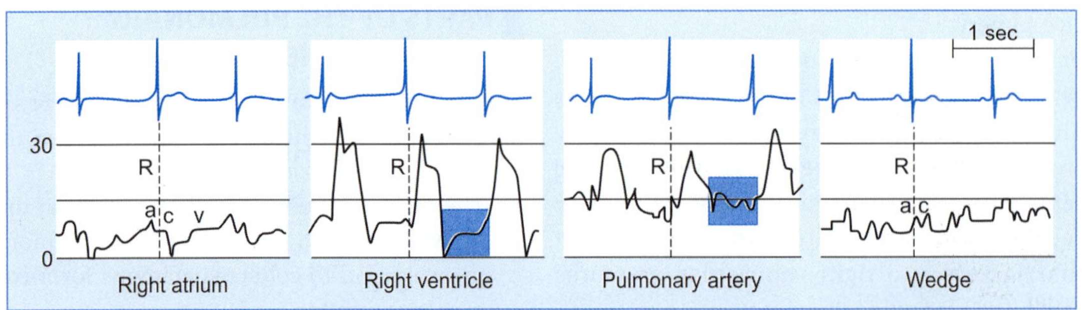

Fig. 2: Pressure tracings recorded from the right atrium, right ventricle, pulmonary catheter, and on pulmonary artery occlusion.

TABLE 1: Normal cardiovascular pressures recorded from pulmonary artery catheterization (PAC).

	Pressure	
	Average (mm Hg)	***Range (mm Hg)***
Right ventricle		
Peak systolic	25	15–30
End-diastolic	6	1–7
Pulmonary artery		
Peak systolic	25	15–30
End-diastolic	9	4–12
Mean	15	9–19
Pulmonary artery wedge pressure		
Mean	9	4–12

to the left or right. Additionally, the pulmonary artery port can be inflated with 1–2 mL of cold sterile saline to stiffen the catheter. The catheter is further advanced until it enters the pulmonary artery, usually around 40–45 cm. As the catheter enters the pulmonary artery, the diastolic pressure will increase (from near-zero in the right ventricle), while the systolic pressure remains similar to that in the right ventricle.

The catheter is then advanced very gradually, watching the monitor for a wedged pressure reading. When wedged, the waveform resembles a CVP tracing, showing a pressure close to the pulmonary artery diastolic pressure. This is known as the pulmonary artery occlusion pressure (PAOP), also referred to as pulmonary capillary wedge pressure (PCWP), and it is always lower than the pulmonary artery diastolic pressure. The balloon is deflated and then reinflated in 0.5 cc increments while monitoring for wedging. If wedging occurs before the balloon reaches full capacity (1.5 cc), the catheter is pulled back 3–4 cm with the balloon deflated until proper wedge tracing is recorded at full inflation. The catheter should then be fixed in place, ensuring that the balloon remains deflated. The balloon inflation syringe should never be left attached to the inflation port, and the lock on the balloon inflation port should only be used during catheter insertion, not at any other time.

Ideally, the tip of the PAC should be located in Zone 3 of the lung, where pulmonary arterial pressure exceeds pulmonary venous pressure, and alveolar pressure is the lowest. This position is optimal for recording PAOP, as all other external pressures are lower than the intra-arterial pressure, allowing for accurate measurements without interference. If the catheter tip is located outside of Zone 3, this can be suspected based on a lateral chest radiograph showing significant respiratory variation in PAOP and increases in PAOP due to positive end-expiratory pressure (PEEP). On the chest X-ray, the tip of the PAC should lie below the level of the left atrium, within 2 cm of the cardiac silhouette. The respiratory variation in PAOP should be less than 50% of the static airway pressure. Blood aspirated from the distal port of the catheter should have values nearly equivalent to arterial blood gas values.

PAOP should be measured at end-expiration, regardless of the ventilation mode—whether spontaneous or controlled—as all intrathoracic pressures equal (in spontaneous breathing) or approximate (in mechanical ventilation) atmospheric pressure at end-expiration. During spontaneous ventilation, pleural and alveolar pressures decrease during inspiration and increase during expiration. In contrast, during controlled mechanical ventilation, both pleural and alveolar pressures rise during inspiration and fall during expiration.

The effects of PEEP on PAOP can vary and depend on lung compliance. PEEP increases intrapleural pressure, which lead to an overestimation of measured PAOP compared to transmural or filling pressures. However, the clinical significance of PEEP's effect on PAOP is minimal if the catheter is correctly positioned in Zone 3.

Wedge pressure will underestimate the left ventricular end in the following conditions:
1. Diastolic dysfunction
2. Aortic regurgitation
3. Pulmonary regurgitation
4. Right bundle branch block
5. Post pneumonectomy

Wedge pressure will overestimate the left ventricular end-diastolic pressure in the following conditions:
1. Pulmonary artery hypertension
2. Pulmonary veno-occlusive disease
3. Tachycardia
4. Mitral stenosis
5. Mitral regurgitation

COMPLICATIONS OF PULMONARY ARTERY CATHETERIZATION

- *Complications during insertion of PAC:*
  - Arrhythmias
  - Right bundle branch block, complete heart block
  - Catheter misplacement, knotting
  - Vessel or valve rupture

- *Complications due to catheter:*
  - Infection
  - Thromboembolism
  - Pulmonary infarction
  - Pulmonary artery rupture
- *Misinterpretation of data:*
  - Improper leveling and zeroing
  - Improper location of the tip (other than zone 3)
  - Overestimation or underestimation due to improper filling of the balloon.[4]

MEASURING CARDIAC OUTPUT WITH THERMODILUTION

Cardiac output can be measured with the use of PAC by using the thermodilution method, which is based on Fick's principle. A bolus of 5 mL or 10 mL saline at room temperature (21°C) is injected smoothly and at a constant rate through the proximal port (CVP port) into the right atrium which mixes with the blood. The blood temperature in the right ventricle is lowered by this bolus. the temperature change is detected over time by a thermistor near the catheter tip, which generates a temperature-time curve.

Generally, three such readings are taken and averaged and are deemed to be the cardiac output of the patient. Various factors influence the accuracy of the measurement, which include the presence of intracardiac shunts, tricuspid regurgitation, pulmonary regurgitation, respiratory cycle influence, and the speed of injection of the saline. **Tables 2 and 3** shows different derived hemodynamic and oxygen transport parameters derived from PAC.

Continuous Cardiac Output Measurement

Newer catheters are capable of measuring continuously instead of intermittent bolus technique. They consist of copper thermal filament which is embedded 30 cm proximal to the tip such that it is approximately in the right ventricle. It heats blood in the right ventricle which is detected by the thermistor at the catheter tip. The change in temperature over time is computed and cardiac output is measured. The cardiac output values are updated every 30–60 seconds and an average value is displayed.

PULMONARY ARTERY CATHETER IN CLINICAL PRACTICE: THE EVIDENCE FROM THE LITERATURE

Following its introduction in the 1970s, the use of pulmonary artery catheters (PAC) increased incrementally over the following decade. Few observational studies

TABLE 2: Derived hemodynamic parameters.

Parameter	*Physiologic significance*	*Formula*	*Normal value*
SVR	Reflects impedance of the systemic vasculature	80 × (MAP – CVP)/CO	800–1,500 dynes/cm^5
PVR	Reflects impedance of pulmonary circuit	80 × (mPAP – PCWP)/CO	20–130 dynes/cm^5
CI	Allows for meaningful comparison between patients	CO/BSA	2.5–4.2 L/min/m^2
SVI	Reflects fluid status and ventricular performance	CI/HR × 1,000	40–60 mL/beat/m^2
LVSVI	Estimates of work of the left ventricle, reflect the contractile state	(MAP – PCWP) × SVI × 0.0136	45–60 g/m^2
RVSWI	Estimates of work done by the right ventricle and RV performance	(mPAP – CVP) × SVI × 0.0136	5–10 g/m^2

(BSA: body surface area; CI: cardiac index; CO: cardiac output; CVP: central venous pressure; HR: heart rate; LVSVI: left ventricular stroke work index; MAP: mean arterial pressure; mPAP: mean pulmonary artery pressure; PCWP: pulmonary capillary wedge pressure; PVR: pulmonary vascular resistance; RVSWI: right ventricular stroke work index; SVI: stroke volume index; SVR: systemic vascular resistance)

TABLE 3: Oxygen transport parameters.

Parameter	*Symbol*	*Formula*	*Normal value*
Mixed venous oxygen saturation	SvO_2	Measured variable	70–75%
Oxygen delivery	DO_2	1.34 × Hb × SaO_2 × CO	500–600 mL/min/m^2
Oxygen uptake	VO_2	1.34 × Hb × (SaO_2 – SvO_2) × CO	110–160 mL/min/m^2
Oxygen–extraction ratio	O_2ER	VO_2/DO_2	20–30%

(CO: cardiac output; DO_2: oxygen delivery; Hb: hemoglobin; O_2ER: oxygen extraction ratio; SaO_2: hemoglobin arterial oxygen saturation; SvO_2: venous oxygen saturation)

conducted on patients with acute myocardial infarction challenged the use of PAC in managing these patients, revealing no significant outcome benefits but an increase in the length of hospital stays.[6,7] Connors et al. published a retrospective study in 1998 involving a propensity-matched cohort, reporting that 30-day mortality was higher in patients treated with a pulmonary catheter. Their data suggested that PAC use in critically ill patients was associated with increased healthcare costs and longer intensive care unit (ICU) stays, even after adjusting for underlying risk factors. Critiques of this study primarily focused on its retrospective design, issues with propensity matching, and concerns about the similarity of illness severity between the two groups, suggesting that those who had a PAC inserted were sicker compared to the control group.[8]

Similar findings emerged from other studies that investigated PAC use during aortic surgeries, which indicated that routine PAC use was not beneficial and might even lead to increased intraoperative complications.[9] Murdoch and colleagues, who examined PAC and mortality in critically ill patients, found that PAC use was not predictive of death after propensity matching. They concluded that while mortality was greater in patients receiving a PAC, it was not directly related to the PAC itself.[10]

A randomized controlled trial among critically ill patients compared survival and clinical outcomes between those treated with PAC and those without. The study found no difference in mortality between the groups; however, patients in the PAC group received more fluids and experienced higher rates of renal failure and thrombocytopenia.[11] Another multicenter observational cohort study assessed the impact of PAC on outcomes and discovered that PAC use was not an independent risk factor and did not correlate with increased mortality.[12]

The PAC-Man trial (Pulmonary Artery Catheters in Management of Patients in Intensive Care) evaluated whether PAC use affected hospital mortality in multiple ICUs. The trial concluded that there was no clear evidence of benefit or harm associated with managing critically ill patients using PAC.[13]

The ESCAPE trial (Evaluation Study of Congestive Heart Failure and Pulmonary Artery Catheterization Effectiveness) aimed to determine whether PAC use is safe and improves clinical outcomes for patients hospitalized with severe symptomatic and recurrent heart failure. The study found that decisions regarding vasodilator and diuretic therapy based on PAC data combined with clinical judgment were not superior to decisions made based solely on clinical judgment concerning mortality or length of hospital stay.[14]

A systematic review and meta-analysis comparing patients who received PAC with those who did not, noted a higher rate of vasodilator and inotropic agent use in the PAC group but found no difference in mortality between the groups. The review concluded that among critically ill patients, PAC use neither increased overall mortality nor hospital stay duration, nor did it provide significant benefits.[15]

A multicenter randomized clinical trial with a 2 × 2 design, which compared PAC versus central venous pressure monitoring (CVP) and liberal versus conservative fluid management in patients with acute respiratory distress syndrome (ARDS), reported that PAC use did not confer any benefit. The study found that conservative fluid management was more effective than a liberal strategy.[16]

CONCLUSION

The pulmonary artery catheter (PAC) was once an essential tool for intensivists, used to characterize and manage hemodynamics in critically ill patients. However, it has largely been replaced by less invasive monitoring techniques like transpulmonary thermodilution and echocardiography. Studies have not demonstrated improved patient outcomes with the use of PAC. While it may not be suitable for most critically ill patients, the PAC still offers benefits for certain subsets and remains the gold standard for measuring cardiac output.

It's important to note that simply using a specific monitoring device does not guarantee improved outcomes. Expertise in the insertion process, accurate data acquisition, and the optimal application of the device by an experienced intensivist are crucial for effectively managing complex patients.

REFERENCES

1. Chatterjee K. The Swan-Ganz catheters: past, present, and future. A viewpoint. Circulation. 2009;119(1):147-52.
2. Greenberg SB, Murphy GS, Vender JS. Current use of the pulmonary artery catheter. Curr Opin Crit Care. 2009;15(3):249-53.
3. Cecconi M, De Backer D, Antonelli M, Beale R, Bakker J, Hofer C, et al. Consensus on circulatory shock and hemodynamic monitoring. Task force of the European Society of Intensive Care Medicine. Intensive Care Med. 2014;40(12):1795-815.

4. Evans DC, Doraiswamy VA, Prosciak MP, Silviera M, Seamon MJ, Rodriguez Funes V, et al. Complications associated with pulmonary artery catheters: a comprehensive clinical review. Scand J Surg. 2009;98(4):199-208.
5. Teboul JL, Pinsky MR, Mercat A, Anguel N, Bernardin G, Achard JM, et al. Estimating cardiac filling pressure in mechanically ventilated patients with hyperinflation. Crit Care Med. 2000;28(11):3631-6.
6. Gore JM, Goldberg RJ, Spodick DH, Alpert JS, Dalen JE. A community-wide assessment of the use of pulmonary artery catheters in patients with acute myocardial infarction. Chest. 1987;92:(4)721-7.
7. Zion MM, Balkin J, Rosenmann D, Reicher-Reiss H, Kaplinsky E, Behar S. Use of pulmonary artery catheters in patients with acute myocardial infarction. Analysis of experience in 5,841 patients in the SPRINT Registry. SPRINT Study Group. Chest. 1990;98(6):1331-5.
8. Connors AF Jr, Speroff T, Dawson NV, Thomas C, Harrell FE Jr, Wagner D, et al. The effectiveness of right heart catheterization in the initial care of critically ill patients. SUPPORT Investigators. JAMA. 1996;276(11):889-97.
9. Valentine RJ, Duke ML, Inman MH, Grayburn PA, Hagino RT, Kakish HB, et al. Effectiveness of pulmonary artery catheters in aortic surgery: a randomized trial. J Vasc Surg. 1998;27(2):203-12.
10. Murdoch SD, Cohen AT, Bellamy MC. Pulmonary artery catheterization and mortality in critically ill patients. Br J Anaesth. 2000;85(4):611-5.
11. Rhodes A, Cusack RJ, Newman PJ, Grounds RM, Bennett ED. A randomised, controlled trial of the pulmonary artery catheter in critically ill patients. Intensive Care Med. 2002;28(3):256-64.
12. Sakr Y, Vincent JL, Reinhart K, Payen D, Wiedermann CJ, Zandstra DF, et al. Use of the pulmonary artery catheter is not associated with worse outcome in the ICU. Chest. 2005;128(4):2722-31.
13. Harvey S, Harrison DA, Singer M, Ashcroft J, Jones CM, Elbourne D, et al. Assessment of the clinical effectiveness of pulmonary artery catheters in management of patients in intensive care (PAC-Man): a randomised controlled trial. Lancet. 2005;366(9484):472-7.
14. Binanay C, Califf RM, Hasselblad V, O'Connor CM, Shah MR, Sopko G, et al. Evaluation study of congestive heart failure and pulmonary artery catheterization effectiveness: the ESCAPE trial. JAMA. 2005;294(13): 1625-33.
15. Shah MR, Hasselblad V, Stevenson LW, Binanay C, O'Connor CM, Sopko G, et al. Impact of the pulmonary artery catheter in critically ill patients: meta-analysis of randomized clinical trials. JAMA. 2005;294(13): 1664-70.
16. Wiedemann HP, Wheeler AP, Bernard GR, Thompson BT, Hayden D, deBoisblanc B, et al. Comparison of two fluid-management strategies in acute lung injury. N Engl J Med. 2006;354(24):2564-75.

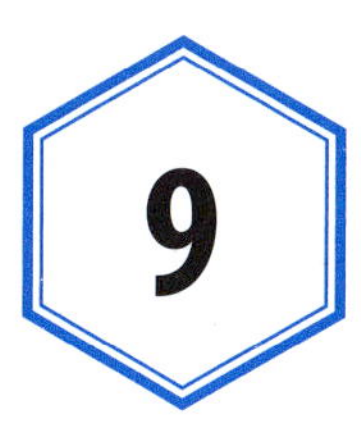

Transpulmonary Thermodilution

Alexandra Beurton, Jean-Louis Teboul, Xavier Monnet

INTRODUCTION

Several techniques of hemodynamic monitoring have emerged in the early 2000's as alternatives to the pulmonary artery catheter (PAC).[1] Transpulmonary thermodilution (TPTD) and pulse contour analysis are among the ones that are the most frequently used today in critically ill patients.[2] A task force of the European Society of Intensive Care Medicine has recommended the use of advanced hemodynamic monitoring in severe shock that does not respond to initial treatment and suggested that TPTD devices, along with PAC, should be used for this purpose.[2] The two devices that are available (PiCCO, Pulsion Medical Systems, Feldkirchen, Germany, and Volume View, Edwards Life Sciences, Irvine, CA, USA) measure cardiac output but also provide several other valuable pieces of hemodynamic information regarding cardiac preload and contractile function, lung edema and permeability.

In this chapter, we describe the way the different indices provided by TPTD are measured, review their clinical interest, and list their potential limitations.

MEASUREMENT OF CARDIAC OUTPUT

Principle of Measurement

Transpulmonary thermodilution requires a specific arterial catheter, which is usually inserted through the femoral artery, and a standard central venous catheter usually placed in the superior vena cava region. At the tip of the arterial catheter, a thermistor senses the decrease in blood temperature after the injection of a cold saline bolus through the venous catheter. The calculation of cardiac output is performed by the analysis of the thermodilution curve using a modified Stewart-Hamilton algorithm. The results of three thermodilution measurements must be averaged.

Accuracy for Measuring Cardiac Output with Transpulmonary Thermodilution

It is now well established that, compared to the PAC and the Fick method, TPTD is accurate for measuring cardiac output and tracking its changes.[3-5] When three measurements of thermodilution are averaged, the least significant change of the technique, i.e., the smallest change in cardiac output that can be trusted as being significant, is 12%,[6] which is similar to that of the PAC.[7]

Caution should be taken during thermodilution to respect the volume of injection (15–20 mL saline), the bolus temperature (<8°C), the absence of leaks in the circuit, and the regularity of the speed of injection. Overestimation of cardiac output might appear with boluses at room temperature,[8] but therapeutic hypothermia does not affect the precision of the measurement.[8]

The cold bolus of saline can be injected through a port-a-cath.[8] The venous catheter should be inserted in the femoral vein, contralateral to the arterial catheter of course, without altering the measurement of cardiac output.[9,10] The thermistor-tipped catheter could be inserted in the axillary, brachial, or radial arteries with dedicated catheters.

Limitations

The measurement of cardiac output with TPTD remains accurate during venovenous hemofiltration,[8] even for high blood pump flows,[8] and it is not necessary to stop renal replacement therapy to perform the measurement.[11] In fact, the blood flow in the extracorporeal circuit is likely too small compared to cardiac output. Nevertheless, TPTD is unreliable during extracorporeal membrane oxygenation (ECMO). It has been shown that the measurement of cardiac output remains valid in the cases of valvular disease of cardiomyopathy or atrial fibrillation.[4] It has been suspected that, in case of a large volume of extravascular lung water (EVLW), the loss of temperature might be marked and the measurement of cardiac output is less reliable.[12] Nevertheless, if it exists, this phenomenon is likely negligible. Finally, the main drawback of TPTD for measuring cardiac output is that it only provides intermittent measurements.

Calibrated Pulse Contour Analysis

Besides TPTD, the pulse index continuous cardiac output (PiCCO) and VolumeView devices measure cardiac output in real time through pulse contour analysis of the pressure curve obtained from the arterial catheter. This method is based on the principle that the amplitude of the systolic part of the arterial curve and its geometrical features are in relationship with stroke volume.[13] The advantage is that it provides a real-time estimation of cardiac output, but the main drawback is that this estimation deviates away from the true value over time.

With PiCCO and VolumeView devices, the pulse contour analysis is calibrated by the value obtained by TPTD. At each cold bolus injection, the value of cardiac output provided by thermodilution is used to reset pulse contour analysis. Calibrated devices are more reliable than techniques performing pulse contour analysis without calibration,[13] especially when arterial resistance changes to a significant extent, as under vasopressors.[8] Calibration should be encouraged after a 1-hour calibration-free period.[14] In practice, this does not mean that a calibration should be done every hour in a patient with a TPTD device in place, but rather that, when one looks at cardiac output for interpreting the hemodynamic condition, one should carefully check that the TPTD measurement has been performed <1 hour ago.

The measurement of cardiac output by pulse contour analysis is very precise, more than with TPTD. The least significant change is 2–3% only.[14] Then, pulse-contour analysis is appropriate for testing preload responsiveness with dynamic tests inducing small and short-term changes in cardiac output, such as passive leg raising, the end-expiratory occlusion test, and the recruitment maneuvers.[15-17]

ASSESSMENT OF CARDIAC PRELOAD: THE GLOBAL END-DIASTOLIC VOLUME

Principle of Measurement

Besides cardiac output, TPTD estimates several intrathoracic volumes **(Fig. 1)**. With the PiCCO device,

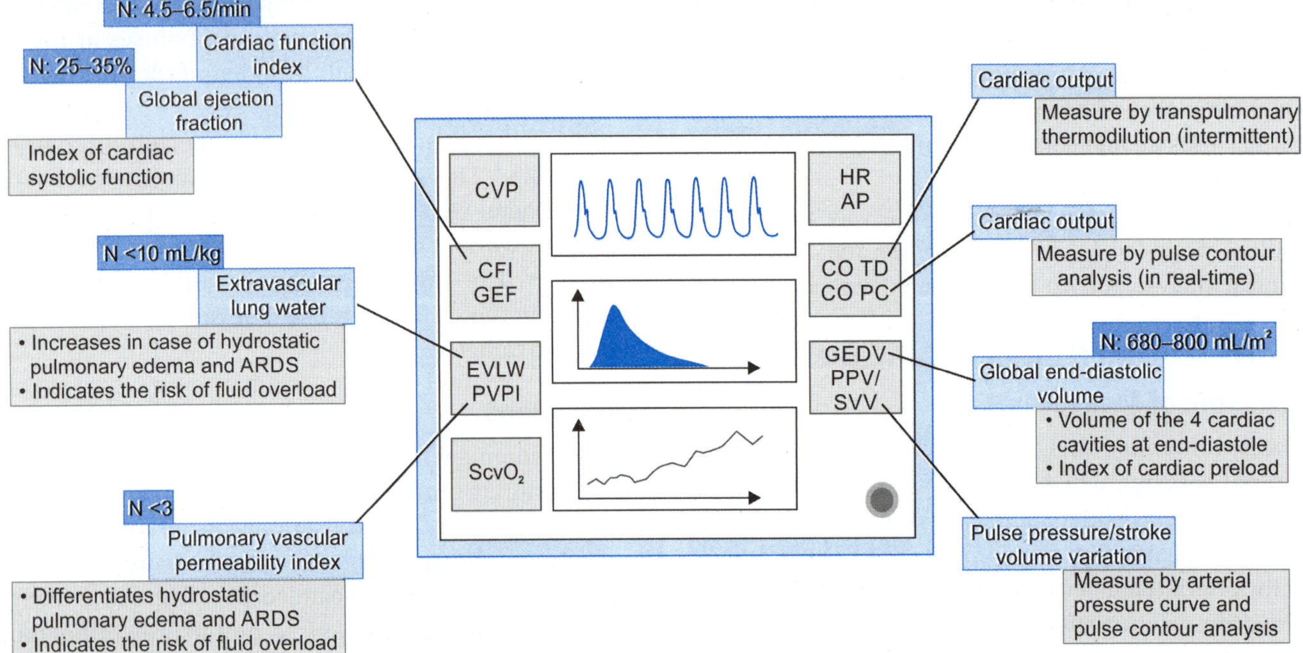

Fig. 1: Hemodynamic variables provided by TPTD and calibrated pulse contour analysis, with their meaning, utility, and normal values (N) (AP: arterial pressure; ARDS: acute respiratory distress syndrome; CFI: cardiac function index; CO: cardiac output; CVP: central venous pressure; EVLW: extravascular lung water; GEDV: global end-diastolic volume; GEF: global ejection fraction; HR: heart rate; PC: pulse contour; PPV: pulse pressure variation; PVPI: pulmonary vascular permeability index; $ScvO_2$: central venous oxygen saturation; SVV: stroke volume variation; TD: thermodilution).

its estimation is based on the analysis of both the thermodilution curve and its logarithmic transformation **(Fig. 2)**. According to the Stewart-Hamilton principle, the total distribution volume of the cold indicator between the injection and detection sites, the intrathoracic thermal volume, is obtained by multiplying cardiac output by the mean transit time of the cold indicator **(Fig. 2)**. According to the Newman principle, the largest distribution volume

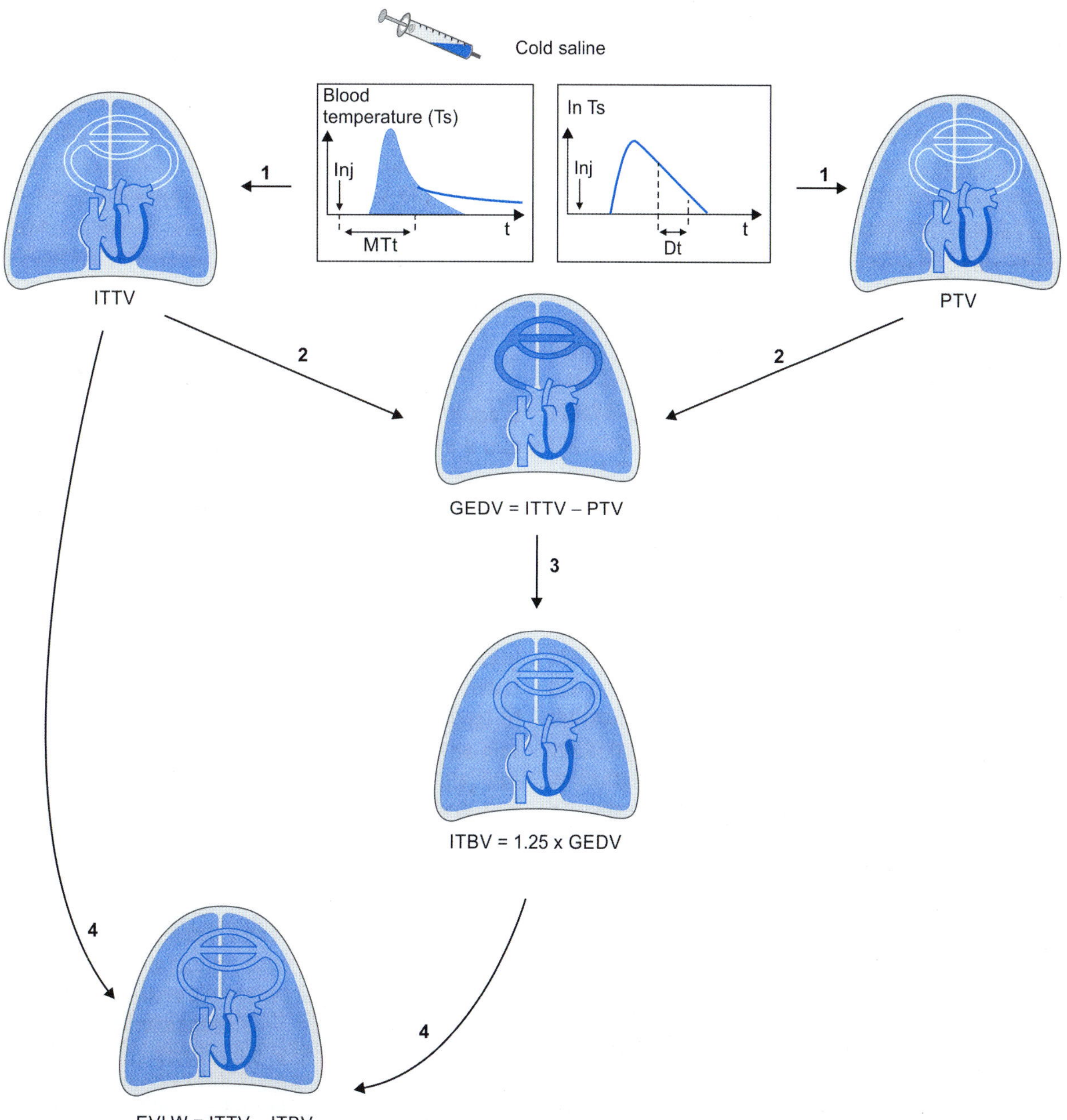

Fig. 2: Assessment of intrathoracic volume by the PiCCO device. With the VolumeView device, the geometrical analysis of the thermodilution curve directly estimates the global end-diastolic volume (Dt: downslope time; EVLW: extravascular lung water; GEDV: global end-diastolic volume; ITBV: intrathoracic blood volume; ITTV: intrathoracic thermal volume; MTt: mean transit time; PiCCO: pulse index continuous cardiac output; PTV: pulmonary thermal volume).
Source: Monnet X, Teboul JL. Transpulmonary thermodilution: advantages and limits. Crit Care. 2017;21(1):147.

of the cold indicator between the injection and detection sites, the total pulmonary volume, is obtained by multiplying cardiac output by the downslope time of the thermodilution curve. Then, subtracting the pulmonary thermal volume from the intrathoracic thermal volume estimates the global end-diastolic volume (GEDV) **(Fig. 2)**. GEDV, indexed for body surface, is the volume of the four cardiac chambers at end-diastole.

The VolumeView device works differently since it assesses GEDV by analyzing the slopes of the up and down parts of the thermodilution curve.[8] Nevertheless, both techniques have been demonstrated to be interchangeable.[8] GEDV is larger than the actual volume of the four cardiac chambers because it includes the cardiac volume, a part of the superior vena cava volume, and the volume of the aorta that is between the bolus injection site and the thermistor. Nevertheless, these vascular volumes are roughly unchanged during changes in cardiac preload. When the cold boluses are injected through the femoral venous catheter, the normal value of GEDV is higher since it includes the volume of the inferior vena cava.[18] A correction of GEDV is applied in such a case using the patient's characteristics.[10]

The smallest change in GEDV that can be accurately detected by TDTP is 12% when three cold boluses are injected.[6]

Clinical Use

Global end-diastolic volume is a "static" marker of cardiac preload.[19] As such, it does not allow the prediction of the response of cardiac output to a fluid bolus. Nevertheless, it is a reliable estimate of cardiac preload. In particular, GEDV reliably tracks the changes in preload induced by volume expansion when compared to echocardiographic measurements, better than the volumetric assessment allowed by some modified versions of the PAC.[8] Assessing cardiac preload by GEDV may also help determine the shock origin when it is unclear.

Limitations

Global end-diastolic volume does not distinguish between left and right cardiac preload. It includes the volume of the four cardiac cavities so that it overestimates the left ventricular preload in the case of right ventricular dilation.[8] As with all TPTD-derived measurements, it is unreliable under ECMO.

ESTIMATION OF LEFT VENTRICULAR SYSTOLIC FUNCTION: THE CARDIAC FUNCTION INDEX AND THE GLOBAL EJECTION FRACTION

Principle of Measurement

Transpulmonary thermodilution estimates the left ventricular systolic function with two indices, the cardiac function index (CFI) and the global ejection fraction (GEF). The CFI is calculated by the PiCCO and VolumeView devices, as the ratio of cardiac output measured by TPTD divided by the GEDV **(Fig. 2)**. The GEF is the ratio of stroke volume to a quarter of the GEDV expressed as a percentage, assuming that the left ventricular end-diastolic volume is a quarter of GEDV. GEF resembles more the left ventricular ejection fraction than CFI.

Studies have shown a good correlation between absolute values of CFI and of the left ventricular ejection fraction measured by echocardiography.[8] In particular, a low CFI accurately detects low values of left ventricular ejection fraction and tracks its changes.[8] The least significant change of CFI is 12% when three boluses are injected.[6]

Clinical Use

There is no doubt that echocardiography is the reference for estimating the cardiac function of hemodynamically unstable patients. Nevertheless, its drawback is that it is tedious and time-consuming, which prevents its frequent repetition at the bedside. The interest of TPTD might be that it easily warns that global cardiac function is impaired. This should be confirmed by echocardiography, which will distinguish between the right and left ventricular dysfunction, analyze the cardiac structure, and find an explanation for the cardiac failure. In a patient who receives inotropes, TPTD systolic function indices also allow one to follow the treatment effect.[8]

Limitations

As the GEDV reflects the volume of the four cardiac chambers, CFI and GEF underestimate the left ventricular systolic function in case of right ventricular dilation. In this case, the GEDV is increased, CFI and GEF are decreased while the left ventricular contractility is unchanged.[8] Furthermore, CFI and GEF depend on left ventricular preload and afterload.[8] In the case of femoral venous access, GEDV is corrected for calculating GEF and CFI,[18] though there is doubt regarding the latter.[20]

EXTRAVASCULAR LUNG WATER AND PULMONARY VASCULAR PERMEABILITY INDEX

Principle of Measurement

Extravascular lung water reflects the volume of the liquid contained in the pulmonary interstitium and the alveoli. It augments because of increased lung permeability, because of elevated hydrostatic pressure in the pulmonary capillaries, or because of both.[21]

Its estimation with the PiCCO device is obtained by subtracting the intrathoracic blood volume from the intrathoracic thermal volume[8] **(Fig. 2)**. The intrathoracic blood volume is estimated by multiplying GEDV by 1.25.[8] It is indexed by the predicted body weight. The estimation of EVLW with the VolumeView is quite different due to its different estimation of GEDV[8] but a good agreement between values provided by both devices has been reported.[8]

Transpulmonary thermodilution allows the estimation of the permeability of the alveolocapillary barrier through the pulmonary vascular permeability index (PVPI). The PVPI is the ratio of EVLW indexed over pulmonary blood volume, i.e., the ratio between the volume of fluid that has leaked toward the extravascular spaces over the volume of fluid that remains in the vessels.[8]

Validation of Extravascular Lung Water and Pulmonary Vascular Permeability Index

Extravascular lung water has been validated in animals but also in humans[22] in comparison with gravimetry, which is considered the gold standard. When three boluses of cold saline are injected, the least significant change in EVLW is 12%.[6] TPTD can detect small and short-term changes in lung water induced by a bronchoalveolar lavage[23] or weaning-induced pulmonary edema.[24] Studies have shown that EVLW predicts mortality in critically ill patients.[25,26] PVPI has been demonstrated to be higher in acute respiratory distress syndrome (ARDS) compared to hydrostatic pulmonary edema and to accurately detect an increase in lung permeability.[27] A PVPI value of three was found to be the best threshold for distinguishing hydrostatic from inflammatory lung edema.[8,27]

Limitations

In the case of pulmonary embolism with occlusion of relatively large vessels, the amount of EVLW is underestimated by TPTD because the diffusion of the cold indicator to the lung tissues irrigated by the occluded artery is impeded.[8] In the case of lung resection, the amount of lung water logically decreases but TPTD may overestimate the remaining volume of EVLW.[28] The type of ARDS may affect the reliability of TPTD for estimating EVLW. In the case of heterogeneous forms of ARDS, the pulmonary blood flow might be redistributed away from the edematous areas, leading to an EVLW underestimation.[8] Pleural effusions of large volume may lead to EVLW overestimation by TPTD because the cold indicator also diffuses into the pleural liquid. Renal replacement therapy and therapeutic hypothermia do not alter the reliability of EVLW measurement, likely because the blood flow in the extracorporeal circuit is not sufficient.[8] Using room temperature boluses results in a slight but significant overestimation of EVLW.[8]

Clinical Use

Definition of Acute Respiratory Distress Syndrome

Although an increase in lung water and the impairment of lung permeability are the hallmarks of ARDS, their estimation by TPTD is not taken into account in the Berlin definition.[29] However, the latter has many drawbacks.[30] The diagnosis requires an accurate interpretation of the chest X-ray, which is difficult in practice. Then, the severity of ARDS depends on the ratio of the arterial oxygen partial pressure over the oxygen-inspired fraction but also on the level of positive end-expiratory pressure. Also, according to the Berlin definition, the increase in lung permeability is suspected on the estimation that the filling pressure of the left ventricle is not elevated, which is obviously rough and indirect. Finally, there is a modest agreement between the pathological findings in ARDS and the Berlin diagnostic criteria, while diffuse alveolar damage is accurately detected through EVLW.[30] All these arguments argue in favor of integrating EVLW in the definition of ARDS,[31] even though the cost of such devices prevents their use as a standard of care for every ARDS patient.

Fluid Management

Reducing the cumulative fluid balance should be a goal of the management of critically ill patients[32] since a positive fluid balance is an independent factor associated with mortality.[33] Then, one needs criteria to decide not to administer fluids. Negative indices of fluid responsiveness are obviously very helpful for this purpose.[32] Also, high

EVLW and PVPI values indicate the risk of fluid infusion, especially in the case of ARDS.[34]

Weaning from Mechanical Ventilation

The increase in EVLW during a spontaneous breathing trial accurately detects the short-term weaning-induced pulmonary edema with good accuracy.[24] TPTD devices should not be set up with the only purpose of making this diagnosis, because their invasiveness is not justified in patients who will be extubated shortly. Nevertheless, if patients are still equipped with such a device, one should check the EVLW value in patients who fail a spontaneous breathing trial.

Other Settings

Some publications have also emphasized how monitoring EVLW and PVPI might be useful in other clinical settings, such as in burn patients for assessing the risk of fluid overadministration,[35,36] in lung transplantation for detecting early graft dysfunction[37] and after pulmonary endarterectomy for detecting pulmonary edema.[38]

INDICATIONS OF TRANSPULMONARY THERMODILUTION

In the perioperative setting, hemodynamic monitoring should be used to detect hypovolemia or low oxygen delivery for early prevention. Advanced hemodynamic monitoring should be preferred over less invasive devices in complex situations, such as during cardiac and prolonged major surgery,[39] or when major vasomotor tone changes are expected, as during liver surgery.[40]

In the critical care setting, current consensual recommendations state that cardiac output should be monitored in patients who do not respond to initial resuscitation, and suggest that the PAC or TPTD devices should be used for this purpose.[2,41] First, this is justified by the fact that the estimation of cardiac output from clinical examination in general, as it was recently confirmed[42] and from the arterial pressure in particular, is only rough. Second, only sophisticated devices can answer all the questions that arise during the resuscitation of complex and severely ill patients.[43] Nevertheless, it seems that this is less common than recommended in practice.[44]

Monitoring with a TPTD device or a PAC has never been demonstrated to improve the outcome of critically ill patients. In fact, such a demonstration would require that a therapeutic algorithm is attached to the use of the device. Otherwise, no prognosis improvement could be demonstrated, as it has been the case with PAC. Nevertheless, summarizing the treatment of diseases so complex as septic or cardiogenic shock in one single algorithm is impossible, due to the number of factors that are taken into account when making decisions in such patients. Finally, in our opinion, we do not necessarily need studies demonstrating that their use improves prognosis for using these monitoring devices. No study has demonstrated that using echocardiography improves the prognosis of circulatory failure, and there is no doubt that it is absolutely useful.

The choice between the PAC and TPTD devices mainly depends on the team's experience. However, they answer the questions that are asked during circulatory failure quite differently. Fluid responsiveness is at best predicted by dynamic tests, which are very easily performed with calibrated pulse-contour analysis, and which cannot be done with the PAC intermittent estimation of cardiac output. An advantage of PAC is to allow for the measurement of the mixed venous oxygen saturation, while only the central venous blood can be sampled with TPTD devices. PVPI and EVLW directly assess the pulmonary risk of fluid administration while with the PAC, a given value of pulmonary artery occlusion pressure may correspond to different degrees of risk depending on lung capillary permeability. Regarding the estimation of cardiac contractility, both types of devices provide indirect indicators of its impairment, through decreases in CFI and GEF with TPTD, and through a combination of a decreased cardiac output and increased pulmonary occlusion arterial pressure with PAC. Finally, a unique advantage of PAC is to provide a direct estimation of pulmonary vascular resistance. This explains why it is suggested that PAC might be preferred in case of right ventricular dysfunction and acute pulmonary hypertension.[2,41] The rate of complications is similar with both types of devices.

Echocardiography has no equivalent for a complete assessment of cardiac structure and function, but its main drawback is that it does not allow easy and continuous monitoring. In this regard, it should be used combined with TPTD, during intermittent assessments. In addition, TPTD measurements may trigger recourse to echocardiography, if GEF or CFI suddenly decreases. Opposing the use of echocardiography to TPTD alone probably makes no sense.[45]

COMPLICATIONS OF TRANSPULMONARY THERMODILUTION

The main risk resides in arterial injuries, especially when the femoral route is used. This is due to quite large diameter of the catheter, which sometimes requires artery dilatation before its insertion. This may result in arterial dissection or thrombosis, pulse loss and limb ischemia, or hematoma at insertion, or removal of the catheter. Even though this risk is small,[46] the rate of complications is similar to the one of PAC, and TPTD must be considered as an invasive device. TPTD is contraindicated in cases of vascular prostheses. In patients with severe arteriopathy or risk of bleeding, the risk/benefit ratio should be cautiously evaluated.

CONCLUSION

Beyond cardiac output, TPTD devices provide many indices, which allow a complete hemodynamic assessment that may help clinicians facing a patient with acute circulatory failure. Their main advantages reside in the real-time measurement of cardiac output with calibrated pulse contour analysis and in the estimation of lung water and permeability. The latter may be particularly useful for guiding fluid therapy in patients with hemodynamic instability. Because of their cost and invasiveness, TPTD devices are indicated in patients with acute circulatory failure who do not respond to initial treatment, and/or with associated ARDS, in whom fluid management can be particularly tricky. In those clinical situations, the combination of TPTD with echocardiography may help clinicians answer all the questions that are asked by the clinical situation.

REFERENCES

1. De Backer D, Bakker J, Cecconi M, Hajjar L, Liu DW, Lobo S, et al. Alternatives to the Swan-Ganz catheter. Intensive Care Med. 2018;44(6):730-41.
2. Cecconi M, De Backer D, Antonelli M, Beale R, Bakker J, Hofer C, et al. Consensus on circulatory shock and hemodynamic monitoring. Task force of the European Society of Intensive Care Medicine. Intensive Care Med. 2014;40(12):1795-815.
3. Vetrugno L, Bignami E, Barbariol F, Langiano N, De Lorenzo F, Matellon C, et al. Cardiac output measurement in liver transplantation patients using pulmonary and transpulmonary thermodilution: a comparative study. J Clin Monit Comput. 2019;33(2):223-31.
4. Hilty MP, Franzen DP, Wyss C, Biaggi P, Maggiorini M. Validation of transpulmonary thermodilution variables in hemodynamically stable patients with heart diseases. Ann Intensive Care. 2017;7(1):86.
5. Sakka SG, Reuter DA, Perel A. The transpulmonary thermodilution technique. J Clin Monit Comput. 2012;26(5):347-53.
6. Monnet X, Persichini R, Ktari M, Jozwiak M, Richard C, Teboul JL. Precision of the transpulmonary thermodilution measurements. Crit Care. 2011;15(4):R204.
7. Stetz CW, Miller RG, Kelly GE, Raffin RA. Reliability of the thermodilution method in the determination of cardiac output in clinical practice. Am Rev Respir Dis. 1982;126(6):1001-4.
8. Monnet X, Teboul JL. Transpulmonary thermodilution: advantages and limits. Crit Care. 2017;21(1):147.
9. Schmidt S, Westhoff T, Hofmann C, Schaefer JH, Zidek W, Compton F, et al. Effect of the venous catheter site on transpulmonary thermodilution measurement variables. Critical Care Med. 2007;35(3):783-6.
10. Saugel B, Umgelter A, Schuster T, Phillip V, Schimid RM, Huber W. Transpulmonary thermodilution using femoral indicator injection: a prospective trial in patients with a femoral and a jugular central venous catheter. Crit Care. 2010;14(3):R95.
11. Geith S, Stecher L, Rabe C, Sack S, Eyer F. Sustained low efficiency dialysis should not be interrupted for performing transpulmonary thermodilution measurements. Ann Intensive Care. 2018;8(1):113.
12. Pohl T, Kozieras J, Sakka SG. Influence of extravascular lung water on transpulmonary thermodilution-derived cardiac output measurement. Intensive Care Med. 2008;34(3):533-7.
13. Jozwiak M, Monnet X, Teboul JL. Pressure Waveform Analysis. Anesth Analg. 2018;126(6):1930-3.
14. Hamzaoui O, Monnet X, Richard C, Osman D, Chemla D, Teboul JL. Effects of changes in vascular tone on the agreement between pulse contour and transpulmonary thermodilution cardiac output measurements within an up to 6-hour calibration-free period. Crit Care Med. 2008; 36(2):434-40.
15. Monnet X, Teboul JL. Assessment of fluid responsiveness: recent advances. Curr Opin Crit Care. 2018;24(3):190-5.
16. Monnet X, Teboul JL. Passive leg raising: five rules, not a drop of fluid! Crit Care. 2015;19(1):18.
17. Monnet X, Osman D, Ridel C, Lamia B, Richard C, Teboul JL. Predicting volume responsiveness by using the end-expiratory occlusion in mechanically ventilated intensive care unit patients. Crit Care Med. 2009;37(3):951-6.
18. Huber W, Gruber A, Eckmann M, Elkmann F, Klein I, Lahmer T, et al. Comparison of pulmonary vascular permeability index PVPI and global ejection fraction GEF derived from jugular and femoral indicator injection using the PiCCO-2 device: a prospective observational study. PLoS ONE. 2017;12(10):e0178372.
19. Michard F, Alaya S, Zarka V, Bahloul M, Richard C, Teboul JL. Global end-diastolic volume as an indicator of cardiac preload in patients with septic shock. Chest. 2003;124(5):1900-8.

20. Herner A, Heilmaier M, Mayr U, Schmid RM, Huber W. Comparison of cardiac function index derived from femoral and jugular indicator injection for transpulmonary thermodilution with the PiCCO-device: a prospective observational study. PLoS ONE. 2018;13(7):e0200740.
21. Jozwiak M, Teboul JL, Monnet X. Extravascular lung water in critical care: recent advances and clinical applications. Ann Intensive Care. 2015;5(1):38.
22. Tagami T, Kushimoto S, Yamamoto Y, Atsumi T, Tosa R, Matsuda K, et al. Validation of extravascular lung water measurement by single transpulmonary thermodilution: human autopsy study. Crit Care. 2010;14(5):R162.
23. Dres M, Teboul JL, Guerin L, Anguel N, Amilien V, Clair MP, et al. Transpulmonary thermodilution enables to detect small short-term changes in extravascular lung water induced by a bronchoalveolar lavage. Crit Care Med. 2014;42(8):1869-73.
24. Dres M, Teboul JL, Anguel N, Guerin L, Richard C, Monnet X. Extravascular lung water, B-type natriuretic peptide, and blood volume contraction enable diagnosis of weaning-induced pulmonary edema. Crit Care Med. 2014;42(8):1882-9.
25. Jozwiak M, Silva S, Persichini R, Anguel N, Osman D, Richard C, et al. Extravascular lung water is an independent prognostic factor in patients with acute respiratory distress syndrome. Crit Care Med. 2013;41(2):472-80.
26. Gavelli F, Shi R, Teboul JL, Azzolina D, Mercado P, Jozwiak M, et al. Extravascular lung water levels are associated with mortality: a systematic review and meta-analysis. Crit Care 2022;26(1):202.
27. Anguel N, Monnet X, Osman D, Castelain V, Richard C, Teboul JL. Increase in plasma protein concentration for diagnosing weaning-induced pulmonary oedema. Intensive Care Med. 2008;34(7):1231-8.
28. Roch A, Michelet P, D'journo B, Brousse D, Blayac D, Lambert D, et al. Accuracy and limits of transpulmonary dilution methods in estimating extravascular lung water after pneumonectomy. Chest. 2005;128(2):927-33.
29. Ranieri VM, Rubenfeld GD, Thompson BT, Ferguson ND, Caldwell E, Fan E, et al. Acute respiratory distress syndrome: the Berlin Definition. JAMA. 2012;307(23):2526-33.
30. Tagami T, Ong MEH. Extravascular lung water measurements in acute respiratory distress syndrome: why, how, and when? Curr Opin Crit Care. 2018;24(3):209-15.
31. Tagami T, Sakka SG, Monnet X. Diagnosis and treatment of acute respiratory distress syndrome. JAMA. 2018; 320(3):305.
32. Malbrain MLNG, Van Regenmortel N, Saugel B, De Tavernier B, Van Gaal PJ, Joannes-Boyau O, et al. Principles of fluid management and stewardship in septic shock: it is time to consider the four D's and the four phases of fluid therapy. Ann Intensive Care. 2018;8(1):66.
33. Sakr Y, Rubatto Birri PN, Kotfis K, Nanchal R, Shah B, Kluge S, et al. Higher Fluid Balance Increases the Risk of Death from Sepsis: Results from a Large International Audit. Crit Care Med. 2017;45(3):386-94.
34. Monnet X, Teboul JL. My patient has received fluid. How to assess its efficacy and side effects? Ann Intensive Care. 2018;8(1):54.
35. Gong C, Zhang F, Li L, He F, Liu GC, Zhu SH, et al. The variation of hemodynamic parameters through PiCCO in the early stage after severe burns. J Burn Care Res. 2017;38(6):e966-72.
36. Soussi S, Deniau B, Ferry A, Levé C, Benyamina M, Maurel V, et al. Low cardiac index and stroke volume on admission are associated with poor outcome in critically ill burn patients: a retrospective cohort study. Ann Intensive Care. 2016;6(1):87.
37. Pottecher J, Roche AC, Dégot T, Helms O, Hentz JG, Schmitt JP, et al. Increased extravascular lung water and plasma biomarkers of acute lung injury precede oxygenation impairment in primary graft dysfunction after lung transplantation. Transplantation. 2017;101(1):112-21.
38. Stéphan F, Mazeraud A, Laverdure F, Camous J, Fadel E. Evaluation of reperfusion pulmonary edema by extravascular lung water measurements after pulmonary endarterectomy. Crit Care Med. 2017;45(4):e409-17.
39. Vincent JL, Rhodes A, Perel A, Martin GS, Della Rocca G, Vallet B, et al. Clinical review: update on hemodynamic monitoring—a consensus of 16. Crit Care. 2011;15(4):229.
40. Biais M, Nouette-Gaulain K, Cottenceau V, Cottenceau V, Vallet A, Cochard JF, et al. Cardiac output measurement in patients undergoing liver transplantation: pulmonary artery catheter versus uncalibrated arterial pressure waveform analysis. Anesth Analg. 2008;106(5):1480-6.
41. Teboul JL, Saugel B, Cecconi M, De Backer D, Hofer CK, Monnet X, et al. Less invasive hemodynamic monitoring in critically ill patients. Intensive Care Med. 2016;42(9):1350-9.
42. Eyeington CT, Lloyd-Donald P, Chan MJ, Eastwood GM, Young H, Peck L, et al. Rapid response team review of hemodynamically unstable ward patients: the accuracy of cardiac index assessment. J Crit Care. 2019;49:187-92.
43. Monnet X, Teboul JL. Cardiac output monitoring: throw it out... or keep it? Crit Care. 2018;22(1):35.
44. Cecconi M, Hofer C, Teboul JL,Pettila V, Wilkman E, Molnar Z, et al. Fluid challenges in intensive care: the FENICE study: a global inception cohort study. Intensive Care Med. 2015;41(9):1529-37.
45. Vignon P, Begot E, Mari A, Silva S, Chimot L, Delour P, et al. Hemodynamic assessment of patients with septic shock using transpulmonary thermodilution and critical care echocardiography: a comparative study. Chest. 2018;153(1):55-64.
46. Belda FJ, Aguilar G, Teboul JL, Pestaña D, Redondo FJ, Malbrain M, et al. Complications related to less-invasive haemodynamic monitoring. Br J Anaesth. 2011;106(4): 482-6.

CHAPTER

Arterial Pressure-based Cardiac Output Measurements

Daniel De Backer, Simone Giglioli

INTRODUCTION

Monitoring of cardiac output is one of the most important aspects of hemodynamic monitoring. Cardiac output is a key determinant of tissue perfusion and is thus used to classify the different types of shock[1] as well as to trigger therapeutic interventions.[2]

Unfortunately, clinicians are not good in estimating cardiac output based on clinical signs.[3,4] In addition, even when a low cardiac output is suspected based on clinical signs, identification of its cause requires further hemodynamic evaluation.[5] While echocardiography is now recommended as the first modality to evaluate the cardiovascular system in shock states,[6] cardiac output using continuous techniques is often desired in order to evaluate the effects of the various interventions.[7] While the pulmonary artery catheter has widely been used for this purpose in the past,[8] its use has decreased over time[9] and less invasive alternatives are now suggested.[10] Among these alternatives, arterial pressure cardiac output measurements are among the most popular. In this chapter we will review the various techniques, their advantages, and limitations.

WHAT IS THE LINK BETWEEN ARTERIAL PRESSURE AND CARDIAC OUTPUT?

Even though arterial pressure is generated by the irruption of stroke volume in the aorta at each systole, the link between arterial pressure and cardiac output is not obvious. In critically ill patients, the correlation between mean arterial pressure (MAP) and cardiac output is at best weak.[11] In simulated hemorrhage, changes in MAP could not detect changes in stroke volume.[12] During fluid administration, changes in MAP were not related with changes in cardiac output.[13,14] The lack of relationship between MAP and cardiac output is likely to be due to the impact of vascular tone on the diastolic component of arterial pressure.

Pulse pressure may be a more direct surrogate of stroke volume. In volunteers submitted to simulated hemorrhage, there was an excellent correlation between pulse pressure and stroke volume.[12] Similarly in cardiac surgical patients, clamping the inferior vena cava was associated with a proportional decrease in stroke volume, assessed by esophageal Doppler, and pulse pressure.[15] Unfortunately, pulse pressure does not track changes correctly in stroke volume during norepinephrine infusion[13] or fluid administration.[14] Nevertheless, over one respiratory cycle, pulse pressure variations correlate with stroke volume variations.[16]

Altogether, these data suggest that arterial pressure trace is the result of a complex relationship between stroke volume, vascular tone, and aortic elastance. There are several ways to get around these issues and to derive cardiac output from arterial traces **(Figs. 1 and 2)**.[17] *Obtaining a good quality arterial signal is required.*[18]

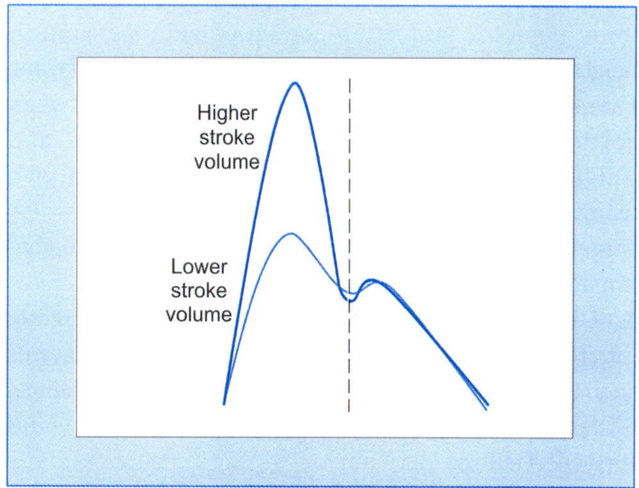

Fig. 1: Relationship between stroke volume and arterial pressure waveform.

Note: In conditions of unchanged arterial impedance and vascular tone, any change in stroke volume is associated with a change in arterial pressure waveform before the dicrotic notch.

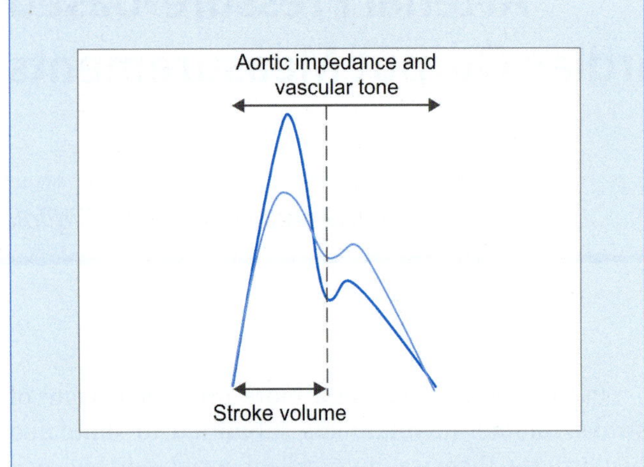

Fig. 2: Factors influencing arterial pressure waveform.
Note: To derive stroke volume from an arterial pressure waveform, arterial impedance can be derived from biometric variables and vascular tone should be estimated by a dedicated software. When the latter is not feasible, the alternative is to use an external calibration.

NONCALIBRATED TECHNIQUES

There are essentially two types of noncalibrated techniques, those taking only into account aortic impedance and those estimating vascular tone in addition to taking into account aortic impedance.

Noncalibrated Techniques not Taking into Account Vascular Tone

These noncalibrated methods estimate aortic impedance from biometric and anthropometric data (age, gender, height, and weight). Using aorta obtained from cadavers, Langewouter[19,20] described the relationship between aortic impedance and age and gender, height, and weight. These data were recently confirmed in vivo using echocardiography in patients submitted to cardiac surgery.[20] Interestingly, aortic atheromatosis had moderate impact on impedance.

Different proprietary algorithms, based on slightly different assumptions, are used by the different devices such as the Modelflow (Finometer®PRO, Finapres Medical Systems, Netherlands), LiDCOrapid (LiDCO, UK), and ProAQT (Getinge, Germany).

While these devices perform adequately in perioperative patients with preserved vascular tone, these devices may be in trouble in more extreme conditions. In particular, in patients with septic shock, these devices may be less reliable with broad limits of agreement with more invasive techniques.

Accordingly, these devices are mostly useful in perioperative settings when cardiac output and vascular tone are usually close to the usual normal range. More importantly, perhaps, in these patients trends are more important than the absolute value. In many instances, these devices have been validated in the perioperative setting and provide relatively accurate measurements.[21] However, in more extreme conditions, such as in septic shock or in low cardiac output states, these devices may provide erroneous information and more accurate devices are required.[22,23]

Noncalibrated Techniques Attempting to Take into Account Vascular Tone

Two devices are currently the FloTrac/Vigileo (Edwards Lifesciences, US) and the PRAM (Vygon, Italy) systems. These use different concepts of analyzing the arterial waveform. Both devices can be attached to radial or femoral arterial lines.

The FloTrac/Vigileo applies some statistical analysis to the arterial waveform. Cardiac output is computed as: pulse rate . APsd . χ

The stroke volume is computed from the standard deviation of arterial pressure (APsd) over several beats. Chi (χ) is the factor representing arterial impedance and vascular tone. Chi was determined using a large human database of simultaneous collection of arterial pressure curves and cardiac output measurements using the reference bolus thermodilution with a pulmonary artery catheter in different clinical conditions. Chi is influenced on the one hand for the impedance component by biometric variables (age, gender, etc.) and on the other hand, for the vascular tone component, by shape variables such as kurtosis and skewness. Initially, Chi was updated every 10 minutes, but this interval was decreased to 1 minute in the subsequent versions. In critically ill patients, most of which were submitted to surgery, the use of this device was associated with a good agreement and precision compared to bolus thermodilution.[24] In addition, changes in thermodilution cardiac output were adequately tracked by changes in arterial pressure derived cardiac output. However, in a subsequent study also including patients with various alterations in vascular tone, it was reported that the agreement was poor in patients with systemic vascular resistances below

800 dynes/sec cm,[5] while it was satisfactory in patients with higher values of systemic vascular resistance.[25] The computation algorithm was adapted, after expanding the database in order to include more patients with low vascular resistance. The adapted algorithm (version 3 and beyond) was shown to provide adequate agreement and precision in patients with septic shock, compared to both intermittent and continuous thermodilution cardiac output measurements.[26]

The PRAM uses a complex algorithm to estimate the deviation from equilibrium induced by irruption of stroke volume into the aorta.[27] While there may be some aspects which are operator dependent (such as the precise recognition of the dicrotic notch) that may interfere with reliability, PRAM has been shown to be accurate in critically ill patients.[28-30] In addition, the system provides interesting additional measurements based on the analysis of the arterial waveform and that do correlate with cardiac function and performance.[31] In addition, this device can also reconstruct the central arterial waveform, which is interesting to evaluate left ventricular afterload.[32]

The limitation of the two techniques is that acute changes in vascular tone, such as those induced by boluses of vasopressor agents, impair the reliability of these devices.[33] Sufficient time should elapse to allow the device to recompute the new vascular tone.

CALIBRATED TECHNIQUES

To derive stroke volume from an arterial pressure waveform in calibrated techniques, the device does not attempt to compute vascular tone. At a given time, the calibration is performed, and it is assumed that any subsequent change in arterial waveform is related to changes in stroke volume. In calibrated techniques, the calibration is obtained either by transpulmonary thermodilution for the PiCCO device (Getinge, Germany) or by lithium dilution for the LiDCO (LiDCO, UK) device. The PiCCO device requires the insertion of a dedicated catheter, equipped with a thermistor, often inserted in femoral arteries even though brachial arteries can also be used. The LiDCO device can be adapted to any existing arterial line.

Both techniques provide reliable measurements of cardiac output,[34] even in hyperdynamic/vasoplegic conditions.[35] Importantly, both transpulmonary thermodilution and lithium dilution require recalibration at regular intervals (usually 6 hours), but calibration should be performed more frequently when there are important deviations in arterial tone.[36,37]

ROLE OF ADDITIONAL MEASUREMENTS

Transpulmonary thermodilution computes the global end-diastolic volume, a reflection of the dimension of the heart and cardiac preload, extravascular lung water, permeability index, and a cardiac function index. Altogether, these can be used both for diagnostic purposes and for decision making in patients management. A full review of these indices is provided elsewhere.[38]

In complex cases, it is often considered that these indices are particularly valuable.[39-42]

CONCLUSION

Cardiac output measurements can reliably be obtained from the arterial pressure waveform, especially when the software takes into account vascular tone and not only aortic impedance, or when external calibration is performed. The choice of the hemodynamic monitoring tool should be based on the interest for additional measurements and patient's condition.

REFERENCES

1. Vincent JL, De Backer D. Circulatory shock. N Engl J Med. 2013;369(18):1726-34.
2. De Backer D. Detailing the cardiovascular profile in shock patients. Crit Care. 2017;21(Suppl 3):311.
3. Connors AF, McCaffree DR, Gray BA. Evaluation of right-heart catheterization in the critically ill patient without acute myocardial infarction. N Engl J Med. 1983;308(5):263-7.
4. Hiemstra B, Koster G, Wiersema R, Hummel YM, van der Harst P, Snieder H, et al. The diagnostic accuracy of clinical examination for estimating cardiac output in critically ill patients: the Simple Intensive Care Studies-I. Intensive Care Med. 2019;45(2):190-200.
5. De Backer D, Vieillard-Baron A. Clinical examination: a trigger but not a substitute for hemodynamic evaluation. Intensive Care Med. 2019;45(2):269-71.
6. Cecconi M, De Backer D, Antonelli M, Beale R, Bakker J, Hofer C, et al. Consensus on circulatory shock and hemodynamic monitoring. Task Force of the European Society of Intensive Care Medicine. Intensive Care Med. 2014;40(12):1795-815.
7. Teboul JL, Saugel B, Cecconi M, De Backer D, Hofer CK, Monnet X, et al. Less invasive hemodynamic monitoring in critically ill patients. Intensive Care Med. 2016;42(9):1350-9.
8. De Backer D, Fagnoul D, Herpain A. The role of invasive techniques in cardiopulmonary evaluation. Curr Opin Crit Care. 2013;19(3):228-33.

9. De Backer D, Vincent JL. The pulmonary artery catheter: is it still alive? Curr Opin Crit Care. 2018;24(3):204-8.
10. De Backer D, Bakker J, Cecconi M, Hajjar L, Liu DW, Lobo S, et al. Alternatives to the Swan-Ganz catheter. Intensive Care Med. 2018;44(6):730-41.
11. Wo CC, Shoemaker WC, Appel PL, Bishop MH, Kram HB, Hardin E. Unreliability of blood pressure and heart rate to evaluate cardiac output in emergency resuscitation and critical illness. Crit Care Med. 1993;21(2):218-23.
12. Convertino VA, Cooke WH, Holcomb JB. Arterial pulse pressure and its association with reduced stroke volume during progressive central hypovolemia. J Trauma. 2006;61(3):629-34.
13. Monnet X, Letierce A, Hamzaoui O, Chemla D, Anguel N, Osman D, et al. Arterial pressure allows monitoring the changes in cardiac output induced by volume expansion but not by norepinephrine. Crit Care Med. 2011;39(6):1394-9.
14. Pierrakos C, Velissaris D, Scolletta S, Heenen S, De Backer D, Vincent JL. Can changes in arterial pressure be used to detect changes in cardiac index during fluid challenge in patients with septic shock? Intensive Care Med. 2012;38(3):422-8.
15. Marquez J, McCurry K, Severyn DA, Pinsky MR. Ability of pulse power, esophageal Doppler and arterial pulse pressure to estimate rapid changes in stroke volume in humans. Crit Care Med. 2008;36(11):3001-7.
16. De Backer D, Taccone FS, Holsten R, Ibrahimi F, Vincent JL. Influence of respiratory rate on stroke volume variation in mechanically ventilated patients. Anesthesiology. 2009;110(5):1092-7.
17. Kouz K, Scheeren TWL, de Backer D, Saugel B. Pulse wave analysis to estimate cardiac output. Anesthesiology. 2021;134(1):119-26.
18. Saugel B, Kouz K, Meidert AS, Schulte-Uentrop L, Romagnoli S. How to measure blood pressure using an arterial catheter: a systematic 5-step approach. Crit Care. 2020;24(1):172.
19. Langewouters GJ, Wesseling KH, Goedhard WJ. The pressure dependent dynamic elasticity of 35 thoracic and 16 abdominal human aortas in vitro described by a five component model. J Biomech. 1985;18(8):613-20.
20. Langewouters GJ, Wesseling KH, Goedhard WJ. The static elastic properties of 45 human thoracic and 20 abdominal aortas in vitro and the parameters of a new model. J Biomech. 1984;17(6):425-35.
21. Heerman JR, Segers P, Roosens CD, Gasthuys F, Verdonck PR, Poelaert JI. Echocardiographic assessment of aortic elastic properties with automated border detection in an ICU: in vivo application of the arctangent Langewouters model. Am J Physiol Heart Circ Physiol. 2005;288(5):H2504-11.
22. Monnet X, Vaquer S, Anguel N, Jozwiak M, Cipriani F, Richard C, et al. Comparison of pulse contour analysis by Pulsioflex and Vigileo to measure and track changes of cardiac output in critically ill patients. Br J Anaesth. 2015;114(2):235-43.
23. Grensemann J, Defosse JM, Willms M, Schiller U, Wappler F, Sakka SG. Validation of radial artery-based uncalibrated pulse contour method (PulsioFlex) in critically ill patients: A observational study. Eur J Anaesthesiol. 2017;34(11):723-31.
24. Biais M, Mazocky E, Stecken L, Pereira B, Sesay M, Roullet S, et al. Impact of Systemic Vascular Resistance on the Accuracy of the Pulsioflex Device. Anesth Analg. 2017;124(2):487-93.
25. McGee W, Horswell J, Janvier G. Validation of a continuous cardiac output measurement using arterial pressure waveforms. Crit Care. 2005;9:P62.
26. Biais M, Nouette-Gaulain K, Cottenceau V, Vallet A, Cochard JF, Revel P, et al. Cardiac output measurement in patients undergoing liver transplantation: pulmonary artery catheter versus uncalibrated arterial pressure waveform analysis. Anesth Analg. 2008;106(5):1480-6.
27. De Backer D, Marx G, Tan A, Junker C, Van Nuffelen M, Hüter L, et al. Arterial pressure-based cardiac output monitoring: a multicenter validation of the third-generation software in septic patients. Intensive Care Med. 2011;37(2):233-40.
28. Romagnoli S, Franchi F, Ricci Z, Scolletta S, Payen D. The Pressure Recording Analytical Method (PRAM): Technical Concepts and Literature Review. J Cardiothorac Vasc Anesth. 2017;31(4):1460-70.
29. Franchi F, Silvestri R, Cubattoli L, Taccone FS, Donadello K, Romano SM, et al. Comparison between an uncalibrated pulse contour method and thermodilution technique for cardiac output estimation in septic patients. Br J Anaesth. 2011;107(2):202-8.
30. Scolletta S, Romano SM, Biagioli B, Capannini G, Giomarelli P. Pressure recording analytical method (PRAM) for measurement of cardiac output during various haemodynamic states. Br J Anaesth. 2005;95(2):159-65.
31. Scolletta S, Bodson L, Donadello K, Taccone FS, Devigili A, Vincent JL, et al. Assessment of left ventricular function by pulse wave analysis in critically ill patients. Intensive Care Med. 2013;39(6):1025-33.
32. Scolletta S, Herpain A, Romano SM, Taccone FS, Donadello K, Lubicz B, et al. Estimation of central arterial pressure from the radial artery in patients undergoing invasive neuroradiological procedures. BMC anesthesiology. 2019;19(1):173.
33. Meng L, Phuong TN, Alexander BS, Laning K, Chen G, Kain ZN, et al. The impact of phenylephrine, ephedrine, and increased preload on third-generation Vigileo-FloTrac and esophageal doppler cardiac output measurements. Anesth Analg. 2011;113(4):751-7.
34. Hadian M, Kim HK, Severyn DA, Pinsky MR. Cross-comparison of cardiac output trending accuracy of LiDCO, PiCCO, FloTrac and pulmonary artery catheters. Crit Care. 2010;14(6):R212.

35. Costa MG, Della RG, Chiarandini P, Mattelig S, Pompei L, Barriga MS, et al. Continuous and intermittent cardiac output measurement in hyperdynamic conditions: pulmonary artery catheter vs. lithium dilution technique. Intensive Care Med. 2008;34(2):257-63.
36. Cecconi M, Fawcett J, Grounds RM, Rhodes A. A prospective study to evaluate the accuracy of pulse power analysis to monitor cardiac output in critically ill patients. BMC Anesthesiol. 2008;8:3.
37. Hamzaoui O, Monnet X, Richard C, Osman D, Chemla D, Teboul JL. Effects of changes in vascular tone on the agreement between pulse contour and transpulmonary thermodilution cardiac output measurements within an up to 6-hour calibration-free period. Crit Care Med. 2008;36(2):434-40.
38. Monnet X, Teboul JL. Transpulmonary thermodilution: advantages and limits. Crit Care. 2017;21(1):147.
39. Saugel B, Kouz K, Scheeren TWL, Greiwe G, Hoppe P, Romagnoli S, et al. Cardiac output estimation using pulse wave analysis-physiology, algorithms, and technologies: a narrative review. Br J Anaesth. 2021;126(1):67-76.
40. Kouz K, Scheeren TWL, de Backer D, Saugel B. Pulse wave analysis to estimate cardiac output. Anesthesiology. 2021;134:119-26.
41. Saugel B, Kouz K, Meidert AS, Schulte-Uentrop L, Romagnoli S. How to measure blood pressure using an arterial catheter: a systematic 5-step approach. Crit Care. 2020;24(1):172.
42. Scolletta S, Herpain A, Romano SM, Taccone FS, Donadello K, Lubicz B, et al. Estimation of central arterial pressure from the radial artery in patients undergoing invasive neuroradiological procedures. BMC anesthesiology. 2019;19(1):173.

Noninvasive Cardiac Output Monitoring

VR Srivats, Suhail S Siddiqui, Atul Prabhakar Kulkarni

INTRODUCTION

Circulatory shock and the need for hemodynamic monitoring is one of the most common indications for admission into the intensive care unit (ICU). Cardiac output (CO) is a crucial determinant of oxygen delivery to tissues.[1] Fluid bolus increases the cardiac preload and increases the CO. Fluid resuscitation is the initial therapy for patients with hemodynamic compromise. However, not all patients are fluid responsive. Fluid responsiveness (FR) is defined as the ability of the left ventricle to increase its stroke volume (SV) in response to fluid administration. Almost half the patients admitted to the ICU are not fluid responsive. Excess fluid administration can lead to venous congestion and can lead to adverse consequences. The current consensus statements on circulatory shock recommend measurement of CO and SV during resuscitation of patients not responding to initial therapy to evaluate and titrate the response to fluids and/or vasoactive agents. CO monitoring has also been recommended in perioperative patient management in high-risk surgical patients.[2]

Various instruments with different principles have been devised for the measurement of CO. Pulmonary artery thermodilution with pulmonary artery catheter introduced in 1970, has been considered the reference method for decades.[3] There is a decrease in its use due to its invasiveness, associated complications, and no overall benefit in critically ill patients.[4-6] Due to technological advancements, it is now possible to measure the CO and assess FR using minimally invasive or noninvasive techniques. These techniques are associated with fewer complications, but at the expense of accuracy, precision, and dynamic response.

Each equipment operates by a specific principle, and it is imperative to know the basic principles of these monitors, and the appropriate clinical setting where to use them. An ideal CO monitor would be accurate, precise, operator independent, reliable in various physiological and pathological conditions, with fast response time, noninvasive, continuous, easy to use, cheap, and without complications.[7,8]

Research has shown that use of minimally invasive CO monitoring combined with a goal-directed fluid administration protocol in the high-risk perioperative setting is associated with favorable outcomes in surgical patients.[1] The evidence for use of these equipment in the sicker cohort of ICU patients is less robust.

CLASSIFICATION

The CO monitors can be classified **(Fig. 1)** based on their:

- Invasiveness
- Principles in which they operate
- Whether they measure the CO continuously or intermittently

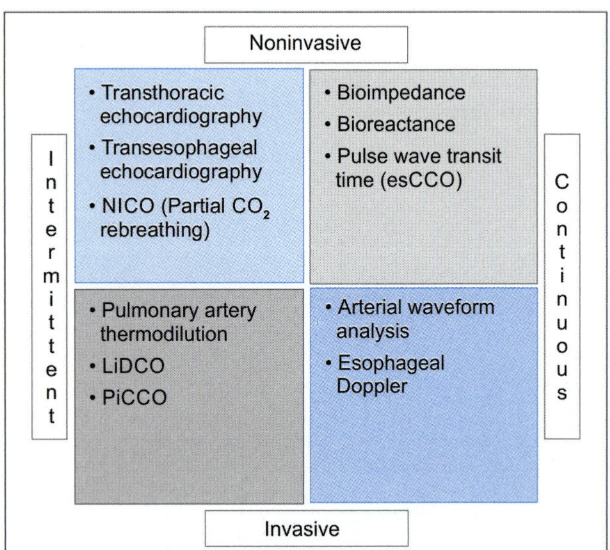

Fig. 1: Classification of cardiac output devices based on their invasiveness. (esCCO: estimated continuous cardiac output; LiDCO: lithium dilution cardiac output; NICO: noninvasive cardiac output; PiCCO: pulse index continuous cardiac output)

FICK'S PRINCIPLE AND DIFFERENTIAL FICK PARTIAL REBREATHING METHOD

In 1870, Adolf Fick, a German physician, described the first method to estimate CO.[9] He stated that the uptake of oxygen by a tissue is the product of the amount of oxygen delivered to the tissue times the difference in oxygen content between the blood entering and leaving the tissue. Considering the entire body to be the tissue and the blood entering as the CO, we get the equation as:

$$VO_2 = CO\,(CaO_2 - CvO_2) \quad (1)$$

Rearranging equation (1) CO can be calculated as the ratio between oxygen consumption (VO_2) and arteriovenous difference in oxygen (A-VDO_2) **(Fig. 2)**.

Fick's principle equation:

$$CO = \frac{VO_2}{(CaO_2 - CvO_2)} \quad (2)$$

Where, CO: cardiac output; VO_2: oxygen uptake; CaO_2 and CvO_2 are the oxygen contents of arterial and venous blood, respectively. This requires measurement oxygen uptake (VO_2), which is cumbersome as compared to carbon dioxide elimination (VCO_2) which is relatively easier. The above principle is invasive as it requires both arterial and central venous blood gas concentration of oxygen.[8,10]

The above principle, based on law of conservation of mass, also holds true for any gas which is eliminated through the lungs, e.g., CO_2. Fick's principle can be applied to CO_2 to measure the CO noninvasively. Fick's equation for measuring CO using CO_2:

$$CO = \frac{VCO_2}{(CaCO_2 - CvCO_2)} \quad (3)$$

A partial rebreathing method has been devised to measure the partial pressure of mixed venous CO_2. The CO measurement is obtained by using the above formula. The value of VCO_2 is computed from CO_2 content of exhaled gases. The CO_2 concentration in the arterial blood ($CaCO_2$) is estimated from the partial pressure of end tidal CO_2 ($EtCO_2$) in the expired gas and modified in accordance with CO_2 dissociation curve. The above equation (equation 3) can further be solved for partial rebreathing (where there are phases of rebreathing and nonrebreathing alternately) method as follows:

During nonrebreathing (NR) period

$$CO = \frac{VCO_2\,NR}{(CaCO_2\,NR - CvCO_2\,NR)} \quad (4)$$

During rebreathing (R) period

$$CO = \frac{VCO_2\,R}{(CaCO_2\,R - CvCO_2\,R)} \quad (5)$$

Supposing the CO remains unchanged during nonrebreathing and rebreathing period the above equations (3) and (4) can be combined as:

$$CO = \frac{VCO_2\,NR - VCO_2\,R}{(CaCO_2\,NR - CvCO_2\,NR) - (CaCO_2\,R - CvCO_2\,R)} \quad (6)$$

Due to high solubility of CO_2 in the blood, it diffuses rapidly leaving no difference between $CvCO_2$ of rebreathing

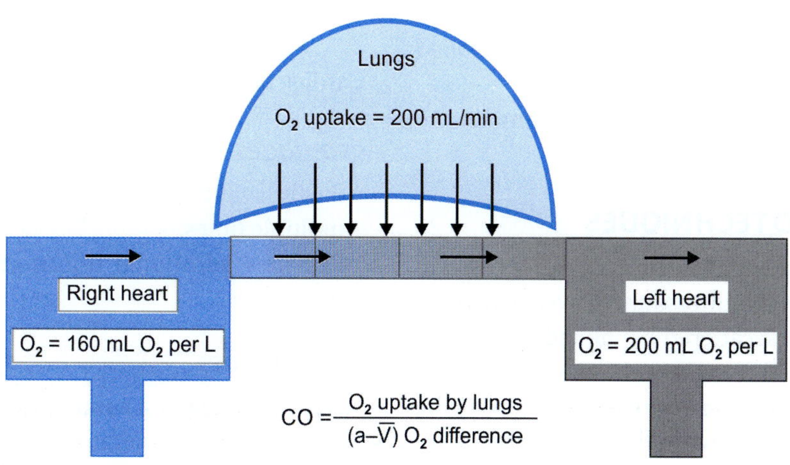

Fig. 2: Fick's principle.

versus nonrebreathing phase which will cancel out in the equation yielding the equation given below and thereby omitting the need of central venous blood:

$$CO = \frac{\Delta VCO_2}{\Delta CaCO_2} \quad (7)$$

NONINVASIVE CARDIAC OUTPUT DEVICE

The noninvasive cardiac output (NICO®) (Novametrix Medical Systems, Wallingford, Conn, United States) is a noninvasive CO monitor based on the Fick's principle using intermittent partial rebreathing of CO_2, which is accomplished by incorporating a rebreathing loop for phasic rebreathing, with CO_2 sensors and transducer within. VCO_2 is calculated from the CO_2 content within the minute ventilation. The arterial CO_2 content ($CaCO_2$) is estimated from partial pressure of $EtCO_2$ multiplied by a correction factor (S), i.e., the slope of the CO_2 dissociation curve.

The device measures the VCO_2, $PaCO_2$, and $EtCO_2$ during periods of normal breathing and rebreathing. The measured variables during rebreathing and nonrebreathing phases are processed by the formula and the nonshunted (blood flow which takes part in pulmonary gas exchange) CO is calculated.

The system measures the nonshunted portion of cardiac output (Q_{PCBF}) and total cardiac output (Q_{CO}) which will be calculated by adding the shunted portion of cardiac output (Q_{shunt}) to nonshunted portion. In NICO, the proprietary algorithm calculates shunted portion of CO noninvasively by arterial oxygen saturation using pulse oximeter probe and fraction of inspired oxygen.

Limitations

- Can be used only in intubated patients on controlled mechanical ventilation.
- Poor agreement of measured CO when compared to thermodilution techniques.[11-12]

DOPPLER-BASED TECHNIQUES

The ultrasound and the Doppler principle can be used to calculate the CO. Here, the ultrasound waves which are sent by the probe is backscattered by the red blood cells traveling in the artery. The backscattered waves are at a different frequency depending on the direction of the blood flow. The difference between the two frequencies is called the Doppler frequency shift and is proportional to the velocity of the blood flow as described in the equation below:

$$V = \frac{CF}{2FoCos\phi}$$

Where:

- V is blood flow velocity;
- C is speed of the ultrasound waves;
- F is Doppler frequency shift;
- Fo is emitted frequency from ultrasound device; and
- $Cos\phi$ is cosine of angle (ϕ) of insonation.

The following devices measure the cardiac output based on the Doppler principle.

- Transesophageal echocardiography (TEE)
- Transthoracic echocardiography (TTE)
- Esophageal Doppler (CardioQ-ODM)
- The ultrasound CO monitor

Transthoracic Echocardiography

A routine echocardiography machine or point of care ultrasound machine is required to measure the CO. CO is measured based on the continuity equation. There are two parameters required to calculate the CO—left ventricle outflow tract (LVOT) area and the left ventricle velocity time integral (LVOT VTi). The LVOT diameter is calculated from the parasternal long axis after zooming into the LVOT. LVOT area is then calculated from the diameter.

$$\text{LVOT area} = 3.14 \times \frac{\text{LVOT diameter}}{4}$$

The next step is to measure the LVOT VTi. A parasternal five-chamber view of the heart is obtained. A pulsed wave Doppler gate is placed across the LVOT. The ejection wave is traced and the VTi is calculated.

$$\text{Stroke volume (SV)} = \text{LVOT area} \times \text{LVOT VTi}$$

$$\text{Cardiac output (mL/min)} = \text{Stroke volume} \times \text{Heart rate}$$

Advantages

- Easily available, noninvasive, and can be repeated multiple times.
- Provides additional information regarding cardiac functions.

Disadvantages

- Does not provide a continuous CO monitoring.
- Requires skilled operator.
- Poor echo window can hinder CO measurement.

Transesophageal Echocardiography

A specialized probe is placed in the esophagus which provides high-quality image of the cardiac chambers and the major vessels. The principle of measuring the CO is similar to TTE. The LVOT diameter is measured in the mid-esophageal long axis view. The LVOT VTi is measured in the deep transgastric view where the Doppler signals are in line with the LVOT flow.

Advantages

- Provides detailed assessment of the cardiac functions.

Disadvantages

- Does not provide a continuous CO monitoring.
- Requires skilled operator.
- Equipment is costly and the procedure requires sedation.

Esophageal Doppler

A specialized Doppler probe is placed in the esophagus. Doppler signals sent from the probe are reflected off the red blood cells flowing in the descending aorta. The Doppler shift is picked up by the probe and analyzed using fast Fourier transformation. This is displayed in the monitor as a spectral density display of the distribution of blood flow velocity in the y-axis against time in the x-axis.

This technology was introduced by Abbott Medical in 1990. The first generation was called the esophageal Doppler monitor, the ODMII. Subsequently, it has undergone modifications and the current generation introduced in 2009 is the CardioQ-ODM. It has a proprietary algorithm which converts aortic flow velocity to SV.

Each CardioQ-ODM probe is of 50 cm length coil of steel wrapped in silicone and the tip of the probe contains a piezoelectric crystal which sends ultrasound waves. The probe is of 19 French size and can be placed orally or nasally, after lubrication, till it reaches the lower end of the esophagus. It is then rotated until the transducer faces the descending aorta and a characteristic waveform is seen on the screen, and audible Doppler sound is heard through the monitor speaker. The Doppler signals are obtained at a depth of 35–40 cm, if inserted orally. Each probe is a single use and should be discarded after each use. There are two knobs on the monitor that can help adjust the gain of the waveform and the volume of the audio. The patient's data including age, height, and weight needs to be entered in the monitor initially.

The aortic Doppler waveform has a characteristic appearance which help in its accurate placement which is a prerequisite for proper measurement. An ideal waveform appears triangular with the spectral display confined to the peripheral edge of the triangular waveform. There is an absence of signal in the central part of the waveform. If the probe position is not optimal the waveform shows evidence of spectral dispersion. These values are used in the proprietary nomogram to calculate the aortic cross-sectional area, and this can be used to calculate the SV from the stroke distance.

Based on the characteristics of the waveform several parameters of the cardiovascular functions can be assessed.[13] The *peak velocity* of the waveform (height) is an approximate estimate of afterload and contractility. The slope of the upstroke called the *mean acceleration* is measure of contractility. The duration of aortic blood flow called the *flow time* is an estimate of preload. Smaller flow time indicates hypovolemia. The area under the curve is the *stroke distance* and is an estimate of the SV. Increase in afterload is indicated by a reduction in waveform height and width.[14]

Advantages

- Minimally invasive
- Very low incidence of complication

Disadvantages

- The device assumes that a fixed percentage of the CO is directed toward the descending aorta which may not be in all cases.
- Repositioning essential before every measurement.
- Position changes can alter values.[15]
- The presence of Ryle's tube may interfere with the measurement.
- Training is required for accurate measurement.[16]

Bioimpedance and Bioreactance

Bioimpedance and bioreactance are completely noninvasive methods to detect the CO. Bioimpedance technology was first described in aeronautical medicine nearly 50 years ago.[17] Impedance is *a measure of the opposition to electrical flow.* It works on the principle that electrical conductivity and impedance of the thorax changes with respect to the changes in the intrathoracic volume. This change in the intrathoracic volume is caused by SV during every cardiac cycle. By estimating the changes in the electric characteristics, it is possible to measure the cardiac output. With every systole, the volume of the aorta increases, and there is an increase in the iron content in the thorax, which decreases the impedance. The change in the impedance is proportional to the changes in aortic volume and this is used to calculate the CO. The cardiac chambers are electrically isolated by the cardiac muscle and hence do not affect the electrical changes.[18]

Bioimpedance device consists of four pairs of electrodes which are attached to the skin on the base of neck and lower part of the thorax on either side. The two pairs on each side are placed in a straight line. In one pair, a single electrode injects a high-frequency current of known amplitude and the other electrode detects the returning current. The device measures the current changes from each side separately and averages the result.

Stroke volume is calculated as the product of the ventricular ejection time (VET) and the slope of the initial change of the aortic volume obtained from the first derivative of the impedance signal (dZ/dt max).[19] The bioimpedance monitor only calculates the relative changes in CO, a calibration factor (CF) is added to obtain the absolute values of SV.[19]

$$SV = VET \times \frac{dZ}{dt\ max} \times CF$$

Bioimpedance devices measure the *change in amplitude* of the return current whereas the *bioreactance* device measure the *change in phase* of the return current. Because change in phase is associated with high signal to noise ratio, bioreactance devices are prone to less error. In addition to SV, CO and total water content including extravascular lung water is calculated.

The devices which use the bioimpedance technology include NCCOM (BoMed Medical, Irvine, CA, USA), BioZ (Cardiodynamics, San Diego, CA, USA), NICCOMO (MEDIS, Limenau, Germany), ICON (Osypka Cardiotronic, Berlin, Germany), ICG (Philips Medical Systems, Andover, MA, USA), NICOMON (Larsen and Toubro Ltd., Mumbai, India), and PHYSIOFLOW (Manatec Biomedical, Paris, France). The only device using bioreactance technology is the NICOM (Cheetah Medical, MA, USA).[18] It has been upgraded to the latest version as Starling SV hemodynamic monitoring system after being acquired by Baxter.

Advantages

- Completely noninvasive
- Cheaper
- Provides a continuous measurement of CO.
- The response time is fast in Starling SV monitors and they can be used to measure CO changes with passive leg raise (PLR) test.

Limitations

- Affected by electric noise such as cautery and ventilator.
- Obesity, anemia, and hypertension can give erroneous reading.
- Less reliable in critically ill patients compared to operating room.[20-22]

Pulse Wave Transit Time

This method noninvasively measures the CO using pulse wave transit time (PWTT) with the help of a pulse oximeter and electrocardiography (ECG) which are continuously recorded. It works based on the relationship between PWTT and SV. PWTT is the time taken from the appearance of R wave of the ECG to the rise point of pulse waveform in the pulse oximeter **(Table 1)**. This PWTT period can be divided into three intervals:

1. Preejection period (PEP)
2. Pulse wave transit time through elastic artery (T1)
3. Pulse wave transit time through peripheral arteries (T2)[23]

Estimated continuous cardiac output (EsCCO) (Nihon Kohden, Japan) is the only device which uses the above technology. It uses a proprietary algorithm to use PWTT and its components to measure the CO. CO using EsCCO is given by the following formula:

$$CO = k \times (\alpha \times PWTT + \beta) \times HR$$

Where α is obtained from past experimental subjects and β is calculated from patient demographics (age, height, weight, and gender).[24]

Advantages

- Completely noninvasive
- Cheaper
- No additional sensors or special training required.

Limitations

- Not validated in critically ill patients.[25,26]
- Not responsive to measure CO changes produced by PLR.[27]

TABLE 1: Pulse wave transit time.

Parameter	*Description*	*Interpretation*
Preejection period (PEP)	Time from the electrocardiography (ECG) R wave to the rise point of the aortic root pressure wave	• Affected by cardiac contractility and preload • PEP decreases if preload or contractility increases
T1 wave	Time from the rise point of the aortic pressure wave to the rise point of the radial artery pressure wave	• Affected by arterial compliance • Decreases when blood pressure (BP) increases
T2 wave	Time from the rise point of the radial artery pressure wave to the rise point of the pulse oximeter wave in the finger	Reflects vascular resistance

CONCLUSION

Several noninvasive cardiac devices have become available in the past two decades. They have their own advantages and shortcomings. It is imperative to know the principle behind their function and appropriate clinical context where to use them. Though none of the devices showed any outcome benefits, these devices can be used to guide hemodynamic response in appropriate situations.

REFERENCES

1. Saugel B, Vincent JL, Wagner JY. Personalized hemodynamic management. Curr Opin Crit Care. 2017;23(4):334-41.
2. Vincent JL, Pelosi P, Pearse R, Payen D, Perel A, Hoeft A, et al. Perioperative cardiovascular monitoring of high-risk patients: a consensus of 12. Crit Care. 2015;19(1):224.
3. Swan HJ, Ganz W, Forrester J, Marcus H, Diamond G, Chonette D, et al. Catheterization of the heart in man with use of a flow-directed balloon-tipped catheter. N Engl J Med. 1970;283(9):447-51.
4. Sandham JD, Hull RD, Brant RF, Knox L, Pineo GF, Doig CJ, et al. A randomized, controlled trial of the use of pulmonary-artery catheters in high-risk surgical patients. New Engl J Med. 2003;348(1):5-14.
5. Harvey S, Harrison DA, Singer M, Ashcroft J, Jones CM, Elbourne D, et al. Assessment of the clinical effectiveness of pulmonary artery catheters in management of patients in intensive care (PAC-Man): a randomised controlled trial. Lancet. 2005;366(9484):472-7.
6. Binanay C, Califf RM, Hasselblad V, O'Connor CM, Shah MR, Sopko G, et al. Evaluation study of congestive heart failure and pulmonary artery catheterization effectiveness: the ESCAPE trial. JAMA. 2005;294(13):1625-33.
7. Mehta Y, Arora D. Newer methods of cardiac output monitoring. World J Cardiol. 2014;6(9):1022-9.
8. Geerts BF, Aarts LP, Jansen JR. Methods in pharmacology: Measurement of cardiac output. Br J Clin Pharmacol. 2011;71(3):316-30.
9. Fick A. Ueber die Messung des Blutquantums in den Herzventrikeln. Sitzungsberichte der Physiologisch-Medizinosche Gesellschaft zu Wuerzburg. 1870;2:16.
10. Jaffe MB. Partial CO_2 rebreathing cardiac output operating principle of the NICO system. J Clin Monit Comput. 1999;15(6):387-401.
11. Nilsson LB, Eldrup N, Berthelsen PG. Lack of agreement between thermodilution and carbon dioxide-rebreathing cardiac output. Acta Anaesthesiol Scand. 2001;45(6):680-5.
12. Tachibana K, Imanaka H, Takeuchi M, Takauchi Y, Miyano H, Nishimura M. Noninvasive cardiac output measurement using partial carbon dioxide rebreathing is less accurate at settings of reduced minute ventilation and when spontaneous breathing is present. Anesthesiology. 2003;98(4):830-7.
13. Singer M, Bennett ED. Noninvasive optimization of ventricular filling by esophageal Doppler. Crit Care Med. 1991;19(9):1132-7.
14. Singer M. Oesophageal Doppler. Curr Opin Crit Care. 2009;15(3):244-8.
15. Freund PR. Transesophageal Doppler scanning versus thermodilution during general anesthesia. An initial comparison of cardiac output techniques. Am J Surg. 1987;153(5):490-4.
16. Lefrant JY, Bruelle P, Aya AG, Saïssi G, Dauzat M, de La Coussaye JE, et al. Training is required to improve the reliability of esophageal Doppler to measure cardiac output in critically ill patients. Intensive Care Med. 1998;24(4):347-52.
17. Kubicek WG, Karnegis JN, Patterson RP, Witsoe DA, Mattson RH. Development and evaluation of an impedance cardiac output system. Aerosp Med. 1966;37(12):1208-12.
18. Nguyen LS, Squara P. Non-invasive monitoring of cardiac output in critical care medicine. Front Med (Lausanne). 2017;4:200.
19. Fellahi JL, Fischer MO. Electrical bioimpedance cardiography: an old technology with new hopes for the future. J Cardiothorac Vasc Anesth. 2014;28(3):755-60.
20. Teboul JL, Saugel B, Cecconi M, De Backer D, Hofer CK, Monnet X, et al. Less invasive hemodynamic monitoring in critically ill patients. Intensive Care Med. 2016;42(9):1350-9.
21. Saugel B, Cecconi M, Hajjar LA. Noninvasive cardiac output monitoring in cardiothoracic surgery patients: available methods and future directions. J Cardiothorac Vasc Anesth. 2019;33(6):1742-52.

22. Sanders M, Servaas S, Slagt C. Accuracy and precision of non-invasive cardiac output monitoring by electrical cardiometry: a systematic review and meta-analysis. J Clin Monit Comput. 2020;34(3):433-60.
23. Sugo Y, Sakai T, Terao M, Ukawa T, Ochiai R. The comparison of a novel continuous cardiac output monitor based on pulse wave transit time and echo Doppler during exercise. Conf Proc IEEE Eng Med Biol Soc. 2012;2012:236-9
24. Ishihara H, Okawa H, Tanabe K, Tsubo T, Sugo Y, Akiyama T, et al. A new non-invasive continuous cardiac output trend solely utilizing routine cardiovascular monitors. J Clin Monit Comput. 2004;18(5-6):313-20.
25. Bataille B, Bertuit M, Mora M, Mazerolles M, Cocquet P, Masson B, et al. Comparison of esCCO and transthoracic echocardiography for non-invasive measurement of cardiac output intensive care. Br J Anaesth. 2012;109(6):879-86.
26. Ishihara H, Sugo Y, Tsutsui M, Yamada T, Sato T, Akazawa T, et al. The ability of a new continuous cardiac output monitor to measure trends in cardiac output following implementation of a patient information calibration and an automated exclusion algorithm. J Clin Monit Comput. 2012;26(6):465-71.
27. Biais M, Berthezène R, Petit L, Cottenceau V, Sztark F. Ability of esCCO to track changes in cardiac output. Br J Anaesth. 2015;115(3):403-10.

CHAPTER

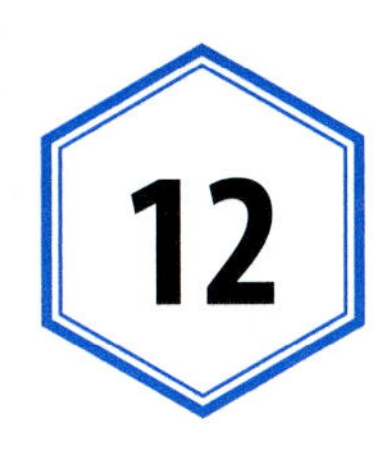

Bioimpedance and Bioreactance Cardiac Output Measurement

Atul Prabhakar Kulkarni, Ruchira Wasudeo Khasne

INTRODUCTION

Cardiac output (CO) is one of the most important macrohemodynamic variables and its measurement provides diagnostic valuable information. A trend obtained during measurement is immensely important in assessing patient response and to make further decisions regarding therapeutic measures. Bioimpedance (Z) is a method to estimate body composition such as fat and muscle mass on passing a weak electric current (I) through the body. Impedance, that is resistance, is calculated by measuring voltage (V). The pulsatile changes occurring in the intrathoracic blood volume (during ejection of blood from heart and in diastole) induce changes in the electrical conductivity of the thorax. By measuring electrical resistance, stroke volume (SV) and continuous cardiac output (CCO) are derived. In the era of less invasive or noninvasive monitoring devices, the use of noninvasive technologies are desirable to monitor CCO.[1] In this technique, SV actually serves as an electrical contrast medium and is being continuously assessed by these devices.

Decades ago, this technique was used during space exploration by astronauts in 1960s by National Aeronautics and Space Administration (NASA). In 1966, Kubicek had proposed use of this (impedance) technology to measure CO,[2] and since mid-90s there is a renewed interest in medical field to assess CO using thoracic electrical bioimpedance (TEB) and thoracic bioreactance (TBR). These techniques have advantage particularly in the setting of anesthesiology, cardiology, and perioperative medicine. It has yet not found the niche in the plethora of other devices available to measure CO in the critically ill patients. The main reason is discordant and disappointing results. Besides that, concern of accuracy and precision has been questioned in a meta-analysis published recently.[3] In this review, we are going to discuss the basic principles, advantages, conditions where it is preferred, and the limitations of this technology.

BASIC PRINCIPLES OF THORACIC BIOIMPEDANCE AND THORACIC BIOREACTANCE

Various bioimpedance-based technologies, such as electrical impedance plethysmography, impedance cardiography, electric cardiometry, integral rheography, or thoracic bioimpedance, etc., have come up. TEB and TBR systems are fundamentally based on the same general physical model, which links the change in aortic volume with that of chest impedance. The basic principle is that the ejection of blood causes changes in intrathoracic blood volume and if high-frequency but low-magnitude current (I) is passed through the thorax via skin electrodes, its conductivity changes accordingly. The higher the fluid content, the lower is impedance, as fluid is a good conductor of electricity. This technique analyzes thoracic fluid content (TFC) and the changes in electrical conductivity. In each cardiac cycle (systole and diastole), with ejection of blood, the volume of blood in the thorax changes and this can be measured electrically after passing a electric current.[4] Traditional bioimpedance systems use "amplitude modulation" [the amplitude (signal strength) of the carrier wave varies in proportion to the signal being transmitted] as signal, whereas bioreactance systems use "frequency modulation" and "phase shifts." Frequency modulation is the modulation of a wave by variation of its frequency, to carry a signal. The phase angle is the angle by which a waveform is displaced in the x-axis, i.e., it is the characteristic of the single waveform and it is termed as phase angle of that waveform. In phase shift, the second waveform is shifted X° in phase in relation to the reference (first) waveform on the x-axis. When the second waveform shifts by 90°, in a trigonometric sine waveform, it is shifted by a quarter of total waveform **(Fig. 1)**. Theoretically, frequency modulation, used in TBR, due to its easier electric noise filtration, seems to be superior.

TERMS OF METROLOGY IN MEDICINE TO ASSESS THE QUALITY CRITERIA[5]

Every device should be reviewed for following metrologic quality criteria for CO measurement, although they are not standardized in medicine. Hence, validation of these devices is often limited to metrologic parameters for measurements such as accuracy, precision, trueness, reproducibility, and repeatability, and parameters for devices such as step response time, etc. Terms of metrology in medicine are as follows:

- *Accuracy:* Closeness of agreement between a measurement value and a true value of the measured. Assessment is by measurement error, percentage error (PE).
- *Precision:* Closeness of agreement between replicate measurements on the same or similar objects under specified conditions. Assessment is by random measurement error, which qualifies, imprecision [Standard deviation (SD), coefficient of variation].
- *Reproducibility:* Precision under a set of conditions that includes different locations, operators, measuring systems, and replicate measurements on the same or similar objects (for different devices and different patients). Assessment is by random measurement error (SD, coefficient of variation).
- *Repeatability:* Precision under conditions that includes the same measurement procedure, same device, and on same patient replicate measurements on the same or similar objects over a short period of time.
- *Trueness:* Closeness of agreement between the average of an infinite number of replicate measurements and the true or reference value. Systematic measurement error qualifies as untrueness (Bias = Mean measured value – True value)
- *Step response change:* Delay between physiological change and its indication.

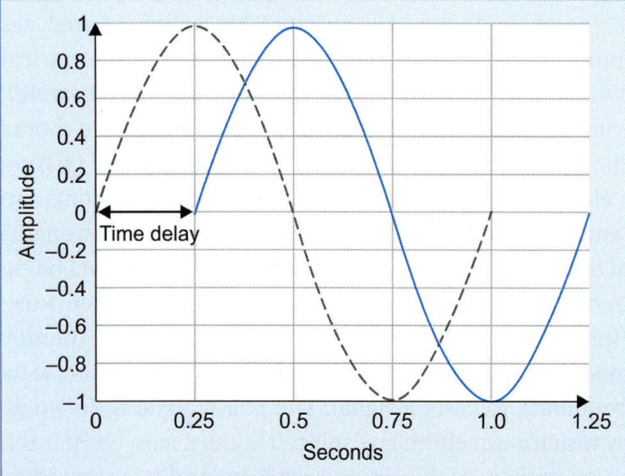

Fig. 1: The phenomenon of phase shift. Blue wave is the reference wave. (See text for explanation.)

Source: Adapted from Baxter. Starling fluid management system. [online] Available from https://www.cheetah-medical.com/how-it-works/ bioreactance [Last accessed September, 2024).

ADVANTAGES OF THORACIC BIOIMPEDANCE

- Completely noninvasive
- Cost-effective
- Continuous, automated, real-time CO measurement
- Simple tool
- Speed of implementation and fast response time
- Can be used as an ambulatory monitoring technique
- Operator-independent
- No external calibration required such as pulse index contour cardiac output (PiCCO) and LiDDCO
- Good inter- and intraobserver reproducibility

HEMODYNAMIC PARAMETERS GIVEN BY THORACIC BIOIMPEDANCE DEVICES

With the aid of software, various hemodynamic parameters (measured or calculated variables—see in the following text) are derived and then integrated into a modern concept of global noninvasive hemodynamic monitoring as per **Table 1**.[6]

TECHNOLOGY DESCRIPTION OF THORACIC BIOIMPEDANCE

NICCOMO, Physio-Flow, BioZ.com, [BioZ (Cardiodynamics, USA), Aesculon (Osypka Medical, Germany)].

This technique is based on the hypothetical assumption that thorax as a cylinder is perfused with fluid and with specific resistivity. Standard bioimpedance systems apply six electrodes, which are placed, two on either side of neck and four in lower thorax on the patient. High-frequency electric current (I) of known amplitude and frequency (frequency ranging between 20 and 100 kHz and the

TABLE 1: Measured and calculated variables by thoracic bioimpedance device.

		Definitions	***Clinical application***
Measured variables	Heart rate (HR)		Usual clinical use
	Left ventricular ejection time (LVET)	It is the period of time during which blood flows across the aortic valve *Range:* 0.35 ± 0.08 s	Heart rate, preload, afterload, and left ventricular contractility all affect the LVET. Mitral incompetence and left heart failure lead to shortening of LVET
	Pre-ejection period (PEP)	It is the time between the depolarization (QRS on the ECG) of the left ventricle and the start of ejection of blood, i.e., opening of cardiac valves	Used to calculate other variables
	Noninvasive blood pressure (NIBP)		Usual clinical application
	Acceleration index	Peak acceleration of blood flow in the aorta	A decrease indicates a decrease in the cardiac performance, e.g., CAD
	Velocity index	Peak velocity of blood flow in the aorta	Used mainly for patients with aortic stenosis
	Intrathoracic fluid content (ITFC)	It is the sum of intravascular, intra-alveolar, and interstitial fluids in the chest	Similar to intrathoracic thermal volume (ITTV) with transpulmonary thermodilution (TPTD)
Calculated variables	Stroke volume (SV)		Usual clinical application
	Cardiac output	Is the product of SV and HR (SV × HR)	Usual clinical application
	Systemic vascular resistance	[Blood pressure/cardiac output (BP/CO)]	Usual clinical application
	Left ventricular work index	It is the work done by the left ventricle to eject the stroke volume	Usual clinical application
	Systolic time ratio (STR) (PEP/LVET)	It is used to differentiate between the patients with preserved versus impaired left ventricular function	Similar to difference between ejection fraction with preserved ejection fraction (HfpEF) and those without preserved ejection fraction
	Systolic time ratio index (STRI)	Index of STR	Similar to STR

(CAD: coronary artery disease; ECG: electrocardiogram)

current amplitude between 1 and 5 mA) flows from outermost to innermost electrodes, and the voltage (V) received by electrodes is measured. The electric current preferentially flows through the liquid media (thoracic blood vessels and heart chambers) and continuous recording of the electrical impedance of the thorax is calculated. Average of two or more different circuits is used. The ratio between voltage (Vo) in volts and current (Io) in amplitudes of oscillating current in ampere is generically referred to as impedance that is (Zo), expressed as (Vo/Io). This ratio (Vo/Io) is a measure of the steady-state transthoracic impedance (Zo), when there is "no blood flow", and thus baseline chest fluid is estimated, which closely correlates with TFC. The TEB is indirectly proportional to the content of TFC such as tissue fluid volume, pulmonary and venous blood, and the aortic blood volume, contribute to the TEB measurement. Changes in thoracic impedance Z(t) may be mostly due to variations of aortic blood volume. Decrease in intrathoracic blood volume during systole is associated with transient increase in the impedance (inverse relation) and there is cyclic reduction of the electrical impedance during diastole. Any change in CO will change the amount of aortic blood and is further reflected in a change in TEB. Conditions associated with increase in the aortic blood volume that is presence of blood flow through the aorta, increase in water and iron in the thorax, and Z decreases over time, i.e., Z(t), proportionally from Zo. Thus, any changes in chest impedance and/or reactance are closely linked with variations in the aortic blood volume. Since these changes only indicate relative changes in CO, a calibration factor (CF) is necessary.

Several electrode configurations are mentioned in the literature but the most popular one is a "tetrapolar-band" electrode configuration, where two outer-band electrodes are placed around the base of the neck and two inner-band electrodes around the upper abdomen at the level of xiphisternum, and the injected current used is 4 mA at 100 kHz frequency. Additionally, "band electrodes" are modified to "spot electrodes" to improve measurements.

Following are the assumptions and mathematical simplifications that are necessary to derive the SV from the change in impedance (ΔZ) on flow of alternating current (AC). Structures such as thoracic cavity, aorta, blood volume in veins, ventilation, and myocardial wall thickness are considered with few assumptions. Impedance law is applied to aorta, which is considered as a conductor. Thus, impedance (Z) is expressed as:

$$\rho L/A$$

Where, ρ = Specific resistivity; L = Length; and A = Cross-sectional area of the tube.

For both TEB and TBR-based systems, same assumptions are applicable which are as follows:

- The thorax is considered as a cylinder (for calculations used by software).
- Thorax is considered as a unique chamber in parallel with the aorta.
- Aorta is a cylinder with a constant length.
- Blood volume of veins, which are low-pressure vessels, is relatively constant.
- The effect of ventilation on the blood flow can be averaged.
- The thickness of myocardial walls electrically isolates intraventricular blood volumes.
- On emitting and receiving AC across and around the chest, a change in thoracic impedance is due to a change in blood flow.
- The resistivity of blood is considered to remain constant for the calculations; however, whenever there is any deviation in hemoglobin (Hb) concentration (Hb out of the normal range but stable), it can be corrected.
- It is assumed that resistivities of thoracic tissue and blood are similar.

Each of these assumptions may lead to individual discordances. To limit the impact of these assumptions and to improve the reliability of CO estimation, several approaches have been suggested; one such being, truncated cone instead of a cylinder, to model the thorax. Thus, a multivariate CF is required using a reference method based on age, gender, height, weight, body surface area, and body mass index. Additionally, hematocrit and pulmonary artery pressure should be considered. Again, the CF derived from a specific population may raise the question whether it can be generalized. Thus, uncertainty remains among clinicians about the reliability of TEB-and/or TBR-derived CO, as effects of these assumptions are still unclear.

Limitations

- Several physical, anatomical hypotheses, and numerous mathematical assumptions are made.
- There is need for initial calibration with independent reference or an autocalibration process. CF value is determined, which is created to adjust the indications obtained by the tested device to the reference values.
- There is no association between aortic systolic deformation and the SV in conditions such as aortic dissection and aortic prosthesis.
- Conditions such as hematocrit, elevated pulmonary arterial pressure (for which, CFs exist), or physical abnormalities such as obesity and dehydration make this device unreliable.
- Limitations due to difficulty in acquiring signals such as movement of patient and electrical interference [electronical environment is heavier in operation theater (OT) or intensive care unit (ICU) due to the number of devices, e.g., electrocautery]. Higher the level of noise, less is the chance that bioimpedance would be accurate because of an unfavorable signal/noise ratio, temperature, and humidity. Presence of arrhythmias (arrhythmias may lead to inaccuracy due to an irregular R-R interval), improper electrode placement, and internal or external pacemakers all reduce accuracy of this technique.
- Pathological conditions, such as hemodynamic instability, pleural effusions, pulmonary edema, increase the electrical conductivity of the thorax, and thus there is reduction in impedance. Hypovolemia or left ventricular failure (cause small changes in SV) makes calculations difficult.
- Lack of consistent accuracy shown by the evidence is due to the inherently low signal-to-noise ratio.

FORMULAS FOR CALCULATING THE STROKE VOLUME BY IMPEDANCE CARDIOGRAPHY

Different formulae for calculating the SV have been proposed and modified and derivation of SV calculation by various equations is as follows:

- Kubicek equation, Stramek equation, Stramek-Bernstein equation, and new equation—N Bernstein equation are used.
    - *Kubicek equation:* Oldest equation described in 1966 assumed that the adult thorax acts as a cylinder.[2] It is expressed as follows:

$$SV_{Kubicek} = \rho \frac{L^2}{Z_0^2}\left(-\frac{dZ}{dt}\right)_{max} T_{lvet} \quad (1)$$

    where,

    SV: Stroke volume (cm^3 or mL)

    L: Distance between the voltage sensing electrodes (cm)

    Z_0: Basal impedance (Ω)

    $\left(-\frac{dZ}{dt}\right)_{max}$: Maximum value of rate of change in impedance (Ω/s)

    T_{lvet}: Left ventricular ejection time(s)
    - *Stramek equation:* Proposed equation assuming adult thorax acts as a truncated cone and blood resistivity is eliminated from the equation (ρ is not considered)

$$SV = \frac{L_0^3}{4.25 \times z_0} \cdot \left(\frac{dZ}{dt}\right)_{max} \cdot LVET \quad (2)$$

    Where, L_0: The distance between the inner electrodes (cm). It is equal to 17% of the subject height H (cm) ($L_0 = 0.17 \times H$).
    - *Stramek-Bernstein equation:* Recent modification of Stramek equation by introducing a new term that is related to the ideal body weight led to Stramek-Bernstein equation,[7] a more simplified version where correction factor δ is introduced, which is a dimensionless parameter (scalar quantity) related to the ideal body weight W (kg).

$$SV = \delta \,. \frac{(0.17 \times H)^3}{4.25 \times z_0} \left(\frac{dZ}{dt}\right)_{max} \cdot LVET \quad (3)$$

    Where, SV: Stroke volume;

    LVET: Left ventricular ejection time;

    k: Constant estimated from a patient nomogram incorporating the main morphologic characteristics (height, sex, and age);

    Z_0: Represents the baseline impedance of the thorax;

    $(dZ/dt)_{max}$: Maximum impedance change during the cardiac cycle.
    - *Bernstein equation*: It is modification of the Stramek-Bernstein formula.[8] Calculation of the SV is even more reliable (better correlation and greater accuracy) when Z_0 is greater than 15 ohms $(dZ/dt)_{max}$ greater than 0.3.

$$SV = \frac{V_{ITBV}}{\varepsilon^2} \cdot \sqrt{\frac{\left(\frac{dZ}{dt}\right)_{max}}{Z_0}} \cdot LVET \quad (4)$$

    Where, ITBV: Intrathoracic blood volume and it is related to the body weight W (kg);

    ε: Dimensionless index of transthoracic aberrant conduction (for all $z_0 < 20\ \Omega$, $0 < \varepsilon < 1$, and for all $z_0 \geq 20\ \Omega$, $\varepsilon = 1$)

Evidence

Earlier studies have shown varied results despite of development of complex algorithms but recent publications have shown conflicting results regarding the accuracy of CO measurement with TEB. Studies with positive articles were mostly conducted outside the ICU settings and trend of CO changes was preferred over absolute values. Only cardiac surgical patients have shown to have good correlation intraoperatively.[8,9] Those who are hospitalized in ICU and postoperative care units, these discrepancies are more frequently observed and their metrologic performance has been challenged with the PE >50%[10,11] as mentioned in **Table 2**. The PE is considered to be acceptable when it is <30%, as previously recommended by Critchley and Critchley.[12] This criterion has been used by ample number of studies performed later. Majority of studies have employed bias and precision statistics, as described by Bland and Altman.[13] The limits of agreement have been derived [bias ±1.96 standard deviation (SD)] which are expressed as a proportion of the mean CO (PE). However, accuracy and precision assessed with a Bland Altman graph does not statistically determine superiority of one device over another. PE has been found to be increasing as per recent studies. In 1999, PE for TEB was found to be 37% and now as per this it has increased to 42%. Accuracy and precision have been questioned in one meta-analysis (47 studies) by Peyton[14] which reviewed the published data on four different minimally invasive methods such as pulse contour analysis, esophageal Doppler, partial carbon dioxide rebreathing, and TEB use during surgery and critical care. Out of these studies, 13 studies (*n* = 435 total number of pooled measurements) have shown mean weighted bias of −0.10 L/min with mean of ±0.11 and precision of 1.14 L/min with PE of 42.9%

TABLE 2: Clinical conditions with correlation of thoracic bioimpedance (TEB) to estimate cardiac output (CO).

Clinical condition	*Correlation*	*Limitation*
Cardiac surgical patients, Sageman et al.[16]	Good correlation intraoperatively	Postoperative period, sternal wires, and arrhythmias may cause inaccuracy in readings[17]
Critically ill patients, Raue W et al.[18]	• TEB is found to be inaccurate • Showed a lower correlation compared to studies done on non-ICU patients. The overall correlation coefficient was 0.81 and decreased a little when it came to ICU patients ($p = 0.003$)[19]	Results are not encouraging Factors such as electric noise and body motion exist in patients with increased lung water
Volume overload, Critchley LA et al.[10]	The accuracy is worsened as the degree of increase in volume overload	Heart failure results in increased pulmonary edema and pleural effusion, which affects conduction leading to incongruity
During cardiac catheterization, Barin E[20] Marik PE[21]	Poor correlation of CO determined by TEB compared to thermodilution in cardiac catheterization has been reported	

(CO: cardiac output; ICU: intensive care unit)

(±3.6%). Thus, TEB, even after meeting 30% limits, did not achieve agreement with bolus thermodilution. Therefore, its use is limited in clinical practice. Few studies with use of TEB compared with pulmonary artery catheter (PAC) or PiCCO have been mentioned in **Table 3**, with bias and PE. Thus, with such a wide PE, and unacceptable level of agreement, these noninvasive CO devices cannot be used interchangeably with the gold standard, the thermodilution methods.[3] The factors which added to this discrepancy are as follows:

- Studies have been conducted with (1) different generations of monitors using different physiological models and equations, thus difficult to compare, and (2) in setting of wide range of patient profiles (healthy to heart failure), in ambulatory patients at home, in laboratories, during surgery, and in an ICU.
- Reference method is at times different, although pulmonary artery thermodilution is the most commonly used reference method.
- Use of different statistical tools.
- Level of different methodological requirement varies from simple correlation coefficient to the polar plot method, linear regression, Bland and Altman method, and the PE of Critchley and Critchley.
- Lack of accuracy due to inherently low signal-to-noise ratio.
- Methodological problems in terms of the "gold" standard used and the sample size.

During comparison of cardiac index measurement with thoracic bioimpedance cardiography (ICG) (NICOM™ device) and transthoracic Doppler echocardiography (TTE) in 25 resting healthy volunteers,[15] the observations were as follows:

- There was a weak but statistically significant relationship between cardiac index by TTE and cardiac index by ICG ($r = 0.36$; $p = 0.002$).
- Agreement between cardiac index by TTE and cardiac index by ICG was 0.94 L/min^2/m^2 [95% confidence interval (CI): 0.77–1.11].
- Precision was 0.72 L/min^2/m^2.
- Limits of agreement was – 0.47–2.35 L/min^2/m^2
- PE was found to be 53% (acceptable is <30% or less)

They underwent hemodynamic load challenge by application of positive end-expiratory pressure (PEEP) ±10 cmH$_2$O and lower body positive pressure by means of medical antishock trousers (MASTs) inflated to +30 cmH$_2$O in the abdominal compartment. No statistically significant relationships were found between percent changes in cardiac index by TTE and cardiac index by ICG after applications of PEEP +10 cmH$_2$O ($r = 0.21$; $p = 0.31$) and MAST ($r = 0.22$; $p = 0.30$). Thus, TEB was not found to be interchangeable with 2D Echo with PE of 53% and absolute values of cardiac index measurement have been weakly correlated in healthy volunteers and also TEB failed to detect changes in CO reliably with the PEEP manipulations (addition of 10 cmH$_2$O of PEEP). Thus, ICG is erratic for monitoring changes in cardiac index during hemodynamic load challenge in resting healthy volunteers.

TABLE 3: Studies comparing TEB with PAC and PiCCO with respect to bias and PE.

Authors	Device type/ device name	Reference method (RM)	Setting	Mean CO of RM (SD) [range (L/ min)]	Bias (SD) (L/ min)	PE (%) limits of agreement (1.96 ± SD)/mean CO of the reference method
Bernstein and colleagues[8] (*n* = 106)	TEB (ICG)	PAC	Cardiac surgery patients	5.97 (1.41)	0.1 (0.94)	31
Critchley and colleagues[10] (*n* = 24)	TEB (NICOM™)	PAC	ICU patients	6.7 (3.6–12.9)	–1.49	62
Engoren and colleagues[22] (*n* = 46)	TEB (BIOZ)	PAC	ICU	6.3 (2.2)	–1 (1.33)	41.3
Heringlake and Colleagues[15] (*n* = 29)	TEB Aesculon	PAC	Cardiac surgery patients operating room/ICU	4.65 (NC)	0.02 (1.73)	73.1
Mekis and colleagues[23] (n = 16)	TEB Aesculon	PAC	Cardiac surgery patients operating room/ICU	NR (2.2–7.5)	±0.21 (0.78)	Not reported (NR)
Raue and colleagues[18] (*n* = 30)	TEB Aesculon	PiCCO	ICU patients	7.04 (NR)	–0.3 (1.9)	52.9
Sharma and colleagues[24] (*n* = 46)	TEB NICOMON ™	PAC	ICU patients	4.56 (NC)	0.02 (0.84)	36.2
Squara and colleagues[25] (*n* = 20)	Bioreactance NICOM™	PiCCO	ICU patients	4.23 (NR)	0.22 (0.85)	39.5
Zoremba and Colleagues[11] (*n* = 25)	TEB Aesculon	PAC	ICU patients	5.25 (NR)	0.05 (0.71)	26.5

[CO: cardiac output; ICG: impedance cardiography, Phillips; ICU: intensive care unit; NC: not calculated; NICOM™: bioreactance based noninvasive cardiac output monitoring system; NICOMON™: NICOMON™ (Larsen and Toubro Ltd., Mysore, India); PAC: pulmonary artery catheter; PE: percentage error; PiCCO: pulse index contour cardiac output; TEB: thoracic electrical bioimpedance]

New generation noninvasive monitoring devices have improved the performance in the past few years with subsequent modifications in technique, refined algorithms. However, further developments are warranted to improve the accuracy and to make these devices useful in routine practice.[26]

THORACIC BIOREACTANCE

Thoracic bioreactance (NICOM™ device, Cheetah medical, Portland, Oregon) is a modification of TEB. It is an improvised version of TEB, based on similar assumptions and simplifications with better signal-to-noise ratio. It measures "bioreactance" or the phase shift in voltage (V) across the thorax **(Fig. 1)**. This phase shift is exclusively dependent on pulsatile flow and TBR signals which are closely related to aortic blood flow. It is less dependent on intravascular and extravascular lung water like TEB. As the underlying thoracic fluid is relatively static, fluids as well as phasic shifts, both do not contribute to the signals. TBR technique does not use the static impedance (Zo) and does not depend on the distance between the electrodes for the calculations of SV. Besides that, it contains highly sensitive phase detector, which continuously captures thoracic phase shifts too. These modifications in TBR device allow accurate determination of CO in patients with arrhythmias, and it averages the signal over 1 minute which makes the calculations more reliable.

NICOM™ consist of high-frequency (75 kHz) sine wave generator and four dual electrode patches (each patch consisting of two electrodes). These patches are placed two on either side of the body to establish electric contact. Each patch, one electrode is used by the high-frequency current generator to inject the high-frequency sine wave into the body, whereas the other electrode is used by the voltage input amplifier. The patches on a given side of the body are paired, so the current is passed between the outer electrodes of the pair, and voltage is recorded from between the inner electrodes. CO is derived noninvasively from each side of the body, and the final calculation of CO is arrived at by averaging these two signals. Human thorax is described as electric circuit with a resistor (R) and a capacitor (C), which together create the thoracic impedance (Zo). The values of R and C determine the two components of impedance: the amplitude (a), the magnitude of the impedance (measured in ohms), and phase (phi), the direction of the impedance (measured in degrees). Values of R and C are modified due to pulsatile nature of the blood ejected from the heart causing changes in amplitude and the phase of Zo instantaneously. Phase shifts can occur only because of pulsatile flow. NICOM™ signal captures pulsatile aortic blood flow. It does not capture thoracic fluid and changes in it, which is static, and it does not induce any phase shifts. SV is calculated with following formula:

$$SV = C \times VET \times d\Phi/dt_{max}$$

Where, C: Capacitor; VET: Ventricular ejection time calculated by NICOM™; and $d\Phi/dt_{max}$: It is the peak rate of change of phase shift which is proportional to the peak aortic flow during each beat.

Advantages

- Ease of use in intubated patients.
- It can be used in emergency room, ICU, and operating room.
- Electrocautery interference is less with NICOM™ signal. Limitation is that if the electrocautery is on for >40 seconds in a minute, the CO for that particular minute is not displayed.
- NICOM™ assessment of the CO in ventilated and nonventilated patients is alike.
- It can compute the CO in patients with atrial and ventricular arrhythmias.
- It is very easy to set up with a high degree of acceptability by nursing staff.

Evidence

Cardiac output derived by TBR has not found to be acceptable in more heterogeneous populations of patients but in homogeneous population, good precision (allows a resolution <20%), and step response time close to 1 minute, suggest its utility. A given patient is considered as his own reference, such as for pacemaker optimization, or hemodynamic challenges, etc. As per current literature, there is a good agreement between TBR and other reference techniques. Few studies are quoted in **Table 4**.

Limitations

- Thoracic bioreactance needs initial calibration with independent reference or an autocalibration process, and CF value is determined.
- The method by which the CF is derived in specific populations is usually not reported and that can add to discrepancies in results of different studies.[27]
- The CF is based on various preliminary internal measurements, demographic, and some morphologic parameters based on which other parameters are derived (i.e., body surface area or body mass index). Hematocrit is also used to optimize the CF.
- Thoracic bioreactance has shown decrease in accuracy during low-flow state and when electrocauterization is being used.

CONCLUSION

Extensive range of novel monitoring devices has come up in the market in last few decades, which measure TFC, SV, and CCO. The biggest benefit of this technology is its noninvasive nature and low cost. It can be useful at the bedside to measure CCO without need to monitor arterial pressure. TBR is an improved form of TEB which is based on similar assumptions and simplifications but gives better signal-to-noise ratio. These are promising technologies which are totally safe with acceptable precision, with good resolution, and fast step response time to assess CCO with good correlation particularly in operation room. It is more useful for tracking changes in CO rather than measuring absolute values. However in ICU, TEB is not considered as accurate enough to estimate CO. The available evidence is conflicting regarding validation of these devices and even metrological performance remains controversial. Clinician should be aware of the limitations of each of these devices while interpreting the measurements. These devices need initial calibration through either an independent reference or an autocalibration process. Additional studies are warranted to demonstrate their role in improving the quality of care by focusing or better understanding of the signal composition and better extraction of the aortic expansion signal. Till date, validation studies are discordant.

TABLE 4: Comparison of thoracic bioreactance (TBR) with other techniques.

Author, year	*Device type/device name*	*Reference monitor*	*Study group*	*Reported bias*	*Result*
Spiess BD et al.[17] ($n = 47$)	NICOM™	PAC	Cardiac index measured four times after anesthesia induction with the mediastinum open immediately after cardiopulmonary bypass at the end of the case	Cardiac index TEB and PAC had an overall correlation of $r = 0.71$ ($p < 0.0001$). The Bland–Altman statistics showed a mean difference of –0.28 L/min/m^2 and precision of 0.67 L/min/m^2	• The best correlation was observed after anesthesia induction, and the lowest correlation was at the end of the case • Mediastinal opening and cardiopulmonary bypass had little or no effect on the correlation between technologies
Squara P et al.[25] ($n = 20$)	NICOM™	PiCCO PC coupled to transpulmonary thermodilution (PiCCO TD)	Following cardiac surgery, hemodynamic variables are monitored at baseline, during a lung recruitment maneuver (20 cmH_2O of PEEP), and following withdrawal of PEEP with baseline PiCCO TD as reference and accuracy is evaluated and estimated precision	• At baseline, CO values were comparable for all three devices. Limits of agreements with PiCCO TD were 1.52 L/min for NICOM™ and 1.77 L/min for PiCCO PC, NS • The 95% statistical power gives an equivalence with a threshold of 0.52 L/min for NICOM™ versus PiCCO PC • The CO precision was 6 ± 3% and 6 ± 5% for NICOM™ and PiCCO PC, respectively, NS. When PEEP was applied, CO was reduced by 33 ±12%, 31 ± 14%, and 32 ±13%, for NICOM™, PiCCO PC, and PiCCO TD, respectively (NS) • Time response was 3.2 ± 0.7 minute for NICOM™ versus 2 ± 0.5 minute for PiCCO PC (NS)	Study has shown comparable CO and SV monitoring capabilities with acceptable accuracy, precision, and responsiveness
Kupersztych–Hagege E[28] ($n = 48$)	Cardiac index by NICOM™ and before and after 500 mL saline expansion and PLR test before volume expansion and measure the changes and compared with PiCCO	Cardiac index by PiCCO	In critically ill patients, before PLR, and before and after volume expansion	• The bias between PiCCO and NICOM™ was 0.9 (– 2.2–4.1) L/min^2/m^2. PE was 82% • Nonsignificant correlation between the changes in cardiac index by PiCCO and by NICOM™ induced by volume expansion ($p = 0.24$) AUROC of PLR-induced changes in cardiac index by NICOM™ in predicting fluid responsiveness did *not* differ significantly from 0.5 ($p = 0.77$)	• NICOM™ cannot accurately estimate the CO in critically ill patients • It cannot predict fluid responsiveness through the PLR test

Contd...

Contd...

Author, year	***Device type/device name***	***Reference monitor***	***Study group***	***Reported bias***	***Result***
Squara et al.[29] (*n* = 110)	NICOM™	PAC	After cardiac surgery, intensive care unit	• Out of 65,888 pairs of cardiac output measurements. During periods of stable PAC-CCO the correlation was $r = 0.82$; bias was + 0.16 ± 0.52 L/min (+4.0 ± 11.3%), and relative error was 9.1% ± 7.8%. In 85% of patients, the relative error was <20%. During periods of increasing output, intraclass correlation was positive in 96%. Corresponding values during periods of decreasing output were 90% with NICOM™ and 84% with PAC NICOM™ found to have better precision. Time responsiveness of the bioreactance: 3 minutes faster ($p < 0.01$). Amplitude response is also comparable • Sensitivity for detecting significant CO directional changes is 93% and specificity was 93%.	• Precision of the NICOM™ system found to be better than that of PAC • Device can also track the changes in CO accurately. CO by NICOM™ has acceptable accuracy precision
Raval et al.[30] (*n* = 111) At five centers	NICOM™	PAC	Cardiac catheterization laboratories, cardiac care units, and intensive care units	Both devices CO changes are correlated ($r = 0.78$, $p < 0.0001$) and did not differ significantly from each other ($p = 0.55$). Results in the cardiac catheterization laboratory were similar ($r = 0.71$, $p < 0.001$; $p = 0.28$ NICOM™ versus PAC)	Compared to TD, NICOM™ derived noninvasive CO measurement allows clinicians to get information about CO to guide the therapy with acceptable accuracy in challenging clinical environments
Rich et al.[31] (*n* = 50)	NICOM™	CO by thermodilution and Fick method. Baseline and after adenosine vasodilator challenge	In patients with pulmonary hypertension	• CO measured by NICOM™ is more precise than by thermodilution (3.5 ± 0.3% versus 9.6 ± 6.1%, $p < 0.001$) • Bland–Altman analyses comparing NICOM™ to thermodilution and Fick revealed bias and 95% limits of agreement that is comparable to those comparing Fick to thermodilution. All three CO methods are comparable to detect an increase in CO in response to adenosine challenge	CO measured via NICOM™ is precise and reliably measures CO at rest and changes in CO with vasodilator challenge in patients with PH

(AUROC: area under receiver operating curve; CO: cardiac output; NICOM™: NICOM™ bioreactance based *n*oninvasive cardiac output monitoring system; NS: *n*onsignificant; PAC: pulmonary artery catheter; PH: pulmonary hypertension; PEEP: positive end-expiratory pressure; PiCCO: pulse index contour cardiac output; PLR: passive leg raising; PE: percentage error; SV: stroke volume; TEB: thoracic bioimpedance)

Definitely future research is needed for better understanding the signal composition to minimize bias. Further technological modifications may make these devices preferred modalities in hemodynamic monitoring in future.

REFERENCES

1. Funk DJ, Moretti EW, Gan TJ. Perioperative setting. Anesth Analg. 2009;108(3):887-97.
2. Kubicek WG, Karnegis JN, Patterson RP, Witsoe DA, Mattson RH. Development and evaluation of an impedance cardiac output system. Aerosp Med. 1966;37(12):1208-12.
3. Joosten A, Desebbe O, Suehiro K, Murphy LS, Essiet M, Alexander B, et al. Accuracy and precision of non-invasive cardiac output monitoring devices in perioperative medicine: a systematic review and meta- analysis. Br J Anaes. 2017;118(3):298-310.
4. Shoemaker WC, Belzberg H, Wo CC, Milzman DP, Pasquale MD, Baga L, et al. Multicenter study of noninvasive monitoring systems as alternatives to invasive monitoring of acutely ill emergency patients. Chest. 1998;114(6):1643-52.
5. Squara P, Imhoff M, Cecconi M. Metrology in medicine: from measurements to decision, with specific reference to anesthesia and intensive care. Anesth Analg. 2015;120(1):66-75.
6. Mansouri S, Alhadidi T, Chabchoub S, Salah RB. Impedance cardiography: recent applications and developments. Biomed Res. 2018;29(19):3542-52.
7. Bernstein D. A new stroke volume equation for thoracic electrical bioimpedance: theory and rationale. Crit Care Med. 1986;14(10):904-9.
8. Bernstein DP, Lemmens HJM. Stroke volume equation for impedance cardiography. Med Biol Eng Comput. 2005;43(4):443-50.
9. Simon R, Desebbe O, Hénaine R, Bastien O, Lehot JJ, Cannesson M. Comparison of ICG thoracic bioimpedance cardiac output monitoring system in patients undergoing cardiac surgery with pulmonary artery cardiac output measurements. Ann Fr Anesth Reanim. 2009;28(6):537-41.
10. Critchley LA, Calcroft RM, Tan PY, Kew J, Critchley JA. The effect of lung injury and excessive lung fluid, on impedance cardiac output measurements, in the critically ill. Intensive Care Med. 2000;26(6):679-85.
11. Zoremba N, Bickenbach J, Krauss B, Rossaint R, Kuhlen R, Schälte G. Comparison of electrical velocimetry and thermodilution techniques for the measurement of cardiac output. Acta Anaesthesiol Scand. 2007;51(10):1314-9.
12. Critchley LA, Critchley JA. A meta-analysis of studies using bias and precision statistics to compare cardiac output measurement techniques. J Clin Monit Comput. 1999;15(2):85-91.
13. Bland JM, Altman DG. Statistical methods for assessing agreement between two methods of clinical measurement. Lancet. 1986;1(8476):307-10.
14. Peyton PJ, Chong SW. Minimally invasive measurement of cardiac output during surgery and critical care: A meta-analysis of accuracy and precision. Anesthesiology. 2010;113(5):1220-35.
15. Heringlake M, Handke U, Hanke T, Eberhardt F, Schumacher J, Gehring H, et al. Lack of agreement between thermodilution and electrical velocimetry cardiac output measurements. Intens Care Med. 2007;33(12):2168-72.
16. Sageman WS, Riffenburgh RH, Spiess BD. Equivalence of bioimpedance and thermodilution in measuring cardiac index after cardiac surgery. J Cardiothorac Vasc Anesth. 2002;16(1):8-14.
17. Spiess BD, Patel MA, Soltow LO, Wright IH. Comparison of bioimpedance versus thermodilution cardiac output during cardiac surgery: evaluation of a second-generation bioimpedence device. J Cardiothorac Vasc Anesth. 2001;15(5):567-73.
18. Raue W, Swierzy M, Koplin G, Schwenk W. Comparison of electrical velocimetry and transthoracic thermodilution technique for cardiac output assessment in critically ill patients. Eur J Anaesthesiol. 2009;26(2):1067-71.
19. Fuller HD. The validity of cardiac output measurement by thoracic impedance: a meta-analysis. Clin Invest Med. 1992;15(2):103-12.
20. Barin E, Haryadi DG, Schookin SI, Westenskow DR, Zubenko VG, Beliaev KR, et al. Evaluation of a thoracic bioimpedance cardiac output monitor during cardiac catheterization. Crit Care Med. 2000;28(23):698-702.
21. Marik PE, Pendelton JE, Smith R. A comparison of hemodynamic parameters derived from transthoracic electrical bioimpedance with those parameters obtained by thermodilution and ventricular angiography. Crit Care Med. 1997;25(9):1545-50.
22. Engoren M, Barbce D. Comparison of cardiac output determined by bioimpedance, thermodilution, and the Fick method. Am J Crit Care. 2005;14(1):40-5.
23. Mekis D, Kamenik M, Starc V, Jeretin S. Cardiac output measurements with electrical velocimetry in patients undergoing CABG surgery: a comparison with intermittent thermodilution. Eur J Anaesthesiol. 2008;25(3):237-42.
24. Sharma V, Singh A, Kansara B, Karlekar A. Comparison of transthoracic electrical bioimpedance cardiac output measurement with thermodilution method in post coronary artery bypass graft patients. Ann Card Anaesth. 2011;14(2):104-10.
25. Squara P, Rotcajg D, Denjean D, Estagnasie P, Brusset A. Comparison of monitoring performance of Bioreactance vs. pulse contour during lung recruitment maneuvers. Crit Care. 2009;13(4):R125.

26. Nguyen LS, Squara P. Non-invasive monitoring of cardiac output in critical care medicine. Front Med (Lausanne). 2017;4:200.
27. Fellahi J, Caille V, Charron C, Deschamps-Berger PH, Vieillard-Baron A. Noninvasive assessment of cardiac index in healthy volunteers: a comparison between thoracic impedance cardiography and Doppler echocardiography. Anesth Analg. 2009;108(5):1553-9.
28. Kupersztych-Hagege E, Teboul JL, Artigas A, Talbot A, Sabatier C, Richard C, et al. Bioreactance is not reliable for estimating cardiac output and the effects of passive leg raising in critically ill patients. Br J Anaesth. 2013;111(6):961-6.
29. Squara P, Denjean D, Estagnasie P, Brusset A, Dib JC, Dubois C. Noninvasive cardiac output monitoring (NICOM): a clinical validation. Intensive Care Med. 2007;33(7): 1191-4.
30. Raval NY, Squara P, Yalamanchili K, Yalamanchili K, Winklmaier M, Burkhoff D. Multicentre evaluation of noninvasive cardiac output measurement by bioreactance technique. J Clin Monit Comput. 2008;22(2):113-9.
31. Rich JD, Archer SL, Rich S. Noninvasive cardiac output measurements in patients with pulmonary hypertension. Eur Respir J. 2013;42(1):125-33.

CHAPTER

Pulse Wave Transit Time for Cardiac Output Measurement (Estimated Continuous Cardiac Output Device)

Natesh Prabu R, Kandaswamy N

INTRODUCTION

Cardiac output (CO) monitoring is essential in patients who remain hypotensive despite ongoing resuscitative measures, particularly in patients with complex hemodynamic disturbances, such as patients with acute respiratory distress syndrome (ARDS) associated with right ventricular failure.[1] Monitoring and measuring stroke volume (SV) and thus CO in patients with inadequate or partial response to initial resuscitation will help evaluate and choose further therapies. These may include infusion of fluid, vasopressors, and/or inotropes. CO measurement also helps diagnose and track the hemodynamic response to therapeutic interventions. In recent years, there has been a rapid shift in monitoring CO from pulmonary artery catheters to minimally invasive to noninvasive techniques. CO monitors should accurately measure CO in a reproducible manner. It should also be able to track changes in CO accurately following interventions. Even though the interest in monitoring CO has increased in recent years, no specific monitoring device has been found to influence outcomes in critically ill patients.[2] Newer monitors have come up with different techniques to measure CO, but none has shown a benefit in critically ill patients.[3] Although invasive CO monitoring is considered superior and recommended in critically ill patients, there is growing interest in less invasive and noninvasive technologies to monitor CO.[1] Many such noninvasive CO measuring devices are available based on various principles such as bioimpedance and bioreactance, respiratory-derived CO monitoring technique, pulse wave transit time (PWTT), ultrasound CO monitoring, multimodal algorithmic estimation, and inductance thoracocardiography.[4] Recent interest in estimated continuous cardiac output (esCCO) monitoring, i.e., using PWTT [(esCCO), Nihon Kohden, Japan] is due to its use of only electrocardiography (ECG) and plethysmography since both are routinely used in the care of critically ill patients. In this chapter, we will review PWTT technology and its clinical applications.

PULSE WAVE TRANSIT TIME: UNDERSTANDING THE BASICS

Pulse Wave Velocity

When the heart pumps blood during systole, the ejection of blood distends the elastic vessels and generates a pressure wave that travels along the arterial tree. The velocity of the pulse wave is influenced by increasing age and stiffness of the arterial wall. With increased stiffness, the velocity increases. Analyzing the pulse wave gives a lot of information regarding the elastance of the vessel. So, it is a measure of arterial stiffness.

Pulse wave transit time is the time required for a pulse pressure wave to travel between two points, i.e., between the ECG R-wave peak to the rise point of the pulse oximeter wave. PWTT consists of three subtime periods. It consists of a pre-ejection period (PEP) and pulse wave arrival time from the ascending aorta to the peripheral pulse-oximetry (SpO_2) probe site, i.e., the pulse transit time through an elastic artery (T1), and the pulse transit time through peripheral resistance arteries (T2), i.e., (PWTT = PEP + T1 + T2). Practically, PWTT is calculated as the time from the ECG R-wave peak to the rise point of the pulse oximeter wave. The rise point of the pulse wave is defined as the point at which the differentiated pulse wave reaches 30% of its peak amplitude **(Fig. 1)**.

Pre-ejection period: Time from the ECG R-wave to the rise point of the aortic root pressure wave.

- Increased cardiac contractility—short PEP
  T1: Time from the rise point of the aortic pressure wave to the rise point of the radial artery pressure wave.
- It depends on arterial compliance.

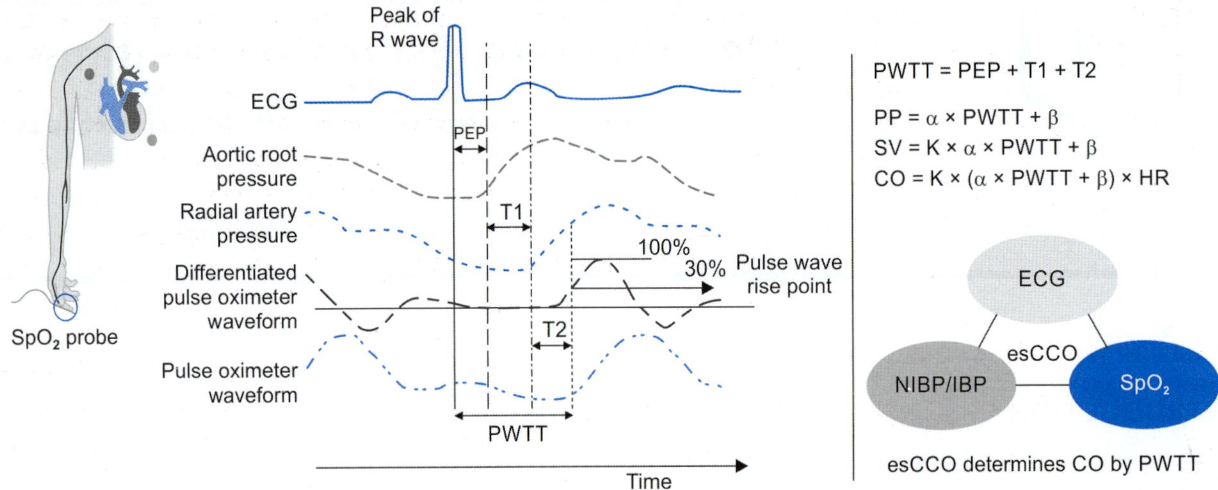

Fig. 1: The principles of pulse wave transit time and esCCO. (CO: cardiac output; ECG: electrocardiography; esCCO: estimated continuous cardiac output; HR: heart rate; IBP: invasive blood pressure; NIBP: noninvasive blood pressure; PEP: pre-ejection period; PP: pulse pressure; PWTT: pulse wave transit time; SpO_2: peripheral pulse oximetry (waveform); SV: stroke volume; T: time)
Source: With permission from Nihon Kohden, Tokyo, Japan.

- Lesser compliance, increasing blood pressure—T1 shortens. T2*:* Time from the rise point of the radial artery pressure wave to the rise point of the pulse oximeter wave in the fingertips. This reflects vascular resistance.
- Lower vascular resistance (vasodilation)—T2 shortens

EQUATIONS AND RELATION BETWEEN STROKE VOLUME AND PULSE WAVE TRANSIT TIME

In arterial pulse contour analysis, SV is calculated from the area under the curve of systole or from a relationship with pulse pressure.

SV = K × PP
CO = K × PP × heart rate (HR)
(K—depends on demographics)

Stroke volume, PP, and PWTT are related to each other. A negative correlation exists between PEP and SV.[5]

Stroke volume is inversely proportional to the square of T1. An increase of SV with an increase in blood pressure accompanies shortening T1. Also, SV is inversely proportional to the fourth power of T2. An increase in SV with a decrease in peripheral vascular resistance accompanies the shortening of T2.[6]

$PP = \alpha \times PWTT + \beta$
$SV = K \times \alpha \times PWTT + \beta$
$CO = K \times (\alpha \times PWTT + \beta) \times HR$

where α and β are experimental constants; K—depends on the demographics; CO: cardiac output; PP: pulse pressure; SV: stroke volume.

Pulse wave transit time is suggested as a surrogate for blood pressure and there is a good correlation between PWTT and blood pressure.[7] There is an increase in blood pressure with shorter PWTT and a decrease in blood pressure with longer PWTT. When the three-component wind Kessel model is applied, blood pressure can be associated with blood flow in a complex nonlinear function and hence CO.[8,9] So PWTT is inversely correlated with the SV.[10] When there is increased blood pressure and stiff arteries, PWV increases and PWTT shortens. The change in PWTT (ΔPWTT) predicts the change in blood pressure which correlates with the change in SV (ΔSV), from which CO is derived.

ESTIMATED CONTINUOUS CARDIAC OUTPUT (NIHON KOHDEN, TOKYO, JAPAN)

Estimated continuous cardiac output monitoring, uses PWTT to continuously measure SV and CO using ECG, SpO_2, and either noninvasive blood pressure (NIBP) or invasive blood pressure (IBP). esCCO requires patient calibration information, i.e., demographics and other information. esCCO also requires calibration for the first CO reading. Calibration can be done with either invasive or noninvasive methods, i.e., we can use CO values obtained by noninvasive methods or can use CO obtained by other invasive methods, e.g., thermodilution. CO can be used for calibration and continuous CO can be monitored using esCCO. When CO from another device is not available, it uses blood pressure to get the first CO and later gives CCO.

It is particularly useful when the clinical situation warrants only monitoring continuous CO and there is no need for invasive CO monitoring, i.e., when there is no need for additional parameters given by a thermodilution-based calibrated CO monitoring device. The parameters given by esCCO are esCO, esSV, esSVR (estimated CO, estimated SV, and estimated systemic vascular resistance, respectively), and corresponding indices [estimated Continuous Cardiac Index (esCCI), estimated Stroke Volume Index (esSVI), and estimated Systemic Vascular Resistance Index (esSVRI)]. Interestingly, if PWTT exceeds the threshold, then the machine triggers an additional NIBP measurement that allows early detection and treatment of any sudden changes in blood pressure between programmed noninvasive measurements.

VALIDATION OF PULSE WAVE TRANSIT TIME AND ESTIMATED CONTINUOUS CARDIAC OUTPUT

Every new device is tested for its accuracy (how close is the agreement between a measurement value and a true value of the measured), precision (closeness of agreement between repeated measurements under specified conditions), and tracking ability/step response change (delay between physiological change and its indication by the monitor). In 2004, researchers from Nihon Kohden Corporation compared esCCO with thermodilution continuous cardiac output using pulmonary artery catheter (CCOpa) in elective cardiac surgical patients.[11] Among 1,093 paired sets of measurements, a total of 981 paired sets of data (89.9%) were compared. The bias (mean difference between esCO and CCOpa results) was –0.06 ± 0.82 L/min (SD), and there was a linear correlation between them (r = 0.80, p < 0.0001). The difference between them was 0.00 ± 0.48 L/min at the first 1 hour, which remained unchanged throughout the 20 hours after the start of measurement. The results of the study were encouraging, and the authors concluded that esCO may be a potential noninvasive alternative to CCOpa, even though they were not interchangeable.

Yamada et al. conducted a multicenter study to evaluate the efficacy of noninvasive esCCO.[12] The esCCO was compared with intermittent thermodilution from the pulmonary artery catheter. Both patients from the intensive care unit n = 139/139 patients and the operating room n = 74/74 patients were included. The analysis showed a correlation coefficient of 0.79 (95% confidence limits of 0.756–0.819, p < 0.0001). The bias and precision were 0.13 L/min (95% confidence interval of bias 0.04–0.22 L/min) and 1.15 L/min (95% prediction interval was 2.13–2.39 L/min). So, this study showed that the CO measured by PWTT is accurate and clinically comparable to thermodilution-based CO measurement.[12] But the results may be affected by SVR and require further studies to evaluate its accuracy in different conditions. On the other hand, Ball et al. showed contrasting results questioning the accuracy when compared with pulmonary thermodilution in cardiac surgical patients.[13] This was a small study done intraoperatively in cardiac surgical patients at different time intervals (after induction, sternotomy, cardiopulmonary bypass, and chest closure). The correlation was poor at all times, the composite Pearson R coefficient was 0.62, with a bias of 0.80 (95% limits of agreement), and a percent error of 53%.

A study done in the cardiology laboratory that compared CO measured by esCCO, inert gas rebreathing, and Doppler echocardiography showed acceptable reproducibility and accuracy.[14] Terada et al. compared the tracking ability of esCCO with arterial pulse contour-based CO methods in transplant surgery patients with thermodilution-based methods as reference methods and esCCO methods were shown to have clinically acceptable tracking ability. Similar results were shown in another study done in hepatectomy patients. However, the performance of esCCO was not good when there was altered SVR with vasopressor use.[15] Studies done in critically ill patients did not show encouraging results, particularly regarding the tracking ability of the device. A recent study showed poor tracking ability in critically ill patients when preload or vasomotor tone was altered. In this study, esCCO was compared with transthoracic echocardiography. esCCO showed around 60% error in tracking CO after the passive leg raise test or change in vasomotor tone with vasopressors.[16] Similarly, a study done in critically ill patients with sepsis and septic shock showed a good correlation of measured CO with thermodilution-based CO when there is no shock.[17]

Ehlers et al. compared esCCO by PWTT against the TPTD method in 38 critically ill patients from a mixed intensive care unit (ICU) cohort.[18] They found a bias of 1.76 L/min and a percentage error of 47% for esCCO by PWTT, concluding that the two devices are not interchangeable due to poor precision and reliability of esCCO by PWTT. However, they did not account for systemic vascular resistance, which might have affected the CO calculation by the PWTT method.

Joshi et al. compared esCCO by PWTT and arterial pressure-based cardiac output (APCO) in 50 patients undergoing major abdominal surgeries.[19] They observed that PWTT tends to underestimate the cardiac index by –0.44 L/min/m^2, with wide limits of agreement and a percentage error of 46.29%.

The acceptable percentage error for a CO monitor is up to 30%, and in most studies to date, the percentage error of esCCO by PWTT exceeds this range.[20] Although, these studies are limited by small sample sizes and heterogeneous populations, they reinforce that esCCO is less accurate compared to thermodilution and APCO devices. Current evidence does not support esCCO as being as reliable as invasive methods of CO monitoring in critically ill patients, particularly those with altered vasomotor tone and hyperdynamic circulation.

CLINICAL APPLICATION

Though esCCO is attractive due to its complete noninvasiveness and is simple to use, esCCO has not been validated, especially in critically ill patients. The major limitations include inaccuracy in patients with vasoconstriction, vasoactive agent use, cold peripheries, and arrhythmias.[4] Another potential problem is that it requires an external calibration for initial CO measurement. When an invasive CO monitor is used to calibrate initial CO, then no longer it can be fully noninvasive. Though patient information calibration and automated exclusion algorithms were developed to overcome certain drawbacks, still there are concerns regarding their validity in critically ill patients. The potential clinical applications could be in the following situations:

- General monitoring of patients in the emergency room, operation room, ICU, and general ward
- Continuous hemodynamic monitoring after pulmonary artery or transpulmonary thermodilution catheter removal
- Monitoring hemodynamic trends
- Volumetric parameters may help to optimize fluid status
- Hemodynamic optimization of patients who are ineligible for more aggressive and risky techniques (i.e., pulmonary artery catheter)
- Triage tool for early detection of sudden deterioration.

CONCLUSION

Cardiac output assessed by noninvasive methods is continuously evolving. PWTT may rightly identify patients with low and normal CO, but the accuracy and trending ability need further refinement, particularly in critically ill patients. It cannot be used in patients with arrhythmias, vasoconstriction, or cold peripheries, and it needs further validation in the critically ill patient population. At present, routine use is not encouraged and it needs to be subjected to further studies; but it can be a potential option in surgical and less critically ill patients.

REFERENCES

1. Cecconi M, De Backer D, Antonelli M, Beale R, Bakker J, Hofer C, et al. Consensus on circulatory shock and hemodynamic monitoring. Task force of the European Society of Intensive Care Medicine. Intens Care Med. 2014;40(12):1795-815.
2. Ospina-Tascon GA, Cordioli RL. What type of monitoring has been shown to improve outcomes in acutely ill patients? Intens Care Med. 2008;34(5):800-20.
3. Cecconi M, Rhodes A, Teboul J, De Backer D, Hofer CK, Monnet X, et al. Less invasive hemodynamic monitoring in critically ill patients. Intens Care Med. 2016;42(9):1350-9.
4. Nguyen LS, Squara P. Non-invasive monitoring of cardiac output in critical care medicine. Frontiers in medicine. 2017;4:200.
5. Weissler AM, Harris WS. Systolic time intervals in heart failure in man. Circulation. 1968;37(2):149-59.
6. Sugo Y, Ukawa T, Takeda S, Ishihara H, Kazama T, Takeda J. A novel continuous cardiac output monitor based on pulse wave transit time. Annu Int Conf IEEE Eng Med Biol Soc. 2010;2010:2853-6.
7. Kaur H, Bhutto JK, Choudhary BS. Methods for continuous non-invasive measurement of blood pressure: pulse transit time a review. Asian J Pharm. 2018;12(3):S863.
8. Rang S, de Pablo Lapiedra B, van Montfrans GA, Boums BJ, Wesseling KH, Wolf H. Modelflow: a new method for noninvasive assessment of cardiac output in pregnant women. Am J Obstet Gynecol. 2007;196(3):235.e1-8.
9. Hirschl MM, Binder M, Gwechenberger M, Herkner H, Bur A, Kittler H, et al. Noninvasive assessment of cardiac output in critically ill patients by analysis of the finger blood pressure waveform. Crit Care Med. 1997;25(11):1909-14.
10. Saugel B, Cecconi M, Wagner JY, Reuter DA. Noninvasive continuous cardiac output monitoring in perioperative and intensive care medicine. Br J Anaesth. 2015;114(4):562-75.
11. Ishihara H, Okawa H, Tanabe K, Tsubo T, Sugo Y, Akiyama T. A new non-invasive continuous cardiac output trend solely utilizing routine cardiovascular monitors. J Clin Monit Comput. 2004;18(18-6):313-20.
12. Yamada T, Tsutsui M, Sugo Y, Sato T, Akazawa T, Sato N, et al. Multicenter study verifying a method of noninvasive continuous cardiac output measurement using pulse wave transit time: a comparison with intermittent bolus thermodilution cardiac output. Anesth Analg. 2012;115(1):82-6.

13. Ball TR, Tricinella AP, Kimbrough BA, Luna S, Gloyna DF, Villamaria FJ, et al. Accuracy of noninvasive estimated continuous cardiac output (esCCO) compared to thermodilution cardiac output: a pilot study in cardiac patients. J Cardiothorac Vasc Anesth. 2013;27(6):1128-32.
14. Raissuni Z, Zores F, Henriet O, Dallest S, Roul G. Can we obtain a noninvasive and continuous estimation of cardiac output? Comparison between three noninvasive methods. Int Heart J. 2013;54(6):395-400.
15. Tsutsui M, Araki Y, Masui K, Kazama T, Sugo Y, Archer TL, et al. Pulse wave transit time measurements of cardiac output in patients undergoing partial hepatectomy: a comparison of the esCCO system with thermodilution. Anesth Analg. 2013;117(6):1307-12.
16. Biais M, Berthezène R, Petit L, Cottenceau V, Sztark F. Ability of esCCO to track changes in cardiac output. Br J Anaesth. 2015;115(3):403-10.
17. Permpikul C, Leelayuthachai T. Non-invasive estimated continuous cardiac output (esCCO) during severe sepsis and septic shock resuscitation. J Med Assoc Thai. 2014;97(Suppl 3):S184-8.
18. Ehlers U, Erlebach R, Brandi G, Stretti F, Valek R, Klinzing S, et al. Continuous estimation of cardiac output in critical care: a noninvasive method based on pulse wave transit time compared with transpulmonary thermodilution. Crit Care Res Pract. 2020;2020:8956372.
19. Joshi M, Rathod R, Bhosale SJ, Kulkarni AP. Accuracy of estimated continuous cardiac output monitoring (esCCO) using pulse wave transit time (PWTT) compared to arterial pressure-based CO (APCO) measurement during major surgeries. Indian J Crit Care Med. 2022;26(4): 496-500.
20. Cecconi M, Rhodes A, Poloniecki J, Della Rocca G, Grounds RM. Bench-to-bedside review: the importance of the precision of the reference technique in method comparison studies–with specific reference to the measurement of cardiac output. Crit Care. 2009;13(1):201.

CHAPTER 14

Pressure Recording Analytical Method of Cardiac Output Measurement

Ruchira Wasudeo Khasne, Atul Prabhakar Kulkarni

INTRODUCTION

Hemodynamic monitoring plays a vital role in the management of critically ill patients. Cardiac output (CO) measured by pulmonary artery catheter (PAC) by thermodilution (ThD) technique is considered to be the gold standard, but there have been concerns regarding its utility and safety in clinical practice. Pulse contour methods (PCM) have been gaining a foothold in clinical practice due to their minimally invasive or noninvasive nature. These methods are uncalibrated in nature but measure the stroke volume (SV) and CO, continuously from the arterial pulse wave shape, after simply cannulating a peripheral artery. The pressure recording analytical method (PRAM) is a minimally invasive method based on the complex theory of perturbations with analysis of arterial pressure waveform. PRAM was first described by Romano and Pistolesi in 2002 who recorded pressure signals invasively in the aorta (PRAMa) or noninvasively at the finger (PRAMf) on a beat-to-beat basis.[1] They observed the absolute values of CO by measuring the area-under-the-curve (AUC) of the arterial-pressure waveform which are comparable with other methods such as the Fick method and ThD methods for a desired length of time. PRAM is a patented algorithm installed in the MostCare® system (Vytech, Padua, Italy).[2] It is the only PCM-based method that measures SV without any form of external calibration, central venous cannulation, and user-entered data and can be useful in hemodynamically stable and unstable patients.

ADVANTAGES OF PRESSURE RECORDING ANALYTICAL METHOD

- Minimally invasive
- Simple, quick, and versatile
- Operator-independent
- Immediate response to even in smallest of changes in the hemodynamic variables
- It does not require external calibration or anthropometric normalization
- Internal calibration is done by the morphology of the arterial waveform
- Real-time, beat-to-beat values of CO and sensitivity to the slightest hemodynamic variations
- It does not require precalculated parameters
- As it does not require a central venous pressure (CVP) line, it is devoid of potential complications related to central venous catheterization.

DISADVANTAGES OF PRESSURE RECORDING ANALYTICAL METHOD

- Accuracy yet not proven
- Not validated in most of conditions with abnormal vascular compliance such as septic shock
- Not validated in cardiac surgical hemodynamically unstable patients with atrial fibrillation (AF)
- Not validated to assess stroke volume variations (SVV) fluid responsiveness.

BASIC PRINCIPLE OF PRESSURE RECORDING ANALYTICAL METHOD

The basic principle of this technology is that in any given vessel, the volume changes occur mainly because of the radial expansion of the artery in response to variations in pressure. It converts a pressure-based signal into a flow measurement.[2] The original concept of PCM-based technology assumed that the SV is to be estimated (not measured) by analyzing the relationship between the pulsatile and continuous AUC by the systolic portion of a pressure curve (Asys) divided by the dynamic impedance [Z(t)] determined by physical characteristics of the cardiocirculatory system expressed as below[1] **(Fig. 1)**:

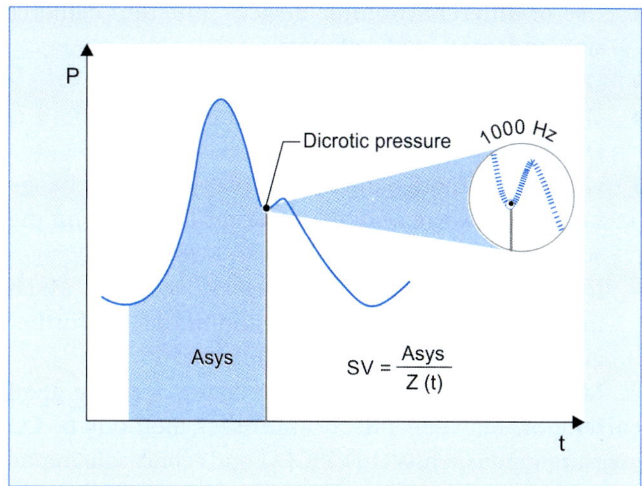

Fig. 1: Arterial-pressure waveform showing Asys, dicrotic pressure, SV, and Z(t). (AUC: area under the curve; SV: stroke volume; Asys: AUC by the systolic portion of a pressure curve AUC by the systolic portion of a pressure curve; Z(t): dynamic impedance)
Source: Vygon India. With permission from How can we help practitioners to make the right clinical choices? [Online] Available from https://hemodynamic-management.vygon.com/ [Last accessed September, 2024].

SV = Asys/Z(t)
SV: Stroke volume
Asys: AUC by the systolic portion of a pressure curve
Z(t): Dynamic impedance

Using PRAM, it is possible to compute dynamic impedance Z(t) directly from the analysis of the pressure-recording signal. It is the key factor that represents the elastic and mechanical characteristics of the cardiovascular system. The major concern while deriving dynamic impedance Z(t) is that it is influenced by a dynamic physical property of the whole arterial tree. It represents the total opposition to the propagation of the pressure wave transmitted along the vessel tree. To overcome this difficulty of measuring dynamic impedance Z(t) in vivo and beat-by-beat, PCM-based technologies are either externally calibrated, internally calibrated (or autocalibrated), and noncalibrated.

Pressure recording analytical method technology is based on an interplay of several physical variables. It needs an arterial line (radial or femoral) and the arterial pressure profile is analyzed at a high frequency of 1,000 Hz to catch all the components of the arterial pressure wave signal. This is a proprietary algorithm-based system that analyzes both the systolic and diastolic phases of pressure tracing. Dicrotic notch (point of separation between systolic and diastolic phase) is identified precisely. SV is obtained from the area under the whole systolic portion of the pressure wave [i.e., from the start of the upstroke (aortic valve opening) to the dicrotic notch (aortic valve closure)] and thus, CO is calculated.

At any given time, volume changes in the vessels occur mainly due to radial expansion of the vessel, because of variations in pressure. The force of blood ejection generated by the left ventricle, arterial impedance counteracting the pulsatile blood inflow, the arterial compliance that permits to elastically storing a portion of the kinetic energy of the cardiac upstroke, peripheral vessel's resistance generating backward reflections of the pressure wave depending on heart rate and relative tightening, bifurcations, and stiffness of downstream arterial vessels: these variables are all interdependent and need to be evaluated simultaneously.[1,2]

Arterial pressure trace contains a series of pressure variations that are registered overtime at a predefined rate. Any arterial tracing comprises of forward wave (F) generated by the left ventricular systole, encountered by the backward (B) waves coming from the periphery which generates a series of specific pressure trace parts as "points of instability" (POI) which is a unique feature of this technology. These points are distributed over both the phases and pressure time changes are analyzed. Identification of POI to estimate the Z[t] beat to beat makes PRAM technology unique compared to other PCM systems. This technology basically analyzes the microscopic pressure tracing oscillations to estimate vascular impedance. This makes the system highly reactive to changes in vascular impedance in abnormal conditions, such as vasodilatation, vasoconstrictions, and aortic counter pulsations.

VARIABLES DERIVED BY PRESSURE RECORDING ANALYTICAL METHOD

- Systemic variables (systolic pressure, diastolic pressure, mean pressure, and pulse pressure are measured with every beat).
- *Dicrotic pressure:* The value of the dicrotic pressure, gauged with precision at 1,000 Hz, provides information about the vascular condition and the ventricle-arterial pairing.
- *SV:* Measured beat-to-beat
- *Cardiac output:* Measured beat-to-beat

- *Systemic vascular resistance (SVR):* It is calculated in Dynes × s/cm^5 with the standard formula: SVR = Mean arterial pressure (MAP) – CVP/CO × 80/CO × 80
- Cardiac power output (CPO)
- Oxygen delivery (DO_2)
- *Cardiac cycle efficiency (CCE):* CCE is an exclusive variable that describes hemodynamic performance in terms of the ratio between hemodynamic work performed and the energy expenditure. It assesses the ability of the cardiovascular system to maintain homeostasis at different energy levels. It provides information about the overall progress of the patient's clinical condition and the effectiveness of the therapies. There is a direct correlation between CCE and left ventricular ejection fraction. Also, its inverse relation with probrain natriuretic peptide (pro-BNP) has also been studied; however, more studies are required for its validation.[2]
- *dP/dt_{max}:* With a sampling rate of 1,000 Hz, the exact value of dP/dT_{max} is displayed on the monitor. Its accurate value in addition to other hemodynamic parameters helps to understand the cardiovascular status of the patient. It is the maximum slope of the systolic portion of the arterial pressure waveform. The maximum pressure variation compared to time (dP/dt_{max}) is linked to the heart's contractility and also to the condition of the vascular system. The velocity of transmission and the reflected waves depend on the relationship between left ventricular function, arterial tone, and its stiffness.
- *Pulse pressure variation (PPV), SVV, and systolic pressure variation (SPV):* To assess the volume status during the respiratory cycle which can be viewed simultaneously. These parameters are calculated according to the operator's needs (default every 15 seconds).
- Dynamic filter which automatically optimizes the quality of the arterial wave to reduce the chances of alteration of the shape of the pressure curve by resonance phenomena.

FACTORS INFLUENCE THE RELIABILITY OF PRESSURE RECORDING ANALYTICAL METHOD

Pressure recording analytical method technology has been subjected to a large validation study because of the following factors which affect the results and induce a large bias with a high percentage of error (PE).

- Use of different monitor devices, different catheter size, and location of catheters
- Different reference methods
- Operators dependency, if the reference method is Doppler echocardiography
- Unstable hemodynamic states may induce a change in pressure wave and affect the results based on the software used.
- In older studies, PE of <30% was well accepted, which interferes with recent studies and makes the further analysis of these studies more difficult.

Many studies, although single center, found a good correlation between PRAM and other methods of CO measurements such as ThD, PiCCO, and echocardiography **(Table 1)**. However, the cardiac index measured by PRAM has not shown any agreement with ThD as per a study including 49 in cardiac surgical unstable patients with AF.[3] The mean difference found to be 0.136 L/min/m^2 [0.43 L/min/m^2 – 0.15 L/min/m^2], with an upper limit of agreement of 1.94 L/min/m^2 and a lower limit of agreement of –1.665 L/min/m^2, respectively.

Another study including 46 CO measurements of PRAM and ThD, CO obtained in 23 postoperative cardiac surgery patients has shown a lack of agreement with this method compared to the ThD method, which questions the reliability of PRAM technology. The Bland-Altman analysis showed a mean difference (bias) of 0.0 l min^1 and limits of agreement (1.96 SD) of 4.53 to –4.54 l min^1 [upper 95% confidence interval (CI), 3.26–5.80; lower 95% CI, –5.8 to –3.27]. PE of 1.96 SD/mean of the reference method was found to be very high (87%). The authors concluded that PRAM CO cannot replace the ThD technique to measure CO.[4] Even in septic shock patients, validation studies against CO by ThD have reported divergent results. One study in 22 patients with septic shock recorded the CO simultaneously by PRAM technique and ThD technique, found a high error rate, and concluded that PRAM was unreliable. Bland–Altman analysis for CO showed a bias of 0.31 L/min, precision (=SD) of 1.97 L/min with a high PE of 62.54%. Bias was 0.21 L/min/m^2, precision of 1.10 L/min/m^2, and PE of 64% for CI. The bias was 5 mL, precision of 24.46 mL, and PE of 70.21% for $\dot{S}V$. Linear regression produced a correlation coefficient r^2 for CO, CI, and SV, of 0.403, 0.306, and 0.3 respectively.[5]

Another limitation of this technology is that, although it measures SVV and it is displayed on the monitor, it is unable to predict fluid responsiveness and track the changes in CO induced by volume expansion. One study

TABLE 1: The correlation between PRAM and other methods for CO measurement.

Study	*Reference method*	*Patients*	*Site of cannulation*	*Correlation*	*Bias (L/min/m^2)*	*% error (PE%)*
Romano SM et al.[1] 2002	Fick method (*n* =18), ThD (*n* =22)	Diagnostic heart catheterization hemodynamically stable (*n* =22)	Aortic catheter (PRAMa) and noninvasively by photoplethysmography (PRAMf)	The Bland-Altman analysis confirmed the agreement between the Fick method and PRAM, and ThD and PRAM Fick method vs PRAMa: $r^2 = 0.88$ PRAMf: $r^2 = 0.94$ ThD vs. PRAMa $r^2 = 0.77$ PRAMf, $r^2 = 0.77$	Fick: –0.012 ThD: –0.154	Not reported
Giomarelli P et al.[7] 2004	ThD	CPB On extracorporeal circulation (*n* =28) 112 measurements	Radial artery	• The Bland–Altman analysis demonstrated that the overall estimates of CO measured by PRAM closely agreed with CO measured by PAC (mean difference, 0.027; SD, 0.43; LoA, –0.83 and +0.89) $R^2 = 0:78$; $p < 0:0001$) found between ThD and PRAM • Highest correlation $R^2 = 0:86$ (at 3 hours after arrival in the ICU) • A lower degree of correlation $R^2 = 0:70$ (at 30 minutes after extracorporeal circulation)	–0.40 with SD 0.59 (30 minutes after CPB) 0.01 with SD 0.33 (3 hours after ICU admission)	
Zangrillo A et al.[8] 2010	ThD	Cardiac surgical unstable patients on intra-aortic balloon pump and/or high doses of inotropic drugs but without atrial fibrillation (*n* =32)	Radial artery	Significant correlation $r = 0.72$, $p < 0.001$	The mean bias between the ThD and PRAM is found to be 0.072 ± 0.41 L/min/m^2 with lower and upper 95% limits of confidence of –0.089 and 0.233 L/min/m^2, respectively	30

Contd...

Contd...

Study	Reference method	Patients	Site of cannulation	Correlation	Bias (L/min/m²)	% error (PE%)
Franchi F et al.[9] 2013	Echocardiography	Blunt trauma admitted in ICU (n =49) 116 measurements	Radial artery	• The correlation between the two methods was 0.94 [95% CI = 0.89–0.97; $p < 0.001$] • Even changes in CO showed a correlation of 0.91 (95% CI = 0.87–0.95; $p < 0.001$) a mean bias of –0.01 L/min with LoA of –0.67–0.65 L/min (lower 95% CI, –0.83 to –0.51; upper 95% CI, 0.48–0.81	Mean bias was –0.06 L/min with LoA of –0.94–0.82 L/min (lower 95% CI, –1.16 to –0.72; upper 95% CI, 0.60 to 1.04)	18
Franchi F et al.[10] 2011	ThD	Septic shock patient with noradrenaline (n =30) 90 paired measurements	Radial artery	Good correlation between the pulse contour method and thermodilution	Mean bias –0.26 (SD 0.98 L/min and 95% LoA –2.22–1.70 L/min	25%
Donati A et al.[11] 2014	PiCCO vigilance	Mixed medical surgical postcardiac surgical (n =32) PiCCO (n =16) vigilance Total 112 measurements	Femoral artery	• The correlation coefficient between PRAM with vigilance-CO and: 0.83 (95% CI, 0.57–0.94; $p < 0.001$ • Similarly, good correlation with PRAM and PiCCO: 0.91 (95% CI, 0.83–0.96; *Pb* 0.0001) • The coefficient of variation for PiCCO was 4% ± 2%, and the coefficient of variation for PRAM was 10% ± 8%	• PRAM and vigilance bias of 0.22 ± 0.55 with LoA between 0.87 and 1.30 L/min. PRAM and PiCCO • The bias was 0.67 ± 0.89 L/min with LoA–1.07 and 2.41 L/min	25%, 25% for PRAM vs vigilance and 28% PRAM vs PiCCO
Scolletta et al.[12] 2016	Echocardiography	Multicenter study with mixed population including septic patients (n =400)	Radial/femoral	A significant correlation was found between echocardiographic cardiac output and MostCare® cardiac output (r = 0.85; $p < 0.0001$)	Ranged from –0.40 to 0.45	Ranged from 13.2 to 47.2%

(CI: confidence interval; CO: cardiac output; CPB: cardiopulmonary bypass; ICU: intensive care unit; LoA: limits of agreements; PRAM: pressure recording analytical method; SD: standard deviation; ThD: thermodilution) involving 35 mechanically ventilated patients who were subjected to fluid challenges and SVV and CO was obtained with the PRAM and compared with echocardiography. They observed that SVV obtained by PRAM cannot predict fluid responsiveness and is unable to track the changes induced by volume expansion. PE between CO by echocardiography and CO by PRAM was 34% at baseline and 33% after volume expansion.[6]

Besides that, PRAM technology has been compared with ThD CO monitoring in patients implanted with a left ventricular assist device (LVAD). There was a good agreement among them, although the sample size was small (n = 12).[13] Also, PRAM demonstrated good agreement with ThD in 32 patients undergoing cardiac surgery during extracorporeal circulation (ECC) on a roller pump and it allowed early recognition of patients with low-flow states during weaning.[14] In one study, the correlation of PRAM with pro-BNP level was evaluated in patients with congestive cardiac failure (CCF) who underwent ultrafiltration. The measurements were found to correlate pro-BNP positively with SVR ($r = 0.96$, $p = 0.002$) and the New York Heart Association (NYHA) class ($r = 0.96$, $p = 0.037$) and negatively with dP/dt_{max} ($r = -0.83$, $p = 0.039$), CCE ($r = -0.93$, $p = 0.011$), and CO ($r = -0.94$, $p = 0.014$). Additional hemodynamic performance has been evaluated by PRAM and they observed that fluid removal was found to be associated with clinical hemodynamic improvement, plasma BNP levels, CPO, CCE, systemic vascular resistances, and dicrotic pressure which was effectively recorded by PRAM technique.[15]

LIMITATIONS

The main concern of this technique is the quality of the recorded arterial signal either due to the factors discussed further. It is a very common scenario in the ICU to have suboptimal arterial tracing which further affects the interpretation of hemodynamic variables by PRAM technology. Any major change in vascular compliance affects its interpretation.

INAPPROPRIATE SIGNAL ACQUISITION DUE TO FOLLOWING FACTORS

- Aortic valve regurgitation, abnormal transmission of the signal during aortic dissection, obstruction to the transmission of the signal (thoracic outlet syndrome, significant stenosis along the arterial tree from the aortic valve to the sampling site).
- Inadequate dynamic response of the transducer and fluid-filled tubing system.
- An inadequate damping of the signal leads to an incorrect estimation of arterial impedance and hence an incorrect value of SV.
- *Underdamped waveforms and resonance of the signal:* As this method analyzes the arterial pressure wave profile, any artifacts that alter the arterial waveform misleads and there is wrong information about the systolic, diastolic, and mean pressures which ultimately affects its validation to measure CO. Thus, it mandates us to check the arterial pressure waveform carefully to avoid errors in hemodynamic waveforms (such as underdamped or overdamped). Romagnoli S et al. observed the impact of underdamping/resonance artefacts which are very common and are difficult to recognize. With conventional catheter transducer systems, high natural frequency is difficult to achieve, because these systems are usually underdamped. Thus, extradamping must be introduced to minimize the distorting effects of this system which often resonates. He observed that all hemodynamic parameters showed clinically acceptable differences in the group without underdamping but the results differed significantly in the group associated with underdamping. They found systolic blood pressure bias, 16.7 mm Hg; CI bias, 0.24 L/min/m^2; dP/dtmax bias, 0.92 mm Hg/ms; and cardiac cycle efficiency bias (CCE bias), 0.018 in this study.[16]
- Another variable is dP/dt_{max} which should be calculated carefully and if it is greater than 1.67 mm Hg/ms in cardiac and vascular surgical patients, it should raise suspicion of the underdamping/resonance of the arterial pressure signal. The damping coefficient of the conventional catheter transducer system is frequently insufficient and resonance artifacts may affect the morphology and amplitude of the recorded pressure wave. This may be helpful to identify the phenomena related to the resonance of the catheter-transducer system which affects the reliability of this technique.

CONCLUSION

The pressure recording analytical method is a minimally invasive technique that is reliable, real-time, and efficient, which is a good alternative particularly when invasive monitoring is not possible to implement, not justified, and is disproportionate. It works well with a wide range of patient types and clinical conditions. It has been validated in cardiac surgical patients who are stable as well as unstable (without AF). High-quality pressure signal acquisition is of primary importance to limit the misleading results by this technique. One must be aware of the misinterpretation of the data which is influenced by inadequately damped arterial signal. Hence, artifacts should be minimized for better interpretation of the results with this technology. As the validation studies (against ThD) have reported divergent results, the clinical application of this technology is still limited. Various factors such as different reference methods, the patient's characteristics, different methodologies, heterogeneous patient population, and high incidence of arterial pressure waveform artifacts preclude us from definitive strong evidence to validate its use. With the invention of better algorithms, further studies are warranted to evaluate the accuracy and limitations of this technology in various clinical settings.

REFERENCES

1. Romano SM, Pistolesi M. Assessment of cardiac output from systemic arterial pressure in humans Salvatore. Crit Care Med. 2002;30(8):1834-41.
2. Romagnoli S, Bevilacqua S, Lazzeri C, et al. Most Care®: a minimally invasive system for hemodynamic monitoring powered by the Pressure Recording Analytical Method (PRAM). HSR Proc Intensive Care Cardiovasc Anesth. 2009;1(2):20-7.
3. Maj G, Landoni G, Barile L, Ciappi F, Dini D, Pratesi C, et al. Cardiac index assessment by the pressure recording analytic method in unstable patients with atrial fibrillation. J Cardiothorac Vasc Anesth. 2011;25(3):476-80.
4. Paarmann H, Groesdonk HV, Hanke T, Hanke T, Heinze H, Heringlake M, et al. Lack of agreement between pulmonary arterial thermodilution cardiac output and the pressure recording analytical method in postoperative cardiac surgery patients. Br J Anaesth. 2011;106(4):475-81.
5. Gopal S, Do T, Pooni JS, Martinelli G. Validation of cardiac output studies from the Mostcare compared to a pulmonary artery catheter in septic patients. Minerva Anestesiol. 2014;81(2):314-23.
6. Biais M, Cottenceau V, Stecken L, Jean M, Ottolenghi L, Roullet S, et al. Evaluation of stroke volume variations obtained with the pressure recording analytic method. Crit Care Med. 2012;40(4):1186-91.
7. Giomarelli P, Biagioli B, Scolletta S. Cardiac output monitoring by pressure recording analytical method in cardiac surgery. Eur J Cardiothoracic Surg. 2004;26(3):515-20.
8. Zangrillo A, Maj G, Scandroglio AM, Scandroglio AM, Nuzzi M, Plumari V, et al. Cardiac index validation using the pressure recording analytic method in unstable patients. J Cardiothorac Vasc Anesth. 2010;24(2):265-9.
9. Franchi F, Falciani E, Donadello K, Zacà V, Silvestri R, Taccone FS, et al. Echocardiography and pulse contour analysis to assess cardiac output in trauma patients. Minerva Anestesiol. 2013;79(2):137-46.
10. Franchi F, Silvestri R, Cubattoli L, Taccone FS, Donadello K, Romano SM, et al. Comparison between an uncalibrated pulse contour method and thermodilution technique for cardiac output estimation in septic patients. Br J Anaesth. 2011;107(2):202-8.
11. Donati A, Carsetti A, Tondi S, Scorcella C, Domizi R, Damiani E, et al. Thermodilution vs pressure recording analytical method in hemodynamic stabilized patients. J Crit Care. 2014;29(2):260-4.
12. Scolletta S, Franchi F, Romagnoli S, Carlà R, Donati A, Fabbri LP, et al. Comparison between Doppler-echocardiography and uncalibrated pulse contour method for cardiac output measurement: a multicenter observational study. Crit Care Med. 2016;44(7): 1370-9.
13. Scolletta S, Miraldi F, Mario S, Muzzi L. Continuous cardiac output monitoring with an uncalibrated pulse contour method in patients supported with mechanical pulsatile assist device. Interact Cardiovasc Thorac Surg. 2011;13(1):52-7.
14. Romano SM, Scolletta S, Olivotto I, Biagioli B, Gensini GF, Chiostri M, et al. Systemic arterial waveform analysis and assessment of blood flow during extracorporeal circulation. Perfus Arnold Ltd. 2006;21(2): 109-16.
15. Giglioli DL, Gensini EC, Scolletta MC, Valente S, Cecchi E, Scolletta S, et al. Cardiac efficiency improvement after slow continuous ultrafiltration is assessed by beat-to-beat minimally invasive monitoring in congestive heart failure patients: a preliminary report. Blood Purif. 2010;29(1):44-51.
16. Romagnoli S, Mario S, Bevilacqua S, Lazzeri C, Gensini GF, Pratesi C, et al. Dynamic response of liquid-filled catheter systems for measurement of blood pressure: precision of measurements and reliability of the Pressure Recording Analytical Method with different disposable systems. J Crit Care. 2011;26(4):415-22.

CHAPTER

Ultrasound Dilution Technique for Cardiac Output Measurement

Jacob George Pulinilkunnathil, Atul Prabhakar Kulkarni

INTRODUCTION

Hemodynamic optimization in critically ill patients in the intensive care unit (ICU) often necessitates accurate quantification and monitoring of the trend of change in the of cardiac output (CO). CO monitoring in the ICU helps in obtaining the diagnosis or differential diagnosis of shock by evaluating the cause of hypotension, pulmonary edema, and cardiac failure, thus aiding in the management of the patient. CO monitoring with the pulmonary artery catheter (PAC) using the Fick principle is considered the gold standard for CO monitoring, although less invasive devices are currently available. The major principles and techniques of CO measurement are the Fick principle and indicator dilution techniques (that include thermodilution, lithium dilution, and pulse dye densitometry), arterial waveform analysis, transthoracic impedance and bioreactance analysis, and also the Doppler principle.[1] Ultrasound dilution technique (UDT) is an old, time-tested technology in the ICU, although its use for the measurement of CO is novel.[2]

UNDERSTANDING ULTRASOUND DILUTION TECHNIQUE

Ultrasound dilution technology derives its information from two technologies: (1) Indicator dilution technology and (2) differential transit-time ultrasound technology. Here, warm isothermic saline is used as the indicator while flow is calculated from differential transit time ultrasound technology.[3]

Differential Transit Time Ultrasound Technology

Differential transit time ultrasound technology uses in-line ultrasonic flow meters, both in upstream and downstream circulation, to measure the time difference between the initial transmission of an ultrasonic signal from the transducer and the time of reception of the signal by a second transducer. This is then compared between upstream and downstream values. At states of no flow, the travel time will be the same in both directions, while it will be faster if measured upstream and slower if measured downstream. The difference between the time taken for upstream and downstream transit provides a measure of volume flow. This is different from the Doppler technology that measures the frequency shift between ultrasound beam and its reflection. Flow rates are derived by mathematical calculation from the frequency shifts.[4]

Principle of Ultrasound Dilution Technology

The ultrasonic velocity of blood is 1560–1590 m/s and is primarily dependent on the protein concentration of the blood. When blood is diluted by a bolus of isotonic saline whose ultrasound velocity is 1,533 m/s, the ultrasound velocity of blood also gets reduced. The changes in ultrasound velocity are sensed and measured and the monitor is able to calculate actual flows from the indicator dilution principle.[4]

Use of Ultrasound Dilution Technique

In Hemodialysis

Many methods have been described to assess vascular access flow rates in hemodialysis. The technique with the most extensive validation and most precise standardization is UDT. It is also used for measuring access recirculation and delivered blood flow.[5]

Ultrasound Dilution Technology for Cardiac Output Monitoring

In concordance with the same principles, isotonic and isothermic (temperature 37°C) saline bolus (0.5–1 mL/kg, maximum 30 mL) is injected into the venous limb of the arteriovenous (AV) circuit at a rate of 6–12 mL/min for 5–6 minutes and the decrease in the velocity of ultrasound in the blood is recorded. The recording requires an extracorporeal disposable AV loop pre-filled with heparinized saline in between arterial and central venous lines, a peristaltic pump to circulate the blood through the AV loop, flow, and dilution sensors on both the venous and arterial sites of the circulation. The decrease in ultrasound velocity is detected by the sensor at the arterial side, and an ultrasound dilution curve is obtained **(Fig. 1)**. CO is calculated with the use of the Stewart–Hamilton equation. This technology has been validated in animal models and also in critically ill pediatric and adult patients, mainly in the surgical population though.

Hemodynamic Parameters Obtained from Ultrasound Dilution Technology

Central blood volume (CBV) is the volume of blood present between the injecting venous site and the recording arterial site. This includes the cumulative volume of blood present in the heart, lungs, and blood vessels.

Total end-diastolic volume (TEDV) is the volume of blood present at the end of diastole in the atria and ventricles and forms the preload volume of the heart.

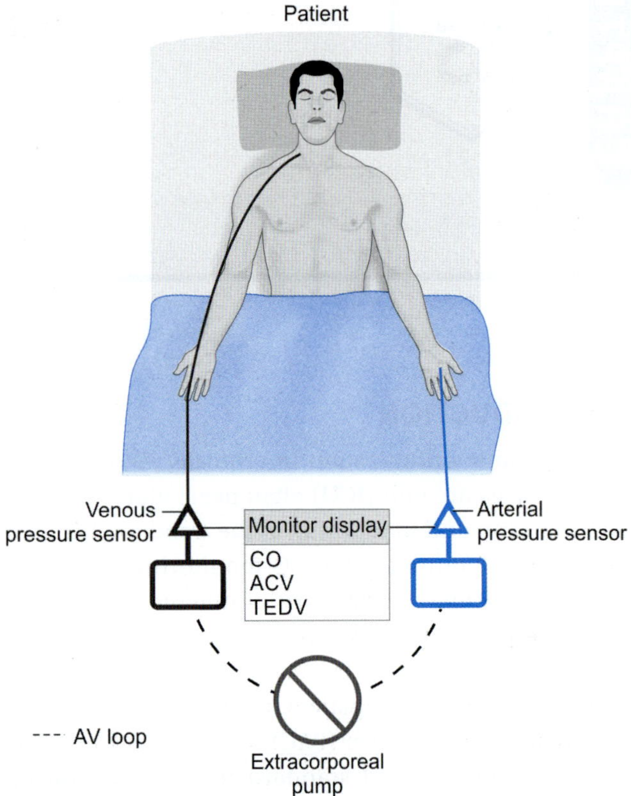

Fig. 1: The setup for measurement of CO using ultrasound dilution technique. (ACV: active circulation volume; AV: arteriovenous; CO; cardiac output; TEDV: total end-diastolic volume)

TABLE 1: Summary of evidence for use of UDT for CO monitoring.

Author, year	*Population*	*Compared to*	*Results*
Nikiforov YV[6] 1996	Adult cardiac surgery patients	PAC thermodilution	Good agreement with PAC
Krivitski[7] 2008	In vitro model	Known volume and flow	Accurately measured even the small flows and volumes required for hemodynamic assessments
Tsutsui[4] 2009	Adult patients undergoing abdominal surgery	PAC thermodilution	Good agreement with PAC
Boehne[8] 2010	Animal model	Perivascular flow of pulmonary artery	Reliable cardiac output measurement
Eremenko[9] 2010	Adult cardiothoracic surgery	PAC thermodilution	Good agreement in postcardiac surgery ICU patients
Galstyan[10] 2010	Adult hematology ICU	Transpulmonary thermodilution PICCO®	CO measurements were interchangeable Measured blood volumes varied significantly
Shih[11] 2011	Dogs	LIDCO®	Comparable
Crittendon III[12] 2012	Pediatrics	PAC thermodilution	Good correlation
Boehne[13] 2014	Pediatrics	Fick principle	Good correlation
Sigurdsson[14] 2019	Pediatrics	CO measured by periaortic flow probe	Comparable

(CO: cardiac output; ICU: intensive care unit; PAC: pulmonary artery catheter; UDT: ultrasound dilution technique)

TABLE 2: Major advantages and limitations of UDT.

Advantages	*Major limitations*
• Reliable CO monitoring • The indicator is safe to use and nontoxic. No blood wastage • Can be used to any patient of any age or any size • It is operator-independent and can be easily performed by any healthcare personnel • Requires no additional invasive lines as it uses existing CVC and arterial lines • Running the test has not been shown to alter systemic or cerebral hemodynamics or worsening of oxygenation • It has been used to identify and quantify and also measure cardiac output in the presence of left-to-right shunts • Provides additional information regarding the quantification of TEDV and ACV also	• Requires heparinization of the extracorporeal circuit when not being used • Requires a central line for venous access Intermittent CO monitoring • Interruption of the arterial pressure tracing during measurement of CO • Repetitive fluid boluses may increase the volume of fluid being administered (significant, especially in pediatrics) • The effect of nonhomogeneous perfused lungs is not clear • Need a disposable extracorporeal loop and pump to run the blood through the circuit • Need calibration of transpulmonary blood volumes and also validation regarding the ability to differentiate hydrostatic pulmonary edema from ARDS

(ACV: active circulating volume; ARDS: acute respiratory distress syndrome; CO: cardiac output; CVC: central venous catheter; TEDV: total end-diastolic volume; UDT: ultrasound dilution technique)

Active circulation volume (ACV) is defined as the amount of blood that undergoes circulation in the major organs. ACV ranges from 30 to 70 mL/kg depending on the volume status of the patient.

Evidence for Use of Ultrasound Dilution Technology for Cardiac Output Monitoring

The evidence on this technology for CO monitoring is limited but growing. A summary of the available evidence is discussed in **Table 1**. The advantages and disadvantages of UDT are summarized in **Table 2**.

CONCLUSION

Ultrasound dilution technology seems an accurate minimally invasive method for CO monitoring in critically ill patients. The requirement of relatively small volumes of nontoxic indicators (normal saline) and many validation studies in pediatrics support the use of this technique in a pediatric population. It however needs further validation in specific patient-populations, such as those with acute respiratory distress syndrome (ARDS), patients with shunts, and hyperdynamic circulation.

REFERENCES

1. Kobe J, Mishra N, Arya VK, Al-Moustadi W, Nates W, Kumar B. Cardiac output monitoring: technology and choice. Ann Card Anaesth. 2019;22(1):6-17.
2. Vincent JL, Rhodes A, Perel A, Martin GS, Della Rocca G, Vallet B, et al. Clinical review: update on hemodynamic monitoring—a consensus of 16. Crit Care. 2011;15(4):229.
3. Lee AJ, Cohn JH, Ranasinghe JS. Cardiac output is assessed by invasive and minimally invasive techniques. Anesthesiol Res Pract. 2011;2011:475151.
4. Tsutsui M, Matsuoka N, Ikeda T, Sanjo Y, Kazama T. Comparison of a new cardiac output ultrasound dilution method with thermodilution technique in adult patients under general anesthesia. J Cardiothorac Vasc Anesth. 2009;23(6):835-40.
5. Krivitski NM, MacGibbon D, Gleed RD, Dobson A. Accuracy of dilution techniques for access flow measurement during hemodialysis. Am J Kidney Dis. 1998;31(3):502-8.
6. Nikiforov YV, Kisluchine VV, Chaus NI. Validation of a new method to measure cardiac output during extracorporeal detoxification. ASAIO J. 1996;42(5):M903-5.
7. Krivitski NM, Kislukhin VV, Thuramalla NV. Theory and in vitro validation of a new extracorporeal arteriovenous loop approach for hemodynamic assessment in pediatric and neonatal intensive care unit patients. Pediatr Crit Care Med. 2008;9(4):423-8.
8. Boehne M, Baustert M, Paetzel V, et al. Comparison of a new cardiac output ultrasound dilution method with thermodilution technique in adult patients under general anesthesia. Pediatr Crit Care Med. 2010;23:1-7.
9. Eremenko AA, Safarov PN. Flow-regulated extracorporeal arteriovenous tubing loop for cardiac output measurements by ultrasound velocity dilution: validation in post-cardiac surgery intensive care unit patients. ASAIO J. 2010;56(6):522-6.
10. Galstyan G, Bychinin M, Alexanyan M, Gorodetsky V. Comparison of cardiac output and blood volumes in intrathoracic compartments measured by ultrasound dilution and transpulmonary thermodilution methods. Intensive Care Med. 2010;36(12):2140-4.

11. Shih A, Giguère S, Vigani A, Shih R, Thuramalla N, Bandt C. Determination of cardiac output by ultrasound velocity dilution in normovolemia and hypovolemia in dogs. Vet Anaesth Analg. 2011;38(4):279-85.
12. Crittendon I, Dreyer WJ, Decker JA, Kim JJ. Ultrasound dilution: an accurate means of determining cardiac output in children. Pediatr Crit Care Med. 2012;13(1): 42-6.
13. Boehne M, Baustert M, Paetzel V, Köditz H, Schoof S, Happel CM, et al. Determination of cardiac output by ultrasound dilution technique in infants and children: a validation study against direct Fick principle. Br J Anaesth. 2014;112(3):469-76.
14. Sigurdsson TS, Aronsson A, Lindberg L. Extracorporeal arteriovenous ultrasound measurement of cardiac output in small children. Anesthesiology. 2019;130(5):712-8.

CHAPTER

Electrical Cardiometry for Cardiac Output Measurement

Shilpushp Jagannath Bhosale, Atul Prabhakar Kulkarni

INTRODUCTION

Hemodynamic assessment is vitally important in assessment of patients in the perioperative patients as well as the critically ill. Cardiac output (CO) monitoring allows the clinicians to fine tune the fluid therapy and vasoactive drug therapy. Noninvasive CO measurement techniques using thoracic bioimpedance have been shown to help in diagnostic evaluation, management, and prognostication in patients with heart failure in the outpatient department.[1] CO monitoring has been the cornerstone of hemodynamic assessment since the introduction of pulmonary artery catheter (PAC), however, the use of PAC and the data provided by the device has failed to improve outcomes and may in fact be associated with complications.[2-9] It is evident that there is a growing need for a reliable and accurate noninvasive CO measurement modality in the intensive care unit (ICU). Electrical cardiometry (EC) is a completely noninvasive method of determination of CO. It is very simple and easy to setup, use, and interpret the data obtained, is cost effective, and allows the continuous measurement of CO at bedside. EC measures CO and other parameters related to cardiac contractility and fluid status by measuring the thoracic electrical bioimpedance (TEB).

There has been renewed interest in this technology, which was first described and used 50 years back to measure noninvasive CO in astronauts in space. It is a based on the modification of the bioimpedance principle, which states that impedance of the thorax (i.e., the resistance to electrical current) is dependent on the amount of fluid in the thoracic compartment. Later Bernstein and Osypka modified the basic bioimpedance equation so that the maximum rate of change of impedance is correlated to the peak aortic blood acceleration. This modification considerably improved the reliability of measurements and was called electrical velocimetry.[10,11] EC considers that the alignment of erythrocytes in the aorta causes a change in the thoracic impedance. This is dependent on the blood flow in the aorta after the aortic valve opening. The mean velocity index is derived from the peak amplitude measurement, which is the index of peak aortic blood flow acceleration over time. The change in the amount of blood volume in the aorta during the cardiac cycle correlates to the observed changes in impedance. Cardiometry considers that the main impedance changes are caused by the flow in the aorta and the impedance of tissues that show a high resistance, such as the lung and the surrounding tissue are not accounted for.

PRINCIPLE OF ELECTRICAL CARDIOMETRY

It is important to realize whether the principle is bioimpedance, bioreactance, or EC. The hemodynamic parameter that is measured can only be as accurate and reliable as the theoretical model. Therefore, understanding the origin of the signal measured is the key to correct modeling to acquire accurate results. Impedance cardiography (ICG) assumes that volumetric changes in the ascending aorta are the origin of the characteristic change in bioimpedance following aortic valve opening. EC works on the bioimpedance principle described by Kubicek and Bernstein.[12]

The impedance principle considers that the myocardial chambers are electrically isolated relative to chest and lungs, and changes in impedance are linked to variation in aortic blood volume. Blood has high electrical conductivity compared with muscle, fat, and air, and hence the current is distributed preferentially to the blood. The theory suggests that there is a change in the red blood cells (RBCs) orientation during each systole, which causes a change in the electrical conductivity of blood. This change in electrical conductivity occurs for the reasons explained here. In diastole, when the flow decreases in the aorta, the RBCs are oriented randomly due to Brownian principle and present a high resistance (and low conductivity) **(Fig. 1)**. During systole, the RBCs align due to shear forces generated in the aorta due to the blood flowing through

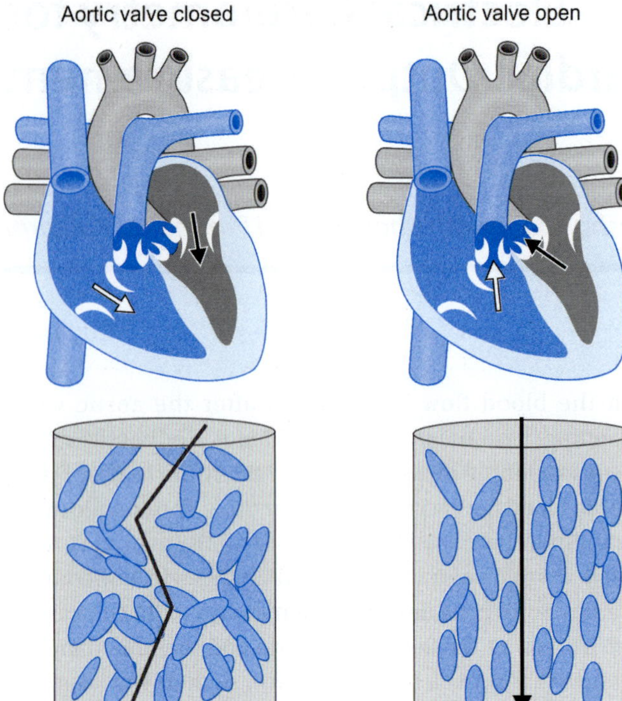

Fig. 1: Impedance change graph during systole and diastole.
Source: Adapted from Markus Osypka 2009, Cardiotronic Inc.

the aorta leading to higher conductivity and drop in the impedance proportional to the increase in the volume of blood. Bernstein and Osypka, in 2001, developed a new model for interpreting the bioimpedance signal and termed it as EC. This change is measured and incorporated in the proprietary algorithm (Cardiotronic, Osypka) to calculate the stroke volume (SV) and thus the CO. EC thus determines an estimate of the SV by measuring the TEB and its changes related to the cardiac cycle.

Monitor Setup

The setup consists of placement of a total of four skin sensor electrodes on the neck and left side of the thorax (two each at thoracic inlet and outlet) as shown in **Figure 1**. This allows continuous measurement of the changes in electrical conductivity within the thorax. A fixed, low amplitude, high frequency (50 kHz) alternating electrical current (AC) is applied via the pair of outer electrodes toward the thorax, and in particular, the ascending and descending aorta. By sending this current through the thorax and aorta, the change in resistance during systole and diastole is measured.

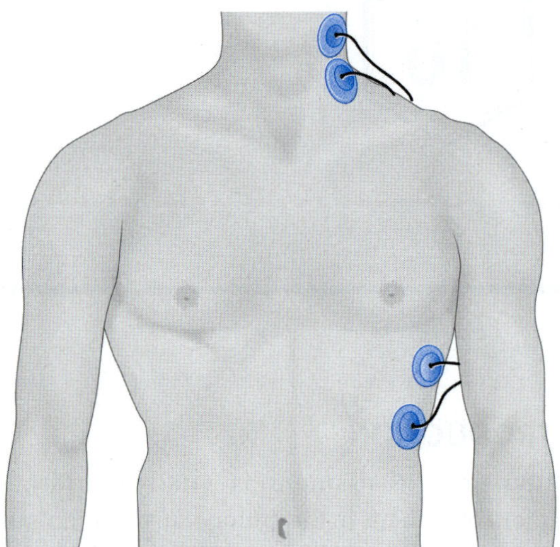

Fig. 2: Electrode placement (thoracic inlet and outlet).
Source: With permission from Osypka.

Mathematics of Measurement of Stroke Volume and Cardiac Output

Thoracic impedance (Z_0) is calculated as the ratio of voltage received and current applied and corresponds to changes in total thoracic fluid content (TFC). By analyzing the rate of change in conductivity before and after aortic valve opening, EC derives the peak aortic acceleration of blood (maximum slope seen in **Figure 2**) and the left-ventricular ejection time (LVET) (flow time). The velocity of the blood flow derived from the peak aortic acceleration is measured.

The rate of change of impedance during this systolic pulsatile flow and time helps calculate the SV. Derivative of the impedance is depicted as dZ/dt_{max} **(Fig. 2)**. SV is calculated as the product of the ventricle ejection time (VET) and slope of the initial change of the aortic volume obtained from the first derivative of the impedance (dZ/dt_{max}). This bioimpedance measured over time is actually derived from all three components in the thorax and expressed as:

$$Z(t) = Z_0 + \Delta ZR + \Delta ZC$$

Where, Z_0 is the baseline impedance due to thoracic fluids and thoracic blood volume, ΔZR is impedance change during respiration, and ΔZC is impedance change related to the systole. The respiratory impedance ΔZR is suppressed, since it is an artifact for measuring systolic change. Thus, measurement of ΔZC over time reveals an impedance waveform that is similar to an arterial blood pressure waveform (*see* **Fig. 3**).

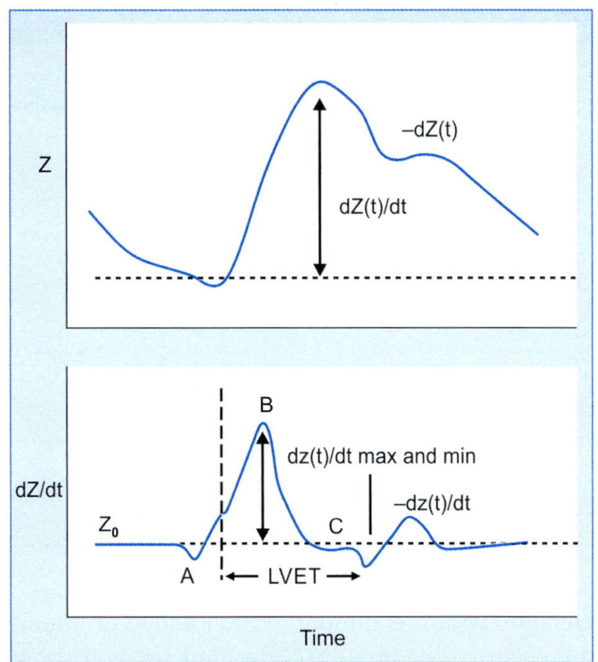

Fig. 3: Bioimpedance and time derivative waveform, highlighted impedance changes. (LVET: left-ventricular ejection time)
Source: Adapted from Markus Osypka 2009, Cardiotronic Inc.

Cardiac output and TFC is computed based on mathematical equations under the assumption that thoracic impedance changes over time are proportional to the SV.

SV = VET × dZ/dt_{max} × CF (correction factor from proprietary database of patients)

It is important to note the inverted change of impedance during systole ΔZC, hence [-dZ(t)], the calculated time derivative -dZ(t) is [-dZ(t)/dt] and is not a physiological signal.

Thus, analyzing the time derivative waveform (**Fig. 3**, -dZ(t)/dt) helps in determining important time points for obtaining the various hemodynamic parameters according to the proprietary algorithm such as opening of aortic valve [Point A: Begining of flow time (FT)/LVET], peak aortic blood acceleration (Point B: Aortic dP/dt_{max}), and closure of aortic valve (Point C: End of FT/LVET).

The baseline resistance and conductivity gives the TFC which represent the total fluids in the chest.[13] The change in conductivity according to the systolic time helps in deriving LVET.

The change from random orientation to alignment of RBCs upon opening of aortic valve generates a characteristic steep increase of conductivity (corresponds to decrease impedance) (**Fig. 3**—black arrows denoting the change of conductivity signal).

The steeper the slope of the -dZ(t) signal, or the higher the peak amplitude of -dZ(t)/dt, the quicker the alignment process and, thus, the higher the contractility of the heart. It is important to note that EC measures impedance rather than conductivity and since impedance is reciprocal to conductivity, we get the characteristic inverted shape of the change-of-impedance [-dZ(t)] but it is read as a change-of-conductivity waveform. It is important to note that velocimetry uses volume of electrically participating tissue (VEPT) that is derived from the body mass index as the patient constant (CP), which necessitates appropriate use of body weight for accuracy in measurements.

Depending on the shape of the impedance waveform and from the Bernstein and Osypka model, various hemodynamic parameters can be derived **(Table 1)**:

- Index of contractility (ICON) which is akin to the ejection fraction on echocardiography, this is derived from peak change of impedance.
- Stroke volume can be calculated as the product of CP, the mean blood velocity, and flow time.
- Mean blood velocity is derived from the measured index for peak aortic acceleration.
- Corrected flow time (FTC) is the flow time corrected for heart rate and, it is directly proportional to the LVET **(Table 1)**.

ELECTRICAL CARDIOMETRY VERSUS IMPEDANCE CARDIOGRAPHY (TRADITIONAL BIOIMPEDANCE)

Electrical cardiometry is often confused with the traditional bioimpedance technology most commonly known as impedance cardiography. EC and ICG both measure impedance change from baseline impedance Z_0 in relation to CO, Z(t) the time of change of impedance from the signal waveform to accurately identify the opening and closing of aortic valve, and the LVET. The methods differ from the phenomenon responsible for the steep increase in bioimpedance during each heartbeat. EC (velocimetry) uses a modified equation based on the maximum rate of change of impedance to assess aortic blood flow and thereby CO.

Though both methods use sensors placed on the thorax, traditional bioimpedance cardiography methods rely on the assumption of periodical volumetric changes in the aorta to determine SV and CO. ICG attributes the decrease in impedance [dZ(t)/dt] to the volumetric expansion of the ascending aorta thus determines the

TABLE 1: Derived hemodynamic parameters from electrical impedance cardiometry (Equations from Bernstein and Osypka).

Parameter	***Equation***	***Abbreviations***
Index of contractility (ICON)	$\frac{\left\lvert \left(\frac{dZ(t)}{dt}\right)_{MIN} \right\rvert}{Z_0} \cdot 1{,}000$	• dZ(t)/dt: Peak amplitude impedance change over time • Z_0: Baseline impedance
Stroke volume (SV)	$SV_{TEB} = C_P \cdot \bar{v}_{FT} \cdot FT$ $SV = V_{EPT} \cdot \sqrt{\frac{\left\lvert \left(\frac{dZ(t)}{dt}\right)_{MIN} \right\rvert}{Z_0}} \cdot FT_C$	• $\bar{v}_{FT}$: Mean blood velocity index • FT: Flow time • C_P: Patient constant in mL • V_{EPT}: Volume of electrically participating tissue
Flow time corrected	$FT_C = \frac{LVET}{\sqrt{T_{RR}}}$	• FT_C: Flow time corrected for heart rate • LVET: Left-ventricular ejection time • T_{RR}: R-R interval
Cardiac output (CO)	$CO = \frac{SV}{1{,}000} \cdot HR$	

peak velocity in contrast to cardiometry that attributes the decrease in impedance to alignment of RBCs during systole and determines peak acceleration. Due to the continuously upgraded algorithm, the EC seems to be superior to bioimpedance cardiography.

ADVANTAGES

Ideally, the noninvasive CO device has to be tested for accuracy, precision, and reliability, where accuracy is how close is the measurement to gold standard, even if taken repeatedly and precision is the consistent reproducibility of the same results when measured multiple times.[14,15] EC has been extensively studied in wide range of patient population and varying conditions, while bioimpedance has been studied in healthy adults. The cardiometry has the advantage of having multiple measures to obtain more accurate values to improve the calibration, and precision and with more data incorporated in the algorithm. The major advantage of use of EC is that it has shown to be reliable and has been approved for use in adults, children, and neonates.[16] The EC is supposed to have higher sensitivity to changes in low conductivity and hence may be more accurate than bioimpedance.

Emerging evidence suggest that the advantage of EC as a trend monitor of noninvasive continuous CO may be used in pediatrics population, especially when there is a dearth of noninvasive CO monitors in children.

Electrical cardiometry parameter, TFC, qualitative parameter of changes in thoracic fluid (calculated as the inverse of the impedance across the thorax), show a good correlation with the amount of fluid added or intended to be used to measure absolute fluid levels. However, dynamic measurements of TFC using EC can reflect directional changes in thoracic fluids, whether increasing or decreasing.[17,18]

The additional advantage of EC is that it measures a circulating blood volume and hemodynamics by providing an estimation of dynamic parameters of cardiac preload [stroke volume variation (SVV)], afterload [systemic vascular resistance (SVR)], and cardiac contractility (ICON), which helps clinicians to target (goal directed) approach.[19]

EVIDENCE FOR CLINICAL USE

Initial studies suggested that the overall agreement of TEB with standard thermodilution methods was poor, while the more recent studies have demonstrated TEB can measure CO with the same clinical accuracy as the thermodilution technique.[20,21] A study done by Gujjar et al. on adult patients with coronary artery disease comparing bioimpedance to radionuclide equilibrium cardiography showed poor correlation (r = 0.67 and agreement –0.42 L/min) and the percentage error of 42%.[22] Another study performed by Bougault et al. compared bioimpedance with Ficks CO in chronic obstructive pulmonary disease (COPD) patients found good correlation (r = 0.71–0.85) but the difference in the CO measured by two methods was almost 2.0 L/min.[23] In more recent studies, the EC (Cardiotronic Osypka, Inc.) has been validated against gold standard thermodilution methods.[24] Tirrota et al. compared the EC to the CO measurement done from arterial and venous catheters and gas analysis and found to have strong correlation between the two methods in pediatric surgical patients.[16]

Lui et al. compared the precision of CO by EC to indirect Fick method during cardiopulmonary exercise test in patients with dyspnea and found that the two measurements were within acceptable limits.[25]

A recent trial of 125 patients with acute circulatory failure compared EC to transthoracic echocardiography (TTE) for assessing fluid responsiveness. They found that the limits of agreement [i.e., bias ±1.96 standard deviation (SD)], were –1.7 L/min and 5.8 L/min in the two groups and the percentage of error between EC and TTE was 56%.[26]

LIMITATIONS

The TEB technology may be unreliable in arrhythmias, pleural and pericardial effusions and concerns have been raised about the accuracy of EC during low flow states or when electrocautery is performed, since it depends on the same TEB principle. Concerns have been raised about the accuracy during low-flow state or when electrocauterization was performed. There are also concerns about the use of TEB technology in conditions such as prosthetic aortic valve or when hematocrit is very low.[26]

Other disadvantages of thoracic bioimpedance technology are clinical conditions which can interfere with the accuracy of final results and the device's algorithms do not always detect them, e.g., aortic regurgitation and poor electrode skin contact.[27]

Since the model is computed from the RBC orientation during pulsatile flow, it may be inaccurate during nonpulsatile flows like extracorporeal membrane oxygenation (ECMO).

Though EC has been reintroduced with improved technology and equations for the mathematical derivation of CO, better understanding of the signal composition and better extraction of the aortic signal is still needed. The automatic calibration process is said to improve the overall agreement and accuracy of this method; however, the results need to be validated in larger clinical studies. Due to these limitations, routine clinical use of EC monitoring device is still not widespread.

CONCLUSION

Electrical cardiometry appears to be an accurate and clinically reliable CO monitor; it is important to understand its limitations. Although widespread application of cardiometry has not been yet seen, it may be useful to monitor the patients in whom other hemodynamic technologies are difficult to use (e.g., pediatric population).[28]

Future role of EC would become clear after more studies demonstrate its accuracy in challenging hemodynamic situations.

REFERENCES

1. Yancy C, Abraham WT. Noninvasive hemodynamic monitoring in heart failure: utilization of impedance cardiography. Congest Heart Fail. 2003;9(5):241-50.
2. Connors AF, Speroff T, Dawson NV, Thomas C, Harrell FE Jr, Wagner D, et al. The effectiveness of right heart catheterization in the initial care of critically ill patients. JAMA. 1996;276(11):889-97.
3. Shoemaker WC, Kram HB, Appel PL. Therapy of shock based on pathophysiology, monitoring, and outcome prediction. Crit Care Med. 1990;18(1 Pt 2):S19-25.
4. Swan HJ, Ganz W, Forrester J, Marcus H, Diamond G, Chonette D. Catheterization of the heart in man with use of a flow-directed balloon-tipped catheter. N Engl J Med. 1970;283(9):447-51.
5. Sandham JD, Hull RD, Brandt RF, Knox L, Pineo GF, Doig CJ, et al. A randomized, controlled trial of the use of pulmonary-artery catheters in high-risk surgical patients. N Engl J Med. 2003;348(1):5-14.
6. Harvey S, Young D, Brampton W, Cooper AB, Doig G, Sibbald W, et al. Pulmonary artery catheters for adult patients in intensive care. Cochrane Database Syst Rev. 2006;3:CD003408.
7. Schwann NM, Mangano DT. For the Multicenter Study of Perioperative Ischemia Research Group. Pulmonary-artery catheters in high-risk surgical patients. N Engl J Med. 2003;348(20):2035-7.
8. Iberti TJ, Fischer EP, Leibowitz AB, Panacek EA, Silverstein JH, Albertson TE. A multicenter study of physician's knowledge of the pulmonary artery catheter. Pulmonary Artery Study Group. JAMA. 1990;264(22):2928-32.
9. Tuman KJ, McCarthy RJ, Spiess BD, DaValle M, Hompland SJ, Dabir R, et al. Effect of pulmonary artery catheterization on outcome in patients undergoing coronary artery surgery. Anesthesiology. 1989;70(2):199-206.
10. Osypka MJ, Bernstein DP. Electrophysiologic principles and theory of stroke volume determination by thoracic electrical bioimpedance. AACN Clin Issues. 1999;10(3):385-99.

11. Moshkovitz Y, Kaluski E, Milo O, Vered Z, Cotter G. Recent developments in cardiac output determination by bioimpedance: comparison with invasive cardiac output and potential cardiovascular applications. Curr Opin Cardiol. 2004;19(3):229-37.
12. Kubicek WG, Karnegis JN, Patterson RP, Witsoe DA, Mattson RH. Development and evaluation of an impedance cardiac output system. Aerosp Med. 1966;37(12):1208-12.
13. van de Water JM, Mount BE, Chandra KM, Mitchell BP, Woodruff TA, Dalton ML. TFC (thoracic fluid content): a new parameter for assessment of changes in chest fluid volume. Am Surg. 2005;71(1):81-6.
14. Peyton PJ, Chong SW. Minimally invasive measurement of cardiac output during surgery and critical care: a meta-analysis of accuracy and precision. Anesthesiology. 2010;113(5):1220-35.
15. Joosten A, Desebbe O, Suehiro K, Murphy LS, Essiet M, Alexander B, et al. Accuracy and precision of non-invasive cardiac output monitoring devices in perioperative medicine: a systematic review and meta- analysis. Br J Anaesth. 2017;118(3):298-310.
16. Tirotta CF, Lagueruela RG, Madril D, Velis E, Ojito J, Monroe D, et al. Non-invasive cardiac output monitor validation study in pediatric cardiac surgery patients. J Clin Anesth. 2017;38:129-32.
17. Sanidas EA, Grammatikopoulos K, Anastasiadis G, Papadopoulos D, Daskalaki M, Votteas V. Thoracic fluid content and impedance cardiography: a novel and promising noninvasive method for assessing the hemodynamic effects of diuretics in hypertensive patients. Hellenic J Cardiol. 2009;50(6):465-71.
18. Kang WS, Lee JH, Shin HJ, Kim SH, Kim TY, Seo DM, et al. Noninvasive cardiac output monitoring in paediatric cardiac surgery: correlation between change in thoracic fluid content and change in patient body weight. J Int Med Res. 2012;40(6):2295-304.
19. Pranulis M. Impedance cardiography noninvasive hemodynamicmonitoringprovidesasopportunitytodeliver cost effective quality care for patients with cardiovascular disorders. J Cardiovasc Manag. 2000;11(3):13-7.
20. Sageman WS, Amundson DE. Thoracic electrical bioimpedance measurements of cardiac output in postaortocoronary bypass patients. Crit Care Med. 1993;21(8):1139-42.
21. Appel PL, Kram HB, Mackabee J, Fleming AW, Shoemaker WC. Comparison of measurements of cardiac output by bioimpedance and thermodilution in severely ill surgical patients. Crit Care Med. 1986;14(11):933-5.
22. Gujjar AR, Muralidhar K, Bhandopadhyaya A, Sathyaprabha TN, Janaki P, Mahalla BK, et al. Transthoracic electrical bioimpedance cardiac output: comparison with multigated equilibrium radionuclide cardiography. J Clin Monit Comput. 2010;24(2):155-9.
23. Bougault V, Lonsdorfer-Wolf E, Charloux A, Richard R, Geny B, Oswald-Mammosser M. Does thoracic bioimpedance accurately determine cardiac output in COPD patients during maximal or intermittent exercise? Chest. 2005;127(4):1122-31.
24. Raue W, Swierzy M, Koplin G, Schwenk W. Comparison of electrical velocimetry and transthoracic thermodilution technique for cardiac output assessment in critically ill patients. Eur J Anaesthesiol. 2009;26(12):1067-71.
25. Liu YH, Dhakal BP, Keesakul C, Kacmarek RM, Lewis GD, Jiang Y. Continuous non-invasive cardiac output monitoring during exercise: validation of electrical cardiometry with Fick and thermodilution methods. Br J Anaesth. 2016;117(1):129-31.
26. Sharma S, Ramachandran R, Rewari V, Trikha A. Evaluation of electrical cardiometry to assess fluid responsiveness in patients with acute circulatory failure: A comparative study with transthoracic echocardiography. IJCCM. 2024;28(7):651-6
27. Squara P. Bioreactance: a new method for non-invasive cardiac output monitoring. Yearbook of Intensive Care and Emergency Medicine; 2008. pp. 619-30.
28. Suttner S, Schöllhorn T, Boldt J, Mayer J, Röhm KD, Lang K, et al. Noninvasive assessment of cardiac output using thoracic electrical bioimpedance in hemodynamically stable and unstable patients after cardiac surgery: a comparison with pulmonary artery thermodilution. Intensive Care Med. 2006;32(12):2053-8.

CHAPTER

Nexfin Noninvasive Continuous Cardiac Output Monitoring

Shweta Ram Chandankhede, Atul Prabhakar Kulkarni

INTRODUCTION

Cardiac output (CO) measurement is an essential component of the advanced hemodynamic monitor in many patients in coronary and intensive care units (ICUs). It serves as a significant prognostic parameter in critically ill patients. CO is the volume of blood pumped by the heart into the aorta per minute, calculated as the product of stroke volume (SV) and heart rate (HR). It is a crucial parameter in evaluating cardiac function and is fundamental in diagnosing, treating, and determining the prognosis of cardiovascular diseases. Maintaining optimal hemodynamic conditions ensures adequate tissue oxygenation and homeostasis, reducing the rate of complications, especially during critical phase. CO can be measured using either invasive or less invasive techniques.[1]

PURPOSES OF CARDIAC OUTPUT MEASUREMENT

Identifying Types of Circulatory Shock

Types of Circulatory Shock and Cardiac Output Measurement

Cardiac output measurement is crucial for identifying various types of circulatory shock. SV depends on ventriculoarterial (VA) coupling, assessed by the end-systolic elastance (Ees) to arterial elastance (Ea) ratio. A normal Ees/Ea ratio (1–2) supports optimal stroke work and cardiac efficiency.

Different shock types exhibit distinct VA coupling characteristics:

- *Low CO shocks:* Include cardiogenic, hypovolemic, and obstructive shocks, indicating inadequate oxygen delivery.
- *High CO shocks:* Seen in distributive shocks like septic shock, which may feature elevated CO unless there is myocardial depression or cardiac dysfunction.

Guiding Fluid Therapy

In circulatory shock management, fluid administration is critical for enhancing tissue perfusion and oxygenation. Determining the appropriate endpoint for fluid therapy relies on assessing fluid responsiveness. This involves manipulating preload (e.g., through mini volume administration or passive leg raising) and observing changes in CO or SV. The aim is to avoid overloading the heart, ensuring it remains on the responsive portion of the Frank–Starling curve.[2,3]

INVASIVE VERSUS NONINVASIVE METHODS OF CARDIAC OUTPUT MONITORING

Advanced hemodynamic variables can help determine the nature and extent of elements contributing to circulatory shock.[4] While physical examination and simple hemodynamic variables, such as HR and blood pressure, are vital for diagnosing circulatory shock, they are unreliable for assessing a patient's volume status and predicting CO. Biochemical markers, like lactate, are useful in diagnosing circulatory insufficiency but cannot differentiate between different types of shock. Therefore, using more advanced hemodynamic variables, particularly CO, can significantly enhance clinical assessment.[5] Historically, the pulmonary artery catheter (PAC) was used for CO monitoring. However, due to the risk of serious complications from PAC installation, less invasive alternatives have been developed. For instance, transpulmonary thermodilution, which does not require right heart catheterization, is now widely accepted. Additionally, devices that do not require central venous catheterization, or are completely noninvasive, are becoming more prevalent. These devices theoretically meet the criteria of an "ideal" hemodynamic monitoring device.[6]

Although invasive methods are still regarded as the gold standard for hemodynamic evaluation by experts, noninvasive methods are gaining prominence due to their safety and accessibility.

Many newer technologies offer less invasive approaches than the PAC for measuring CO with similar accuracy. A significant recent development in this field is the introduction of uncalibrated continuous CO technologies. These technologies, typically based on pulse contour methods, compute CO values from the blood pressure waveform without using intermittent thermodilution for calibration.

Although the absolute accuracy of some of these technologies may not match that of intermittent thermodilution, they generally provide good tracking accuracy. This makes them valuable tools for assessing hemodynamic events with short time constants, such as fluid loading, passive leg raising, and the initiation of inotropes. An example of this technology is the Nexfin HD, which not only falls into the category of continuous CO monitors but also offers the unique feature of total noninvasiveness.[7,8]

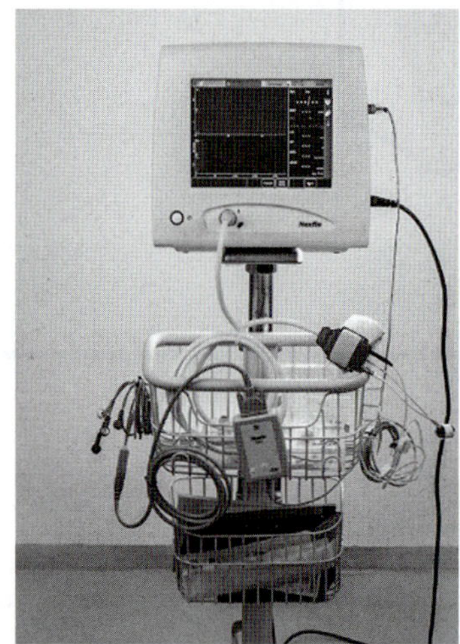

Fig. 1: Nexfin monitor *(For color version, see Plate 1)*.

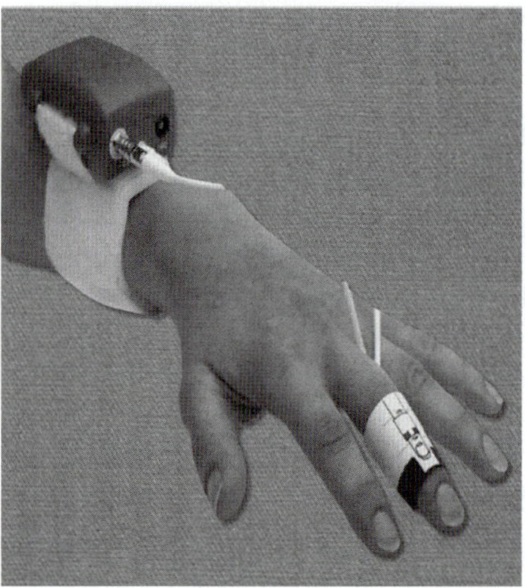

Fig. 2: Finger cuff *(For color version, see Plate 1)*.

THE MONITOR

The Nexfin HD monitor measures continuous CO through an inflatable finger cuff, the sole patient interface. It combines continuous blood pressure monitoring with the Nexfin CO-Trek pulse contour method, based on systolic pressure area and a physiological three-element Windkessel model. CO is calculated without external calibration, though it can be calibrated externally, if needed. The Nexfin HD measures several parameters other than continuous CO like continuous blood pressure (systolic, diastolic, and mean), HR, SV, systemic vascular resistance (SVR), and an index of left ventricular (LV) contractility (dP/dt).[9]

The components of the Nexfin HD include a monitor unit **(Fig. 1)** with an intuitive touch screen and internal data storage, a compact and lightweight wrist unit, and finger cuff sensors in small (S) and medium (M) sizes.

The Nexfin monitor consists of several key components that enable its function:

- *Finger cuff:* A noninvasive cuff placed on the patient's finger to capture arterial pressure waveforms **(Fig. 2)**.
- *Signal processing unit:* Processes the pressure waveforms from the finger cuff to estimate beat-to-beat SV and CO.
- *CO-trek algorithm* An algorithm that transforms finger blood pressure into brachial artery waveforms, which serve as a substitute for aortic pressure in CO calculation.
- *Display unit:* Shows real-time hemodynamic parameters such as CO, SV, and arterial pressure.
- *User interface:* Intuitive controls and display interface for healthcare providers to monitor and interpret data.
- *Data storage and connectivity:* Capabilities for data storage and possibly connectivity for data transfer to electronic medical records or other systems.
- *Power supply:* Typically powered by mains electricity or battery, ensuring continuous operation.

These components work together to provide continuous, noninvasive monitoring of CO and other hemodynamic parameters.

PRINCIPLES OF CONTINUOUS CARDIAC OUTPUT MEASUREMENT USING THE NEXFIN HD

The Nexfin HD measures continuous CO in three steps:[8]

1. Continuous beat-by-beat finger blood pressure measurement.
2. Transformation of this curve into a brachial arterial blood pressure waveform.
3. Calculation of CO from the brachial pressure pulse contour.

Measurement of Continuous Finger Blood Pressure

To measure continuous beat-by-beat blood pressure, a cuff is wrapped around the middle phalanx of the 2nd, 3rd, or 4th finger. This cuff includes an LED emitter-detector to measure the diameter of finger arteries **(Fig. 3)**. The cuff pressure adjusts to keep the artery diameter constant throughout the cardiac cycle, generating a real-time arterial pressure waveform. Initial calibration takes 1–2 minutes, after which the Nexfin uses an auto-calibration algorithm ("Physiocal") for periodic recalibration. The system adjusts pressure at three levels to maintain accuracy, with calibration intervals varying from 5 to 70 beats depending on signal stability. A "heart reference system" (HRS) corrects for height differences between the cuff and heart, allowing free hand movement.[8]

Transformation of Finger Blood Pressure to Brachial Artery Waveform

The Nexfin HD addresses the influence of measurement site on pulse contour algorithms by transforming finger blood pressure into a brachial artery waveform. Using a transfer function based on extensive clinical data, it corrects for the brachial-finger pressure gradient. This transformation allows the brachial pressure waveform to serve as a reliable substitute for aortic pressure in continuous CO measurement, eliminating the need for upper arm cuff calibration.[7]

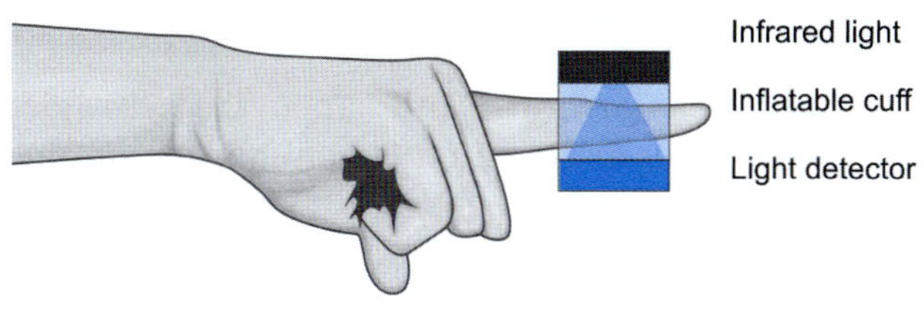

Fig. 3: Finger inflatable cuff with infrared light source and light detector.

Calculation of Continuous Cardiac Output from Brachial Arterial Pressure

The Nexfin HD calculates continuous CO using pulse contour algorithms that originated from Otto Frank's two-element Windkessel model. These algorithms utilize the relationship between cardiac systole and arterial input impedance to estimate SV and arterial pressures. Initially described by Wesseling and colleagues in 1983, the corrected characteristic impedance (cZ) method integrates the systolic arterial pressure pulse area, adjusting for mean arterial pressure (MAP) and HR. This approach required patient-specific calibration and did not fully account for compliance changes or extreme vascular conditions. To improve accuracy, Wesseling later developed the Modelflow method in 1993, which simulates a physiological, age-dependent three-element Windkessel model to better describe aortic arterial input impedance and LV afterload.[8,10-12]

Characteristic Impedance and Nexfin CO-trek Algorithm

Characteristic impedance reflects the combined effects of aortic compliance (C) and inertance (L) during left heart ejection into the proximal aorta. It is calculated as $\sqrt{(L/C)}$, where inertia opposes ejection and compliance facilitates it. Total arterial compliance (Cw) sums the elastic storage capacities of major arteries, primarily the aorta. Total peripheral resistance (Rp) sums all small artery, arteriole, and capillary resistances during diastole.[8]

The Nexfin CO-trek algorithm, introduced in 2007, calculates beat-to-beat SV using an updated pulse contour method. It integrates the systolic pressure-time integral akin to the cZ method, using reconstructed brachial arterial pressure as a proxy for aortic pressure input. Afterload is determined from a three-element Windkessel model incorporating patient-specific parameters (age, gender, height, and weight). This model adjusts for varying arterial pressure levels and computes SV by dividing the pressure-time integral by resulting impedance (Zin).[12,13]

ASSESSMENT OF VALIDITY OF THE NEXFIN HD

The Nexfin HD's CO-trek algorithm has limited published validation studies. However, previous pulse contour methods such as cZ and Modelflow have been extensively validated in high-risk surgical and intensive care settings. Studies in cardiac and liver transplant surgeries showed excellent correlation with thermodilution CO, a gold standard method involving multiple injections over the ventilatory cycle for accuracy.[13]

In a study involving coronary artery bypass graft (CABG) surgery patients, the Modelflow method demonstrated superior accuracy in absolute values and tracking changes in CO compared to other algorithms. Another study compared Modelflow with FloTrac and transesophageal ultrasonic systems in ICU patients, finding Modelflow to have the best precision and smallest limits of agreement (LA).[14]

Studies have shown a good correlation between Nexfin HD and PAC measurements in severely ill patients, despite retrospective data analysis and concurrent norepinephrine use. The Nexfin HD was noted for its safety, ease of use, and potential to provide rapid hemodynamic insights in critical situations, serving as a bridge to more invasive monitoring, if needed.[15]

In another study, CO measured by the Nexfin CO-trek was compared with the inert gas rebreathing method during exercise. It revealed a strong correlation between the two methods, particularly converging well for higher CO values.[16]

In a study comparing noninvasive continuous arterial waveform analysis (Nexfin) with transthoracic Doppler echocardiography (TTE) for CO monitoring, the findings suggest that despite the known precision limits of ±30% with Doppler echocardiography, there is reasonable agreement between the noninvasive CO measurements obtained with Nexfin and TTE.[17]

In another study by Bubenek Turconi et al., the Nexfin provided reliable tracking of preload-induced changes in CO in stable patients following cardiac surgery, despite moderate vasopressor and inotropic therapy. While it showed limited accuracy compared to PACs, its noninvasiveness, quick setup, and user-friendly design made it suitable for perioperative CO monitoring.[18]

In a study by Ameloot et al., Nexfin, a noninvasive continuous hemodynamic monitoring device, was validated against continuous pulse contour and intermittent transpulmonary thermodilution-derived CO measurements in critically ill patients. The study found that Nexfin demonstrated moderate to strong correlation with CO measurements obtained from pulse index continuous cardiac output (PiCCO), an invasive method. Despite a noted high percentage error (PE), Nexfin proved effective in monitoring CO changes over time, highlighting its utility in evaluating treatment effects in diverse ICU patient populations.[19]

In critical care settings, Nexfin's CO trending was less reliable, with 84% concordance and challenges in some patients. Finger plethysmography detects distal arterial waveforms, potentially offering better reliability in CO trend analysis during anesthesia.[20,21]

ADVANTAGES[22]

- *Patient safety:*
  - Eliminates arterial cannulation and associated complications.
  - Avoids injections of drugs, dyes, or tracers.
  - Provides real-time continuous monitoring for precise correlation with clinical events.
  - Enables early detection of instability.
  - Uses a comfortable noninvasive finger cuff for patients.
- *Streamlined patient management:*
  - Saves time and reduces morbidity by avoiding invasive procedures.
  - Streamlines care with continuous monitoring and precise diagnostics.
  - Facilitates accurate and adjustable treatment.
  - Reduces nursing time spent on manual measurements and data recording.
- *Immediate diagnostic feedback:*
  - Provides instant assessment of diagnostic test or intervention outcomes.
- *Optimized management:*
  - Enhances management of blood pressure, CO, pharmacological treatment, or pacemaker settings.
- *Early warning system:*
  - Detects sudden hemodynamic changes in real-time, alerting to potential serious clinical events.
- *Immediate response capability:*
  - Enables prompt and accurate clinician interventions based on continuous monitoring, optimizing patient outcomes.
- *Cost efficiency:*
  - Enables sophisticated hemodynamic monitoring noninvasively, reducing the need for expensive ICU resources or costly echocardiographic procedures.

- *Lower acuity setting:*
  - Provides monitoring in a more comfortable and less costly environment compared to traditional intensive care settings.
- *Ease of use:*
  - Simple application of the finger cuff in seconds.
  - Intuitive, portable monitor that is easy to operate.
- *Patient comfort:*
  - Comfortable technology that accommodates patient motion, suitable for awake patients, exercise, and transport.
- *Flexible monitoring:*
  - The monitor enables blood pressure and CO measurements for spot checks or extended periods, adaptable to various settings.
  - Ideal for inpatient care, clinical offices, laboratories, and specialized diagnostic tests such as syncope evaluations, pacemaker optimization, and exercise testing.

LIMITATIONS OF NEXFIN IN INTENSIVE CARE UNIT SETTINGS[19]

- *Accuracy and precision:* Nexfin's broad LA lead to potentially clinically unacceptable variability in CO measurements, with true values often ranging widely around calculated values.
- *Reliability issues:* Nexfin's reliability diminishes in patients with hypothermia or conditions like cardiogenic shock, where it tends to overestimate CO, compared to more invasive methods like PiCCO.
- *Complementary monitoring needed:* Nexfin cannot replace invasive arterial lines, essential for continuous monitoring of blood gases and lactate, crucial in critical care management.
- *Calibration challenges:* In unstable patients, varying conditions of preload, afterload, or contractility necessitate frequent recalibration of CO devices.
- *Practical limitations:* Nexfin may fail to record measurements due to finger hypoperfusion in a notable percentage of patients, limiting its applicability.
- Limitations of the Nexfin system include incompatibility with severe peripheral vasoconstriction, highly edematous fingers, regurgitant aortic valve conditions, and proximal aortic aneurysms. Continuous CO monitoring using the finger cuff is restricted to a maximum of 8 hours per finger. With the latest system featuring two finger cuffs, continuous use is limited to a maximum of 72 hours.[23]

UTILITY OF NEXFIN CONTINUOUS CARDIAC OUTPUT MONITORING[8,9]

- Nexfin provides continuous CO monitoring without the need for invasive procedures, broadening its applicability across diverse patient populations.
- Useful cardiology for tilt-tests to detect orthostatic hypotension, diagnosis, and management of syncope.
- Nexfin enables real-time monitoring during various diagnostic and therapeutic challenges such as passive leg raising, fluid challenges, and exercise.
- In perioperative care, especially for high-risk patients, Nexfin's noninvasive approach is advantageous. It avoids complications associated with invasive methods while supporting continuous hemodynamic optimization and monitoring.
- Useful in neurology patients with autonomic dysfunction.

CONCLUSION

Nexfin continuous CO monitoring represents a significant advancement in hemodynamic monitoring, offering real-time and noninvasive assessment of cardiac function across a wide spectrum of clinical settings. Its ability to provide continuous, accurate data, without the need for invasive procedures, makes it particularly valuable in optimizing patient care, from perioperative management to critical care scenarios. While acknowledging its limitations in certain clinical contexts, Nexfin's versatility and reliability in tracking hemodynamic changes underscore its role as a valuable tool for enhancing patient safety and clinical outcomes. Definitive recommendations for the routine clinical use of the Nexfin system will be well-supported once phase III studies confirm its clinical utility and outcomes across various patient subgroups and surgical contexts. As technology continues to evolve, Nexfin stands at the forefront of noninvasive monitoring solutions, promising continued advancements in cardiovascular care.

REFERENCES

1. McGuinness S, Parke R. Using cardiac output monitoring to guide perioperative haemodynamic therapy. Curr Opin Crit Care. 2015;21(4):364-8.
2. Huang SJ. Measuring cardiac output at the bedside. Curr Opin Crit Care. 2019;25(3):266-72.
3. Monnet X, Marik PE, Teboul J-L. Prediction of fluid responsiveness: an update. Ann Intensive Care. 2016; 6(1):1-11.

4. Perel A, Saugel B, Teboul J-L, Malbrain ML, Belda FJ, Fernández-Mondéjar E, et al. The effects of advanced monitoring on hemodynamic management in critically ill patients: a pre and post questionnaire study. J Clin Monit Comput. 2016;30(5):511-8.
5. Hiemstra B, Eck RJ, Keus F, van der Horst ICC. Clinical examination for diagnosing circulatory shock. Curr Opin Crit Care. 2017;23(4):293-301.
6. Clement RP, Vos JJ, Scheeren TWL. Minimally invasive cardiac output technologies in the ICU: putting it all together. Curr Opin Crit Care. 2017;23(4):302-9.
7. Camporota L, Beale R. Pitfalls in hemodynamic monitoring based on the arterial pressure waveform. Crit Care. 2010;14(2):124.
8. Perel A, Settels JJ. Totally non-invasive continuous cardiac output measurement with the Nexfin CO-Trek. In: Vincent JL (Ed). Annual Update in Intensive Care and Emergency Medicine, Volume 1. Berlin, Heidelberg: Springer; 2011.
9. Perel A, Wesselink WA, Settels J. The Nexfin Monitor—A totally non-invasive cardiac output monitor. In: Gullo A (Ed). Anaesthesia, Pharmacology, Intensive Care and Emergency Medicine A.P.I.C.E. Milano: Springer; 2011. pp. 103-8.
10. Truijen J, van Lieshout JJ, Wesselink WA, Westerhof BE. Noninvasive continuous hemodynamic monitoring. J Clin Monit Comput. 2012;26(4):267-78.
11. Wesseling KH, de Wit B, Weber JA, Smith NT. A simple device for continuous measurement of cardiac output. Adv Cardiovasc Phys. 1983;5:16-52.
12. Wesseling KH, Jansen JRC, Settels JJ, Schreuder JJ. Computation of aortic flow from pressure in humans using a nonlinear, three-element model. J Appl Physiol. 1993;74(5):2566-73.
13. Jansen JRC, Schreuder JJ, Mulier JP, Smith NT, Settels JJ, Wesseling KH. A comparison of cardiac output derived from the arterial pressure wave against thermodilution in cardiac surgery patients. Br J Anaesth. 2001;87(2):212-22.
14. de Wilde RBP, Schreuder JJ, van den Berg PCM, Jansen JR. An evaluation of cardiac output by five pulse contour techniques during cardiac surgery. Anaesthesia. 2007;62(8):760-8.
15. Stover JF, Stocker R, Lenherr R, Neff TA, Cottini SR, Zoller B, et al. Noninvasive cardiac output and blood pressure monitoring cannot replace an invasive monitoring system in critically ill patients. BMC Anesthesiol. 2009;9:6.
16. Bartels SA, Stok WJ, Bezemer R, Boksem RJ, Van GJ, Cherpanath TG, et al. Noninvasive cardiac output monitoring during exercise testing: Nexfin pulse contour analysis compared to an inert gas rebreathing method and respired gas analysis. J Clin Monit Comput. 2011;25(5):315-21.
17. van der Spoel AG, Voogel AJ, Folkers A, Boer C, Bouwman RA. Comparison of noninvasive continuous arterial waveform analysis (Nexfin) with transthoracic Doppler echocardiography for monitoring of cardiac output. J Clin Anesth. 2012;24(4):304-9.
18. Bubenek-Turconi SI, Craciun M, Miclea I, Perel A. Noninvasive continuous cardiac output by the Nexfin before and after preload-modifying maneuvers: a comparison with intermittent thermodilution cardiac output. Anesth Analg. 2013;117(2):366-72.
19. Ameloot K, Van De Vijver K, Broch O, Van Regenmortel N, De Laet I, Schoonheydt K, et al. Nexfin noninvasive continuous hemodynamic monitoring: validation against continuous pulse contour and intermittent transpulmonary thermodilution derived cardiac output in critically ill patients. Scientific World Journal. 2013;2013:519080.
20. Monnet X, Picard F, Lidzborski E, Mesnil M, Duranteau J, Richard C, et al. The estimation of cardiac output by the Nexfin device is of poor reliability for tracking the effects of a fluid challenge. Crit Care. 2012;16(5):R212.
21. Taton O, Fagnoul D, De Backer D, Vincent JL. Evaluation of cardiac output in intensive care using a non-invasive arterial pulse contour technique (Nexfin((R)) compared with echocardiography. Anaesthesia. 2013;68(9):917-23.
22. BMEYE. BMEYE monitor series. [online] Available from https://medaval.ie/docs/specs/BMEYE-Nexfin-Specs.pdf [Last accessed October, 2024].
23. Kerstens MK, Wijnberge M, Geerts BF, Vlaar APJ. Non-invasive cardiac output monitoring techniques in the ICU. Netherlands Journal of Critical Care. 2018;26(3):104-10.

SECTION

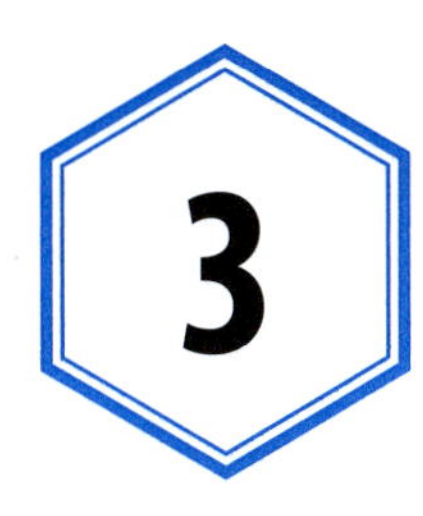

Downstream Parameters and Others

Clinical Assessment of a Patient with Shock

Jacob George Pulinilkunnathil, Jigeeshu Vasistha Divatia, Atul Prabhakar Kulkarni

INTRODUCTION

Clinical examination of a patient in shock is a fount of information, which often goes ignored due to fascination of the intensivists toward more glamorous monitors, gadgets, and tests. Careful clinical examination can help in ascertaining presence of a problem, gauge response to therapy, stratify the risk of developing complication, and prognosticate likely outcome. The patient in shock offers various windows to look at the tissue perfusion, such as, altered mentation, cold, clammy peripheries, and decreased urine output. Early identification of these clinical signs is of paramount importance for diagnosing shock at an early stage **(Fig. 1)**.

EXAMINATION OF SKIN IN SHOCK

Skin is the largest organ in the body; which is easily visible, readily accessible, and provides vital information in patients with shock. Basic clinical examination including inspection of color for mottling, palpation for temperature gradients, and capillary refill time (CRT), can provide in-depth knowledge of local microcirculatory perfusion. As examination of the skin is easy, noninvasive, rapidly diagnostic, and highly informative regarding the microcirculation, experts have suggested integrating the skin perfusion parameters in defining and treating shock.

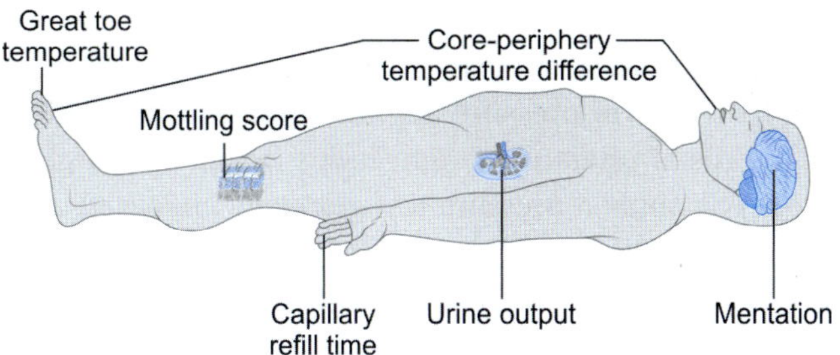

Fig. 1: Windows for assessment of circulation.

Examination of the skin in patients with shock is detailed in the following text.

TEMPERATURE DIFFERENCE

Cutaneous circulation lacks autoregulation unlike other organs and is under neurohumoral control. Therefore, in cases of circulatory insufficiency, the capillaries undergo immediate vasospasm as blood is shunted to the vital organs. These patients rapidly lose temperature and are usually hypothermic. Thus, measuring the temperature can provide early useful information regarding the patient status and prognosis. Temperature monitoring at the bedside is easily available, requires no sophisticated tools, and causes no/minimum discomfort to the patient. Therefore, the value for temperature monitoring is strongly emphasized in clinical examination of patients with shock.

The first study measuring the temperature gradients between rectal temperature and surface temperature in patients with shock was carried out as early as 1967.[1] Later studies showed that the decline in toe temperature significantly correlated with drop in cardiac index and values of cardiac index <2 L/min/m^2 was associated with toe temperatures <27°C.[2] Further studies showed that irrespective of the etiology of shock, increase in toe temperature correlated well with lactate clearance and improvement in cardiac output. The temperature gradient from forearm-to-fingertip has also been evaluated as a marker of vasoconstriction in shock and a temperature gradient cutoff of 4°C has been considered as marker for severe vasoconstriction.[3,4] Accurate measurement of temperature is not mandatory and simple subjective assessment of patient's temperature as warm or cool has also been shown to accurately identify patients with reduced cardiac output, tissue hypoperfusion, and high lactate levels.[5]

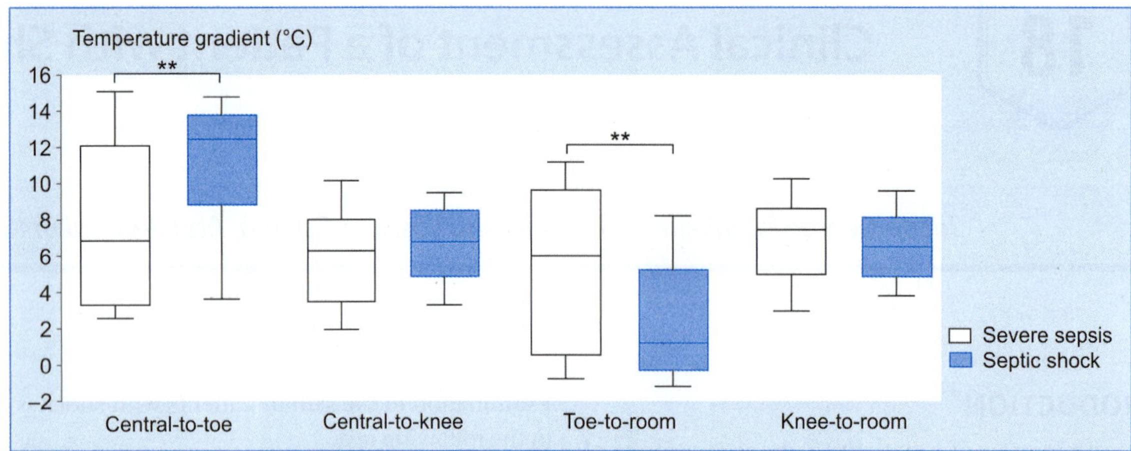

Fig. 2: Temperature gradients measured at 6 hours in patients with severe sepsis or septic shock.
**$p < 0.01$.
Source: Adapted from Bourcier S, Pichereau C, Boelle PY, Nemlaghi S, Dubée V, Lejour G, et al. Toe-to-room temperature gradient correlates with tissue perfusion and predicts outcome in selected critically ill patients with severe infections. Ann Intensive Care. 2016;6(1):63. Permits unrestricted use, distribution, and reproduction in any medium, provided you give appropriate credit to the original author(s) and the source, provide a link to the Creative Commons license, and indicate if changes were made. © The Author(s) 2016 (http://creativecommons.org/licenses/by/4.0/).

Numerous studies have confirmed the correlation of skin temperature not only to suboptimal hemodynamic variables but also to predictors of intensive care unit (ICU) outcome **(Fig. 2)**. Temperature gradient between toe and ambient temperature <3°C is found to be a significant predictor of mortality.[6] The temperature gradient has been shown not only to predict poor cardiac output state, but also to herald recovery, even before the oxygen partial pressure starts to increase.[7,8]

CAPILLARY REFILL TIME

Capillary refill time is another valuable, noninvasive, inexpensive, and quick test available at the bedside for assessing the tissue perfusion in critically ill patients. It was proposed as a parameter for assessing shock as early as 1947.[9] A firm pressure is applied to the distal phalanx of the index finger till it blanches and the time taken for normal color to return is measured. The normal value of CRT varies according to age, gender, pressure applied, presence of ambient light, temperature, choice of limb, etc. CRT is usually performed in the upper limb, positioned above heart level as normal values may be normally obtained in lower limbs or due to passive venous filling. In pediatrics, CRT can be measured by applying pressure to the sternum also. The normal values of CRT measured by chronometer is suggested to be 2.9 seconds in adult women and 4.5 seconds in elderly.[10] Ideally, CRT should be measured at the bedside by applying a uniform pressure of 3–7 N for 2 seconds and the response time should be measured with a chronometer.[11] Prolonged CRT is a marker of tissue hypoperfusion and has also been proven to be a predictor of mortality in critically ill patients.[12] Similar studies in sepsis patients have shown that CRT was highly reproducible, correlated well with other parameters of tissue hypoperfusion and with illness severity and CRT dynamics help in assessing prognosis.[13] Apart from diagnosing hypoperfusion, CRT can also be used to aid in resuscitation. In a recent trial that looked upon CRT versus lactate for resuscitating patients with shock, the authors found a trend toward mortality in favor of CRT as compared to resuscitation with lactate levels.[14] However, other parameters such as mechanical ventilation-free days and renal replacement-free days were similar between the groups. The researchers had standardized measurement of CRT as a firm pressure applied to the ventral surface of the distal phalanx of right index finger with a glass slide. The applied pressure was gradually increased until the skin blanched and they maintained the pressure for 10 seconds. A CRT >3 seconds was taken as abnormal. With improvement in technology, newer devices may come up with automated CRT measuring technologies. A pilot study using a quantitative CRT with help of a device using the principle of pulse oximeter principle, found that CRT times >6–8 seconds correlated well with tissue hypoperfusion and hyperlactatemia.[14,15]

MOTTLING SCORE

Mottling of the skin due to heterogeneous vasoconstriction of the microcirculation is classically described as an erythematous-violaceous hue of the skin that starts around the knees and progressively spreads bidirectionally. This is usually due to the presence of high density of noradrenergic receptors located in knee region causing vasospasm and tissue hypoperfusion with reduced tissue oxygen saturation. Mottling of skin is a common occurrence in patients with sepsis and has an incidence ranging from 46 to 70%. Skin mottling can be quantified from a score of 0–5 based on the area of mottling with a score of 0 indicating no mottling while a score of 5 suggestive of severe mottling spreading beyond the groin fold. As it is a sign of tissue hypoperfusion, skin mottling is strongly correlated with lactate levels and 14-day mortality **(Fig. 3)**.

The area of laser Doppler scanning superposed to the area of mottling score classification can give additional information such as quantification of perfusion in areas of mottling and sequential measures can help to follow up the results of resuscitation **(Fig. 4)**.[16]

Peripheral perfusion index (PPI) is the ratio of pulsatile blood flow to nonpulsatile blood flow. It is calculated from pulse oximetry based upon the amount of infrared light that is getting absorbed. The amount of light absorbed has both pulsatile component and nonpulsatile components.

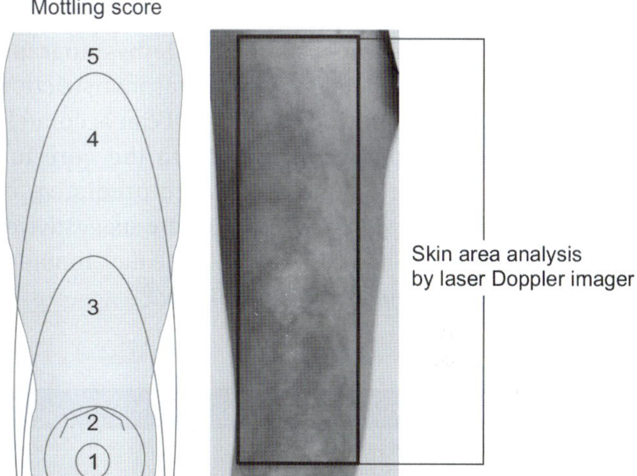

Fig. 3: Mottling score based on mottling area extension on legs. [Score 0: No mottling; Score 1: Modest mottling area (coin size) localized to the center of the knee; Score 2: Moderate mottling area that does not exceed the superior edge of the kneecap; Score 3: Mild mottling area that does not exceed the middle thigh; Score 4: Severe mottling area that does not exceed the fold of the groin; and Score 5: Extremely severe mottling area that exceeds the fold of the groin]. *(For color version, see Plate 1).*

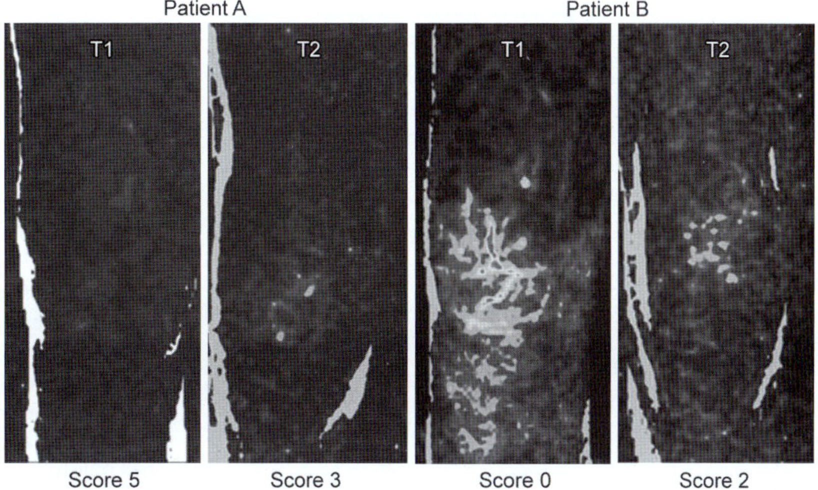

Fig. 4: Examples of laser Doppler images. In patient A, the mottling score decreased from 5 to 3 (improved), whereas in patient B mottling score increased (worsened) from 0 to 2. *(For color version, see Plate 2).*

Source: Adapted from Ait-Oufella H, Bourcier S, Alves M, Galbois A, Baudel JL, Margetis D, et al. Alteration of skin perfusion in mottling area during septic shock. Ann Intensive Care. 2013;3(1):31.

The pulsatile component occurs due to changes in the arterial blood volume and arterial flow, while the nonpulsatile part of absorption is contributed to by the venous blood and extravascular tissues. The advantage is that it can be estimated from the pulse oximeter trace. The drawbacks include dependence on a good plethysmograph trace and provision of highly selective regional perfusion. Factors affecting plethysmograph trace such as tissue edema or severe vasoconstriction may impede the data provided by PPI. PPI can accurately predict tissue hypoperfusion, similar to the core-toe temperature gradient. Values <1.4 were predictive of poor tissue perfusion while values >3.5 were suggestive of severe vasodilatation and could predict the development of hypotension following spinal anesthesia.[17,18]

URINE OUTPUT

Oliguria is an early manifestation of shock, and monitoring urine output can be used as an important sign of hypovolemia. Urine flow rate per minute has been evaluated and found to be an accurate predictor of hypovolemia in spinal surgeries and in trauma victims. The urine flow rate variability has also been shown to be a sensitive and early predictor of hypotension and hypovolemia in trauma patients. However, the applicability of it in critically ill patients need further validation as other factors such as intrinsic renal disease, postrenal obstruction, drugs can all affect the urine output.[19,20] A summary of monitoring peripheral perfusion is given in **Table 1**.

TABLE 1: Peripheral perfusion monitoring.

Method of clinical assessment	*Parameter monitored*	*Advantages*	*Disadvantages*
Examination	Mentation	Easy to assess even before clinical examination	Confounded by the presence of drugs and toxins
	Urine output	Easy and relatively cheap, universal in all critically ill patients	Confounded by obstruction, intrinsic kidney disease, endogenous release of antidiuretic hormone as a stress response, nephrotoxic drugs, etc.
Palpation	Temperature	Easily measured and cheap, available universally, minimal patient discomfort	• Subjective measurements such as cold or warm may not be helpful in prognosis. Accurate estimation of temperature is required, which can be time consuming in busy units • Body temperature can be affected by ambient room temperature, application of warmers or blankets during transport, etc. • It does not give a real time monitoring of perfusion • Temperatures of extremities are highly susceptible to ambient temperature changes • Subjective difference of the application of pressure can vary the results • Duration for which pressure is applied can also affect the result • Accurate assessment of CRT is significantly affected by the presence of nail polish • Exact duration of pressure application needs to be accurately measured preferably with a chronometer
	Temperature gradient	A temperature difference >4°C between forearm-finger or 7°C between core temperature and toe temperature has been shown to be associated with increased morbidity and mortality	
	Capillary refill time (CRT)	Time-tested practice to assess perfusion. Values >4.5 have been shown to be associated with increased mortality	

Contd...

Contd...

Method of clinical assessment	***Parameter monitored***	***Advantages***	***Disadvantages***
	Skin mottling	Has been extensively studied and validated as a marker of tissue perfusion. Well delineated scoring systems with good interobserver coherence exist and a score of 4 or above is associated with increased mortality	• Difficult to appreciate in dark skin • Does not give a time frame or duration of hypoperfusion • Cannot predict organ dysfunction, i.e., mottling scores indicate organ damage but cannot predict organ damage
Plethysmography	Perfusion index	Universally available, noninvasive and cheap, minimal discomfort to patients, values <1.4% suggest hypoperfusion and values >3.5 are suggestive of extreme vasodilation	• Affected by plethysmographic trace and patient motion • Need specialized equipment which are costly • No standardized data regarding normal values to be adopted are available. Regional circulation cannot be generalized to the whole body
Near infrared spectroscopy	Microcirculation	Noninvasive, and provides quantitative information regarding the microcirculation	

HEMODYNAMIC COHERENCE

Is Resuscitation Guided by Clinical Assessment of Perfusion of the Hemodynamic End Point?

As aforementioned, a good clinical examination can give a fair idea of the tissue hypoperfusion. However, at the bedside, resuscitation targeting an improvement in these parameters may not be fruitful, and at times can be counterproductive. This is because the changes in macrocirculation and microcirculation during disease states may not run parallel to each other. Thus, understanding the concept of hemodynamic coherence during resuscitation and detection of resuscitation incoherence at the earliest is of paramount importance as it will probably help to avoid futile treatment by providing targeted resuscitation.

As resuscitation for shock is ongoing, the macrocirculatory and microcirculatory function declines. The aim of shock resuscitation is improvement of circulation at both levels. Resuscitative efforts are based on the assumption that the microcirculation and macrocirculation are in coherence, and improving one will always improve the other. This may not be the case, and decoupling of the macrocirculation and microcirculation can arise before, during, and after resuscitation as mentioned in **Figure 5**.[21] Hence, understanding the possibility of hemodynamic incoherence, identifying it early by way of monitoring of microcirculation or downstream parameters such as lactate or venous to arterial carbon dioxide (avCO_2) content makes good sense at the bedside to avoid over-resuscitation or to time active deresuscitation.

- *Type 1:* Heterogeneous perfusion of the microcirculation is typically seen in septic patients with a mix of obstructed capillaries and perfused capillaries resulting in a heterogeneous oxygenation of the tissue.
- *Type 2:* Hemodilution resulting in the loss of red blood cell (RBC)-filled capillaries and increasing diffusion distance between RBCs in the capillaries and the tissue cells.
- *Type 3:* Stasis of microcirculatory RBC flow induced by altered systemic variables [e.g., increased arterial vascular resistance (R) and/or increased venous pressures causing tamponade].
- *Type 4:* Alterations involve edema caused by capillary leak syndrome which results in increased diffusive distance and reduced ability of the oxygen to reach the tissue cells. *Red,* well-oxygenated RBC and tissue cells; *purple,* RBC with reduced oxygenation; *blue,* reduced tissue cell oxygenation. This hemodynamic incoherence at the tissue level can lead to or further complicate tissue hypoxia at cellular levels.

Thus, even after resuscitation, four clinical scenarios can be recognized at the bedside **(Fig. 6)**.[22]

- *Type 1:* Due to a macrocirculation-microcirculation decoupling.
- *Type 2:* Compensated shock

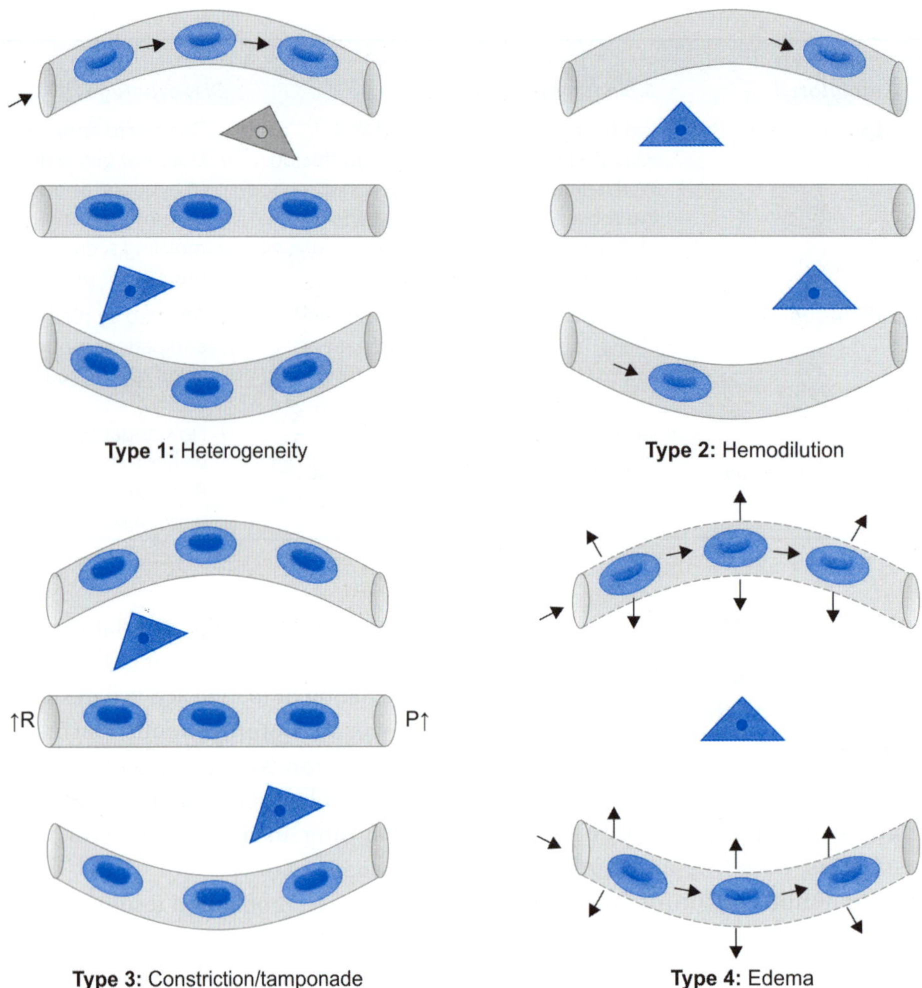

Fig. 5: Mechanisms of microcirculatory alterations with loss of hemodynamic coherence causing tissue hypoxia.
Source: Adapted from Ince C. Hemodynamic coherence and the rationale for monitoring the microcirculation. Crit Care. 2015; 19(Suppl 3):S8.

- *Type 3:* Cytopathic shock
- *Type 4:* Combined cytopathic shock with microcirculatory dysfunction.

At the bedside these changes can be summarized as given in **Table 2**.

CONCLUSION

Peripheral perfusion is a marker of the adequacy of coherence between macrocirculation and microcirculation. Apart from attaining a prespecified goal of a fixed mean arterial pressure or venous pressure for optimizing macrocirculation, other parameters of microcirculatory perfusion and cellular hypoxia need to be assessed frequently to make necessary adjustments in patient management at the bedside. Monitoring regional circulation at the bedside may not give a picture of global circulation as various regions may have variation in microcirculatory adaptations for changes in macrocirculation.[23] Hence, apart from clinical assessment of shock, monitoring regional microcirculation and global markers of microcirculation should also be taken into account.

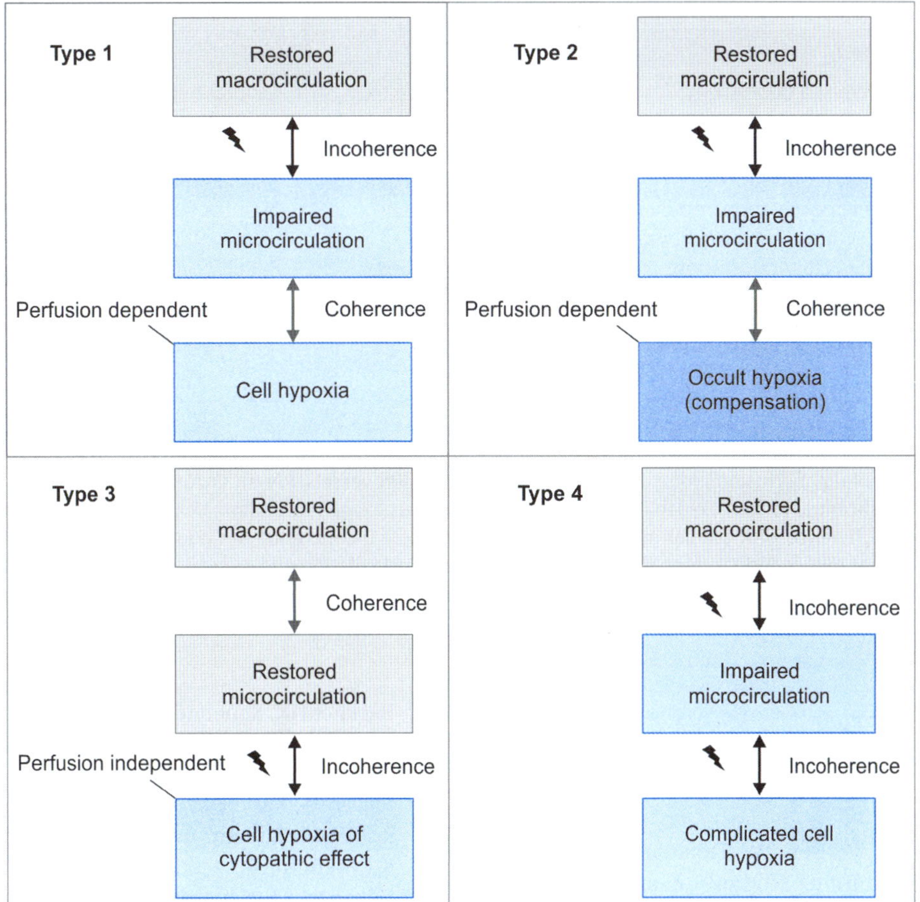

Fig. 6: Resuscitation incoherence at the bedside.

Source: Adapted from He HW, Long Y, Liu DW, Ince C. Resuscitation incoherence and dynamic circulation-perfusion coupling in circulatory shock. Chin Med J (Engl). 2019;132(10):1218-27.

TABLE 2: Classification of incoherent resuscitation as appreciated clinically.

Item	***Type 1***	***Type 2***	***Type 3***	***Type 4***
Macro: Maintained		MAP ≥65 mm Hg (or usual level) $ScvO_2$ ≥70%	$Pv\text{-}aCO_2$ ≤6 mm Hg CI >2.2 L/m^2	
Micro: Normal	• Severely impaired microcirculation with macro-micro decoupling • CRT >5 s, PI <0.6 • PPV <60%, MFI <2 • Mottling score >2 cold extremities, UO <0.3 mL/kg/min	• Mildly impaired. • CRT 2–5 s, PI 0.6–1.4 • PPV 60–80%, MFI 2–3 • Mottling score 0–2 • Cold extremities, • UO 0.3–0.5 mL/kg/min	• Normal microcirculation • CRT £2 s, PI ^{3}1.4 • PPV ≥80%, MFI ^{3}3 • Mottling score 0 • Warm extremities, • UO >0.5 mL/kg/min	• Severely impaired microcirculation and micro-macro decoupling CRT >5 s, PI <0.6 • PPV <60%, MFI <2 • Mottling score >2 cold extremities, UO <0.3 mL/kg/min

Contd...

Contd...

Item	*Type 1*	*Type 2*	*Type 3*	*Type 4*
Cellular hypoxia	• Hypoxia dependent on microcirculatory perfusion. Abnormalities may reduce once microcirculation improves • Lactate >2 mmol/L P(v-a)CO_2/C(a-v)O_2 >1.6, etc.	• Compensatory due to mechanisms • Circulatory maintaining cellular do not oxygen demand. However, if demand macro-rises, hypoxia ensues. microcirculation can help Lactate <2 mmol/L P(v-a)CO_2/C(a-v)O_2 <1.6, etc.	• Cellular hypoxia cytopathy. Changes affect the cells. No manipulation of or Lactate >2 mmol/L • P(v-a)CO_2/C(a-v)O_2 >1.6, etc.	• Microcirculatory abnormalities mask an underlying cytopathy. Even after correction of microcirculation, tissue hypoxia does not improve due to coexisting mitochondrial dysfunction • P(v-a)CO_2/C(a-v)O_2 <1.6, etc.

[CI: cardiac index; CRT: capillary refill time; MFI: microvascular flow index; Macro: macrocirculation; MAP: mean arterial pressure; Micro: microcirculation; PI: peripheral perfusion index; PPV: proportion of perfused vessels; P(v-a)CO_2/C(a-v)O_2: central venous arterial carbon dioxide difference/arterial-central venous oxygen index; ScvO_2: central venous oxygen saturation; UO: urinary output; Types of incoherences: Type 1. macro-micro incoherence with cellular hypoxia; Type 2. macro-micro incoherence but compensated resulting in normal cellular function; Type 3. persistent mitochondrial cytopathy despite restored macrocirculation and microcirculation; Type 4. Incoherence between microcirculation and mitochondria that is often masked by macro-micro circulatory incoherence].

REFERENCES

1. Joly HR, Weil MH. Temperature of the great toe as an indication of the severity of shock. Circulation. 1969;39(1):131-8.
2. Ruiz CE, Weil MH, Carlson RW. Treatment of circulatory shock with dopamine. Studies on survival. JAMA. 1979;242(2):165-8.
3. Sessler DI. Skin-temperature gradients are a validated measure of fingertip perfusion. Eur J Appl Physiol. 2003;89(3-4):401-2.
4. House JR, Tipton MJ. Using skin temperature gradients or skin heat flux measurements to determine thresholds of vasoconstriction and vasodilatation. Eur J Appl Physiol. 2002;88(1-2):141-5.
5. Kaplan LJ, McPartland K, Santora TA, Trooskin SZ. Start with a subjective assessment of skin temperature to identify hypoperfusion in intensive care unit patients. J Trauma. 2001;50(4):620-7.
6. Henning RJ, Wiener F, Valdes S, Weil MH. Measurement of toe temperature for assessing the severity of acute circulatory failure. Surg Gynecol Obstet. 1979;149(1):1-7.
7. Vincent JL, Moraine JJ, van der Linden P. Toe temperature versus transcutaneous oxygen tension monitoring during acute circulatory failure. Intensive Care Med. 1988;14(1):64-8.
8. Bourcier S, Pichereau C, Boelle PY, Nemlaghi S, Dubée V, Lejour G, et al. Toe-to-room temperature gradient correlates with tissue perfusion and predicts outcome in selected critically ill patients with severe infections. Ann Intensive Care. 2016;6(1):63.
9. Beecher HK, Simeone FA. The internal state of the severely wounded man on entry to the most forward hospital. Surgery. 1947;22(4):672-711.
10. Pickard A, Karlen W, Ansermino JM. Capillary refill time, is it still a useful sign? Anesth Analg. 2011;113(1):120-3.
11. Kawaguchi R, Nakada T, Oshima T, Shinozaki M, Nakaguchi T, Haneishi H, et al. Optimal pressing strength and time for capillary refilling time. Crit Care. 2019;23(1):4.
12. Mrgan M, Rytter D, Brabrand M. Capillary refill time is a predictor of short-term mortality for adult patients admitted to a medical department: an observational cohort study. Emerg Med J. 2014;31(12):954-8.
13. Ait-Oufella H, Bige N, Boelle PY, Pichereau C, Alves M, Bertinchamp R, et al. Capillary refill time exploration during septic shock. Intensive Care Med. 2014;40(7):958-64.
14. Hernández G, Ospina-Tascón GA, Damiani LP, Estenssoro E, Dubin A, Hurtado J, et al. Effect of a resuscitation strategy targeting peripheral perfusion status vs serum lactate levels on 28-day mortality among patients with septic shock: The ANDROMEDA- SHOCK randomized clinical trial. JAMA. 2019;321(7):654-64.
15. Morimura N, Takahashi K, Doi T, Ohnuki T, Sakamoto T, Uchida Y, et al. A pilot study of quantitative capillary refill time to identify high blood lactate levels in critically ill patients. Emerg Med J. 2015;32(6):444-8.
16. Oi Y, Sato K, Nogaki A, Matsumoto J, Abe T, Morimura N. Association between venous blood lactate levels and differences in quantitative capillary refill time. Acute Med Surg. 2018;5(4):321-8.
17. Ait-Oufella H, Bourcier S, Alves M, Galbois A, Baudel JL, Margetis D, et al. Alteration of skin perfusion in mottling

area during septic shock. Ann Intensive Care. 2013; 3(1):31.

18. Lima AP, Beelen P, Bakker J. Use of a peripheral perfusion index derived from the pulse oximetry signal as a noninvasive indicator of perfusion. Crit Care Med. 2002; 30(6):1210-3.
19. Duggappa DR, Lokesh M, Dixit A, Paul R, Raghavendra Rao RS, Prabha P. Perfusion index as a predictor of hypotension following spinal anaesthesia in lower segment caesarean section. Indian J Anaesth. 2017;61(8):649-54.
20. Shamir MY, Kaplan L, Marans RS, Willner D, Klein Y. Urine flow is a novel hemodynamic monitoring tool for the detection of hypovolemia. Anesth Analg. 2011; 112(3):593-6.
21. Brotfain E, Klein Y, Toledano R, Koyfman L, Frank D, Shamir MY, et al. Urine flow rate monitoring in hypovolemic multiple trauma patients. World J Emerg Surg. 2017;12:41.
22. Ince C. Hemodynamic coherence and the rationale for monitoring the microcirculation. Crit Care. 2015; 19(Suppl 3):S8.
23. He HW, Long Y, Liu DW, Ince C. Resuscitation incoherence and dynamic circulation-perfusion coupling in circulatory shock. Chin Med J (Engl). 2019;132(10):1218-27.

CHAPTER

Early Goal-directed Therapy, $ScvO_2$, and PCO_2 Gap

Rahul Pandit, Gurudas Sadanand Pundpal

INTRODUCTION

Sepsis and septic shock remain a leading cause of mortality across the world. Despite several years of understanding the pathophysiology, sepsis cascade, and complications, an effective treatment to reduce mortality substantially remains elusive. Though we have made several gains in the last couple of decades, there is still a quest to understand it fully and treat it effectively.

By the late 90s it was clear that sepsis causes an inflammatory cytokine cascade affecting multiple systems and having a very narrow single-prong approach was not effective. The concept of systemic inflammatory response syndrome (SIRS) was well understood.[1] It was clear that the SIRS due to infection could sometimes be self-limiting, however, it could progress on to severe sepsis and septic shock.[2] This essentially produced an imbalance between the oxygen demand and supply at the tissue level, producing global tissue hypoxia and shock. This deterioration was noted to happen quickly, almost akin to the golden hour concept in trauma. Hence, began the search for a group of therapies, if bundled together in a timely fashion, which would then be effective in counteracting the various effects of this cytokine cascade.

EARLY GOAL-DIRECTED THERAPY

The first such protocol-driven treatment approach was published by Rivers et al.[3] in 2001, where Rivers attempted to identify these patients in the emergency department by following a series of simple bedside tests or examinations which included two out of four criteria for SIRS, a systolic blood pressure <90 mm Hg after 20–30 mL/kg of crystalloid fluid challenge or a blood lactate measurement of 4 mmol/L or more. They were then randomized to receive standard care or protocol-based care for 6 hours, in the emergency department itself. The important aspect was identifying parameters that correlated or represented shock or the onset of shock, and then having a goal-based therapy to achieve certain physiological targets achieved within a time frame.

Lactate is produced due to anaerobic glycolysis, (1,400–1,500 mmol of lactate/day in an adult daily), and most of it is cleared by the liver and kidneys. Due to tissue or cellular hypoxia lactate is overproduced due to an increase in anaerobic glycolysis. The production of lactate overwhelms the clearance in sepsis and shock, compounded by liver and renal dysfunction, lactate levels rise quickly in shock. By identifying rising lactate and low blood pressure Rivers et al. were able to demonstrate that patients treated in an early protocol-based bundle of interventions had better organ function and recovery as compared to standard care.

The bundled care, apart from lactate measurement included, the insertion of the central venous catheter, with a fiberoptic tip to measure mixed central venous oxygen saturation ($ScvO_2$), targeting a mean arterial pressure (MAP) of 65 mm Hg or more, intravenous crystalloid boluses, use of vasopressors or inotropes; and blood transfusion to maintain a hematocrit of 30%. This single-center study paved the way for protocol-based treatment for sepsis. In particular, early goal-directed therapy (EGDT) formed the cornerstone of the treatment of early sepsis.

In 2004, the International Surviving Sepsis Campaign[4] (SSC) adopted this EGDT protocol and prepared a surviving sepsis bundle to be followed while treating patients with sepsis and septic shock. It consists of tasks to be completed within the first 3 hours and the first 6 hours of presentation.

To be completed within 3 hours:

- Measure lactate level
- Obtain blood cultures before administration of antibiotics
- Administration of broad-spectrum antibiotics
- Administration of 30 mL/kg crystalloids.

To be completed within 6 hours:

- Apply vasopressors to maintain MAP >65 mm Hg
- In the event of persistent hypotension despite volume resuscitation or initial lactate >4:
  - Measure central venous pressure (CVP)
  - Measure $ScvO_2$
- Remeasure lactate if initial lactate was high. Targets—CVP > 8 mm Hg, $ScvO_2$ >70%.

The following two surviving sepsis guidelines[5,6] also included a large aspect of EGDT; however, the results of several other similar single-center trials and adherence to surviving sepsis guidelines were found to be inconsistent across the world.[7] The other aspect was the significant difference in the patient-population in other hospitals and countries as compared to the Rivers study. There was increasing evidence of volume overload, such as acute pulmonary edema, abdominal compartment syndrome, etc., high inotropic requirements causing arrhythmias and myocardial necrosis along with excess oxygen delivery in the EGDT group. EGDT was only validated in emergency department patients and not in intensive care unit (ICU) patients, also none of the oxygen delivery endpoints were validated and hence utility of $ScvO_2$ was questioned, compounded with adverse effects of blood transfusion. All this compared with varying baseline mortality in sepsis led to a series of multicenter trials that looked at replicating EGDT.

Between 2014 and 2015, three large randomized controlled trials (RCTs) to retest the effect of EGDT on the outcome of patients with severe sepsis and septic shock were conducted. The trials were conducted in different parts of the world, ProCESS (Protocolized Care for Early Septic Shock)[8] trial in the United States, the ARISE (Australasian Resuscitation in Sepsis Evaluation)[9] trial in Australia, and the ProMISE (Protocolized Management of Sepsis)[10] trial in England. Unfortunately, all three trials conducted in different geographical locations failed to demonstrate any mortality benefit. There was no demonstrable treatment effect in any subgroup of patients. However, it was noticed that the usual care of septic patients had improved considerably in the last decade and a half and hence perhaps there was no demonstrable treatment effect. Also, it was clear that appropriate antibiotics along with source control and hemodynamic resuscitation now formed the cornerstone of sepsis management.

In summary, in sepsis management early antibiotic therapy, and targeted and adequate resuscitation seem to help most patients. Use of EGDT with the early placement of a central venous catheter, monitoring $ScvO_2$, and hematocrit-targeted red blood cell (RBC) transfusion did not show any added benefit over usual care of septic shock and severe sepsis.

CENTRAL VENOUS OXIMETRY AND VENOARTERIAL CARBON DIOXIDE TENSION DIFFERENCE (PCO_2 GAP)

The function of the cardiovascular system is to deliver adequate oxygen and other nutrients to tissue as per demand. When the cardiovascular system is unable to fulfill the tissue demands shock occurs. The focus of primary pathophysiology responsible for multiorgan dysfunction is shifting from macrocirculatory to microcirculatory dysfunction. One of the most important factors determining organ dysfunction in shock is sustained tissue hypoxia. So, it is imperative to diagnose and treat tissue hypoxia in its initial stages. Unfortunately, parameters, such as pulse, blood pressure, blood gas, and CVP are poor predictors of tissue hypoxia. Tissue perfusion and oxygenation are assessed by measurement of lactate level, but some trials have given conflicting evidence about the use of lactate to offer survival benefits. This led to a search for new simple parameters for the assessment of the adequacy of oxygen delivery and perfusion at the tissue level. Mixed venous oxygen saturation,[11,12] a marker of global tissue oxygenation, and venoarterial carbon dioxide tension [partial pressure of carbon dioxide (PCO_2) gap], a marker of the adequacy of global tissue perfusion; are helpful guides in the optimization of resuscitation in patients with septic shock.

Physiology

Whole-body oxygen delivery (DO_2) is a product of cardiac output (CO) and arterial oxygen content.

$$DO_2 = CO \times CaO_2$$

Arterial O_2 content is, the sum of oxygen bound to hemoglobin and dissolved in the blood.

$$CaO_2 = (Hb \times 1.34 \times SaO_2) + (PaO_2 \times 0.0031)$$

Oxygen consumption (VO_2) is the product of CO and the difference between arterial and venous oxygen content.

$$VO_2 = CO \times (CaO_2 - CvO_2) \text{ So, } CvO_2 = CaO_2 - VO_2/CO$$

As oxygen dissolved into the blood is miniscule, it can be neglected:

$$\text{So, Hb} \times 1.34 \times SvO_2 = \text{Hb} \times 1.34 \times SaO_2 - VO_2/\text{CO. } SvO_2 \sim VO_2/\text{CO.}$$

Thus, SvO_2 is directly proportional to the ratio of VO_2 to CO.

Pathophysiology

During physiological conditions increase in oxygen demand or consumption (VO_2) is met by an increase in CO, and thus SvO_2 is maintained within its normal range of 65–75%. Whenever there is an oxygen demand-supply mismatch, tissue extracts more oxygen resulting into a fall in SvO_2. Thus, low SvO_2 is an indicator of demand-supply mismatch, but normal or supranormal SvO_2 does not guarantee adequate tissue oxygenation, e.g., in case of tissue death or tissue dysfunction leading to poor oxygen extraction may result into high SvO_2 despite tissue hypoxia.

Low SvO_2 can result from two scenarios:

1. *Low O_2 delivery:* Anemia, hypoxia, hemorrhage, and hypovolemia
2. *Increased O_2 consumption:* Pain, fever, and agitation, increased metabolic demand.

Causes of increased SvO_2:

- *Increased O_2 delivery:* Oxygen therapy, blood transfusion, inotropes, and increased CO.
- *Decreased O_2 consumption:* Sedation and hypothermia
- Decreased O_2 extraction due to cell death or shunting (sepsis).

Clinical Uses of Mixed Venous Oxygen Saturation

Sepsis and Septic Shock

Rivers et al. demonstrated that in patients with septic shock EGDT-guided treatment including SvO_2 lead to a 16% reduction in 28 days of mortality.

Cardiac Failure

In patients with cardiac failure in the early stage, SvO_2 is a good prognostic marker. Persistently low SvO_2 is a marker of poor prognosis.

Trauma

Scalea[13] and colleagues demonstrated that in the management of the initial stages of traumatic shock, SvO_2 correlated well with the degree of blood loss. That persistently low SvO_2 in the first 24 hours. In patients with traumatic brain injury, it was associated with poor outcomes and was shown by Di Filippo and colleagues in 2009.

Major Surgery

In cardiac surgery, SvO_2 has high predictive value in the diagnosis of impending substantial hemodynamic instability. SvO_2 <70% is a poor prognostic marker in cardiac surgery and may predict the development of arrhythmias.

Can central $ScvO_2$ be used as a surrogate for SvO_2?

In critical care practice nowadays, the popularity of pulmonary venous catheters is declining. As a central venous catheter is used commonly if $ScvO_2$ can be used as a surrogate for SvO_2, it would be more convenient. While the blood sample collected from the pulmonary artery catheter is true mixed venous blood; that collected from the central venous catheter is representative of the upper body as the central venous catheter lies in the superior vena cava. Under physiological conditions $ScvO_2$ is less than SvO_2 by 2–3%; due to higher oxygen extraction; by the brain compared to the lower body. But in cases of shock, the blood supply to brain is maintained, with compromised perfusion of splanchnic and renal circulation. So, more oxygen is extracted from lower body structures, thus $ScvO_2$ is greater than SvO_2 during a state of shock. So, in case of shock, there is a poor correlation between SvO_2 and $ScvO_2$.[14] Larger randomized trials are needed before making recommendations regarding the use of $ScvO_2$ as a surrogate for SvO_2.

Disadvantages of SvO_2 (mixed venous oximetry):

- Measurements of SvO_2 need the placement of a pulmonary artery catheter, which is rarely used in patients with septic shock.
- A low value of SvO_2 is a predictor of tissue hypoxia, but a normal or high value of SvO_2 does not rule out tissue hypoxia.
- As SvO_2 is a marker of global tissue oxygenation, local tissue hypoxia can be masked due admixture of highly oxygenated venous blood from other parts of the body.
- SvO_2 is a marker of tissue hypoxia but not of tissue perfusion, so even with normalization of SvO_2, underperfusion of tissue may lead to the progression of organ dysfunction and death.

To conclude, low SvO_2 is an early warning sign of oxygen demand-supply mismatch. A low value of SvO_2 should warn clinicians to take corrective action to optimize tissue O_2 delivery. However, normal or supranormal values of SvO_2 do not rule out tissue hypoxia.

VENOARTERIAL CARBON DIOXIDE TENSION DIFFERENCE (PCO_2 GAP)

Diagnosis of tissue hypoperfusion and optimization of tissue perfusion is a crucial step in the management of shock in its initial stages to avoid organ dysfunction. Venous arterial carbon dioxide tension difference is a good marker for the evaluation of the adequacy of global tissue perfusion and it helps to take measures to optimize tissue perfusion even after optimization of O_2-derived parameters. Variations in partial pressure of CO_2 occur at a faster pace compared to changes in lactate level, thus it is a more attractive marker of tissue perfusion especially in the early stages of shock.

Physiology of Carbon Dioxide Transport in Blood

Transport of CO_2 in blood occurs in three forms. Dissolved in the blood, bicarbonate, and bound to proteins as carbamino compounds, out of which bicarbonate is the major form of CO_2 in the body. Dissolved CO_2 and carbamino compounds comprise approximately 5% each.

Bicarbonates are formed when CO_2 combines with H_2O to form H_2CO_3, which dissociates to form HCO_3 and H^+ ions. Normally, CO_2 is excreted through the lungs, and the amount of CO_2 production and elimination is approximately equal.

Pathophysiology

According to Fick's principle, CO_2 production (VCO_2) is equal to the product of venoarterial CO_2 content difference ($CvCO_2 - CaCO_2$) and CO. In a physiological range, partial pressure of CO_2 and CO_2 content of blood have a linear relationship, i.e.:

$$PCO_2 = CCO_2 \times k \text{ (k is constant)}$$
$$\text{So, } VCO_2 = k \times CO \times P\text{ (v-a) } CO_2$$
$$\text{So, } P\text{ (v-a) } CO_2 = VCO_2/CO \times k.$$

So, under physiological conditions, P (v-a) CO_2 has an inverse relation to CO, i.e., P (v-a) CO_2 increases with decreasing CO and vice versa. The normal value of P (v-a) CO_2 ranges between 2 and 6 mm Hg.

Factors influencing venoarterial CO_2 difference: Aerobic versus anaerobic CO_2 production.

- *Aerobic CO_2 production:* During aerobic energy production oxidative phosphorylation leads to the production of ATP and CO_2. The amount of CO_2 produced is proportionate to oxygen consumption. $VCO_2 = R \times VO_2$, where R is the respiratory quotient. In aerobic energy production value of R varies between 0.7 and 1, but it is never >1. So, during aerobic CO_2 production P (v-a) CO_2 can increase with increasing VCO_2 unless there is an increase in CO to the same extent.
- *Anaerobic CO_2 production:* In the presence of tissue hypoxia, there is an increased lactate production, leading to excessive H^+ ion generation. H^+ ions combine with bicarbonate to produce CO_2 and H_2O. So, during the anaerobic pathway of energy production, there is excessive CO_2 production compared to VO_2, leading to an increase in venoarterial PCO_2 difference, provided CO remains static.
  - *Cardiac output:* P (v-a) CO_2 is directly related to CO_2 production and inversely related to CO as per Ficks principle. So, under physiological conditions P (v-a) CO increases with a fall in CO, provided VO and VCO_2 are in a steady state. Many experimental and clinical studies confirmed the relation between CO and P (v-a) CO_2. Vallet et al.[15] conducted an experiment in a canine model, in which they showed that when hypoxia was induced by reducing blood flow to a single limb (ischemic hypoxia), it resulted in a rise in P (v-a) CO_2, on the other hand when hypoxia was induced by reducing oxygen concentration and maintaining normal blood flow (hypoxic hypoxia) P (v-a) CO_2 did not rise significantly. P (v-a) CO_2 is a marker of tissue perfusion, but not of tissue hypoxia. Clinical studies also demonstrated a correlation between P (v-a) CO_2 and CO. Mencher et al.[16] demonstrated that in patients with septic shock, CO was significantly lower in patients with P (v-a) CO_2 value >6 mm Hg, compared to those with P (v-a) CO_2 < 6 mm Hg. Blood lactate levels were similar in both groups. They also demonstrated that volume expansion-related fall in P (v-a) CO_2 with a rise in CO was seen only in patients with high initial P (v-a) CO_2. So, they concluded that high P (v-a) CO_2 in patients with septic shock was related to a

decrease in systemic blood flow. Ospina-Tascón et al.[17] demonstrated that in patients with septic shock within an initial 6 hours, P (v-a) CO_2 value >6 mm Hg was associated with severe multiorgan failure and high mortality. Thus, P (v-a) CO_2 has very good sensitivity to diagnose tissue hypoperfusion but has poor sensitivity to diagnose tissue hypoxia. The normal value of P (v-a) CO_2 does not rule out tissue hypoxia.

Can ΔPCO_2 be used as a surrogate for P (v-a) CO_2?
For measurements of P (v-a), CO_2 requires a pulmonary artery catheter, but it is rarely used nowadays. The central venous catheter is commonly inserted in patients with septic shock. ΔPCO_2, that is central venous-arterial carbon dioxide difference can be used instead of P (v-a) CO_2. It is calculated as a difference in partial pressure of CO_2 between central venous blood, collected from a central venous catheter and arterial blood. There is good agreement between P (v-a) CO_2 and ΔPCO_2 in patients with septic shock.

A recent prospective study showed that in patients with early septic shock, those who had ΔPCO_2 <6 mm Hg after resuscitation, had a low SOFA score and a greater decrease in lactate level, compared to those who had high ΔPCO_2 levels.[6] Another retrospective study demonstrated that in patients with septic shock after resuscitation, normalization of both $ScvO_2$ and ΔPCO_2 was associated with better prognosis and better lactate clearance.

How to use ΔPCO_2 in clinical settings?
While managing septic shock ΔPCO_2 should be used as a marker of tissue perfusion, but not as an indicator of tissue oxygenation.

- In a state of septic shock ΔPCO_2 >6 mm Hg, is an indicator of tissue hypoperfusion even after normalization of macrocirculatory and downstream parameters, such as MAP, CVP, and SvO_2 or lactate. This should prompt the treating clinician to take measures to increase CO.
- On the other hand, ΔPCO_2 <6 mm Hg is suggestive of adequacy of CO and tissue perfusion, and increasing CO should not be a priority. But one needs to be aware that ΔPCO_2 is a marker of global tissue perfusion and the normal value of ΔPCO_2 does not rule out localized tissue hypoperfusion.

To conclude, ΔPCO_2 is an important marker of tissue perfusion and adequacy of CO in patients with septic shock and should be measured from the beginning of resuscitation. Even normal $ScvO_2$ (>70%), ΔPCO_2 >6 mm Hg is suggestive of low tissue perfusion and low CO, and need for measures to improve CO, rather than increasing oxygen delivery by RBC transfusion or increasing arterial oxygen saturation. However, further randomized trials are needed before making recommendations for clinical use of these parameters.[18]

CONCLUSION

The use of $ScvO_2$ and $PaCO_2$ gap in critical care offers valuable insights into a patient's hemodynamic and metabolic status. $ScvO_2$ provides an indication of tissue oxygenation, while the $PaCO_2$ gap helps assess the adequacy of circulation and ventilation. An elevated $PaCO_2$ gap can indicate poor perfusion or oxygen delivery, potentially signaling early signs of sepsis or shock. Monitoring these parameters together enables clinicians to identify and manage critical conditions more effectively, guiding therapeutic interventions and improving patient outcomes.

REFERENCES

1. Rangel-Frausto MS, Pittet D, Costigan M, Hwang T, Davis CS, Wenzel RP. The natural history of the systemic inflammatory response syndrome (SIRS). A prospective study. JAMA. 1995;273(2):117-23.
2. Beal AL, Cerra FB. Multiple organ failure syndrome in the 1990s. systemic inflammatory response and organ dysfunction. JAMA. 1994;271(3):226-23.
3. Rivers E, Nguyen B, Havstad S, Ressler J, Muzzin A, Knoblich B, et al. Early goal-directed therapy in the treatment of severe sepsis and septic shock. N Engl J Med. 2001;345(19):1368-77.
4. Dellinger RP, Carlet JM, Masur H, Gerlach H, Calandra T, Cohen J, et al. Surviving Sepsis Campaign Management Guidelines Committee. Surviving Sepsis Campaign guidelines for the management of severe sepsis and septic shock. Crit Care Med. 2004;32(3):858-73.
5. Dellinger RP, Levy MM, Carlet JM, Bion J, Parker MM, Jaeschke R, et al. Surviving Sepsis Campaign: International guidelines for the management of severe sepsis and septic shock: 2008. Intensive Care Med. 2008;34(1):17-60.
6. Dellinger RP, Levy MM, Rhodes A, Annane D, Gerlach H, Opal SM, et al. Surviving Sepsis Campaign: International guidelines for management of severe sepsis and septic shock, 2012. Intensive Care Med. 2013;39(2):165-228.
7. McKenna M. Controversy swirls around early goal-directed therapy in sepsis: pioneer defends ground-breaking approach to deadly disease. Ann Emerg Med. 2008;52(6):651-4.

8. ProCESS Investigators; Yealy DM, Kellum JA, Huang DT, Barnato AE, Weissfeld LA, et al. A randomized trial of protocol-based care for early septic shock. N Engl J Med. 2014;370(18):1683-93.
9. ARISE Investigators; ANZICS Clinical Trials Group, Peake SL, Delaney A, Bailey M, Bellomo R, et al. Goal-directed resuscitation for patients with early septic shock. N Engl J Med. 2014;371(16):1496-506.
10. Mouncey PR, Osborn TM, Power GS, Harrison DA, Sadique MZ, Grieve RD, et al. Trial of early, goal-directed resuscitation for septic shock. N Engl J Med. 2015;372(14):1301-11.
11. Reinhart K, Rudolph T, Bredle DL, Hannemann L, Cain SM. Comparison of central-venous to mixed-venous oxygen saturation during changes in oxygen supply/demand. Chest. 1989;95(6):1216-21.
12. Hayes MA, Timmins AC, Yau EH, Palazzo M, Hinds CJ, Watson D. Elevation of systemic oxygen delivery in the treatment of critically ill patients. N Engl J Med. 1994;330(24):1717-22.
13. Scalea TM, Holman M, Fuortes M, Baron BJ, Phillips TF, Goldstein AS, et al. Central venous blood oxygen saturation: an early, accurate measurement of volume during hemorrhage. J Trauma. 1988;28(6):725-32.
14. Pearse R, Dawson D, Fawcett J, Rhodes A, Grounds RM, Bennett ED. Changes in central venous saturation after major surgery, and association with outcome. Crit Care. 2005;9(6):R694-9.
15. Vallet B, Teboul JL, Cain S, Curtis S. Venoarterial CO(2) difference during regional ischemic or hypoxic hypoxia. J Appl Physiol (1985). 2000;89(4):1317-21.
16. Mecher CE, Rackow EC, Astiz ME, Weil MH. Venous hypercarbia associated with severe sepsis and systemic hypoperfusion. Crit Care Med. 1990;18(6):585-9.
17. Ospina-Tascón GA, Bautista-Rincón DF, Umaña M, Tafur JD, Gutiérrez A, García AF, et al. Persistently high venous-to-arterial carbon dioxide differences during early resuscitation are associated with poor outcomes in septic shock. Crit Care. 2013;17(6):R294.
18. Mallat J, Pepy F, Lemyze M, Gasan G, Vangrunderbeeck N, Tronchon L, et al. Central venous-to-arterial carbon dioxide partial pressure difference in early resuscitation from septic shock: a prospective observational study. Eur J Anaesthesiol. 2014;31(7):371-80.

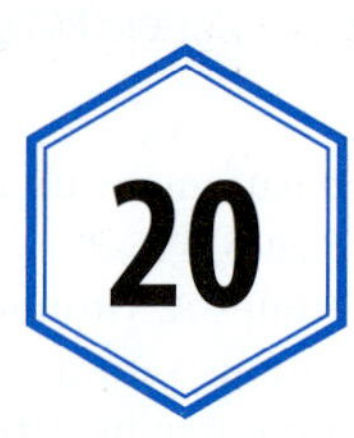

Lactate Monitoring in Critically Ill Patients

Nishanth Baliga

INTRODUCTION

Lactate is a metabolic byproduct of glycolysis. Approximately 1,300 to 1,500 mmol of lactate is produced daily by various organs, including erythrocytes (red blood cells), skeletal muscle cells, the brain, intestines, skin, and perivenous hepatocytes. About 70% of lactate is metabolized by the liver, while the remainder is processed by the kidneys and other organs. The normal blood lactate concentration ranges from around 0.8 to 1 mEq/L. Elevated blood lactate levels, known as hyperlactatemia, can occur in critically ill patients, reflecting an imbalance between lactate production in different organs and its utilization or uptake. Hyperlactatemia can lead to an increase in hydrogen ions, resulting in a decrease in pH, a condition referred to as lactic acidosis.[1,2]

METABOLISM OF LACTATE

Lactate plays a critical role in energy production pathways in the human body, particularly during glycolysis and oxidative phosphorylation. Glycolysis, which occurs in the cytoplasm, converts glucose into two molecules of pyruvate while generating two ATP molecules. Under aerobic conditions, pyruvate is further converted to acetyl coenzyme A (acetyl-CoA), which then enters the Krebs cycle in the mitochondria. This process, along with oxidative phosphorylation, ultimately produces 36 ATP molecules. Therefore, one molecule of glucose generates a total of 38 ATP molecules under aerobic conditions.[3,4] **(Flowchart 1)**.

Flowchart 1: Metabolism of glucose through glycolysis and oxidative phosphorylation.

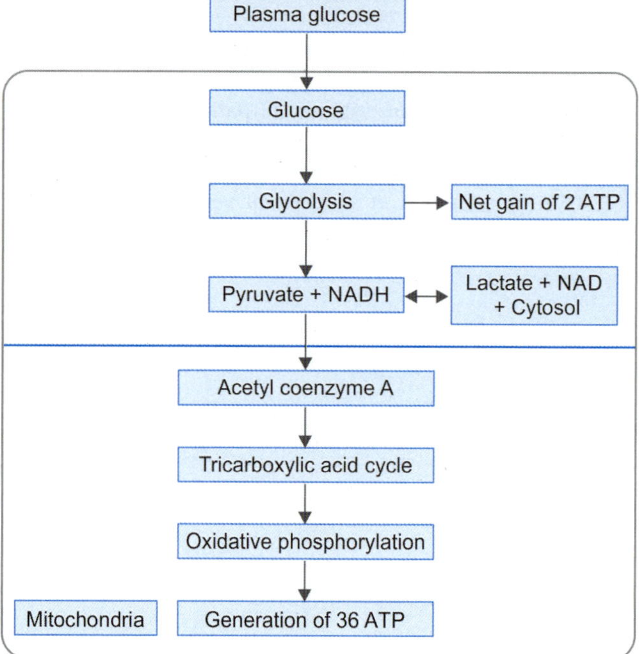

(ATP: adenosine triphosphate; NAD: nicotinamide adenine dinucleotide; NADH: nicotinamide adenine dinucleotide hydrogen)

During times of stress, the glycolysis process may be accelerated, leading to an accumulation of excess pyruvate. When the capacity of the Krebs cycle to metabolize pyruvate is exceeded, the surplus pyruvate is converted into lactate, allowing glycolysis to continue. Upon recovery, lactate can be converted back into pyruvate through the action of the enzyme lactate dehydrogenase (LDH), generating 18 ATP per molecule of lactate. Thus, during periods of high energy demand, such as cellular stress, lactate serves as an essential buffer that enables glycolysis to proceed.[5] **(Flowchart 2)**.

In anaerobic conditions, pyruvate combines with nicotinamide adenine dinucleotide hydrogen (NADH) and hydrogen ions (H^+) to form lactic acid and NAD^+ through the action of LDH. In aqueous solutions, lactic acid almost completely dissociates into lactate and hydrogen ions. The interconversion of pyruvate and lactate occurs in the cytosol and is catalyzed by LDH. Lactate is

Flowchart 2: Lactate metabolism in steady state, stress, and recovery phase.

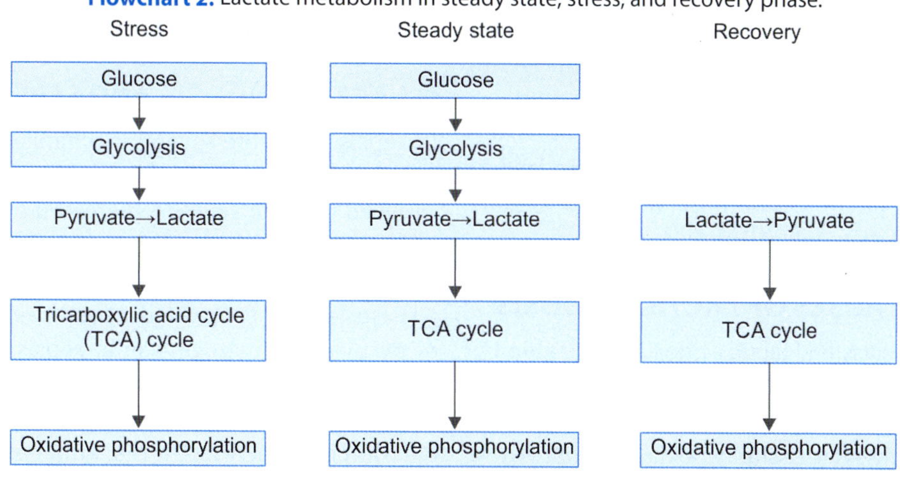

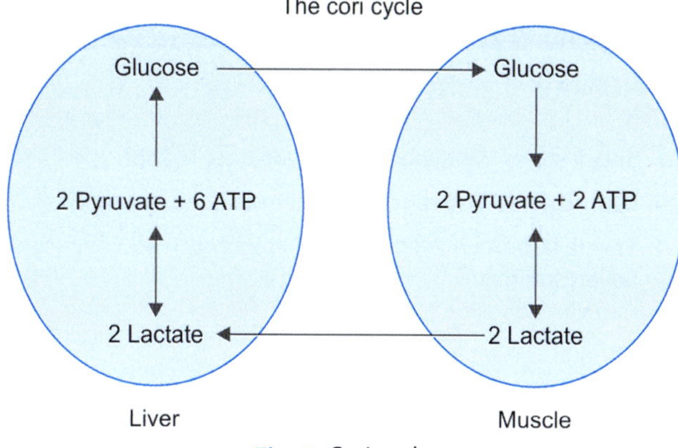

Fig. 1: Cori cycle.

then transported to the liver, where it acts as a substrate for gluconeogenesis and is converted back into glucose. This glucose can return to the muscles, allowing for the regeneration of lactate. This metabolic process is known as the Cori cycle[6] **(Figure 1)**.

Lactate functions as an intermediate fuel that can be readily exchanged among various tissues, facilitated by a family of membrane-bound monocarboxylate transporters (MCTs). The shuttling of lactate between astrocytes, neurons, cardiac muscle, and skeletal muscle is well-documented. This process differs from the renal and hepatic Cori cycle by being energy efficient, resulting in no loss of ATP.[7]

HYPERLACTATEMIA AND LACTIC ACIDOSIS

Hyperlactatemia occurs when lactate production exceeds its utilization, with a serum level greater than 2 mmol/L indicating this condition. In cases of more severe hyperlactatemia, defined as lactate levels between 3 and 5 mmol/L, there is an accumulation of hydrogen ions (H^+) due to the hydrolysis of ATP to ADP. These hydrogen ions are typically neutralized by the body's buffering systems to help maintain pH. However, continued production of hydrogen ions can outpace these buffering mechanisms, leading to metabolic acidosis. The combination of hyperlactatemia and acidosis is known as lactic acidosis, which is typically referenced when blood lactate exceeds 5 mmol/L and pH drops below 7.35.

Hyperlactatemia generally develops due to increased lactate production compared to its clearance. Factors that elevate lactate production or reduce its clearance can contribute to this condition. The most common cause of hyperlactatemia is a decrease in the utilization of pyruvate in the oxidative phosphorylation or gluconeogenesis pathways, leading to increased conversion of pyruvate to lactate, particularly in the absence of oxygen. Therefore, tissue hypoxia is a primary mechanism behind hyperlactatemia. Additionally, alterations in microcirculatory perfusion can limit oxygen availability, which can also elevate lactate levels.

Hyperlactatemia can arise from excessive aerobic glycolysis, a process stimulated by factors other than tissue hypoxia. In response to cellular stress, aerobic glycolysis becomes an effective but inefficient way to rapidly generate ATP, leading to stimulation of glycolysis at about four times the normal rate. Common triggers for this increased glycolysis include stress, exercise, and catecholamines. Exogenous administration of catecholamines, such as epinephrine, results in a dose-dependent rise in lactate levels, caused both by enhanced glycolysis and the stimulation of sarcolemmal Na-K ATPase. Other conditions that can elevate catecholamine levels, such as trauma, hemorrhagic or cardiogenic shock, and pheochromocytoma, can also contribute to hyperlactatemia through similar mechanisms. Moreover, excessive stimulation of phosphofructokinase can lead to hyperlactatemia, a phenomenon observed in conditions like respiratory and metabolic alkalosis.

TYPES AND CAUSES OF LACTIC ACIDOSIS

Cohen and Woods classified lactic acidosis into **(Table 1)**:

- Type A, in which tissue hypoxia results in faster production than removal.
- Type B, in which overt tissue hypoxia does not play a role. Type B has been further subdivided depending on whether it is caused by underlying disease (B1), drugs and toxins (B2), or inborn errors of metabolism (B3).[8]

LACTIC ACIDOSIS AND SEPSIS

In sepsis, there are several mechanisms that can lead to lactic acidosis. Septic shock leading to tissue hypoperfusion can lead to lactic acidosis. Increased pyruvate production may occur in sepsis due to catecholamine-induced increases in aerobic glycolysis and stimulation of Na-K ATPase, leading to elevated lactate levels. Direct inhibition of pyruvate dehydrogenase in sepsis prevents pyruvate from entering the Krebs cycle and subsequent oxidative phosphorylation. Additionally, there may be reduced clearance of lactate by the kidneys and liver due to hypoperfusion.[9]

TABLE 1: Classification, mechanism, and causes of lactic acidosis.

Types	*Mechanism*	*Causes*
Type A	Poor tissue oxygen delivery a. Systemic hypoperfusion	• Shock states like hypovolemic, cardiogenic, septic shock
	b. Local hypoperfusion	• Gastric necrosis, splanchnic ischemia
	c. Systemic hypoxia	• Severe hypoxaemia (PaO_2 <30-40 mm hg) • Severe anemia • Carbon monoxide toxicity
	d. Local tissue hypoxia- more demand than supply	• Strenuous exercise • Trembling • Seizures
Type B1	Systemic diseases where adequate tissue oxygenation and normal hemodynamics is present	
	a. Defect in Lactate clearance	Liver and kidney diseases
	b. Epinephrine induced β2-adrenoceptor stimulation	• Exogenous epinephrine administration • Catecholamine secreting pheochromocytoma
	c. Increased glycolytic activity of tumor (Warburg effect)	Lymphoma/leukemia
	d. Impairment of pyruvate dehydrogenase activity	• Thiamine deficiency • Sepsis
Type B2	Associated with drugs and toxins	
	a. Impairment of pyruvate dehydrogenase activity, suppression of hepatic gluconeogenesis	Metformin
	b. Interference with oxidative phosphorylation	Nucleoside reverse-transcriptase inhibitors, salicylates, cyanide, propofol
	c. Toxic alcohols which interfere with oxidative phosphorylation	Methanol, ethylene glycol, diethylene glycol
	d. Normal products of metabolism	Propylene glycol
Type B3	Associated with inborn errors of metabolism due to deficiency of certain specific enzymes involved in lactate metabolism either gluconeogenesis or pyruvate oxidation	• Pyruvate carboxylase deficiency • Glucose-6-phosphate dehydrogenase (G6PD) • Fructose-1,6-diphosphatase • Pyruvate dehydrogenase deficiency

MEASUREMENT OF LACTATE

Lactate exists in two optical isomers: D-lactate and L-lactate. In humans, L-lactate is about 100 times more common than D-lactate. However, elevated levels of D-lactate may occur due to bacteria in the human colon when exposed to large amounts of unabsorbed carbohydrates in conditions such as short bowel syndrome, mesenteric ischemia, and jejunoileal bypass surgery. Because humans lack the enzymes to metabolize D-lactate, it can accumulate and result in metabolic acidosis. This accumulation can also lead to neurological symptoms, such as encephalopathy and seizures. Routine measurements of lactate typically assess only the L-lactate isomer, which may lead to falsely low blood lactate readings. D-lactate should be suspected in high-risk patients who present with unexplained high anion gap metabolic acidosis.

Normal lactate levels range from 0.5 to 2 mmol/L. Lactate can be measured using either the LDH method or the lactic oxidase method. Point-of-care analyzers commonly use enzymatic amperometry with lactate oxidase that generates H_2O_2, which is detected by an electrode. Serum lactate is measured by biochemistry machines that use the LDH method. In ethylene glycol poisoning, a metabolite called glyoxylate can be misidentified by amperometry using lactic oxidase, resulting in falsely elevated lactate levels. This discrepancy in lactate measurement from the two techniques is referred to as the "lactate gap." Therefore, in these patients, lactate should be measured by the LDH method in a biochemistry lab rather than by point-of-care analyzers.

USE OF LACTATE MEASUREMENT IN CLINICAL PRACTICE

Lactate monitoring is extremely useful in critically ill patients, especially those experiencing shock, after major or cardiac surgeries, trauma, or sepsis. The most common cause of hyperlactatemia in critically ill patients is tissue hypoperfusion, particularly in those with shock. Initial compensatory mechanisms in the body can mask obvious signs of hypoperfusion. Key vital signs may change only when these compensatory mechanisms fail. In patients with occult shock, lactate measurement can help identify those with impaired tissue perfusion and oxygenation. Among various markers of tissue hypoperfusion, lactate is more sensitive than clinical parameters such as the temperature of the great toe, core-peripheral temperature gradients, and capillary refill time. Early identification of patients showing compensated shock through lactate levels can prevent delayed or inadequate resuscitation.

Lactate can also serve as a prognostic marker in critically ill patients encompassing diverse populations such as those with sepsis, general intensive care unit (ICU) patients, trauma cases, and postsurgical patients. An initial lactate level is a reasonable predictor of outcomes, especially when hyperlactatemia is due to tissue hypoperfusion. Higher initial lactate levels correlate with a higher expected mortality rate. Conversely, if tissue hypoperfusion is unlikely to be the cause of hyperlactatemia, it is crucial to assess other factors such as accelerated glycolysis, metabolic interference, and decreased lactate clearance.[10]

Serum lactate is used to identify a subset of sepsis patients who exhibit profound circulatory, cellular, and metabolic abnormalities associated with higher mortality rates. The Sepsis-3 consensus definition describes septic shock as a subset of sepsis in which vasopressors are necessary to maintain a mean arterial pressure of more than 65 mm Hg, despite adequate fluid resuscitation and serum lactate levels exceeding 2 mmol/L.[11]

The 2021 Surviving Sepsis Campaign guidelines provided a weak recommendation for using lactate as a marker of tissue hypoperfusion to guide fluid administration during resuscitation in patients with hyperlactatemia.[12]

Lactate is a complex molecule that functions as a substrate, energy source, biomarker, and modulator of cellular bioenergetics during stress periods. Hyperlactatemia can arise from multiple mechanisms, including cellular hypoperfusion leading to anaerobic glycolysis, stress-related accelerated glycolysis, mitochondrial dysfunction due to defective pyruvate metabolism, or impaired clearance. In hyperlactatemia cases not related to hypoperfusion, fluid resuscitation may be potentially harmful.[13] Studies comparing lactate to mixed venous oxygen saturation, capillary refill time, and temperature gradients as resuscitation targets have found no outcome differences, suggesting that lactate-guided fluid therapy for patients in shock may not be beneficial.[14,15]

Administering intravenous fluids that contain lactate as a buffer, such as Ringer's lactate, does not appear to raise blood lactate levels because the liver metabolizes lactate into bicarbonate. An increase in serum lactate levels due to exogenous administration of balanced salt solutions may only occur in patients with hypoperfusion or liver dysfunction.

Several treatments for hyperlactatemia and lactic acidosis have been attempted. For example, administering sodium bicarbonate to correct acidosis and improve pH levels did not lead to any significant change in patient outcomes. Likewise, the use of dichloroacetate to reduce lactate production was not found to be beneficial. Although renal replacement therapy using a bicarbonate buffer has shown a reduction in plasma lactate levels, there were no corresponding improvements in clinical outcomes.

In patients with hyperlactatemia, it is essential to identify and address the underlying cause of the elevated lactate levels rather than simply focusing on reducing lactate production, improving metabolism, or increasing lactate clearance.[16]

CONCLUSION

Lactate monitoring is crucial for managing critically ill patients in the ICU. Hyperlactatemia, which is often observed in these patients, can result from various mechanisms and underlying causes. It serves as a useful screening tool for identifying patients with occult shock, which is linked to higher mortality rates. Additionally, lactate levels can act as a biomarker for diagnosing septic shock. Monitoring lactate is important for risk stratification, as hyperlactatemia is associated with increased mortality and morbidity in a diverse range of critically ill patients. Although lactate is being investigated as a resuscitation target, recent data suggest that there may not be an improvement in outcomes for those in the lactate-guided group. Further research is needed to explore this topic more thoroughly.

REFERENCES

1. Vincent JL, Quintairos E, Silva A, Couto L Jr, Taccone FS. The value of blood lactate kinetics in critically ill patients: a systematic review. Crit Care. 2016;20(1):257
2. Phypers B, Tom Pierce JM. Lactate physiology in health and disease. Contin Educ Anaesth Crit Care Pain. 2006;6(3):128-32.
3. Luft FC. Lactic acidosis update for critical care clinicians. J Am Soc Nephrol. 2001:17:S15-9.
4. Bakker J, Nijsten MW, Jansen TC. Clinical use of lactate monitoring in critically ill patients. Ann Intensive Care. 2013;3(1):12.
5. Kraut JA, Madias NE. Lactic acidosis. N Engl J Med. 2014;371(1):2309-19.
6. Li X, Yang Y, Zhang B, Lin X, Fu X, An Y, et al. Lactate metabolism in human health and disease. Sig Transduct Target Ther. 2022;7(1):305.
7. Brooks GA. Lactate shuttles in nature. Biochem Soc Trans. 2002;30(2):258-64.
8. Seheult J, Fitzpatrick G, Boran G. Lactic acidosis: an update. Clin Chem Lab Med. 2017;55(3):322-33.
9. Suetrong B, Walley KR. Lactic Acidosis in Sepsis: It's Not All Anaerobic: Implications for Diagnosis and Management. Chest. 2016;149(1):252-261.
10. Fuller BM, Dellinger RP. Lactate as a hemodynamic marker in the critically ill. Curr Opin Crit Care. 2012;18(3):267-72.
11. Singer M, Deutschman CS, Seymour CW, Shankar-Hari M, Annane D, Bauer M, et al. The Third International Consensus Definitions for Sepsis and Septic Shock (Sepsis-3). JAMA. 2016 23;315(8):801-10.
12. Evans L, Rhodes A, Alhazzani W, Antonelli M, Coopersmith CM, French C, et al. Surviving sepsis campaign: international guidelines for management of sepsis and septic shock 2021. Intensive Care Med. 2021; 47(11):1181-247.
13. Hernandez G, Bellomo R, Bakker J. The ten pitfalls of lactate clearance in sepsis. Intensive Care Med. 2019;45(1):82-5.
14. Jones AE, Shapiro NI, Trzeciak S, Arnold RC, Claremont HA, Kline JA. Lactate clearance vs central venous oxygen saturation as goals of early sepsis therapy: a randomized clinical trial. JAMA 2010;303(8):739-46.
15. Hernández G, Ospina-Tascón GA, Damiani LP, Estenssoro E, Dubin A, Hurtado J. Effect of a Resuscitation Strategy Targeting Peripheral Perfusion Status vs Serum Lactate Levels on 28-Day Mortality Among Patients With Septic Shock. JAMA. 2019;321(7):654-664
16. Kraut JA, Madias NE. Lactic Acidosis: Current Treatments and Future Directions. Am J Kidney Dis. 2016;68(3): 473-82.

CHAPTER

Biomarkers Used in Hemodynamic Monitoring

Babu Abraham, Ebenezer Rabindrajan

INTRODUCTION

The term "biomarker" was coined in 1989. The aim was to identify biological markers, which are measurable, quantifiable, and able to assess the health and physiology of patients in terms of disease risk and diagnosis. They are indicators of biological states or conditions, which can be measured and evaluated to examine normal processes, pathological states, or responses to therapeutic interventions.[1] Biomarkers can be used in different scenarios and be grouped as predictors of future disease development—"antecedent biomarkers," aid with diagnosing subclinical disease—"screening biomarkers," help with recognizing clinically manifest disease—"diagnostic biomarkers," help with defining disease severity—"staging biomarkers," predicting disease evolution and the response to therapy—"prognostic and therapeutic biomarkers" and help with inclusion/exclusion and outcome criteria for clinical trials Assays of the biomarker must be accurate and easily reproducible for them to be able to play these roles.

This chapter will discuss those biomarkers that have been in use in clinical practice, look at the evidence for their use, and review a few that are in the pipeline.

BIOMARKERS FOR MONITORING HEART FUNCTION

The three elements of hemodynamics are heart, blood flow, and organ perfusion. Multiple biomarkers have been studied to assess the accuracy of diagnosis, prediction of prognosis, and monitoring of response to therapy of pathological processes that affect hemodynamics. Failure of the first element of hemodynamics, the heart, clinically known as heart failure (HF), is a complex entity. American College of Cardiology Foundation/American Heart Association (ACCF/AHA) guidelines define it as a structural or functional impairment of ventricular filling or ejection of blood, which leads to clinical symptoms such as dyspnea and fatigue and signs, such as edema and crepitations. Advanced therapies for cardiac disorders like ischemic heart disease, valvular heart disease, and arrhythmias have led to an increased survival and this has partly contributed to HF being an increasing problem worldwide.[2] HF is broadly classified into a reduced ejection fraction heart failure (HFrEF), previously called *systolic failure*, and heart failure with preserved ejection fraction (HFpEF), previously called diastolic failure. Diagnosis of HF in the critical care unit is very often confounded by the presence of illness that causes dyspnea, fatigue, edema, and crepitations on auscultation and radiological findings of pulmonary edema. Multiple biomarkers have been evaluated to help with the diagnosis, prognosis, and guiding of therapy of HF **(Table 1)**.

NATRIURETIC PEPTIDES

Natriuretic peptides are one of the most studied biomarkers that are used for hemodynamic monitoring and have a role in salt and water handling, pressure regulation, and modulating myocardial structure and function. There are two types of natriuretic peptides, (1) B-type natriuretic peptide (BNP) and (2) N-terminal proBNP (NT-proBNP). The prohormone, proBNP gets cleaved and forms a biologically active 32 amino acid BNP along and a biologically inert 76 amino acid NT-proBNP. Both BNP and NT-proBNP are released from the myocardium, when there is an end-diastolic ventricular wall stress from either an increase in volume or pressure. The elimination of BNP and NT-pro BNP from the body is different. Around 25% of BNP is excreted unmodified by the kidneys. The remaining part is eliminated after binding to the NPR-C receptor or through enzymatic degradation by neprilysin. NT-proBNP is passively excreted by the kidneys. Due to their different clearance, NT-proBNP has

TABLE 1: Biomarkers in heart failure.

Myocardial insult		***Neurohormonal activation***		***Remodeling***	
Myocyte stretch	NT-prong, BNP MR-proANP	Renin-angiotensin system	Renin-angiotensin II, aldosterone	Inflammation	C-reactive protein, tumor necrosis factor α, Interleukins, etc.
Myocardial injury	Troponin T Troponin I	Sympathetic nervous system	Norepinephrine, chromogranin A	Hypertrophy/ fibrosis	Matrix metalloproteinases, collagen propeptides, galectin 3, and soluble ST2
Oxidative stress	Myeloperoxidase MR-proADM	Arginine vasopressin system	Arginine vasopressin	Apoptosis	GDF-15

(GDF: growth differentiation factor; NT: N-terminal; MR-proADM: mid-regional proadrenomedullin; ST2: suppression of tumorigenicity-2)

a longer half-life (120 vs. 20 minutes) and higher plasma concentrations (approximately six times) than BNP.

B-type natriuretic peptide has diuretic, natriuretic, and hypotensive effects. It acts by inhibiting the renin-angiotensin system, endothelin secretion, and systemic/renal sympathetic activity. Increased secretion of BNP, seen in cases of HF is a compensatory mechanism as it partially counteracts the effects of norepinephrine, endothelin, and angiotensin II, which limits the degree of vasoconstriction and prevents sodium retention.

Role in Diagnosis of Acute Heart Failure

The most common way to diagnose HF is with a combination of classical signs and symptoms, electrocardiogram (ECG), chest X-ray, and echocardiography. The sensitivity, specificity, and diagnostic accuracy of these tools are very variable.[3] BNP and NT-proBNP have been studied extensively as a biomarker for the diagnosis of HF.

In normal healthy individuals, BNP production is minimal with its level being 10 pg/mL.[2] In the Breathing Not Properly Study, in patients presenting to the emergency department with breathlessness, a BNP cutoff of 100 pg/mL was able to diagnose acute HF with a sensitivity of 90% and a specificity of 76%.[4,5] The high sensitivity of BNP gives it a very high negative predictive value in the emergency department. The recommended cut-off of BNP in the diagnosis of acute HF is >400 pg/mL.[5]

N-terminal proBNP has a diagnostic accuracy similar to that of BNP. The ProBNP Investigation of Dyspnea in the Emergency Department (PRIDE) study and The International Collaborative of NT-proBNP (ICON) study confirmed good diagnostic accuracy and a good correlation with symptom severity and NT-proBNP concentrations.[6,7] The positive predictive value improved with age stratification (NT-proBNP ≥450 pg/mL for age <50 years, ≥900 pg/mL for age 50–75 years, and ≥1,800 pg/mL for age >75 years) with a sensitivity of 90% and specificity of 84% for the diagnosis of acute HF.[5] Low concentrations of NT-proBNP also have a good negative predictive value to exclude the diagnosis of acute HF.

Both these natriuretic peptides are equally efficacious in diagnosing HFrEF and HFpEF since the biological trigger for their release is common.[8] Levels of BNP and NT-proBNP are usually raised in both these conditions, with a lower concentration and reduced sensitivity in HFpEF.[9] To support the diagnosis of HFpEF, the recommended values are BNP ≥100 pg/mL and NT-proBNP ≥800 pg/mL.[5]

Drug therapy with β-blockers, angiotensin-converting enzyme inhibitors, angiotensin II receptor blockers,[10] and aldosterone antagonists, as well as following cardiac resynchronization therapy, have been shown to decrease concentrations in BNP and NT-proBNP.[11-14] Levels of these biomarkers need to be interpreted with caution in the presence of confounders, such as age, obesity, presence of renal, and pulmonary diseases **(Table 2)**.

Despite the fact that their levels can be affected by multiple comorbidities both BNP and NT-proBNP measurements are recommended for the diagnosis of acute decompensated HF, especially in the setting of clinical uncertainty.[5]

Role in Prognosis and Risk Stratification of Heart Failure

In acute HF, both BNP and NT-proBNP levels at baseline have a strong correlation to patient outcome. BNP levels, measured in the emergency room, showed a linear relationship to in-hospital mortality.[5] This is true for both HFrEF and HFpEF. In addition, elevated BNP is also associated with increased morbidity, with patients more likely to require intensive care admission, mechanical

TABLE 2: Indications for the use of biomarkers in the ACC/AHA 2017 and ESC 2016 guidelines for heart failure management.

Biomarker	Guidelines	Indication	Recommendation class	Level of evidence
BNP or NT-proBNP	ESC	Diagnosis	I	A
	ACC/AHA		IIa	C
	ACC/AHA	Prognostic stratification at admission (acute HF)	I	A
		Prognostic stratification at discharge (acute HF)	IIa	B
		Screening/prevention	IIa	B
MR-proANP	ESC	Diagnosis	I	A
hs-TnI/T	ESC	Diagnostic support (acute HF)	I	C
	ACC/AHA	Prognostic stratification at admission (acute and chronic HF)	I	A
sST2, galectin-3	ACC/AHA	Prognostic stratification (acute and chronic HF)	IIb	B

(ACC/AHA: American College of Cardiology/American Heart Association; BNP: brain natriuretic peptide; ESC: European Society of Cardiology; hs-TnI/T high-sensitivity-troponin I/T; HR: heart rate; MR-proANP: midregional proatrial natriuretic peptide; NT-proBNP: N-terminal pro-B-type natriuretic peptide; sST2: soluble suppression of tumorigenesis-2)

TABLE 3: Effect on BNP levels—impact of certain conditions.

Increased levels	Decreased levels
• Heart failure • Valvular heart disease • Coronary artery disease • Myocardial trauma • Myocarditis • Arrhythmia—atrial fibrillation • Pulmonary embolism • COPD—with Pulmonary hypertension • Stroke—ischemic and hemorrhagic • Sepsis • Burns • Renal failure • Anemia • Cirrhosis • Hyperaldosteronism	Obesity

ventilation, and having longer length of hospital stay. Predischarge BNP and NT-proBNP levels have a stronger correlation to a postdischarge outcome rather than the baseline or percentage of change in these peptides during hospitalization. The discharge BNP level is an important factor that predicts mortality and hospital readmission **(Table 3)**.[5]

In chronic HF, an elevated BNP and NT-proBNP usually parallel with other clinical parameters of HF and are suggestive of worse clinical outcomes. An increase in BNP by 100 pg/mL has been seen to be associated with a 35% increase in relative risk of mortality.[5]

Role in Guiding Heart Failure Therapy

In-Hospital Management of Acute Heart Failure

B-type natriuretic peptide and NT-proBNP levels both improve with treatment during acute HF hospitalization and a decrease in these natriuretic peptide levels by 25–40% is typically seen with successful therapy. The effectiveness of BNP or NT-proBNP targeted therapy in-hospitalized acute HF is not very clear.

Out-of-Hospital Management of Chronic Heart Failure

Multiple studies have explored the role of the natriuretic peptide-targeted therapy in outpatient management of chronic HF, and they have shown contradicting results with a lack of consistent evidence for improvement in mortality or cardiovascular outcomes. Monitoring BNP levels in patients with cardiovascular risk factors and actively intervening medically, when the BNP level is >50 pg/mL, was shown to decrease the combined rates of HF.[15] A meta-analysis combining many of these studies found a substantial improvement in mortality with HF management with a decreasing trend in natriuretic peptide levels.[16] The lack of clear evidence led to the 2017 Heart Failure Guideline Update not issuing a guideline recommendation for the use of natriuretic peptide-guided therapy. A recent large multicenter, randomized controlled National Heart, Lung, and Blood Institute (NHLB)-funded study called Guide-IT trial, comparing NT-proBNP guided therapy versus usual guideline guided medical therapy in patients with HFrEF, had to be terminated prematurely due to lack of any difference in either the primary or secondary outcomes.[17] This study highlighted the fact that strict adherence to guideline-based treatment protocols would provide the same outcome benefit as that of biomarkers-guided therapy.[17] Based on the available evidence natriuretic peptide-guided therapy cannot be recommended for routine management of outpatient chronic HF patients at this point of time.

Cardiac Troponins

Cardiac troponins (Tn), both T (TnT) and I (TnI) are myofibrillar proteins, that are released in response to myocyte injury and have been evaluated extensively in several clinical studies. They have been incorporated into main guidelines, as a proven diagnostic and prognostic marker for acute myocardial infarction and acute coronary syndrome.[18] However, they also get released in HF in the absence of an acute coronary event. Raised Tn in asymptotic stages A and B, HF has prognostic implications in that it adds to standard risk factors to predict higher chances of new-onset symptomatic HF. A negative Tn helps in identifying patients at lower risk. In symptomatic acute and chronic HF, elevated levels of Tn are associated with poor prognosis with patients experiencing a higher incidence of impaired hemodynamics, progressive decline of left ventricular systolic function, and increased mortality. Decreasing levels of Tn with treatment is associated with a better prognosis.[5] The ACCF/AHA guidelines recommend measuring Tn in acute HF to rule out acute coronary syndrome and for risk stratification.[19]

High-sensitivity Troponin

These are newer assays of TnT and TnI that are more sensitive and precise enough to detect even lower levels of the biomarker. They are not new or novel troponin isoforms. Depending on the assay used high-sensitivity troponin (hsTn) will detect troponins in >50–95% of healthy subjects.[20] The abnormal level or the upper reference limit of a given assay is taken as the 99th percentile of the level found in normal healthy individuals. As hsTn is not a new isoform, it has all the diagnostic and prognostic properties of Tn, with higher analytic precision at lower concentrations, greater clinical sensitivity, and an ability to assess smaller changes in Tn levels with greater accuracy at shorter time intervals.[21,22] The Journal of the American College of Cardiology (JACC) scientific expert panel has recently published recommendations for transitioning from traditional Tn assay to hsTn assay.[23]

Soluble Suppressor of Tumorigenicity-2

Soluble soluble suppression of tumorigenesis (sST2) belongs to the family of the interleukin (IL)-1 receptor-like family of proteins. When there is mechanical stress on the fibroblasts and cardiomyocytes, it gets released and gets expressed in a transmembrane form (ST2L) and a soluble circulating form (sST2). Current assays measure sST2, which has been evaluated in multiple studies. An increase in sST2 levels leads to acceleration of tissue fibrosis, decreased cardiac function, and myocardial fibrosis. It has been found to be associated with adverse outcomes in HF, myocardial infarction, pulmonary disease, infection, and rheumatologic disorders, which reflect increased inflammation and fibrosis. In acute HF, its level is seen to correlate with the New York Heart Association (NYHA) classification, left ventricular ejection fraction, and BNP/NT-proBNP levels. Its concentration is not affected by any of the factors that affect the levels of natriuretic peptides. An increase in the levels in sST2 is associated with increased mortality.[5] Serial measurements of its level add value to the baseline and post-therapy level has a better predictive value for mortality and postdischarge outcomes. The prognostic ability of sST2 has been seen to be additive to that of NT-proBNP. An elevation of both these biomarkers had the highest 1-year mortality.[5] sST2 has a similar prognostic performance in HFrEF and HFpEF and is superior to galectin-3. In HFpEF sST2 levels >32 ng/mL predict poor prognosis. It lacks disease specificity and, therefore, is not a great marker for the diagnosis of HF. Additionally, sST2 has been shown to independently predict reverse remodeling and has been incorporated into the ST2-R2 scoring system.

There is little evidence at the moment for its use in assessing prognosis in chronic HF and its measurement should be limited to risk stratification in acute HF. β-blockers and mineralocorticoid antagonists have been found to abolish the risk associated with elevated sST2 in HF. Its role in guided therapy as a biomarker like NT-proBNP is still unclear.[24,25]

NEWER BIOMARKERS IN HEART FAILURE

Galectin 3

Galectin 3 (Gal 3), a member of the galectin family, is expressed in the heart, kidney, blood vessels, and macrophages at low levels. It plays a role in pathological remodeling by inducing fibroblast proliferation and collagen deposition. On exposure to injury or stress, Gal 3 production is substantially increased. It is considered as a marker of myocardial fibrosis.[26] Increased levels of Gal 3 may be associated with increased mortality in patients with chronic HF. This association is less significant than found with other biomarkers like the natriuretic peptides or sST2[5] and it is largely influenced by renal function.

PRIDE study compared NT-proBNP to Gal 3 and found the latter to be a stronger prognostic marker for 60-day mortality in patients with HF. Galectin-3 is a good predictor of re-hospitalization for HF within 1 to 4 months, as demonstrated by a meta-analysis on 902 patients with acute HF. The combination of Gal 3 and NT-proBNP was better at predicting poor prognosis in patients with acute HF.[27] The role of Gal 3 in guiding therapy for HF is not clear.

Growth Differentiation Factor-15

Growth differentiation factor-15 (GDF-15) is a stress response cytokine produced in cardiomyocytes, which is released in the setting of oxidative stress or in response to stimulation with cytokines or angiotensin II.[28] In acute coronary syndromes (ACSs), both ST segment elevated and non-ST segment elevated, GDF 15 levels are found to be strong predictors of mortality.[29] GDF-15 levels are elevated substantially in HF and worse outcomes have been noted with raised GDF-15 levels and both acute and chronic HF.[30] However, more studies would be required before it can be recommended for routine clinical use.

Midregional Proatrial Natriuretic Peptide

Increased atrial wall stretch leads to a rise in the production of atrial natriuretic peptide (ANP). However, due to its very short half-life of only 2–5 minutes, its detection in serum becomes difficult.[31] The 126 amino acid prohormone of ANP, called proANP, has a longer half-life and can be measured in the serum. Mid-regional proatrial natriuretic peptide (MR-proANP) has been shown to have both diagnostic and prognostic implications in multiple HF studies and they could have an increased predictive effect when combined with BNP or NT-proBNP levels.[32,33] In the PRIDE study the performance of MR-proANP was almost at par with that of NT-proBNP for the diagnosis of acute HF (AUC 0.90 vs. 0.94, $p = 0.001$). European Society of Cardiology (ESC) guidelines recommend the use of MR-proANP, as an alternative to BNP or NT-proBNP, for discriminating acute HF from noncardiogenic causes of dyspnoea (class I, LOE A)

Midregional Proadrenomedullin

Adrenomedullin was first found in pheochromocytoma cells in the adrenal medulla and has potent vasodilatory effects.[34] It has been found in various organs including the heart, where it increases myocardial contractility through a cyclic AMP-independent mechanism. It induces nitric oxide synthesis in conditions where cytokine production is increased.[35] Elevated levels of midregional proadrenomedullin (MR-proADM) were seen in HF and correlated with decreasing left ventricular ejection fraction, increasing pulmonary artery pressures, and the presence of diastolic dysfunction and restrictive filling patterns.[36] In the PRIDE study, MR-proADM was a better predictor of 1-year mortality than MR-proANP and NT-proBNP, which were better at prognostication after 1 year from the diagnosis of acute HF.[33]

OTHER BIOMARKERS THAT HAVE BEEN STUDIED IN HEART DISEASE

D-dimer

D-dimer, a degradation product of fibrin, has been well studied and is recommended as a marker for the diagnosis of hypercoagulability and venous thrombosis.[37,38] It has got a very high negative predictive value and elevated levels have been associated with the risk of thrombotic events[39] in patients with a prior history of vascular disease.[40] It has been shown to have a strong positive association with cancer.[41] Various studies have looked at D-dimer levels as a prognostication marker in HF and an elevated D-dimer at hospital admission in patients with HF has at times shown a higher risk of in-hospital deaths and worse event-free survival after 1 year.[42] This finding has not been consistent and no recommendation for its use in routine clinical practice can be made.

Procalcitonin

Procalcitonin (PCT) is a protein that is expressed on parenchymal tissues. It is formed in response to bacterial infection, either by endotoxin or through the action of cytokines (e.g., IL-6). It has been studied as a surrogate marker of infection. In patients with acute HF, it has been reported that elevated PCT concentration (>0.21 ng/mL) had a worse outcome if not treated with antibiotics while those with low PCT values (<0.05 ng/mL) had a better outcome when they did not receive antibiotic therapy.[43] However, more studies would be required before its use can be recommended for initiating antibiotic therapy in HF patients.

BIOMARKERS FOR MONITORING FUNCTION OF BLOOD VESSELS

Injury to blood vessels, mainly to the endothelium and its lining leads to vascular leak, edema formation, and an increase in platelet and leukocyte adhesion. These changes have been seen in all forms of shock and are considered to be the forerunner of organ failure. Many biomarkers, to help diagnose and treat endothelial injury early have been studied.

Endothelial Glycocalyx

This is a mesh-like structure, made of proteoglycans and glycoproteins that line the endothelial lumen of all blood vessels. It is a dynamic interface between blood and vessel wall, which is essential for vascular homeostasis, and regulation of vessel permeability, and its negative charge acts as a barrier that inhibits leukocyte adhesion. Exposure to sheer and oxidative stress causes damage to endothelial glycocalyx (EG), which leads to loss of vascular barrier function, increased vascular permeability, adherence of monocytes to endothelial cells, leukocyte recruitment, and increased platelet aggregation.[44] There is a high association between shedding of EG and mortality in various disease processes including trauma, sepsis, and cardiogenic shock (CS).[45] At present, damage to EG is assessed by estimating serum levels of its breakdown products, syndecan 1 and heparan sulfate. Studies looking at syndecan 1 levels have not shown a consistent pattern and further investigations will be required before it can be recommended for routine clinical use. The technical difficulties in evaluating endothelial dysfunction may have created a vicious cycle of poor understanding and poor attention. Despite difficulties with visualization and volume quantification of eGC, progress in laboratory techniques has increased awareness of eGC roles in the control of endothelial dysfunction by way of shear stress transduction, control of endothelial permeability, and protection of endothelium from inflammatory cells, enzymes, or cytokines with untoward effects. Meanwhile, new techniques to visualize the EG are being studied using a handheld video microscope.[46]

Soluble Thrombomodulin

Soluble thrombomodulin (sTM) is an endothelial cell transmembrane glycoprotein, which is released only when there is endothelial disruption. It also has procoagulant properties. High sTM levels in patients with sepsis have been shown to predict risk for multiple organ failure and mortality better than syndecan 1.[47] Following an acute coronary event its levels are seen to be high in those patients who have multivessel coronary artery disease and it is also noted to be a predictor for increased risk of acute kidney failure in such patients.[48]

Angiopoietin 2

Angiopoietin 2 (Ang 2) is released in response to systemic inflammation, and it activates the endothelial cells increasing their permeability, leading to capillary leak and multiorgan failure. Its level in the plasma is increased in many conditions including acute coronary syndrome and CS.[49] Increased Ang-2 levels were associated with poor in-hospital outcomes in the IABP-SHOCK II Trial in CS. It has been shown to play an important role in pulmonary vascular leak in sepsis and has been implicated in the development of ARDS in patients with sepsis.[50] Studies have not been consistent in demonstrating its diagnostic or prognostic value in critically ill patients.

BIOMARKERS FOR MONITORING PERFUSION STATUS

Decreased organ perfusion, defined as shock, has a very high mortality, if not recognized early and managed promptly. Like HF, diagnosis of shock is made based on clinical signs and symptoms that can be mimicked by many associated comorbidities in a critically ill patient. The clinical assessment of shock and the various types of shock are being dealt with in detail in separate chapters. The development of multiorgan failure also worsens mortality. Multiple biomarkers have been evaluated to help improve diagnostic accuracy and early detection of both organ dysfunction and shock. The discussion on biomarkers to detect early individual organ hypoperfusion is beyond the preview of this chapter.

Most of the biomarkers of global hypoperfusion such as serum lactate, mixed/central venous oxygen saturation, and partial pressure of carbon dioxide (pCO_2) gap are being discussed as separate chapters.

Growth Differentiation Factor-15

In addition to its role as a biomarker in HF, GDF-15 has been seen to be substantially elevated in CS and is a marker of poor outcome, which is independent from the baseline arterial lactate level. Combining arterial lactate and GDF-15 improved the prognostic predictive value in shock. However, there are no studies looking at the role of this biomarker in guiding therapy in shock. Unlike NT-proBNP, GDF-15 is not affected by atrial fibrillation, so this biomarker could be particularly useful in these patients when combined with natriuretic peptides.[51]

CONCLUSION

An ideal biomarker that qualifies all the criteria laid down by "The Biomarkers Definition Working Group," is quite difficult to find. There are multiple biomarkers under evaluation for monitoring the components of hemodynamics. They are being aggressively studied, their assays fine-tuned, and it is only a matter of time before many more of them would come to be part of clinical recommendations/guidelines. At present, natriuretic peptides have a clear role in the diagnosis and prognostication of HF, while their role in guiding therapy is still debatable. Troponins have their defined role and very clear guidelines for use in acute coronary events and in acute HF, for disease risk stratification. A guideline for transitioning to hsTn assay is also available. D-dimer too has clear guidelines issued for use in the diagnosis of venous thrombosis. All other biomarkers discussed have their evidence, as discussed, but studies have not been able to show them to be consistently useful and hence they cannot be recommended for regular bedside use. Their role in clinical medicine is still evolving. None of the biomarkers have significantly improved the clinical ability to distinguish between health and disease states. None of them are sensitive or specific enough to be used as therapeutic targets before clinical signs and symptoms appear, so their use to make decisions on initiating or changing therapy in an individual patient should be done only after having made very clear clinical considerations.

REFERENCES

1. Biomarkers Definition Working Group. Biomarkers and surrogate endpoints: preferred definitions and conceptual framework. Clin Pharmacol Therapeutics. 2001;69(3):89-95.
2. Dokainish H, Teo K, Zhu J, Roy A, AlHabib KF, ElSayed A, et al. Global mortality variations in patients with heart failure: results from the International Congestive Heart Failure (INTER-CHF) prospective cohort study. Lancet Glob Health. 2017;5(7):e665-72.
3. Morrison LK, Harrison A, Krishnaswamy P, Kazanegra R, Clopton P, Maisel A. Utility of a rapid B-natriuretic peptide assay in differentiating congestive heart failure from lung disease in patients presenting with dyspnea. J Am Coll Cardiol. 2002;39(2):202-9.
4. Maisel AS, Krishnaswamy P, Nowak RM, McCord J, Hollander JE, Duc P, et al. Rapid measurement of B-type natriuretic peptide in the emergency diagnosis of heart failure. N Engl J Med. 2002;347(3):161-7.
5. Chow SL, Maisel AS, Anand I, Bozkurt B, de Boer RA, Felker GM, et al. Role of biomarkers for the prevention, assessment, and management of heart failure: a scientific statement from the American Heart Association. Circulation. 2017;135(22):e1054-91.
6. Januzzi JL Jr, Camargo CA, Anwaruddin S, Baggish AL, Chen AA, Krauser DG, et al. The N-terminal Pro-BNP investigation of dyspnea in the emergency department (PRIDE) study. Am J Cardiol. 2005;95(8):948-54.
7. Januzzi JL, van Kimmenade R, Lainchbury J, Bayes-Genis A, Ordonez-Llanos J, Santalo-Bel M, et al. NT-proBNP testing for diagnosis and short-term prognosis in acute destabilized heart failure: an international pooled analysis of 1256 patients: The International Collaborative of NT-proBNP Study. Eur Heart J. 2006;27(3):330-7.
8. Krishnaswamy P, Lubien E, Clopton P, Koon J, Kazanegra R, Wanner E, et al. Utility of B-natriuretic peptide levels in identifying patients with left ventricular systolic or diastolic dysfunction. Am J Med. 2001;111(4):274-9.
9. Maisel AS, McCord J, Nowak RM, Hollander JE, Wu AH, Duc P, et al. Bedside B-Type natriuretic peptide in the emergency diagnosis of heart failure with reduced or preserved ejection fraction. Results from the Breathing Not Properly Multinational Study. J Am Coll. Cardiol. 2003;41(11):2010-7.
10. Latini R, Masson S, Anand I, Judd D, Maggioni AP, Chiang YT, et al. Effects of valsartan on circulating brain natriuretic peptide and norepinephrine in symptomatic chronic heart failure: The Valsartan Heart Failure Trial (Val-HeFT). Circulation. 2002;106(19):2454-8.
11. Stanek B, Frey B, Hülsmann M, Berger R, Sturm B, Strametz-Juranek J, et al. Prognostic evaluation of neurohumoral plasma levels before and during beta-blocker therapy in advanced left ventricular dysfunction. J Am Coll Cardiol. 2001;38(2):436-42.
12. Yoshimura M, Mizuno Y, Nakayama M, Sakamoto T, Sugiyama S, Kawano H, et al. B-type natriuretic peptide as a marker of the effects of enalapril in patients with heart failure. Am J Med. 2002;112(9):716-20.
13. Berry C, Murphy NF, De Vito G, Galloway S, Seed A, Fisher C, et al. Effects of aldosterone receptor blockade in patients with mild-moderate heart failure taking a beta-blocker. Eur J Heart Fail. 2007;9(4):429-34.
14. Menardi E, Vado A, Rossetti G, Racca E, Conte E, Deorsola A, et al. Cardiac resynchronization therapy modifies the neurohormonal profile, hemodynamic and functional capacity in heart failure patients. Arch Med Res. 2008;39(7):702-8.
15. Ledwidge M, Gallagher J, Conlon C, Tallon E, O'Connell E, Dawkins I, et al. N Natriuretic peptide-based screening and collaborative care for heart failure: the STOP-HF randomized trial. JAMA. 2013;310(1):66-74.

16. Felker GM, Hasselblad V, Hernandez AF, O'Connor CM. Biomarker-guided therapy in chronic heart failure: a meta-analysis of randomized controlled trials. Am Heart J. 2009;158(3):422-30.
17. Felker GM, Anstrom KJ, Adams KF, Ezekowitz JA, Fiuzat M, Houston-Miller N, et al. Effect of Natriuretic Peptide-Guided Therapy on Hospitalization or Cardiovascular Mortality in High-Risk Patients with Heart Failure and Reduced Ejection Fraction: A Randomized Clinical Trial. JAMA. 2017;318(8):713-20.
18. Amsterdam EA, Wenger NK, Brindis RG, Casey DE Jr, Ganiats TG, Holmes DR Jr, et al. 2014 AHA/ACC guideline for the management of patients with non-ST-elevation acute coronary syndromes: a report of the American College of Cardiology/American Heart Association Task Force on Practice Guidelines. J Am Coll Cardiol. 2014;64(24):e139-228.
19. Eckel RH, Jakicic JM, Ard JD, de Jesus JM, Houston Miller N, Hubbard VS, et al. 2013 AHA/ACC guideline on lifestyle management to reduce cardiovascular risk: a report of the American College of Cardiology/American Heart Association Task Force on Practice Guidelines. J Am Coll Cardiol. 2014;63(25 Pt B):2960-84.
20. Apple FS, Collinson PO; IFCC Task Force on Clinical Applications of Cardiac Biomarkers. Analytical characteristics of high-sensitivity cardiac troponin assays. Clin Chem. 2012;58(1):54-61.
21. Pascual-Figal DA, Casas T, Ordonez-Llanos J, Manzano-Fernández S, Bonaque JC, Boronat M, et al. Highly sensitive troponin T for risk stratification of acutely destabilized heart failure. Am Heart J. 2012;163(6):1002-10.
22. Saunders JT, Nambi V, de Lemos JA, Chambless LE, Virani SS, Boerwinkle E, et al. Cardiac troponin T measured by a highly sensitive assay predicts coronary heart disease, heart failure, and mortality in the Atherosclerosis Risk in Communities Study. Circulation. 2011;123(13):1367-76.
23. Januzzi JL Jr, Mahler SA, Christenson RH, Rymer J, Newby LK, Body R, et al. Recommendations for Institutions Transitioning to High-Sensitivity Troponin Testing: JACC Scientific Expert Panel. J Am Coll Cardiol. 2019;73(9):1059-77.
24. Gaggin HK, Motiwala S, Bhardwaj A, Parks KA, Januzzi JL Jr. Soluble concentrations of the interleukin receptor family member ST2 and β-blocker therapy in chronic heart failure. Circ Heart Fail. 2013;6(6):1206-13.
25. Maisel A, Xue Y, van Veldhuisen DJ, Voors AA, Jaarsma T, Pang PS, et al. Effect of spironolactone on 30-day death and heart failure rehospitalization (from the COACH Study). Am J Cardiol. 2014;114(5):737-42.
26. Chen A, Hou W, Zhang Y, Chen Y, He B. Prognostic value of serum galectin-3 in patients with heart failure: a meta-analysis. Int J Cardiol. 2015;182:168-70.
27. Van Kimmenade RR, Januzzi JL, Ellinor PT, Sharma UC, Bakker JA, Low AF, et al. Utility of amino-terminal pro-brain natriuretic peptide, galectin-3, and apelin for the evaluation of patients with acute heart failure. J Am Coll Cardiol. 2006;48(6):1217-24.
28. de Boer RA, Daniels LB, Maisel AS, Januzzi JL Jr. State of the Art: Newer biomarkers in heart failure. Eur J Heart Fail. 2015;17(6):559-69.
29. Fuernau G. Lactate and other biomarkers as treatment target in cardiogenic shock. Curr Opin Crit Care. 2019;25(4):403-9.
30. Wollert KC, Kempf T. Growth differentiation factor 15 in heart failure: an update. Curr Heart Fail Rep. 2012;9(4): 337-45.
31. Rosenzweig A, Seidman AE. Atrial natriuretic factor and related peptide hormones. Annu Rev Biochem. 1991;60:229-55.
32. Maisel A, Mueller C, Nowak R, Peacock WF, Landsberg JW, Ponikowski P, et al. Mid-region pro-hormone markers for diagnosis and prognosis in acute dyspnea: results from the BACH (Biomarkers in Acute Heart Failure) trial. J Am Coll Cardiol. 2010;55(19):2062-76.
33. Shah RV, Truong QA, Gaggin HK, Pfannkuche J, Hartmann O, Januzzi JL. Mid-regional pro-atrial natriuretic peptide and pro-adrenomedullin testing for the diagnostic and prognostic evaluation of patients with acute dyspnoea. Eur Heart J. 2012;33(17):2197-205.
34. Kitamura K. Adrenomedullin and related peptides. Nihon Yakurigaku Zasshi. 1998;112(3):137-46.
35. Ikeda U, Kanbe T, Kawahara Y, Yokoyama M, Shimada K. Adrenomedullin augments inducible nitric oxide synthase expression in cytokine-stimulated cardiac myocytes. Circulation. 1996;94(10):2560-5.
36. Nishikimi T, Saito Y, Kitamura K, Ishimitsu T, Eto T, Kangawa K, et al. Increased plasma levels of adrenomedullin in patients with heart failure. J Am Coll Cardiol. 1995;26(6):1424-31.
37. Meade TW, Mellows S, Brozovic M, Miller GJ, Chakrabarti RR, North WR, et al. Haemostatic function and ischaemic heart disease: principal results of the Northwick Park Heart Study. Lancet. 1986;2(8506):533-7.
38. Lim V, Le Gal G, Bates SM, Righini M, Haramati LB, Lang E, et al. American Society of Hematology 2018 guidelines for management of venous thromboembolism: diagnosis of venous thromboembolism. Blood Advances. 2018;2(22):3226-56.
39. Zakai NA, Katz R, Jenny NS, Psaty BM, Reiner AP, Schwartz SM, et al. Inflammation and hemostasis biomarkers and cardiovascular risk in the elderly: The Cardiovascular Health Study. J Thromb Haemost. 2007;5(6):1128-35.
40. Kleinegris MC, Ten Cate H, ten Cate-Hoek AJ. D-dimer as a marker for cardiovascular and arterial thrombotic events in patients with peripheral arterial disease. A systematic review. Thromb Haemost. 2013;110(2):233-43.
41. Ay C, Dunkler D, Pirker R, Thaler J, Quehenberger P, Wagner O, et al. High D-dimer levels are associated with poor prognosis in cancer patients. Haematologica. 2012;97(8):1158-64.

42. Bittencourt MI, Rocha RM, Rey HCV, Rangel FOD, Oliveira FT, Salgado CG, et al. Prognostic value of D-dimer in acute heart failure. Crit Care. 2005;9(Suppl 2):P29.
43. Maisel A, Neath SX, Landsberg J, Mueller C, Nowak RM, Peacock WF, et al. Use of procalcitonin for the diagnosis of pneumonia in patients presenting with a chief complaint of dyspnoea: results from the BACH (Biomarkers in Acute Heart Failure) trial. Eur J Heart Fail. 2012;14(3):278-86.
44. Liew H, Roberts MA, MacGinley R, McMahon LP. Endothelial glycocalyx in health and kidney disease: Rising star or false Dawn? Nephrology (Carlton). 2017;22(12):940-6.
45. Frydland M, Ostrowski SR, Møller JE, Hadziselimovic E, Holmvang L, Ravn HB, et al. Plasma Concentration of Biomarkers Reflecting Endothelial Cell- and Glycocalyx Damage are Increased in Patients With Suspected ST-Elevation Myocardial Infarction Complicated by Cardiogenic Shock. Shock. 2018;50(5):538-44.
46. Schött U, Solomon C, Fries D, Bentzer P. The endothelial glycocalyx and its disruption, protection and regeneration: a narrative review. Scand J Trauma Resusc Emerg Med. 2016;24:48.
47. Johansen ME, Johansson PI, Ostrowski SR, Bestle MH, Hein L, Jensen AL, et al. Profound Endothelial Damage Predicts Impending Organ Failure and Death in Sepsis. Semin Thromb Hemost. 2015;41(1):16-25.
48. Liu KL, Lee KT, Chang CH, Chen YC, Lin SM, Chu PH. Elevated plasma thrombomodulin and angiopoietin-2 predict the development of acute kidney injury in patients with acute myocardial infarction. Crit Care. 2014;18(3): R100.
49. Fan PC, Chang CH, Chen YC. Biomarkers for acute cardiorenal syndrome. Nephrology. 2018;23(Suppl 4): 68-71.
50. Hendrickson CM, Matthay MA. Endothelial biomarkers in human sepsis: pathogenesis and prognosis for ARDS. Pulmonary Circulation. 2018;8(2):2045894018769876.
51. Santema BT, Chan MMY, Tromp J, Dokter M, van der Wal HH, Emmens JE, et al. The influence of atrial fibrillation on the levels of NT-proBNP versus GDF-15 in patients with heart failure. Clin Res Cardiol 2020;109(3): 331-8.

CHAPTER

Monitoring Regional Circulation

Jacob George Pulinilkunnathil, Atul Prabhakar Kulkarni

INTRODUCTION

Optimizing organ perfusion is the keystone of hemodynamic monitoring. This in turn depends on preserved macro- and microcirculation. A holistic approach to hemodynamic monitoring should take into consideration the relationship between oxygen demand and oxygen delivery rather than a preconceived target of cardiac output as a goal for hemodynamic monitoring. Routine markers for monitoring the adequacy of circulation at the bedside include clinical examination of skin and monitoring hourly urine output, assessment of mentation, and bedside application of other markers, such as serum lactate, central venous oxygen saturation ($ScvO_2$), central-venous and arterial carbon dioxide gap ($Ca\text{-}vCO_2$-gap). Although there are numerous fallacies for the use of these markers as a surrogate for adequacy of circulation, when incorporated into patient management protocols, they give information regarding the adequacy of cardiac output at a global level and also throw light on the adequacy of microcirculatory impairment. With a need to assess the perfusion of individual organs during critical illness, there has been a renewed interest in the development of sophisticated technologies that give a better idea of regional circulation. This chapter will give a precis of the assessment of regional circulation in critically ill patients, although the practical applications for these technologies are still evolving.

CIRCULATION IN SKIN

Skin is the largest organ in the body and assessment of the circulatory status starts with assessing the perfusion of skin. In a state of shock, due to vasoconstriction, the perfusion to the skin is affected early, as blood is diverted to the vital organs. Due to a lack of autoregulation in cutaneous circulation, cutaneous circulation is affected directly by neurohumoral mechanisms which are in turn responsible for maintaining temperature homeostasis. Thus, skin temperature is strongly associated with cardiac output and has been proposed as a guide for the treatment of shock or to predict mortality. Skin temperature can be recorded by intermittent temperature measurements or maybe in the future, there will be a refinement in technologies such as thermal imagery, infrared thermometers, etc., which may permit continuous skin temperature monitoring. A more prosaic way of measuring skin perfusion is an assessment of capillary refill time and grading of skin mottling. Mottling occurs due to heterogeneous constriction of the microcirculation in the skin and can be assessed in an objective manner (e.g., mottling scores and laser Doppler analysis) to predict the intensive care unit (ICU) outcomes. Capillary refill time of the distal phalanx of the index finger and sternum (in pediatric patients) also has been proposed as a resuscitation goal and as a predictor of outcomes although there is considerable variation in the proposed cut-offs and considerable interobserver variability[1] (For a more detailed description see Chapter 19 "Clinical Assessment of Shock").

CIRCULATION OF THE BRAIN

Cerebral circulation is fundamental for optimal neuronal function and accounts for approximately 15–20% of the total circulation. Assessing the adequacy of cerebral circulation is important at the bedside, especially in high-risk cases such as suspected brain death, subarachnoid hemorrhage, stroke, seizures, etc.

Jugular venous oximetry has been used traditionally to assess and monitor the adequacy of cerebral oxygenation. The jugular bulb drains approximately 70% of blood from the ipsilateral side and approximately 30% of blood from the contralateral hemisphere with negligible (<3%) extracerebral contamination. The venous saturation can be analyzed intermittently by direct aspiration of blood from the jugular bulb, via a central line placed retrogradely, by fiberoptic catheters that provide continuous oximetry values, or by fiberoptic probes in the jugular bulb that provide intermittent values. The value of jugular oximetry is usually in the range of 55–75% which is lower than the mixed venous oxygen values. Further desaturation may be seen in cases of increased cerebral demand as in cases of fever, seizures, or in cases of decreased cerebral blood flow (CBF) [due to embolism, raised intracranial pressure (ICP), systemic hypotension] and also in cases due to migration of the catheter tip, or due to increased extracerebral contamination.[2]

Near-infrared spectroscopy (NIRS) and transcranial Doppler (TCD) are currently the most commonly used methods to assess cerebral circulation. Near-infrared spectroscopy monitors the local alterations in cerebral hemodynamics that occur due to neuronal activity and associated oxygen utilization. Infrared photons are differentially absorbed by oxygenated hemoglobin and deoxygenated hemoglobin and therefore mathematical calculation based on the difference in absorption spectra can give continuous real-time information on cerebral oxygenation. The main drawback of NIRS is the possibility of extracerebral contamination (change in the values obtained due to alteration of signals from extracerebral tissues such as skull and skin) which can mask significant cerebral hypoxia.[3] The threshold value of NIRS below which the hypoxic complications increase, or the duration of hypoxia below a threshold value that produces complications are not clear as of now. Other limitations are the cost of the disposables, and relatively insensitivity to focal ischemia, and lack of depth of penetration by the photons to provide an accurate value of deeper brain tissue **(Figs. 1A and B)**.[1,4,5] The partial pressure of oxygen in brain tissue ($PbtO_2$) as measured with Licox CMP Triple Lumen Monitoring System (Integra NeuroSciences) has also been explored to assess the adequacy of cerebral oxygen delivery and demand. The device consists of a bedside monitor, a display screen, and probes that measure the temperature, intracranial pressure, and brain tissue oxygenation which has to be surgically placed via an intracranial bolt. After calibration, a continuous reading of $PbtO_2$, temperature, and ICP are displayed. The normal values of $PbtO_2$ vary from 25 to 50 mm Hg. Lower values are suggestive of ischemia while very low values below 5 mm Hg suggest irreversible damage and death. The system is compatible with CT scans but not with magnetic resonance imaging (MRI). The main drawback is that Licox provides information regarding regional oxygen measurement and may not correlate with global cerebral perfusion.

Transcranial Doppler measures the velocity of moving red blood cells and calculates the Doppler shift and thus an estimate of CBF can be made at the bedside. This is done by using a low-frequency phase array probe and selecting an acoustic window through the transtemporal window, transfrontal window, transorbital window, or submandibular window **(Figs. 2 and 3)**. A reduced flow below 25–30 cm/s, or a relative reduction of 60–80% flow from the baseline suggests increased chances of cerebral ischemia. However, as the exact vessel diameter cannot be determined, the calculation of exact blood volume is only an assumption. In the ICU, TCD can be used for diagnosing midline shift, vasospasm, raised ICP, absent blood flow suggestive of brain death **(Fig. 4)**, hemorrhage, etc. TCD is operator-dependent, has a steep learning curve, and is affected by the need for a good acoustic window, angulation of the probe, etc., limiting its routine use in the ICU.[6-8]

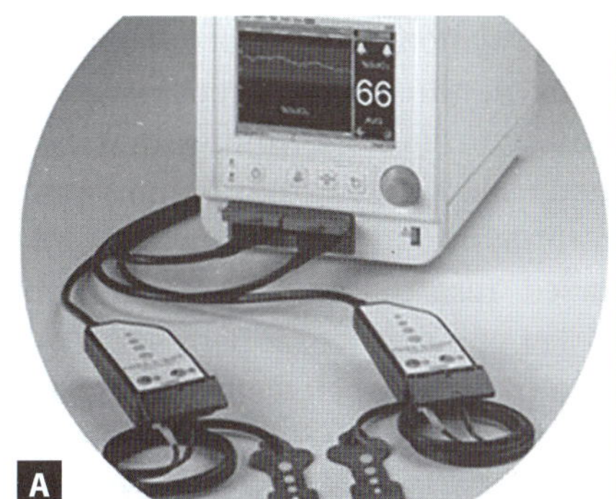

A

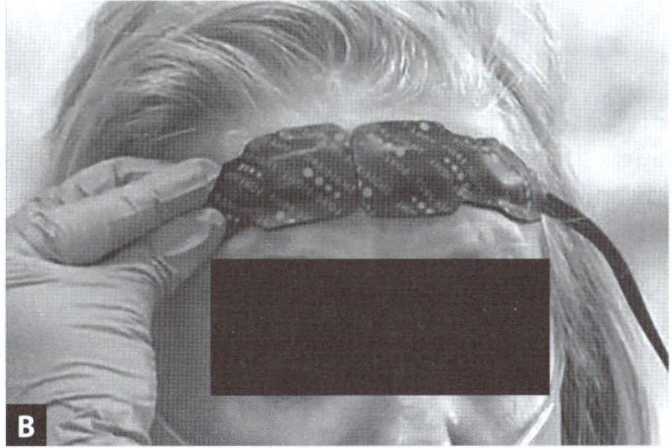
B

Figs. 1A and B: Equipment used for near-infrared spectroscopy *(For color version, see Plate 2)*.
Source: Adapted from Medgadget and Naqvi et al.[4,5]

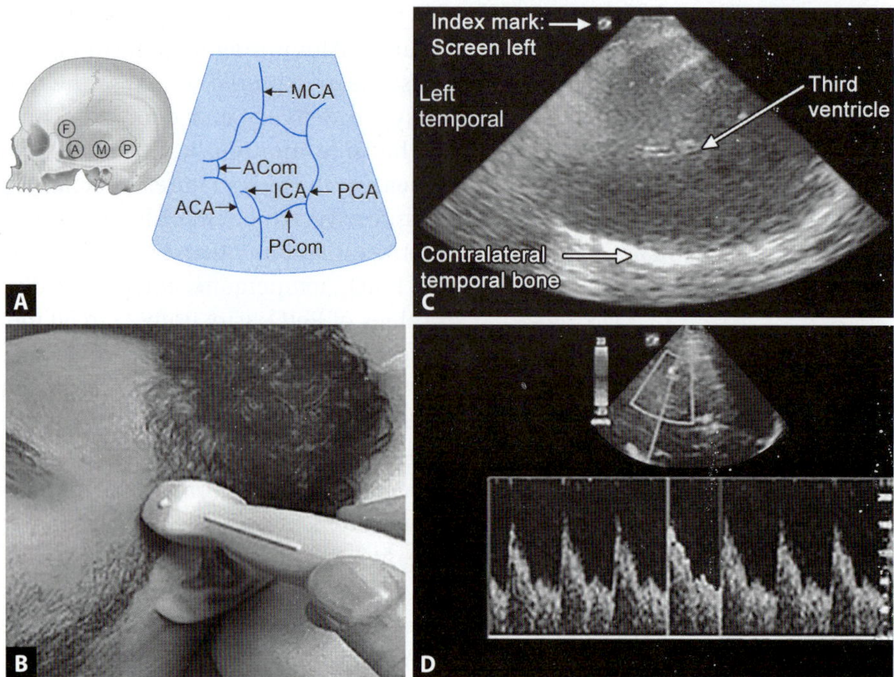

Figs. 2A to D: Transcranial Doppler. Method for the acquisition of TCD: (A) The left side shows the location of the transtemporal window and its various sections: Frontal, anterior, medial, and posterior. The right side illustrates the circle of Willis, with MCA highlighted; (B) Probe index mark orientation toward the patient's anterior/front; (C) Typical 2D image of TCD from transtemporal window with index mark to screen left, with bright echogenic contralateral temporal bone, and anechoic space of midline third ventricle; (D) Typical spectral Doppler velocity waveform from MCA, with steep systolic upstroke and step-down diastolic flow (typical mean velocity of 80 cm/s). (ACom: anterior communicating; A: anterior; ACA: anterior cerebral artery; F: frontal; ICA: internal carotid artery; M: medial; MCA: middle cerebral artery; PCom: posterior communicating; P: posterior; PCA: posterior cerebral artery; TCD: transcranial Doppler)
Source: Adapted from Lau VI, et al.[6]

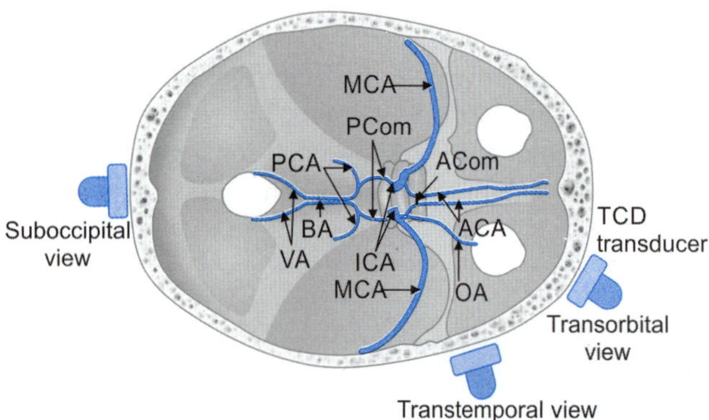

Fig. 3: Various windows for transcranial Doppler. (ACA: anterior cerebral artery; ACom: anterior communicating; BA: basilar artery; ICA: internal carotid artery; MCA: middle cerebral artery; OA: ophthalmic artery; PCA: posterior cerebral artery; PCom: posterior communicating; VA: vertebral artery)
Source: Image adapted from Samagh N, et al.[7]

SPLANCHNIC CIRCULATION

During hypoperfused states, splanchnic circulation is affected early in the course of the disease and is also the last to recover. High gastric residual volumes, ileus, abdominal distention, etc., can be inferred as signs of splanchnic hypoperfusion although they are neither specific nor sensitive and may appear only late in splanchnic hypoperfusion. Assessing bowel edema by ultrasound is highly subjective while X-ray and computed tomography (CT) are associated with harmful effects of radiation and lack actual measurement of blood flow and flow at the microcirculation. The use of contrast can cause contrast-induced nephropathy; direct visualization of ischemic mucosa on upper gastrointestinal (GI) endoscopy is of limited use being intermittent in nature and inability to identify hypoperfusion before the mucosal injury has occurred. Tests that measure absorption and clearance as a marker of gut mucosal permeability [with agents such as chromium 51-labeled ethylenediamine tetraacetic acid (EDTA), urea, lactulose, mannitol, and lactulose/mannitol ratio] have been studied in experimental settings, animal models, and clinical studies, but have not been validated for routine use at the bedside. The other methods that

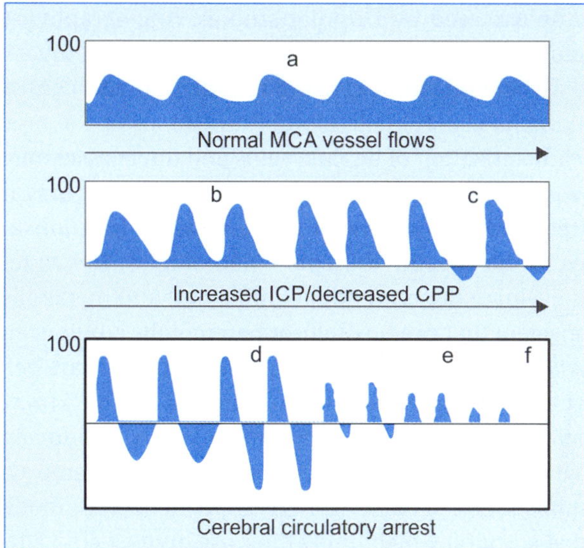

Fig. 4: Progression of intracranial circulatory arrest via transcranial Doppler of middle cerebral artery flows. a—normal systolic upstroke with normal step-down of diastolic flow. b—increased peak systolic flow with decreasing diastolic flow and eventual blunting of diastolic flow. c—diastolic flow reversal. d—biphasic or oscillating flow—where diastolic flow reversal approaches equal size to systolic flow. e—isolated sharp systolic peak flows of <200 milliseconds and small systolic amplitude of <50 cm/s. f—zero flow—where there was previously documented TCD flow. The black box denotes states (d, e, and f) in which cerebral circulatory arrest can be diagnosed. (CPP: cerebral perfusion pressure; ICP: intracranial pressure; MCA: middle cerebral artery)
Source: Adapted from Lau VI, et al.[6]

have been evaluated for assessing splanchnic perfusion are reflectance spectrophotometry, gastric tonometry, sublingual capnometry, indocyanine green (ICG) clearance, Doppler flowmetry of mesenteric vessels, direct estimation of tissue oxygen levels in the colon with the help of oxygen electrodes, etc. The use of radioactive microspheres with postmortem measurement of tissue concentration of microspheres has also been tried, mainly in research as it requires tissue for assessment of perfusion. Of the currently described measures, only gastric tonometry has been studied extensively in critically ill patients.

Reflectance Spectrophotometry

Reflectance spectrophotometry relies on the optical properties of light that is being scattered or absorbed from the mucosa surface of the gut. The instrument consists of two light probes, one that emits light and one that measures the reflected light. Changes in the difference in properties of the light reflect the changes in oxyhemoglobin and deoxyhemoglobin thus reflecting the mucosal oxygenation and perfusion. A spectrum analyzer records the difference in absorption and thus calculates the blood flow across the tissue.[9]

Gastric Tonometry

Gastric tonometry works on the principle that CO_2 levels in the tissues depend upon CO_2 production and CO_2 washout which in turn is significantly affected by regional blood flow assuming normal respiratory status. The bicarbonate levels inside the tissue are the same as that of plasma, while CO_2 is easily diffusible across membranes and follows the laws of passive diffusion according to partial pressures.[10]

In cases of shock, the CO_2 accumulates in tissue due to reduced blood flow and reduced CO_2 clearance. Anaerobic metabolism due to reduced oxygen delivery leads to lactic acidosis and the production of H^+ ions. H^+ ions are buffered with bicarbonate, leading to the accumulation of CO_2, and the tissue CO_2 rises more than what is expected due to a reduction in blood flow. Hence monitoring mucosal CO_2 concentration of the tissues and applying the Henderson-Hasselbalch equation will give an idea of intracellular pH (pHi; a marker of lactic acidosis and anaerobic metabolism) and also an idea about the splanchnic blood flow.[10]

In this technique, a catheter with a semipermeable silicone balloon attached at the tip of the catheter is placed into the stomach (similar to an oronasogastric tube) and the balloon is filled with normal saline. As anaerobic metabolism ensues, the resulting lactic acidosis will cause a drop in intramucosal pH. The H^+ ions thus produced will be buffered by bicarbonate and that will result in an additional increase in CO_2. The CO_2 freely diffuses out from the gastric mucosal cells into the saline-filled balloon and can be measured after a period of equilibrium. After a dwell time for equilibrium, (1–1.5 hours) the partial pressure of carbon dioxide (PCO_2) in the saline is measured using a blood gas analyzer. Assuming that the bicarbonate content of mucosa is the same as blood, and by applying the Henderson-Hasselbalch equation, the gastric intramucosal (pHi) is determined. This method can be used to measure the pH of the stomach or sigmoid colon. Measurements can be made as early as 10 minutes although a dwell time of at least 30 minutes is recommended. An abnormally high value can be obtained in patients with high arterial CO_2, and also by impaired removal of CO_2. Therefore, the usage of high values of tonometer PCO_2 as a surrogate of tissue hypoperfusion needs to be correlated with the clinical scenario. Gastric tonometry is criticized for the assumption that arterial bicarbonate will be similar to intramucosal bicarbonate. Currently, an arterial-to-mucosal PCO_2 gradient >8 mm Hg is suggestive of gut mucosal hypoperfusion, but not necessarily ischemia or hypoxia. Clinically, the pHi has been shown to be a good prognostic indicator in perioperative patients and critically ill patients. However, targeting pHi with gastric tonometry for resuscitation has not been shown to improve outcomes.[11]

Sublingual Capnometry

Although not a part of the splanchnic circulation, sublingual capnometry is also part of the GI tract monitoring as the tongue is developmentally a part of the foregut. Monitoring the changes in sublingual CO_2 is an easily applied tool at the bedside for hemodynamic assessment in shock and does not need interruption of enteral feeds. As already mentioned, the CO_2 content in tissues is determined by the arterial CO_2 content, CO_2 production in tissues, and on tissue perfusion. In shock or hypoperfusion, the CO_2 content increases due to increased CO_2 production and reduced clearance. Measurement of sublingual capnometry thus provides an easy, reliable, and fast method for assessing the adequacy of regional circulation. Studies have shown that sublingual CO_2 can be used as a bedside tool for predicting outcomes. In conjunction with arterial PCO_2, the difference between sublingual CO_2 and arterial PCO_2 is also shown to be a good predictor of microcirculatory flow and outcomes. Potential drawbacks for applying sublingual capnometry in routine monitoring include lack of continuous monitoring, lack of data on the normal value of sublingual CO_2, its variation with different types of shock, interference due to direct stimulation of sublingual flow during measurement of capnometry and by the presence of sublingual drugs or enteral feed which can increase sublingual blood flow and potentially reduce the CO_2 content and role of microbial flora in exogenous CO_2 production. Hemodynamic resuscitation targeting the normalization of sublingual CO_2 has also not translated into clinically useful outcomes.[12]

Hepatic Blood Flow Monitoring

The excretory and synthetic *function* of the liver is dependent on adequate perfusion and maintenance of normal physiology. A gross assessment of blood flow to the liver can be assessed by Doppler studies. Angiography—CT angiography or direct angiography is more invasive and associated with exposure to radiation and contrast, limiting its use. Hepatic blood flow can also be assessed by catheterization of hepatic veins and direct assessment. However, these functions are slow to happen, may not correlate with improving or worsening liver function, and may not be specific to hepatic pathologies. Hence tests that evaluate the excretion, elimination, and metabolism of an agent that can be orally or parenterally administered and not directly influenced by other parameters are being developed. Repetitive measurements of the kinetics of such an agent or its metabolites, such as lidocaine, caffeine, and galactose. have been tried for the same. Oral administration of these agents is dependent on GI motility and absorption which limits their use in most critically ill patients.[1]

Use of Indocyanine Green to Assess Liver Circulation

Indocyanine green is a water-soluble dye that is protein-bound and completely metabolized in the liver. Pharmacokinetics thus depend upon the blood flow through the liver, the hepatocellular uptake, and on the excretion of unconjugated ICG via bile. After administration, ICG appears in the bile for 8 minutes and reaches a maximum concentration in 2 hours.[13] It is neither excreted via the kidney nor does it cross the blood–brain barrier or placental barrier. Based on the pharmacokinetics data, ICG metabolism is then used to determine cardiac output, blood volume, and hepatic blood flow. The rate of plasma disappearance of ICG (ICG-PDR) and the amount of ICG retained after 15 minutes (ICG R15) are the variables used for measuring liver ICG clearance. The normal ICG-PDR values are estimated to be >500 mL/min/m^2 or >18%/min, respectively.[14] As the extraction rate of ICG from blood by the liver is normally high, ICG clearance is dependent on the blood flow through the liver. Thus, ICG monitoring can be used for assessing both intrinsic hepatic function and hepatic blood flow **(Table 1)**. Currently, the LiMON device from Pulsion **(Fig. 5)** and the DDG2001 analyzer from Nihon Kohden are the commercially available devices that provide data on hepatic blood flow using ICG.

CIRCULATION IN KIDNEY

Similar to splanchnic circulation, renal blood flow can be assessed by microsphere distribution methods and

TABLE 1: ICG kinetic variables.

Indocyanine plasma disappearance rate (ICG-PDR)	Reduction of blood concentration of ICG expressed as a percentage from an initial concentration of 100%	18–24%/min
Indocyanine retention rate (ICGR15)	Ratio of concentration of ICG 15 minutes post-injection to the baseline value	<10%
Indocyanine half-life ICG (t1/2)	Time is taken for a 50% reduction in the concentration of indocyanine green from the baseline	3–5 minutes
Indocyanine green plasma clearance (^{Cl}ICG)	Volume of plasma that is cleared off of indocyanine green per unit of time	6–12 mL/min/kg

(ICG: indocyanine green; PDR: plasma disappearance rate)
Source: Modified from Groeneveld AB, Kolkman JJ. Splanchnic tonometry: a review of physiology, methodology, and clinical applications. J Crit Care. 1994;9(3):198-210.[10]

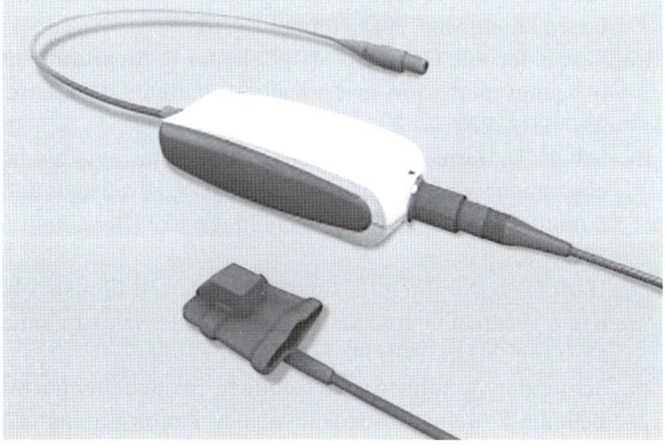

Fig. 5: LiMON probe *(For color version, see Plate 2).*

measuring the concentration in tissues postmortem. This is obviously not suited for practice in critical care, at the bedside. Renal plasma flow is classically estimated by measurement of renal clearance of para-aminohippurate (PAH). PAH is a metabolically inert compound, completely excreted by the kidney, and is neither secreted nor absorbed from the tubules. Thus, the renal clearance of PAH can be used for measuring renal blood flow. So, after an initial bolus and continuous administration of PAH, serial concentrations are measured in plasma and blood, and the blood flow is estimated from plasma clearance of PAH. However, its measurement is cumbersome and depends on intact urine production unless calculated from renal vein samples. Other measures of estimating renal blood flow are thermodilution and xenon washout.

Direct measurement of renal blood flow from intravascular Doppler technique has been described but it has not gained popularity due to its invasive nature. Other techniques that have been described to measure renal flow include nuclear scintigraphy, positron emission tomography, MRI with contrast, cine phase-contrast MRI, arterial spin labeling, blood-oxygen-level-dependent (BOLD), MRI, etc. However, their routine use is limited due to technical issues related to the cost and availability of MRI and shifting of the patients to MRI, retroperitoneal fibrosis associated with gadolinium, etc. Further research in this field may open up more possibilities.

At the bedside, ultrasonography is the most routinely used imaging modality in patients with kidney diseases. It provides information on the size of the kidney, maintenance of cortical thickness and corticomedullary differentiation, the echogenicity and also enables the diagnosis of postrenal acute kidney injury (AKI). Doppler ultrasound can enhance the results of normal ultrasound monitoring and give an estimate of renal blood flow through the kidney. Doppler ultrasound-derived values of renal resistive index (RRI) and renal artery diameter give accurate information regarding renal blood flow. RRI is calculated by measuring the difference between peak systolic velocity and lowest diastolic velocity and dividing it by the peak systolic velocity.[15] Although noninvasive, and available at bedside, it requires repeated measurements and has significant interobserver variation. It is also affected by vessel compliance, heart rate, and rhythm, pressure applied by a transducer, etc. RRI has been shown to have a direct correlation with the occurrence of acute tubular necrosis and predicts the incidence of AKI accurately. Although promising at the bedside, this technique cannot differentiate between a combination of clinical scenarios such as the presence of elevated renal vascular resistance with reduced renal flow versus normal renal vascular resistance but exaggerated flow or from decreased renal vascular resistance with increased flow.[16,17]

The use of contrast (microbubbles from agitated saline as contrast media or commercially available contrast agents) with ultrasound has helped to better delineate the arterial bed and thereby aid in the visualization of the renal microcirculation. It is well tolerated at the bedside and can be used repeatedly to determine changes in renal circulation. Awaiting further studies, contrast-enhanced ultrasound appears to be a potent promising tool to evaluate renal perfusion in critical illness.[17,18]

CONCLUSION

Optimization of organ perfusion requires frequent assessment of the macro- and microcirculation to guide therapy. At the bedside, this is achieved by clinical examination and measurement of lactate, $ScvO_2$, central-venous, and arterial CO_2 gap (cv-a-pCO_2-gap). Assessing regional circulation is likely to help in fine-tuning the therapy further. Noninvasive techniques such as ultrasound and its improvisation seem promising and these too hold the way forward for a holistic approach to the global optimization of hemodynamics.

REFERENCES

1. Huber W, Zanner R, Schneider G, Schmid R, Lahmer T. Assessment of regional perfusion and organ function: less and non-invasive techniques. Front Med (Lausanne). 2019;6:1-15.
2. Schell RM, Cole DJ. Cerebral monitoring: jugular venous oximetry. Anesth Analg. 2000;90(3):559-66.
3. Davie SN, Grocott HP. Impact of extracranial contamination on regional cerebral oxygen saturation: a comparison of three cerebral oximetry technologies. Anesthesiology. 2012;116(4):834-40.
4. Medgadget. (2012). Continuous Near-Infrared Regional Cerebral Perfusion Monitoring Shows Promise in Stroke Patients. [online] Available from https://www.medgadget.com/2012/02/continuous-near-infrared-regional-cerebral-perfusion-monitoring-shows-promise-in-stroke-patients. html/ [Last accessed October, 2023].
5. Naqvi J, Yap KH, Ahmad G, Ghosh J. Transcranial Doppler ultrasound: a review of the physical principles and major applications in critical care. Int J Vasc Med. 2013;2013:629378.
6. Lau VI, Arntfield RT. Point-of-care transcranial Doppler by intensivists. Crit Ultrasound J. 2017;9(1):21.
7. Samagh N, Bhagat H, Jangra K. Monitoring cerebral vasospasm: how much can we rely on transcranial Doppler. J Anaesthesiol Clin Pharmacol. 2019;35(1):12-8.
8. Friedland S, Soetikno R, Benaron D. Reflectance spectrophotometry for the assessment of mucosal perfusion in the gastrointestinal tract. Gastrointest Endosc Clin N Am. 2004;14(3):539-53, ix-x.
9. Groeneveld AB, Kolkman JJ. Splanchnic tonometry: a review of physiology, methodology, and clinical applications. J Crit Care. 1994;9(3):198-210.
10. Heard SO. Gastric tonometry: the hemodynamic monitor of choice (Pro). Chest. 2003;123(5 Suppl):469S-74S.
11. Maciel AT, Creteur J, Vincent J. Tissue capnometry: does the answer lie under the tongue? Intensive Care Med. 2004;30(12):2157-65.
12. Sakka SG. Assessment of liver perfusion and function by indocyanine green in the perioperative setting and in critically ill patients. J Clin Monit Comput. 2018;32(5):787-96.
13. Vos JJ, Wietasch JK, Absalom AR, Hendriks HG, Scheeren TW. Green light for liver function monitoring using indocyanine green? An overview of current clinical applications. Anaesthesia. 2014;69(12):1364-76.
14. Peris A, Barbani F, Spinelli E, Boddi M. Role of renal resistive index to assess renal perfusion in ICU patients. Intern Emerg Med. 2012;7(Suppl 1):S1-2.
15. Schneider AG, Goodwin MD, Bellomo R. Measurement of kidney perfusion in critically ill Patients. Crit Care. 2013;17(2):220.
16. Schnell D, Darmon M. Bedside Doppler ultrasound for the assessment of renal perfusion in the ICU: advantages and limitations of the available techniques. Crit Ultrasound J. 2015;7:8.
17. Harrois A, Duranteau J. Contrast-enhanced ultrasound: a new vision of microcirculation in the intensive care unit. Crit Care. 2013;17(4):449.
18. Schneider A, Johnson L, Goodwin M, Schelleman A, Bellomo R. Bench-to-bedside review: contrast enhanced ultrasonography—a promising technique to assess renal perfusion in the ICU. Crit Care. 2011;15(3):1-8.

CHAPTER

Rationale for the Monitoring of the Microcirculation

Olcay Dilken, Can Ince

INTRODUCTION

Microcirculation is essential in providing oxygen to the tissue, removing waste products, delivering nutrients, and having important immune functions, and other vital functions.[1] It is a vast network of vessels smaller than 20 µm in diameter. Arterioles, venules, and capillaries all together form this network which should be regarded as an organ. By definition, capillaries are microvessels with a diameter of 5–8 µm.[2] Given that a red blood cell (RBC) is approximately 8 µm in diameter, these cells need to deform to enter capillaries and form a single line formation. Flow from capillaries collects into the venules where leukocyte adhesion and rolling also occur in states of infection and inflammation.

Arterioles are upstream from the capillaries and are responsible for controlling the blood flow by the smooth muscle cells, which surround them. Under nonpathological conditions, microcirculation holds approximately 10% of the circulating blood volume. As microcirculation literally exists in every part of the body and has significant functions, its monitoring in critical illness can be regarded as crucial.[3]

HEMODYNAMIC COHERENCE

Shock is a common occurrence in a large number of ICU patients. The fundamental management of these patients has not changed substantially since the 1960s. Fluid therapy along with vasoactive drugs remains the mainstay of therapy.[4] This therapy targets the normalization of macrohemodynamic parameters, such as arterial and venous blood pressures, cardiac output, heart rate, etc. It is the expectation of resuscitation medicine that an improvement in these parameters results in a parallel improvement in microcirculation and tissue perfusion. However, many studies in shock patients have shown that an improvement in macrohemodynamic parameters does not necessarily cause a parallel improvement in microcirculation. This mismatch between the macro- and microcirculation has been termed a loss in hemodynamic coherence.[5] The presence of a loss of hemodynamic coherence has been found to be an independent factor for organ dysfunction and mortality. Moreover, it has been shown that microcirculation is the first circulatory system to be affected by shock and the last one to improve. A persistently altered microcirculation is associated with increased mortality.[6] Four types of microcirculatory alterations associated with a loss of hemodynamic coherence are defined.[5]

As seen from **Figure 1**, Type 1 alterations are associated with flow heterogeneity, where stagnant capillaries and fast-flowing capillaries can be seen next to each other, causing a reduction in the oxygen extraction capacity of the microcirculation due to functional shunting of oxygen transport. Sepsis is a typical Type 1 alteration. Type 2 alterations are caused by a decrease in the O_2-carrying capacity of microcirculatory blood. Fluid resuscitation typically causes hemodilution and thus is an example of Type 2 alteration. Type 3 alterations are seen in microcirculatory stasis caused by the use of excess vasopressors and/or increased venous pressure caused by, for example, fluid overload. Type 4 alterations are defined as a decrease in the functional capillary density of the microcirculation due to leaky capillaries, which occurs in edema, and results in type 4 alteration.[5]

Unlike other hemodynamic monitors, the assessment of the microcirculation provides invaluable mechanistic information regarding the underlying pathophysiology of the disease.

Like other techniques, such as echocardiography and thermodilution cardiac output (CO) measurement, the assessment of the microcirculation requires specialized equipment, experience in making reliable measurements,

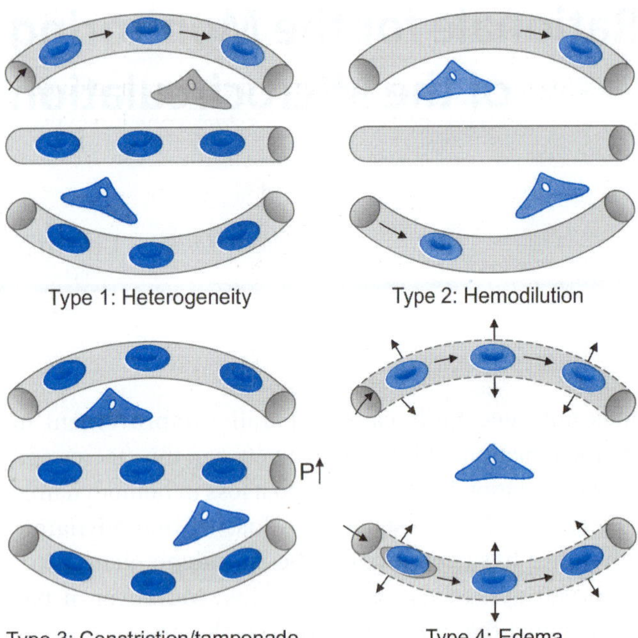

Fig. 1: Microcirculatory alterations associated with loss of hemodynamic coherence. States of loss of hemodynamic coherence where macrocirculatory resuscitation does not necessarily cause an expected parallel improvement in the perfusion of the microcirculation. Type 1: Heterogeneous red blood cell (RBC) flow where flowing RBCs carry oxygen (red RBC) and stagnant RBC (dark red); correspondingly, tissue cells receive oxygen (red tissue cells) or not (blue tissue cells). Type 2: A reduction in the oxygen-carrying capacity of the microcirculation due to hemodilution by, for example, excessive fluid therapy. Type 3: A stagnation in RBC flow in the microcirculation caused due to arterial vasoconstriction [increased vascular resistance (R) and/or raised venous pressures (P)]. Type 4: Increased oxygen diffusion distances due to edema.
Source: Adapted from Ince C.[5]

and knowledge of the pathophysiology of the microcirculation.[3] With the advance of microcirculatory technology, new hand-held vital cameras are now lighter in weight with better optics.[7]

OXYGEN TRANSPORT AND THE MICROCIRCULATION

Oxygen is the key element needed for aerobic respiration to generate adenosine triphosphate (ATP). Oxygen transport to the cells occurs via RBCs that flow in the capillaries. Convection and diffusion of O_2 are the two main determinants of oxygen transport to the parenchymal cells. Oxygen diffusion can be estimated by Fick laws:

- $D*A*(pO_2cap - pO_2mit)/L$ in where D is the diffusion constant, A is the capillary surface area, $pO_2cap - pO_2mit$ is the difference between the capillary and the mitochondrial O_2 tension, and finally, l is the distance between the capillary and the mitochondria **(Fig. 2)**.

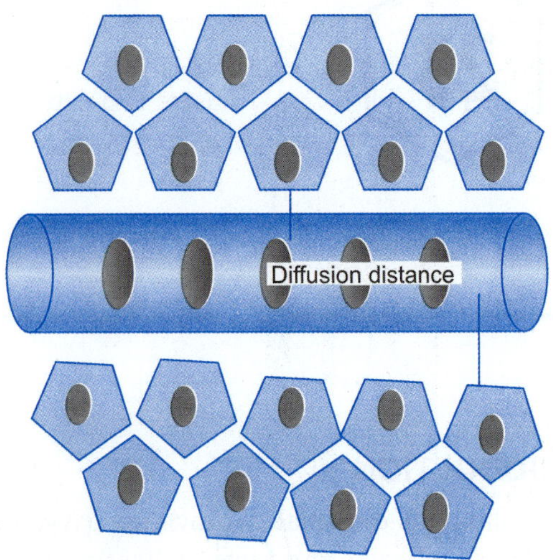

Fig. 2: Diffusion is impaired as the distance increases.

Convection can be estimated by the equation:

- $qO_{2i} = K \times SRi \times SiO_2$ in where K is the single RBCs' total O_2 carrying capacity at 100% saturation, SRi and SiO_2 are the RBC supply rate and oxygen saturation in an individual capillary, respectively.

Convection and diffusion contribute equally to oxygen transport to the tissue cells. Deterioration in either of these components can be compensated for by the other. That is why, monitoring and quantifying these two determinants of oxygen transport is key to quantifying microcirculatory function.[8-10]

MONITORING THE MICROCIRCULATION

Hand-held vital microscopes (HVMs) allow the quantification of capillary density, flow heterogeneity, RBC velocity, leukocyte kinetics, and direct visualization of the region of interest. HVM observations have a limited organ penetration (maximum 0.5 mm) which together with the ease of access and clinical relevance has resulted in the employment of HVM to the sublingual area for measurements.

Hand-held vital microscopes use epi-illumination by green light emitting diodes (LEDs) to illuminate and magnifying lenses at the tip of a light guide to observe the microcirculation of a region of interest. Both the light source and the image recorder including the microscope lens are incorporated in the HVM device.[7] HVMs are used for direct observation of the flowing blood cells in the microcirculation and thereby assess their function in terms of their convective and diffusive capacity. These are quantified as microcirculatory flow index (MFI), percentage of perfused vessels (PPVs), and total vessel density (TVD). These parameters can be calculated by dedicated software.[11,12] In addition, a heterogeneity index is calculated to especially quantify type 1 alterations. Overall, the capacity of perfusion of the tissue depends on the amount, distribution, and diameters of the capillaries.[13]

The MFI is regarded as a semiquantitative measure of perfusion. The recorded image is divided into four quadrants by a vertical and horizontal line and each square is graded from 0 to 3 (0 = no flow, 1 = intermittent flow, 2 = sluggish flow, 3 = continuous flow).

Dominant flow type defines the MFI score per quadrant. The arithmetic average of all quadrants is taken. An MFI <2.6 (along with elevated heart rate) has been found in several studies to be an independent determinant for mortality.[14] Alternatively each vessel is scored, and the mean can be taken for the calculation of MFI.[15]

Total vessel density is calculated as the total length of vessels divided by the area of the region of interest. Each vessel is later categorized according to its flow state in the same manner as MFI, which enables the calculation of PPV.[15]

To graphically quantify RBC kinetics, so-called space-time diagrams (STDs) are used.[3] These STDs also allow the observation of leukocyte kinetics, such as rolling, adhesion, and migration.[16] Its clinical importance however is yet to be determined.

Three generations of HVMs have been developed, orthogonal polarization spectral (OPS), sidestream dark field (SDF), and incident dark field (IDF) imaging. OPS is no longer commercially available, and SDF is outperformed by IDF imaging due to improved technology.[7]

Incident dark field is characterized by high power-illuminating LEDs with very short pulse times (2 milliseconds). These LEDs emit green light, which is absorbed by the hemoglobin (Hb) in the RBCs. A wavelength of 530 nm is used, that is the isosbestic wavelength for Hb by which light is equally absorbed by oxy and deoxyhemoglobin whereby only blood vessels that have RBCs within can be visualized. These RBCs appear as dark globules on a white screen. A five-times magnifying lens is located at the tip of the light guide of the HVM, and the focus is adjusted with a stepping motor inside. This device is also much lighter in weight compared to earlier generation devices reducing the pressure artifacts induced by pressing the device tip. All of these factors are translated into easier and faster bedside usage, faster exporting of the recorded videos, and up to 30% more identifiable vessels in the region of interest.[7]

Similar to other HVMs, IDF also has limitations. Movement artifacts are commonly encountered, and the measurement requires cooperation or sedation of the subject. Pressure artifacts are caused by the weight imposed on the mucosa by the tip of the microscope and it can erroneously result in a deteriorated flow state of the subject. The offline analysis of the recorded images is also quite time-consuming. However, a recently introduced software automatically analyses the images, at approximately 200 times faster speed compared to manual analysis.[17] This advancement now makes HVM as a technique able to make point-of-care measurements allowing microcirculation targeted interventions to be applied feasible. Like many other techniques, such as catheter insertion or heart function imaging with echocardiography, the use of IDF requires a training period and has a learning curve. A guideline is available to optimize the quality of the images acquired.[18]

In addition to HVMs, other techniques are also available which do not require operator experience. Near-infrared spectroscopy (NIRS), is a continuous and noninvasive imaging technique used for the nonquantitative assessment of tissue oxygenation.[19] It can generate real-time information regarding regional perfusion by measuring the oxygenated and deoxygenated Hb. NIRS has found usage in monitoring of the cerebral and muscle oxygenation in cardiac surgery, critically ill patients, trauma and prehospital emergency settings, and especially pediatric patients. A number of limitations also exist with this technique. Firstly, the impact of other molecules such as myoglobin, skin pigmentation, and the scatter of light is not known. Secondly, the deeper tissues such as muscle bounce back most of the signal sent. Finally, the measurement is the sum of the oxygenation of Hb in all of the vascular compartments thus not allowing discrimination between the various vascular segments, especially when there is a volume shift between the various vascular compartments. Tissue oxygenation can be overestimated if a large muscle tissue mass exists in the region of interest since the oxygen affinity of myoglobin is markedly higher than that of Hb.[20,21]

CLINICAL APPLICATION

The paradigm of applying universal treatment modalities derived from large patient groups has shifted to the implementation of personalized medicine based on physiological principles.[22]

Hand-held vital microscopes are one of the tools which incorporate physiology into clinics. Monitoring the sublingual microcirculation may help discriminate patients who are going to benefit from specific therapy in states such as septic shock, perioperative hemodynamic management, and cardiac failure.[22-24] It can also be used to optimize fluid therapy.[25]

It is now well documented that the severity of alterations in the microcirculation associated with adverse outcomes cannot be predicted from macrohemodynamic parameters. Moreover, administering α-adrenergic drugs while improving blood pressure may in fact impair microvascular perfusion.[26] That is why, monitoring the microcirculation should be a part of the hemodynamic assessment of shock management.

Previous generations of HVMs imposed a heavy workload on the operator, such as converting a format of the video, and manually analyzing acquired images. These factors may have limited its widespread use. The newly introduced software may disentangle the time-consuming step of the offline analysis, thus enabling new insights amongst a big number of cases.[17]

CONCLUSION

Measurement of the microcirculation using HVMs offers a unique opportunity for identifying underlying pathophysiology as well as the success of response to therapy. Its ease of applicability has greatly improved due to technological advancement, and it can also be employed by nurses and clinicians at the bedside. However, it should be mentioned that none of the currently applied parameters in critically ill patients, such as cardiac output or global end-diastolic volume, are valuable on their own. As such, microcirculation parameters should be incorporated in other clinical signs or surrogates to contribute to the best available therapy.[3]

REFERENCES

1. Gutterman DD, Chabowski DS, Kadlec AO, Durand MJ, Freed JK, Ait-Aissa K, et al. The Human Microcirculation: Regulation of Flow and Beyond. Circ Res. 2016;118(1): 157-2.
2. Secomb TW, Pries AR. Blood viscosity in microvessels: experiment and theory. Comptes Rendus Phys. 2013; 14(6):470-8.
3. Ince C, Boerma EC, Cecconi M, De Backer D, Shapiro NI, Duranteau J, et al. Second consensus on the assessment of sublingual microcirculation in critically ill patients: results from a task force of the European Society of Intensive Care Medicine. Intensive Care Med. 2018;44(3):281-99.
4. Weil MH, Shubin H. The "VIP" approach to the bedside management of shock. JAMA. 1969;207(2):337-40.
5. Ince C. Hemodynamic coherence and the rationale for monitoring the microcirculation. Crit Care. 2015;19(Suppl 3):S8.
6. Sakr Y, Dubois M-J, De Backer D, Creteur J, Vincent JL. Persistent microcirculatory alterations are associated with organ failure and death in patients with septic shock. Crit Care Med. 2004;32(9):1825-31.
7. Aykut G, Veenstra G, Scorcella C, Ince C, Boerma C. Cytocam-IDF (incident dark field illumination) imaging for bedside monitoring of the microcirculation. Intensive Care Med Exp. 2015;3(1):40.
8. Leach R, Treacher D. The pulmonary physician in critical care • 2: Oxygen delivery and consumption in the critically ill. Thorax. 2002;57(2):170-7.
9. Ince C. The rationale for microcirculatory guided fluid therapy. Curr Opin Crit Care. 2014;20(3):301-8.
10. Sakr Y. Techniques to assess tissue oxygenation in the clinical setting. Transfus Apher Sci Off J World Apher Assoc Off J Eur Soc Haemapheresis. 2010;43(1):79-94.
11. Boerma EC, Mathura KR, van der Voort PHJ, Spronk PE, Ince C. Quantifying bedside-derived imaging of microcirculatory abnormalities in septic patients: a prospective validation study. Crit Care Lond Engl. 2005;9(6):R601-6.
12. Bezemer R, Dobbe JG, Bartels SA, Boerma EC, Elbers PW, Heger M, et al. Rapid automatic assessment of microvascular density in sidestream dark field images. Med Biol Eng Comput. 2011;49(11):1269-78.
13. Trzeciak S, Dellinger RP, Parrillo JE, Guglielmi M, Bajaj J, Abate NL, et al. Early microcirculatory perfusion derangements in patients with severe sepsis and septic shock: relationship to hemodynamics, oxygen transport, and survival. Ann Emerg Med. 2007;49:88-98.e2.
14. Scorcella C, Damiani E, Domizi R, Pierantozzi S, Tondi S, Carsetti A, et al. MicroDAIMON study: Microcirculatory DAIly MONitoring in critically ill patients: a prospective observational study. Ann Intensive Care. 2018;8:64.
15. Pozo MO, Kanoore Edul VS, Ince C, Dubin A. Comparison of different methods for the calculation of the microvascular flow index. Crit Care Res Pract. 2012;2012:102483.
16. Uz Z, van Gulik TM, Aydemirli MD, Guerci P, Ince Y, Cuppen D, et al. Identification and quantification of human microcirculatory leukocytes using handheld video microscopes at the bedside. J Appl Physiol. 2018; 124(6):1550-7.

17. Hilty MP, Guerci P, Ince Y, Toraman F, Ince C. MicroTools enables automated quantification of capillary density and red blood cell velocity in handheld vital microscopy. Commun Biol. 2019;2:217.
18. Massey MJ, Shapiro NI. A guide to human in vivo microcirculatory flow image analysis. Crit Care. 2016;20:35.
19. Scheeren TWL, Schober P, Schwarte LA. Monitoring tissue oxygenation by near infrared spectroscopy (NIRS): background and current applications. J Clin Monit Comput. 2012;26(4):279-87.
20. Nagdyman N, Ewert P, Peters B, Miera O, Fleck T, Berger F. Comparison of different near-infrared spectroscopic cerebral oxygenation indices with central venous and jugular venous oxygenation saturation in children. Paediatr Anaesth. 2008;18(2):160-6.
21. De Backer D, Donadello K, Cortes DO. Monitoring the microcirculation. J Clin Monit Comput. 2012;26(5):361-6.
22. Ince C. Personalized physiological medicine. Crit Care. 2017;21(Suppl 3):308.
23. Legrand M, Ait-Oufella H, Ince C. Could resuscitation be based on microcirculation data? Yes. Intensive Care Med. 2018;44(6):944-6.
24. Lima A, Jansen TC, van Bommel J, Ince C, Bakker J. The prognostic value of the subjective assessment of peripheral perfusion in critically ill patients. Crit Care Med. 2009;37(3):934-8.
25. Uz Z, Ince C, Guerci P, Ince Y, P Araujo R, Ergin B, et al. Recruitment of sublingual microcirculation using handheld incident dark field imaging as a routine measurement tool during the postoperative de-escalation phase-a pilot study in post ICU cardiac surgery patients. Perioper Med (Lond). 2018;7:18.
26. De Backer D, Foulon P. Minimizing catecholamines and optimizing perfusion. Crit Care. 2019;23(Suppl 1):149.

CHAPTER

Intra-abdominal Pressure Monitoring, Intra-abdominal Hypertension, and Abdominal Compartment Syndrome

Shilpushp Jagannath Bhosale, Atul Prabhakar Kulkarni

INTRODUCTION

Intra-abdominal hypertension (IAH) occurs when increased abdominal pressure causes decreased perfusion of the kidneys and other abdominal organs with progressive difficulty in mechanical ventilation and/or hemodynamic compromise. These effects can progress to abdominal compartment syndrome (ACS), a cascade of ischemia and multiple organs dysfunction. ACS is a medical emergency, when increased intra-abdominal pressure (IAP) causes severe organ dysfunction as well as threatens their viability. Its presence carries a high mortality rate. IAH and ACS are two distinct clinical conditions occurring over a spectrum of elevated abdominal pressure and should not be used interchangeably.[1,2] A rapid increase in visceral edema and intra-abdominal volume due to injury to abdominal organs, or other disease processes such as trauma, burn, aortic rupture, and pancreatitis requiring large volume crystalloid resuscitation can be the cause for IAH and so should warrant screening for IAH.[3,4] ACS primarily affects patients, who are already very sick, have received massive intravenous fluid resuscitation in presence of capillary leak and a positive fluid balance. ACS remains under-recognized because the organ dysfunction may be incorrectly attributed to progression of the primary illness.

Though the incidence of IAH and ACS was extremely high earlier, when aggressive intravenous fluid resuscitation was widely practiced there is significant decrease in ACS with increasing awareness nowadays.[5] Early recognition is necessary so that interventions such as sedation, fluid removal, or decompression of bowel, etc., to decrease IAP can be undertaken. However, the clinical benefit of such therapies remains uncertain and surgical decompression remains the standard treatment once ACS is established.[2,6,7]

DEFINITION

Fietsam et al. came up with the term ACS when he described raised IAP, in patients having undergone aortic aneurysm surgery. Patients are manifested with an increase in the peak inspiratory pressures, central venous pressure, and a decrease in urinary output.[8] The World Society of the Abdominal Compartment Syndrome (WSACS) which was founded in 2004 came up with the consensus definitions in 2013 and stated that:

- Intra-abdominal pressure is the steady-state pressure concealed within the abdominal cavity and IAH is a sustained increase in IAP ≥12 mm Hg.
- Abdominal compartment syndrome is defined by a sustained IAP above 20 mm Hg [with or without an abdominal perfusion pressure (APP) <60 mm Hg] with new onset or progressive organ failure.

The IAH is graded as Grade I (12–15 mm Hg), Grade II (16–20 mm Hg), Grade III (21–25 mm Hg), and Grade IV (>25 mm Hg).[6]

Primary IAH or ACS is said to be associated with injury or disease in the abdominal pelvic region that frequently requires early surgical or interventional radiological intervention, while secondary IAH or ACS refers to conditions that do not originate in the abdominopelvic region.[9] Recurrent IAH or ACS refers to the condition in which IAH or ACS redevelops, following treated primary or secondary IAH or ACS.

Normal IAP has been described up to 5–7 mm Hg, but it has been observed that the morbidly obese and pregnant patients may have chronically high IAP (10–15 mm Hg) without adverse effects.[10] For critically ill patients, pressures >12 mm Hg are considered to represent IAH, and pressures >20 mm Hg with new organ dysfunction are termed ACS.

The APP is the difference between mean arterial pressure (MAP) and IAP (APP = MAP – IAP) and it has been suggested as a target for management of IAH. A target APP of at least 60 mm Hg is correlated with improved survival from IAH and ACS.[11] This suggests that higher systemic blood pressure may maintain abdominal organ perfusion when IAP is increased. Abdominal wall compliance initially limits the extent of rise in IAP. Once a critical abdominal girth is reached, the abdominal wall compliance decreases abruptly, leading to rapid rise of IAP and ACS, if untreated. Hence in practice due to individual variations in blood pressure and abdominal wall compliance, ACS is better defined as IAH-induced new organ dysfunction without a strict IAP threshold.[12]

PEDIATRIC-SPECIFIC CONSENSUS DEFINITIONS

Intra-abdominal pressure in critically ill children is approximately 4–10 mm Hg. IAH is defined by a sustained or repeated pathological elevation in IAP >10 mm Hg, while ACS is defined as a sustained elevated IAP of >16 mm Hg associated with new or worsening organ dysfunction that can be attributed to elevated IAP. Omphalocele and gastroschisis have been described to be associated with increased IAP in pediatric population.

INCIDENCE OF INTRA-ABDOMINAL HYPERTENSION/ABDOMINAL COMPARTMENT SYNDROME

Though it is evident that IAH/ACS is independently associated with worse outcomes in medical or surgical patients, the incidence of IAH and ACS is not well characterized due to multiple factors such as underdiagnosis, lack of awareness, or most of the times simply inability to measure the IAP. Most of the times, the organ dysfunction is falsely considered as primary disease process.

The incidence of IAH/ACS is rapidly declining from a high incidence in the old literature that suggested IAH incidence between 32 and 56%, and ACS incidence of about 2–10%.[6] The incidence of ACS in trauma patients seems to be approximately 14%.[13]

PATHOPHYSIOLOGY OF INTRA-ABDOMINAL HYPERTENSION/ABDOMINAL COMPARTMENT SYNDROME

It has been observed that ACS can develop both in nonsurgical and surgical patients. Conditions such as obesity, significant positive fluid balance, prolonged mechanical ventilation, massive blood transfusion, high-organ failure scores, or end-stage liver disease, predispose patients for ACS. Mechanisms for increased IAP and end-organ dysfunction are conditions that decrease abdominal wall compliance, or increase intraluminal contents (such as abdominal collections of fluid, air, or blood) or capillary leak syndromes.

A two hit theory has been proposed for the development of ACS, which suggests that massive volume resuscitation after a "first hit" from any cause (i.e., burns, trauma, pancreatitis, hemorrhagic, or septic shock) can lead to increased IAP, and the "second hit" probably results from the effects of capillary leak, ischemia-reperfusion injury with shock, and the release of cytokines combined with massive increases in total extracellular volume.[14,15] Other contributory factor is the erroneous assessment of fluid responsiveness in IAH as decreased intrathoracic compliance may cause false elevation in pulse pressure variation (PPV) with ventilation or can cause inferior vena cava (IVC) diameter to be less due to compression from increased abdominal pressure prompting the clinician to administrate excessive fluids. The effects on different organ systems caused by IAH/ACS are shown in **Figure 1**.

Acute IAH may lead to an increase in intracranial pressure (ICP), secondary to increase in pleural pressure.[16] Compression of the IVC and aorta can cause decrease in the preload and can increase afterload with consequent reduction in the stroke volume (SV) and cardiac output (CO). Decrease in the extrathoracic compliance can lead to increase in shunt fraction, dead space, and transalveolar pressures. It can also cause hypoperfusion of the splanchnic-hepatic circulation as well as decrease in the renal filtration gradient.[17]

RISK FACTORS

The incidence of IAH in critically ill patients is significantly reduced and routine IAP measurement admitted to the ICU is rarely performed. The WSACS has suggested that IAP monitoring should be done if two or more risk factors as described by it are present.

Understanding the risk factors and the conditions that lead to IAH and ACS is extremely important. Previous studies reported that morbid obesity, sepsis, paralytic ileus, and massive fluid resuscitation are risk factors for development of IAH/ACS.[18,19] Risk factors for development of IAH/ACS have been enumerated in the following text:[2]

- *Diminished abdominal wall compliance:*
    - Abdominal surgery
    - Major trauma, burns
    - Prone positioning

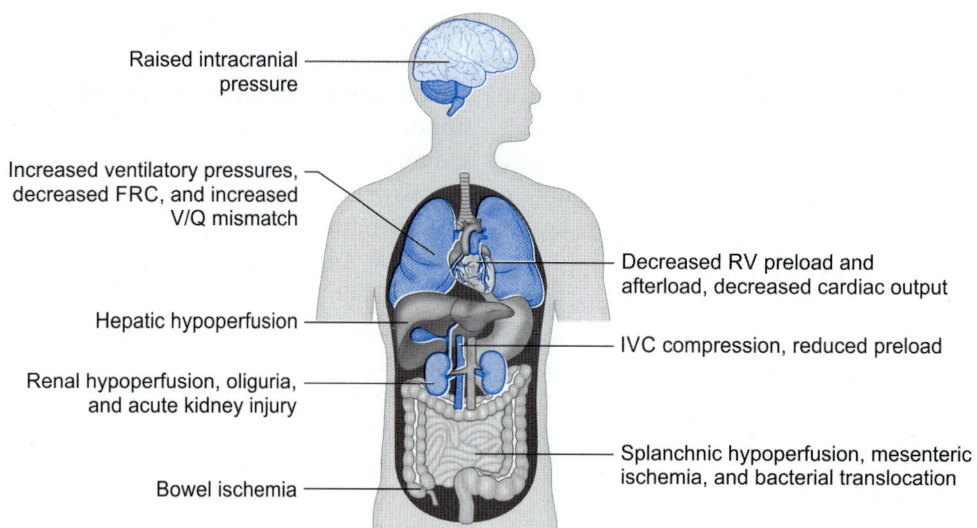

Fig. 1: End-organ effects in abdominal compartment syndrome (ACS). (FRC: functional residual capacity; IVC: inferior vena cava; RV: right ventricular; V/Q: ventilation/perfusion ratio).

- *Increased intraluminal contents:*
  - Gastroparesis/gastric distension/ileus
  - Colonic pseudo-obstruction
  - Volvulus
- *Increased intra-abdominal contents:*
  - Acute pancreatitis
  - Hemoperitoneum or intra-abdominal infection/abscess
  - Intra-abdominal or retroperitoneal tumors
  - Liver dysfunction/cirrhosis with ascites
  - Peritoneal dialysis
- *Others:*
  - Capillary leak/fluid resuscitation
  - Damage control laparotomy
  - Increased APACHE-II (Acute Physiology and Chronic Health Evaluation) or SOFA (Sequential Organ Failure Assessment) score
  - Massive transfusion and fluid resuscitation or positive fluid balance
  - Mechanical ventilation
  - Obesity or increased body mass index
  - Peritonitis
  - Septic shock

DIAGNOSIS OF ABDOMINAL COMPARTMENT SYNDROME

Since treatment can improve organ dysfunction, it is important that the diagnosis be considered in the appropriate clinical situation without delay. Definitive diagnosis of ACS requires measurement of the IAP. This is particularly important for patients who have trauma, have undergone liver transplant, bowel obstruction, pancreatitis, or peritonitis because these conditions are known to be associated with ACS.[18,19]

The key to recognizing ACS in a critically ill patient is demonstrating elevated IAP. The clinical importance of any IAP must be assessed in view of the baseline steady-state IAP for the individual patient. Clinical examination of the abdomen is a poor predictor of ACS, even though patients with ACS have a tender and distended abdomen.[20,21]

Attempts to estimate IAP or diagnose IAH based on changes in abdominal circumference are extremely unreliable. Physical examination has extremely poor sensitivity and accuracy for identifying elevated IAP, even by experienced clinicians.[22] Oliguria, high peak inspiratory pressures, and hemodynamic instability, are also common indicators of ACS. Other findings may include severe metabolic acidosis, mesenteric ischemia, paralytic ileus, raised ICP, etc. Imaging, unfortunately, is not very helpful in the diagnosis of ACS. Chest X-ray (CXR) may show elevated hemidiaphragms, with decreased lung volumes and atelectasis, computed tomography (CT) scan may show nonspecific findings such as bowel wall thickening, or bilateral inguinal herniation or infiltration of the retroperitoneal space, compression of the IVC, and renal vessels.

MEASUREMENT OF INTRA-ABDOMINAL PRESSURE (FIG. 2)

The basic premise in measuring the IAP is the consideration that abdomen with its contents is fluidic in character and behaves in accordance with Pascal's law, hence, the pressure measured at one point in the abdomen can represent pressure throughout the abdomen. The IAP is therefore defined as the steady-state pressure concealed within the abdominal cavity. In clinical practice, the IAP is always measured indirectly by measuring the intravesical bladder pressure through a Foley catheter and this has been shown to correlate well with directly-measured IAP.[10] It has to be noted that IAP increases with inspiration due to the diaphragmatic contraction and decreases with expiration. Other methods of measuring IAP are attaching a manometer to abdominal drains, measuring intragastric pressure via a nasogastric tube or measuring pressure from IVC via catheter placed into femoral vein. These methods have been tried but are not considered reliable.[23,24]

Intra-abdominal pressure can be directly measured with an intraperitoneal catheter attached to a pressure transducer or during CO_2 insufflation in laparoscopic surgery. IAP is measured directly with the Veress needle. Different indirect methods for estimating IAP are used clinically because direct measurements are considered to be too invasive.[25] These techniques include rectal, gastric, IVC, and urinary bladder pressure measurement. Only gastric and bladder pressures are used clinically.[26] The IAP can also be measured via a balloon-tipped gastric catheter.[27] Several other methods for continuous IAP measurement via the stomach, peritoneal cavity (using air-chamber or piezoresistive membranes), and bladder have been validated. Although these techniques seem promising, further clinical validation needs to be done before their general use can be recommended. Bladder pressure is the standard method for the measurement of IAP. It is simple, minimally invasive, reliable, and accurate. To avoid variation in the measurement techniques, WSACS consensus guidelines suggest the standard way for intermittent IAP measurements which is through the bladder catheter with a maximal instillation volume of 25 mL sterile saline into the bladder for priming. IAP expressed in mm Hg is measured at end-expiration in the supine position, after ensuring no abdominal muscle contractions, and the transducer zeroed at the level of midaxillary line at the iliac crest.

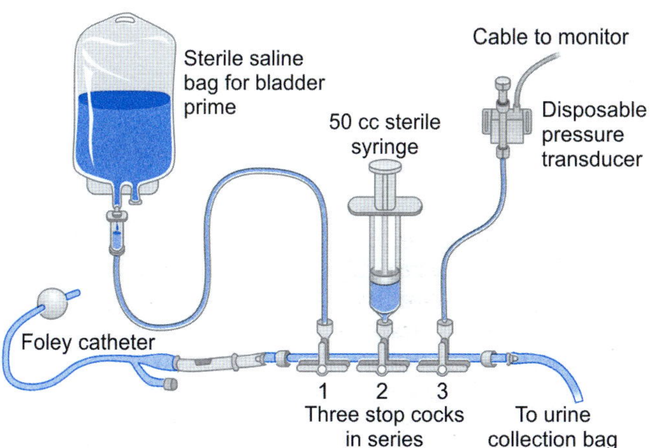

Fig. 2: Measurement of the bladder pressure.

For children, the standard reference for intermittent IAP measurement through the bladder catheter is using 1 mL/kg of instillation volume, since the instillation volume is important (minimum 3 mL to maximum 25 mL sterile saline). Studies have found that 1 mL/kg is reliable for IAP values when compared with higher volumes. Serial measurement of IAP via this method does not appear to lead to increased rates of catheter associated urinary tract infections.[28]

Intermittent measurement of IAP every 4–6 hours is recommended when patients are at risk of developing IAH or ACS, while continuous measurement is preferred in impending or diagnosed IAH/ACS requiring abdominal decompression. APP is also used as a resuscitation end point. Recently continuous IAP measurement commercial kits with Foley manometer are available and used.[29] When an intermittent method is used, measurements should be obtained at least every 4–6 hours, and in patients with evolving organ dysfunction, this frequency should be increased to hourly measurements.

Intra-abdominal pressure measurement should be continued until the risk factors for IAH are resolved with no organ dysfunction and IAP is maintained below 10–12 mm Hg for at least 24–48 hours.

Though WSACS consensus guidelines recommend IAP measurement be performed in sedated patients, where muscle contractions are absent, in awake patients attention should be paid to adequate pain relief during supine positioning and that no muscle contractions are present, especially in chronic obstructive pulmonary disease (COPD) patients, who have forced expiration, which may lead to erroneous readings.

MANAGEMENT OF INTRA-ABDOMINAL HYPERTENSION AND ABDOMINAL COMPARTMENT SYNDROME (SEE FLOWCHART 1)

Management of IAH is essentially supportive care unless ACS mandates abdominal decompression. Procedures like escharotomy release to relieve mechanical limitations due to burn eschars, and percutaneous ascitic drainage can be done in exceptional cases. Supportive care is generally aimed at reduction of intra-abdominal volume and measures to improve abdominal wall compliance.

Simple measures commonly practiced are nasogastric and rectal drainage in patients with bowel distension. Percutaneous drainage (PCD) of ascites or intra-abdominal collections (e.g., hemoperitoneum, intra-abdominal or retroperitoneal abscess, etc.).[30] Abdominal wall compliance can be improved with adequate pain control, sedation, or muscle paralysis, if necessary.[31] Maintaining adequate ventilatory support is crucial, since this condition is associated with high airway pressures. Use of low tidal volume with permissive hypercapnia may be necessary. Optimization of positive end-expiratory pressure (PEEP) may improve oxygenation by reducing the ventilation-perfusion mismatch. Special attention to limiting the amount of fluids may help decrease the risk of developing ACS. However, there is no evidence regarding use of a particular type of fluids or the use of diuretics. Ultrafiltration with continuous renal replacement therapies (RRTs) may result in a significant decrease in IAP.[32]

The WSACS recommendations and suggestions for the management of IAH/ACS have been summarized in the following text.[1]

ABDOMINAL COMPARTMENT SOCIETY CONSENSUS MANAGEMENT STATEMENTS RECOMMENDATIONS[2]

- Measure IAP when known risk for IAH/ACS is present in critically ill or injured patient (Grade 1C).
- Use of trans-bladder technique as the standard IAP measurement technique (Ungraded).
- Use protocolized monitoring and management of IAP (Grade 1C).

Flowchart 1: Algorithm for management.[2]

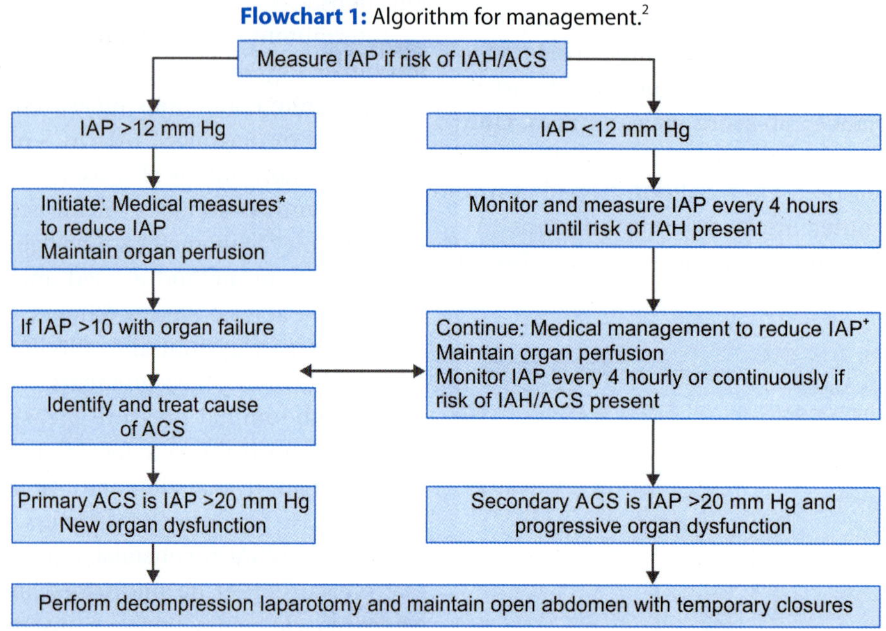

*Medical management of IAH:
- Improve abdominal wall compliance by use of sedation/analgesia/muscle relaxation and avoid head of bed elevation >30°
- Decompress gut by nasogastric/colonic tube, prokinetic use
- Drain abdominal collection or ascites
- Avoid excess fluid administration and/or remove fluid with diuretics and/or ultrafiltration
- Maintain organ perfusion by targeting APP

(IAH/ACS: intra-abdominal hypertension/abdominal compartment syndrome; IAP: intra-abdominal pressure)

- Use protocols to avoid sustained IAH among critically ill or injured patients (Grade 1C).
- Consider decompressive laparotomy in overt ACS in critically ill adults with ACS (Grade 1D).
- In patients with open abdominal wounds, conscious and protocolized efforts be made to obtain an early or at least same-hospital-stay abdominal fascial closure (Grade 1D).
- In critically ill/injured patients with open abdominal wounds, strategies utilizing negative pressure wound therapy should be used (Grade 1C).

SUGGESTIONS

- Ensure optimal pain and anxiety relief for critically ill or injured patients (Grade 2D).
- Brief trials of neuromuscular blockade as a temporary measure for treatment of IAH/ACS (Grade 2D).
- Contribution of body position to elevated IAP to be considered in patients at risk of ACS (Grade 2D).
- Liberal use of enteral decompression with nasogastric or rectal tubes when the stomach or colon are dilated in the presence of IAH/ACS (Grade 1D).
- Neostigmine be used for the treatment of established colonic ileus not responding to other measures (Grade 2D).
- Protocol to avoid a positive cumulative fluid balance in the critically ill or injured patient with, or at risk of IAH/ACS after the acute resuscitation has been completed (Grade 2C).
- Increased ratio of plasma/packed red blood cells for resuscitation of massive hemorrhage (Grade 2D).
- Percutaneous drainage to remove fluid (in the setting of obvious intraperitoneal fluid) in those with IAH/ACS, when this is technically possible (Grade 2C).
- Prophylactic use of the open abdomen in patients undergoing laparotomy for trauma (Grade 2D).
- Bioprosthetic meshes should not be routinely used in the closure of the open abdomen (Grade 2D).
- The WSACS 2013 consensus statement management algorithm is shown in **Flowchart 1**.[2]

SURGICAL DECOMPRESSION

Since mortality among patients who developed ACS is extremely high, ranging from 40 to 100%, it is fairly evident that the only appropriate management is "open abdomen". Open abdomen is a surgical strategy where the incisional defect in the abdominal wall is purposefully left temporarily unrepaired to relieve pressure.[33] However, a temporary cover with towels, sponges, a prosthetic patch, or a translucent cover is left in place to avoid evisceration and heat or fluid losses from the abdominal defect.

Just as there is no consensus on optimal timing of IAP measurement, there is no consensus on timing of decompression. Even though IAH is not an independent predictor of multi-organ failure, decompressing the abdomen prior to the development of ACS is becoming increasingly common and may improve survival. There is no consensus regarding at what level of IAP for surgical decompression should be done, some suggest that surgical decompression is considered when the IAP is 20 mm Hg or greater, regardless of signs of ACS.

The WSACS suggest that surgical decompression cannot be delayed until the development of ACS (Grade 2C). Surgical decompression can be performed in the operating room if the patient is medically stable for transfer or at the bedside in the intensive care unit (ICU). Following decompression, open abdomen can be maintained using temporary abdominal closure techniques such as negative pressure systems and gauze/adhesive dressings which allow dressing and inspection of abdominal contents regularly.[34] Use of a negative pressure system helps to control and quantify fluid losses. Other conditions where the abdomen is left open are damage control surgery in trauma, severe septic abdomen, burns, etc.[35] Though damage control surgery has significantly reduced the incidence of ACS in trauma patients, decompression laparotomy for major burns has not been able to demonstrate mortality benefit probably because the inherent mortality in major burns patient is extremely high.[36] A few retrospective studies have shown reduction in mortality with decompressive laparotomy in burns patients with ACS. There is enough evidence to suggest that delay in surgical decompression after development of ACS can significantly increase the risk of mortality in both trauma and nonsurgical patients. It is hypothesized that surgical decompression improves visceral perfusion and with negative pressure peritoneal cover it can reduce transmission of inflammatory mediators to the bloodstream as well as bacterial translocation, thereby preventing a septic cascade and organ dysfunction. Open abdomen, however, can lead to persistent hypercatabolic state and severe protein loss via peritoneal fluid, enterocutaneous or intestinal fistulae, retraction of the abdominal wall or development of ventral hernias, etc. Hence, continued monitoring is necessary even after surgical decompression. Management of open abdomen can be with temporary covering of the abdominal defect with a negative pressure vacuum system or a prosthetic patch closure.[37]

After resolution of ACS, the open abdomen can be definitively closed with a primary fascial closure or use of skin grafts if lateralization of the abdominal wall occurs.[38,39]

CONCLUSION

It has been widely recognized that intra-abdominal hypertension and abdominal compartment syndrome can be life-threatening condition in critically ill patients. They can cause altered organ perfusion and end-organ damage. The importance of early recognition and timely management of intra-abdominal hypertension and abdominal compartment syndrome has improved the outcomes over recent years.

REFERENCES

1. Kirkpatrick AW, De Waele JJ, De Laet I, De Keulenaer BL, D'Amours S, Björck M, et al. WSACS—The Abdominal Compartment Society. A society dedicated to the study of the physiology and pathophysiology of the abdominal compartment and its interactions with all organ systems. Anaesthesiol Intensive Ther. 2015;47(3):191-4.
2. Kirkpatrick AW, Roberts DJ, De Waele J, Jaeschke R, Malbrain ML, De Keulenaer B, et al. Intra-abdominal hypertension and the abdominal compartment syndrome: updated consensus definitions and clinical practice guidelines from the World Society of the abdominal compartment syndrome. Intensive Care Med. 2013; 39(7):1190-206.
3. Caldwell CB, Ricotta JJ. Changes in visceral blood flow with elevated intraabdominal pressure. J Surg Res. 1987;43(1):14-20.
4. Rubenstein C, Bietz G, Davenport DL, Winkler M, Endean ED. Abdominal compartment syndrome associated with endovascular and open repair of ruptured abdominal aortic aneurysms. J Vasc Surg. 2015;61(3):648-54.
5. Daugherty EL, Hongyan Liang, Taichman D, Hansen-Flaschen J, Fuchs BD. Abdominal compartment syndrome is common in medical intensive care unit patients receiving large-volume resuscitation. J Intensive Care Med. 2007;22(5):294-9.
6. Malbrain ML, Chiumello D, Cesana BM, Reintam Blaser A, Starkopf J, Sugrue M, et al. A systematic review and individual patient data meta-analysis on intra-abdominal hypertension in critically ill patients: the wake-up project. World initiative on Abdominal Hypertension Epidemiology, a Unifying Project (WAKE-Up!). Minerva Anestesiol. 2014;80(3):293-306.
7. Mentula P, Hienonen P, Kemppainen E, Puolakkainen P, Leppäniemi A. Surgical decompression for abdominal compartment syndrome in severe acute pancreatitis. Arch Surg. 2010;145(8):764-9.
8. Fietsam R Jr, Villalba M, Glover JL, Clark K. Intra-abdominal compartment syndrome as a complication of ruptured abdominal aortic aneurysm repair. Am Surg. 1989;55(6):396-402.
9. Balogh Z, McKinley BA, Holcomb JB, Miller CC, Cocanour CS, Kozar RA, et al. Both primary and secondary abdominal compartment syndrome can be predicted early and are harbingers of multiple organ failure. J Trauma. 2003;54(5):848-61.
10. Sanchez NC, Tenofsky PL, Dort JM, Shen LY, Helmer SD, Smith RS. What is normal intra-abdominal pressure? Am Surg. 2001;67(3):243-8.
11. Cheatham ML, White MW, Sagraves SG, Johnson JL, Block EF. Abdominal perfusion pressure: a superior parameter in the assessment of intra-abdominal hypertension. J Trauma. 2000;49(4):621-7.
12. Malbrain ML, De Laet I, De Waele JJ, Sugrue M, Schachtrupp A, Duchesne J, et al. The role of abdominal compliance, the neglected parameter in critically ill patients—a consensus review of 16. Part 2: measurement techniques and management recommendations. Anaesthesiol Intensive Ther. 2014;46(5):406-32.
13. Madigan MC, Kemp CD, Johnson JC, Cotton BA. Secondary abdominal compartment syndrome after severe extremity injury: are early, aggressive fluid resuscitation strategies to blame? J Trauma. 2008;64(2):280-5.
14. Saggi BH, Sugerman HJ, Ivatury RR, Bloomfield GL. Abdominal compartment syndrome. J Trauma. 1998;45(3): 597-609.
15. Trikudanathan G, Vege SS. Current concepts of the role of abdominal compartment syndrome in acute pancreatitis—an opportunity or merely an epiphenomenon. Pancreatology. 2014;14(4):238-43.
16. Deeren DH, Dits H, Malbrain ML. Correlation between intra-abdominal and intracranial pressure in nontraumatic brain injury. Intensive Care Med. 2005;31(11):1577-81.
17. Dalfino L, Tullo L, Donadio I, Malcangi V, Brienza N. Intra-abdominal hypertension and acute renal failure in critically ill patients. Intensive Care Med. 2008;34(4):707-13.
18. Kim IB, Prowle J, Baldwin I, Bellomo R. Incidence, risk factors and outcome associations of intra-abdominal hypertension in critically ill patients. Anaesth Intensive Care. 2012;40(1):79-89.
19. Ke L, Ni HB, Sun JK, Tong ZH, Li WQ, Li N, et al. Risk factors and outcome of intra-abdominal hypertension in patients with severe acute pancreatitis. World J Surg. 2012;36(1):171-8.
20. Sugrue M, De Waele JJ, De Keulenaer BL, DJ, Malbrain ML. A user's guide to intra-abdominal pressure measurement. Anaesthesiol Intensive Ther. 2015;47(3):241-51.

21. Kirkpatrick AW, Brenneman FD, McLean RF, Rapanos T, Boulanger BR. Is clinical examination an accurate indicator of raised intra-abdominal pressure in critically injured patients. Can J Surg. 2000;43(3):207-11.
22. Castillo M, Lis R, Ulrich H, Rivera G,. Ibel C, Kvetan V. Clinical estimate compared to intra-abdominal pressure management. Crit Care Med. 1998;26(Suppl 1):78A.
23. De Keulenaer BL, Regli A, Dabrowski W, Kaloiani V, Bodnar Z, Cea JI, et al. Does femoral venous pressure measurement correlate well with intrabladder pressure measurement? A multicenter observational trial. Intensive Care Med. 2011;37(10):1620-7.
24. Sugrue M, Buist MD, Lee A, Sanchez DJ, Hillman KM. Intra-abdominal pressure measurement using a modified nasogastric tube: description and validation of a new technique. Intensive Care Med. 1994;20(8):588-90.
25. Risin E, Kessel B, Ashkenazi I, Lieberman N, Alfici R. A new technique of direct intra-abdominal pressure measurement: a preliminary study. Am J Surg. 2006;191(2):235-7.
26. Malbrain ML. Different techniques to measure intra-abdominal pressure (IAP): time for a critical reappraisal. Intensive Care Med. 2004;30(3):357-71.
27. Engum SA, Kogon B, Jensen E, Isch J, Balanoff C, Grosfeld JL. Gastric tonometry and direct intra-abdominal pressure monitoring in abdominal compartment syndrome. J Pediatr Surg. 2002;37(2):214-8.
28. Desie N, Willems A, De Laet I, Dits H, Van Regenmortel N, Schoonheydt K, et al. Intra-abdominal pressure measurement using the Foley Manometer does not increase the risk for urinary tract infection in critically ill patients. Ann Intensive Care. 2012;2(Suppl 1):S10.
29. Balogh Z, Jones F, D'Amours S, Parr M, Sugrue M. Continuous intra-abdominal pressure measurement technique. Am J Surg. 2004;188(6):679-84.
30. Ouellet JF, Leppaniemi A, Ball CG, Cheatham ML, D'Amours S, Kirkpatrick AW. Alternatives to formal abdominal decompression. Am Surg. 2011;77 Suppl 1:S51-7.
31. De Laet I, Hoste E, Verholen E, De Waele JJ. The effect of neuromuscular blockers in patients with intra-abdominal hypertension. Intensive Care Med. 2007;33(10):1811-4.
32. Dabrowski W, Kotlinska-Hasiec E, Schneditz D, Zaluska W, Rzecki Z, De Keulenaer B, et al. Continuous veno-venous hemofiltration to adjust fluid volume excess in septic shock patients reduces intra-abdominal pressure. Clin Nephrol. 2014;82(1):41-50.
33. De Waele JJ, Hoste EA, Malbrain ML. Decompressive laparotomy for abdominal compartment syndrome—a critical analysis. Crit Care. 2006;10(2):R51.
34. Quyn AJ, Johnston C, Hall D, Chambers A, Arapova N, Ogston S, et al. The open abdomen and temporary abdominal closure systems—historical evolution and systematic review. Colorectal Dis. 2012;14(8):e429-38.
35. Rotondo MF, Schwab CW, McGonigal MD, Phillips GR 3rd, Fruchterman TM, Kauder DR, et al. "Damage control": an approach for improved survival in exsanguinating penetrating abdominal injury. J Trauma. 1993;35(3):375-82; discussion 82-3.
36. Strang SG, Van Lieshout EM, Breederveld RS, Van Waes OJ. A systematic review on intra-abdominal pressure in severely burned patients. Burns. 2014;40(1):9-16.
37. Regner JL, Kobayashi L, Coimbra R. Surgical strategies for management of the open abdomen. World J Surg. 2012; 36(3):497-510.
38. Chiara O, Cimbanassi S, Biffl W, Leppaniemi A, Henry S, Scalea TM, et al. International consensus conference on open abdomen in trauma. J Trauma Acute Care Surg. 2016; 80(1):173-83.
39. Acosta S, Bjarnason T, Petersson U, Pålsson B, Wanhainen A, Svensson M, et al. Multicentre prospective study of fascial closure rate after open abdomen with vacuum and mesh-mediated fascial traction. Br J Surg. 2011;98(5):735-43.

CHAPTER

Venous Thromboembolism

Shilpushp Jagannath Bhosale, Atul Prabhakar Kulkarni

INTRODUCTION

Deep vein thrombosis (DVT) is one of the most common condition found in critically ill patients and carries extremely high morbidity and mortality risk when complicated with pulmonary embolism (PE).[1] Both DVT and PE are part of the process of venous thromboembolism (VTE) and present extreme diagnostic challenges.[2]

The life-threatening complication of untreated DVT remains pulmonary embolization,[3] however morbidity secondary to post-thrombotic sequelae can also be significant.[4] Generally complications associated with anticoagulant-related bleeding remain unreported and hence unaccounted for. Traditionally, contrast venography has been the gold standard for diagnosis of DVT but has been replaced by ultrasound (US) as the diagnostic modality of choice,[5] however, sometimes venography is used for diagnosis of upper limb or more central DVT or in conjunction with therapeutic procedures. It has been observed that nearly 10–20% of patients develop VTE during their hospitalization[5] and >10% of deaths in these patients are attributed to DVT, which has been reported from autopsy.[6-8]

Deep vein thrombosis can either originate in the calf veins and can progress superiorly or develop in the pelvic or thigh veins and progress inferiorly. The posterior tibial and peroneal veins are more prone to develop thrombosis but the risk of subsequent complications is low, while anterior tibial veins are less susceptible to thrombosis. Though most patients with DVT remain asymptomatic, in some the thrombus may embolize, while in some it may recanalize, or scar with residual obstruction, leading to postthrombotic syndrome. Generally PE is caused by thrombosis originating from lower limbs or pelvic veins, but with increasing incidence of upper limb vessel thrombosis, the clot may originate there.

The cause of DVT can be either inherited, acquired, or both.[9] The condition predisposing to DVT is explained by the classic Virchow's triad, i.e., stasis, hypercoagulability, and injury to the venous wall. Surgery is traditionally recognized as an independent risk factor for VTE, the general risk factors that are identified among medical patients are much more diverse and hence less commonly identified. These are history of prior DVT, elderly patients, patients with diseases such as thrombophilia, malignancy, trauma, estrogen therapy, prolonged immobility, heart failure or severe low flow states, mechanical compression of deep veins, obesity, pregnancy, etc. **(Table 1)**.[10] Apart from these general risk factors, critically ill patients have

TABLE 1: Risk factors for deep vein thrombosis (DVT).

History	*Blood diseases*	*Systemic diseases*
VTE History/malignancy	Thrombophilia	Acute heart failure
Age >60 years	Protein C/Protein S deficiency	Acute MI/stroke
Prolonged immobility	Antithrombin deficiency/Factor V Leiden	Chronic kidney disease
Pregnancy or Estrogen therapy	Hyperhomocysteinemia	Autoimmune diseases
Varicose veins	Hyperfibrinogenemia	
Thrombocytosis	Raised prothrombin/factor VIII levels	

(VTE: venous thromboembolism; MI: myocardial infarction)

other risk factors such as mechanical ventilation, central lines, prolonged sedation, or neuromuscular blockade.[4,5] The other contributing factors are interruption of DVT prophylaxis, or withheld due to bleeding concerns or need for invasive procedures.[7,8]

In these critically ill patients the detection of venous thrombosis is hampered by the patient's lack of symptoms and unreliability of physical signs.[10] There is a strong association between age, sex, and DVT incidence,[11] with linear rise with age, especially in those older than 65 years[1] and it is more common among men.[9]

Mechanical ventilation and intensive care unit (ICU) length of stay remain significant factors associated for DVT despite appropriate thromboprophylaxis.

INCIDENCE AND RISK FACTORS

The incidence of DVT in ICU patients is based on various factors such as patient population, events after ICU admission, clinical suspicion for DVT and methods of screening for VTE, and use of prophylaxis interventions. The mortality rate reported from DVT is about 9% whereas for PE it is about 15%.[12]

In the United States the reported annual incidence of DVT is around 3–6 lakhs cases per year, with the attributable annual mortality of 60,000–100,000 due to PE, while in another study the reported DVT rate was 9 per 10,000 hospital admissions.[13]

Studies of mixed ICU patients have reported nearly 10% DVT on admission,[14-16] while a retrospective study in ICU patients undergoing Doppler US for DVT screening has reported incidence of 33%.[11]

The actual incidence is quite variable depending on diagnostic modalities. The majority of patients with lower extremity DVT remain asymptomatic and hence it is difficult to diagnose DVT, while the exact association of upper extremity DVT with clinically significant PE is not established, but is presumed to be lower than lower-limb DVT.

A large study of over 5,000 patients with DVT diagnosed on US revealed PE in 14.5%. They found unilateral lower limb DVT in 77% patients, bilateral lower limb DVT in 12%, and upper extremity DVT in 11%.[17] It is unclear whether increase in mortality should be attributed to severity of DVT or accompanying disease.[18]

DIAGNOSIS

It is important to have accurate diagnosis of DVT, not only to help prevent a VTE, but also because the treatment for a venous thrombosis is not without risk. DVT remains a diagnostic challenge due to the poor sensitivity and specificity of clinical symptoms and signs.[11] The clinical signs are mainly due to thrombosis and impaired venous drainage along with inflammatory response. However, widespread use of US and awareness of DVT risk factors have increased reported incidence of DVT.[19] It is found that ultrasonography (USG) is more sensitive and specific for the diagnosis of lower-limb DVT in symptomatic patients as compared to nonsymptomatic patients.[12-15] The accuracy of USG for diagnosing DVT in symptomatic patients, with improved US experience and training, is nearly 100%.[20] Another study that compared accuracy of USG to contrast venography in symptomatic patients found US to be able to diagnose proximal DVT (above the calf) with a sensitivity of 100%.[18]

Since the incidence of DVT is high in critically ill patients, it is unclear whether routine screening of DVT using US is recommended although it has been widely practiced.[10]

A complete US examination involves assessment of vein compressibility with B-mode and Doppler evaluation of spectral and color flow signals, respiratory phasicity, and augmentation.

Doppler US comprises color and spectral Doppler that help diagnose indirect evidence of venous occlusion, where monophasic waveform is a reliable indicator of proximal venous obstruction.[21] The other method described is flow augmentation, where the calf is squeezed while simultaneously imaging proximal deep veins with USG. This is routinely practiced but its usefulness remains questionable.[22] The axillary, brachial, basilic, and internal jugular veins can be assessed by compression US but the subclavian vein is not easily compressed since it lies under the clavicle. Therefore, color Doppler with flow augmentation on distal compression method can be used to assess DVT.

The American College of Emergency Physicians has described a point-of-care compression technique for the detection of lower extremity DVT.[23,24] Recent literature describes limited DVT USG examination using two regions (femoral and popliteal) versus a two-point US examination.

Two-point compression-only US examination evaluates thrombosis in the common femoral vein and popliteal veins, while a two-region US examination describes compression-only technique of two-regions (i.e., the femoral veins 1–2 cm above and below the saphenofemoral junction and the popliteal veins including the calf veins confluence.[25,26]

Limited examination techniques rely primarily on compression of the vein by applying pressure by USG transducer. If the vein completely collapses then DVT is ruled out whereas DVT is present if the vein is noncollapsible or partially collapsible. In cases of acute DVT, venous distension with echogenic clot may be seen.[27] The incidence of contralateral DVT is low and it is unclear whether we should routinely scan both lower limbs or only the symptomatic limb.[28,29]

The use of DVT scan in patients with suspected PE without signs of DVT is controversial, since a negative DVT scan does not rule out PE.[30-32] It seems that routine screening may be appropriate when DVT risk is very high but not in patients who have no contraindication to thromboprophylaxis.

It has to be noted that the inferior vena cava (IVC) and iliac veins are difficult to evaluate with US and in some patients duplication of the femoral vein may falsely give negative result, if only the patient limb is examined.[33] Other limitation is that US cannot differentiate acute or chronic DVT. The advantages of US is that it is noninvasive, easily repeatable, and without ionizing radiation.

From the recently published guidelines by the European Society of Cardiology regarding diagnosis and management of acute DVT, the highlights are shown in **Box 1**.[34]

In suspected cases, where USG may be nondiagnostic, computed tomography (CT) and magnetic resonance (MR) venography are useful for imaging. Contrast venography has been the gold standard for diagnosis of DVT, but is largely replaced by US. CT venography (CTV) is invasive, involves the use of ionizing radiation, and transport to radiological suite. CTV however helps in evaluation of the deep veins of the calves, iliac veins, IVC, and the profunda femoris vein, which are not evaluated with USG. CTV can also demonstrate pathological states such as compression of veins from lymph nodes or a mass in the pelvis as possible etiology. Some investigators suggest an adjunctive role for D-dimer testing if the pretest probability of DVT is negative according to Wells scoring systems. Bernardi et al. compared two diagnostic strategies for lower extremity DVT evaluation: (1) serial two-point US plus D-dimer testing, and (2) whole-leg color-coded Doppler US demonstrating the utility of D-Dimer test.[35]

BOX 1: Diagnosis and management of acute deep vein thrombosis (European Society of Cardiology).[34]

- Use of the Wells score to assess pretest probability of deep vein thrombosis (DVT)
- If pretest probability unlikely for DVT, use D-dimer test to rule out DVT
- Perform complete ultrasound examination, if pretest probability or D-dimer is positive
- In isolated DVT with high risk of recurrence, 3 months of anticoagulation is recommended compared to 4–6 weeks in low risk patients, with surveillance ultrasound
- DVT not associated with cancer should be treated with direct oral anticoagulants (DOACs) or warfarin, while patients with cancer should receive low-molecular-weight heparin (LMWH)
- In acute DVT, initial anticoagulation should be either:
  - Apixaban 10 mg twice a day for 7 days, then 5 mg twice a day, or
  - Dabigatran 150 mg twice a day after a 5–10 days lead-in course of LMWH, or
  - Rivaroxaban 15 mg twice a day for 21 days, then 20 mg daily, or
  - Warfarin to target international normalized ratio (INR) 2–3, with LMWH for 5–10 days (until INR >2).
- For secondary prophylaxis against recurrent DVT, patients can be treated with low-dose aspirin, Apixaban 2.5 mg twice a day, or rivaroxaban 10 mg daily
- In DVT associated with pregnancy—LMWH is the recommended anticoagulation for initial and long-term treatment. Anticoagulation to be continued for at least 6 weeks after delivery (for a minimum of 3 months of treatment)

PROPHYLAXIS AND TREATMENT

Ensuring appropriate initiation of prophylaxis remains the most effective method to reduce the burden of thromboembolic disease among critically ill patients.[26] In spite of this, it has been observed that <40% of hospitalized patients receive appropriate prophylaxis.[36]

Routine anticoagulants, such as unfractionated heparin (UFH), low molecular weight heparin (LMWH), or fondaparinux, have been extensively used and studied for thromboprophylaxis; however, antiplatelet agents are not recommended for VTE prophylaxis, as there is no evidence of their efficacy and they increase the risk of bleeding.

With regard to critically ill patients at risk for VTE, increasing use of anticoagulant prophylaxis may be associated with increased rates of bleeding. This anticoagulation related bleeding risk or death caused by bleeding could make use of prophylaxis less attractive.

It has been suggested that prophylaxis can be administered to those with three or more risk factors. The

TABLE 2: American college of chest physicians guidelines for antithrombotic therapy for venous thromboembolism.[38]

Recommendation	*Grade*
In noncancer VTE—direct oral anticoagulants (dabigatran, rivaroxaban, apixaban, or edoxaban) are recommended over vitamin K antagonist therapy and VKA is recommended over LMWH	2C
In cancer associated VTE LMWH is recommended over VKA or any direct oral anticoagulants	2B
Anticoagulants should stop after 3 months of therapy in patients with an acute, proximal deep venous thrombosis (DVT) or PE provoked by surgical or nonsurgical etiology	2B
Anticoagulation should be given for 3 months with a unprovoked VTE and a high risk of bleeding but should be extended without a scheduled stop date in patients with a low or moderate risk of bleeding	2B
Acute VTE treated with anticoagulation, use of an inferior vena cava filter not recommended	1B
In unprovoked proximal DVT or PE upon stopping anticoagulant therapy, the use of aspirin is suggested to prevent recurrent DVT if no contraindications	2B
In acute DVT, routine use of compression stockings to prevent the post-thrombotic syndrome not recommended	2B
In subsegmental PE and no DVT, use of anticoagulation recommended when the risk of VTE recurrence is high	2C
In recurrent VTE LMWH recommended over UFH	2C

(VKA: vitamin K antagonists; DVT: deep vein thrombosis; LMWH: low-molecular-weight heparin; VTE: venous thromboembolism; PE: pulmonary embolism; UFH: unfractionated heparin)

mortality rate of DVT has a strong association with other risk factors such as, cardiovascular disease, cancer, and in patients following surgery or trauma.[37]

The American College of Chest Physicians (ACCP) guidelines recommend prophylaxis for patients with moderate-to-high risk of VTE, by using pharmacological prophylaxis and/or mechanical prophylaxis.[5] The key recommendations are stated in **Table 2.**[38]

Despite the recommendations of international guidelines, it has been observed that physicians often do not prescribe prophylaxis therapy in high-risk situations.[39] The means to improve DVT prophylaxis should include increasing clinicians awareness through training and the implementation of guidelines to assess DVT risk during hospitalization, along with the application of evidence-based guidelines for DVT prophylaxis and treatment in both medical and surgical patients.[5]

Unfractionated heparin has been superseded by LMWHs, as studies have demonstrated their comparable efficacy and improved safety profile. Various trials have validated the use of LMWH or fondaparinux for VTE prophylaxis in medical patients.[40]

There is uncertainty regarding the optimal duration of VTE prophylaxis. A recent trial suggested that prophylaxis with LMWH for 28 days, resulted in a 38% reduction in VTE events but was associated with increase in major bleeding complications.[41]

The newer anticoagulants (apixaban, dabigatran, and rivaroxaban) have become the mainstay in the VTE prophylaxis in mixed medical and surgical patients with encouraging results. They have also shown enormous promise for extended duration prophylaxis in medical patients.[42]

The incidence of heparin-induced thrombocytopenia (HIT), which is described as the immune-mediated phenomenon caused by antibodies against heparin platelet-factor 4 complexes remains uncertain. HIT results in a thrombocytopenia that usually occurs typically 5–10 days after initiation of unfractionated or LMWH, and hence it is recommended to monitor platelet function accordingly. If HIT is suspected or documented, it is recommended to change over to fondaparinux for thromboprophylaxis.[43]

Mechanical prophylaxis such as sequential compression devices (SCDs) and compression stockings that are routinely used have not been rigorously evaluated in critically ill patients.[7,9] Graduated compression stockings (GCSs) or intermittent pneumatic compression (IPC) are used, especially when bleeding risk prevents use of anticoagulants or it is contraindicated.

A study of use of mechanical prophylaxis in patients with ischemic stroke has shown negative results.[44] There is some evidence from surgical studies suggesting the use of GCS and IPC to prevent DVT.[45-47]

The drawback of IPC is that it is cumbersome and may limit mobility, potentially resulting in a paradoxical increase in VTE risk.

Although routine screening would detect many DVTs, in the absence of symptoms or signs, their clinical significance remains questionable. With the current literature still failing to distinguish death with bleeding from death due to bleeding, the risk of bleeding during critical illness may remain underestimated.[48]

REFERENCES

1. Previtali E, Bucciarelli P, Passamonti SM, Martinelli I. Risk factors for venous and arterial thrombosis. Blood Transfus. 2011;9(2):120-38.
2. Cogo A, Lensing AW, Prandoni P, Hirsh J. Distribution of thrombosis in patients with symptomatic deep vein thrombosis. Implications for simplifying the diagnostic process with compression ultrasound. Arch Intern Med. 1993;153(24):2777-80.
3. Kyrle PA, Eichinger S. Deep vein thrombosis. The Lancet. 2005;365(9465):1163-74.
4. Pomero F, Dentali F, Borretta V, Bonzini M, Melchio R, Douketis JD, et al. Accuracy of emergency physician-performed ultrasonography in the diagnosis of deep-vein thrombosis: a systematic review and meta- analysis. Thromb Haemost. 2013;109(1):137-45.
5. Geerts WH, Bergqvist D, Pineo GF, Heit JA, Samama CM, Lassen MR, et al. Prevention of venous thromboembolism: American College of Chest Physicians Evidence-Based Clinical Practice Guidelines (8th Edition). Chest. 2008;133(6 Suppl):381s-453s.
6. Heriot GS, Pitman AG, Gonzales M, McKelvie P. The four horsemen: clinicopathological correlation in 407 hospital autopsies. Intern Med J. 2010;40(9):626-32.
7. Kakkar N, Vasishta RK. Pulmonary embolism in medical patients: an autopsy-based study. Clin Appl Thromb Hemost. 2008;14(2):159-67.
8. Lindblad B, Sternby NH, Bergqvist D. Incidence of venous thromboembolism verified by necropsy over 30 years. BMJ. 1991;302(6778):709-11.
9. Williams MT, Aravindan N, Wallace MJ, Riedel BJ, Shaw AD. Venous thromboembolism in the intensive care unit. Crit Care Clin. 2003;19(2):185-207.
10. Hong KC, Kim H, Kim JY, Kwak KS, Cho OM, Cha HY, et al. Risk factors and incidence of deep vein thrombosis in lower extremities among critically ill patients. J Clin Nurs. 2012;21(13-14):1840-6.
11. Wheeler HB. Diagnosis of deep vein thrombosis. Review of clinical evaluation and impedance plethysmography. Am J Surg. 1985;150(4A):7-13.
12. Cushman M, Tsai AW, White RH, Heckbert SR, Rosamond WD, Enright P, et al. Deep vein thrombosis and pulmonary embolism in two cohorts: the longitudinal investigation of thromboembolism etiology. Am J Med. 2004;117(1):19-25.
13. Beckman MG, Hooper WC, Critchley SE, Ortel TL. Venous thromboembolism: a public health concern. Am J Prev Med. 2010;38(Suppl 4):S495-501.
14. Cook D, Attia J, Weaver B, McDonald E, Meade M, Crowther M. Venous thromboembolic disease: an observational study in medical-surgical intensive care unit patients. J Crit Care. 2000;15(4):127-32.
15. Harris LM, Curl GR, Booth FV, Hassett JM Jr, Leney G, Ricotta JJ. Screening for asymptomatic deep vein thrombosis in surgical intensive care patients. J Vasc Surg. 1997;2(5)6:764-9.
16. Schonhofer B, Kohler D. Prevalence of deep-vein thrombosis of the leg in patients with acute exacerbation of chronic obstructive pulmonary disease. Respiration. 1998;65(3):173-7.
17. Goldhaber SZ, Tapson VF; DVT FREE Steering Committee. A prospective registry of 5,451 patients with ultrasound-confirmed deep vein thrombosis. Am J Cardiol. 2004;93(2):259-62.
18. Lensing AW, Prandoni P, Brandjes D, Huisman PM, Vigo M, Tomasella G, et al. Detection of deep-vein thrombosis by real-time B-mode ultrasonography. N Engl J Med. 1989;320(6):342-5.
19. Spencer FA, Emery C, Lessard D, Anderson F, Emani S, Aragam J, et al. The Worcester Venous Thromboembolism study: a population-based study of the clinical epidemiology of venous thromboembolism. J Gen Intern Med. 2006;21(7):722-7.
20. Fraser JD, Anderson DR. Deep venous thrombosis: recent advances and optimal investigation with US. Radiology. 1999;211(1):9-24.
21. Lin EP, Bhatt S, Rubens D, Dogra VS. The importance of monophasic Doppler waveforms in the common femoral vein: a retrospective study. J Ultrasound Med. 2007;26(7):885-91.
22. Lockhart ME, Sheldon HI, Robbin ML. Augmentation in lower extremity sonography for the detection of deep venous thrombosis. Am J Roentgenol. 2005;184(2):419-22.
23. American College of Emergency Physicians. Emergency ultrasound imaging criteria compendium. Ann Emerg Med. 2006;48(4):487-510.
24. American College of Emergency Physicians. Emergency ultrasound guidelines. Ann Emerg Med. 2009;53(4):550-70.
25. Poppiti R, Papanicolaou G, Perese S, Weaver FA. Limited B-mode venous imaging versus complete color-flow duplex venous scanning for detection of proximal deep venous thrombosis. J Vasc Surg. 1995;22(5):553-7.
26. Pezzullo JA, Perkins AB, Cronan JJ. Symptomatic deep venous thrombosis: diagnosis with limited compression US. Radiology. 1996;198(1):67-70.
27. Lewis BD. The peripheral veins. In: Rumack CM, Wilson SR, Charboneau JW (Eds). Diagnostic Ultrasound, 2nd edition. St. Louis, MO: Mosby; 1998. pp. 943-58.

28. Johnson SA, Stevens SM, Woller SC, Lake E, Donadini M, Cheng J, et al. Risk of deep vein thrombosis following a single negative whole-leg compression ultrasound: a systematic review and meta-analysis. JAMA. 2010;303(5):438-45.
29. Rosen MP, McArdle C. Controversies in the use of lower extremity sonography in the diagnosis of acute deep vein thrombosis and a proposal for a unified approach. Semin Ultrasound CT MR. 1997;18(5):362-8.
30. Turkstra F, Kuijer PM, van Beek EJ, Brandjes DP, ten Cate JW, Büller HR. Diagnostic utility of ultrasonography of leg veins in patients suspected of having pulmonary embolism. Ann Intern Med. 1997;126(10):775-81.
31. Girard P, Sanchez O, Leroyer C, Musset D, Meyer G, Stern JB, et al.; Evaulation du Scanner Spiralé dans l'Embolie Pulmonaire Study Group. Deep venous thrombosis in patients with acute pulmonary embolism: prevalence, risk factors, and clinical significance. Chest. 2005;128(3):1593-600.
32. Katz DS, Loud PA, Bruce D, Gittleman AM, Mueller R, Klippenstein DL, et al. Combined CT venography and pulmonary angiography: a comprehensive review. Radiographics. 2002;22:S3-S24.
33. Quinlan DJ, Alikhan R, Gishen P, Sidhu PS. Variations in lower limb venous anatomy: implications for US diagnosis of deep vein thrombosis. Radiology. 2003;228(2):443-8.
34. Screaton NJ, Gillard JH, Berman LH, Kemp PM. Duplicated superficial femoral veins: a source of error in the sonographic investigation of deep vein thrombosis. Radiology. 1998;206(2):397-401.
35. Mazzolai L, Aboyans V, Ageno W, Agnelli G, Alatri A, Bauersachs R, et al. Diagnosis and management of acute deep vein thrombosis: a joint consensus document from the European Society of Cardiology working groups of aorta and peripheral vascular diseases and pulmonary circulation and right ventricular function. Eur Heart J. 2018;39(47):4208-18.
36. Bernardi E, Camporese G, Büller HR, Siragusa S, Imberti D, Berchio A, et al.; Erasmus Study Group. Serial 2-point ultrasonography plus D-dimer vs whole-leg color-coded Doppler ultrasonography for diagnosing suspected symptomatic deep vein thrombosis: a randomized controlled trial. JAMA. 2008;300(14):1653-9.
37. Cohen AT, Tapson VF, Bergmann JF, Goldhaber SZ, Kakkar AK, Deslandes B, et al.; ENDORSE Investigators. Venous thromboembolism risk and prophylaxis in the acute hospital care setting (ENDORSE study): a multinational cross-sectional study. Lancet. 2008;371(9610):387-94.
38. Heit JA, O'Fallon WM, Petterson TM, Lohse CM, Silverstein MD, Mohr DN, et al. Relative impact of risk factors for deep vein thrombosis and pulmonary embolism: a population-based study. Arch Intern Med. 2002;162(11):1245-8.
39. Kearon C, Akl EA, Ornelas J, Blaivas A, Jimenez D, Bounameaux H, et al. Antithrombotic Therapy for VTE Disease: CHEST Guideline and Expert Panel Report. Chest. 2016;149(2):315-52.
40. Gutt CN, Oniu T, Wolkener F, Mehrabi A, Mistry S, Büchler MW. Prophylaxis and treatment of deep vein thrombosis in general surgery. Am J Surg. 2005;189(1):14-22.
41. Mismetti P, Laporte-Simitsidis S, Tardy B, Cucherat M, Buchmüller A, Juillard-Delsart D, et al. Prevention of venous thromboembolism in internal medicine with unfractionated or low-molecular-weight heparins: a meta-analysis of randomized clinical trials. Thromb Haemost. 2000;83(1):14-9.
42. Hull RD, Schellong SM, Tapson VF, Monreal M, Samama MM, Nicol P, et al. Extended-duration venous thromboembolism prophylaxis in acutely ill medical patients with recently reduced mobility: a randomized trial. Ann Intern Med. 2010;153(1):8-18.
43. Cohen AT, Spiro TE, Buller HR, Haskell L, Hu D, Hull R, et al. Extended duration rivaroxaban thromboprophylaxis in acutely ill medical patients: MAGELLAN study protocol. J Thromb Thrombolysis. 2011;31(4):407-16.
44. Warkentin TE, Pai M, Sheppard JI, Schulman S, Spyropoulos AC, Eikelboom JW. Fondaparinux treatment of acute heparin-induced thrombocytopenia confirmed by the serotonin-release assay: a 30-month, 16-patient case series. J Thromb Haemost. 2011;9(12):2389-96.
45. CLOTS Trials Collaboration; Dennis M, Sandercock P, Reid J, Graham C, Murray G, Venables G, et al. Effectiveness of thigh-length graduated compression stockings to reduce the risk of deep vein thrombosis after stroke (CLOTS trial 1): a multicentre, randomized controlled trial. Lancet. 2009;373(9679):1958-65.
46. Turpie AG, Leizorovicz A. Prevention of venous thromboembolism in medically ill patients: a clinical update. Postgrad Med J. 2006;82(974):806-9.
47. EINSTEIN Investigators; Bauersachs R, Berkowitz SD, Brenner B, Buller HR, Decousus H, Gallus AS, et al. Oral rivaroxaban for symptomatic venous thromboembolism. N Engl J Med. 2010;363(26):2499-510.
48. Agnelli G, Prandoni P, Santamaria MG, Bagatella P, Iorio A, Bazzan M, et al. Three months versus one year of oral anticoagulant therapy for idiopathic deep venous thrombosis: Warfarin Optimal Duration Italian Trial Investigators. N Engl J Med. 2001;345(3):165-9.

SECTION

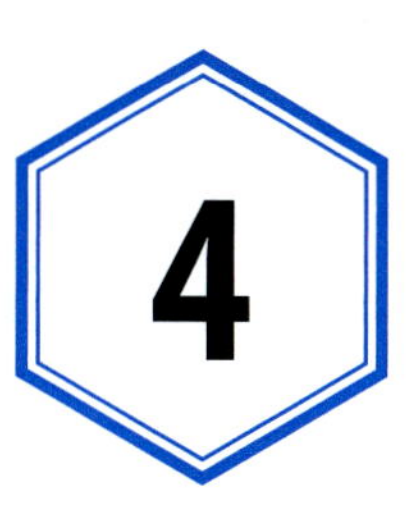

Types of Shock

CHAPTER

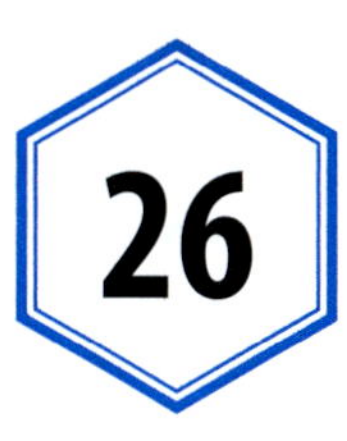

Vasodilatory Shock

Suresh Ramasubban

INTRODUCTION

Shock is a clinical condition of circulatory compromise resulting in decreased delivery of oxygen to tissue/cells or increased oxygen consumption or poor utilization of available oxygen in the tissue resulting in cellular hypoxia ultimately culminating into organ failure. Shock is attributed to almost 33% of admission in the intensive care units (ICUs) worldwide.[1]

Clinically, shock is recognized at the bedside by clinical, hemodynamic, and biochemical parameters. Classically, shock states are characterized by hypotension, though may be relative in patients with chronic hypertension and associated tachycardia. Hemodynamic assessment of tissue perfusion is done at the bedside by looking at the parameters that enable us to peek into the body, i.e., urine output, mental status, and skin condition. Biochemically, lactate levels >1.5 mmol/L point to tissue hypoperfusion, albeit with the caveats attached to lactate interpretation.[2]

Typically, shock has been classified into four major categories, as proposed by Max Henry Weil.[3] Three of the shock states result in profound vasoconstriction, characterized by a cold clammy, mottled skin due to low cardiac output, i.e., hypovolemic, obstructive, and cardiogenic shock. The fourth category which is characterized classically by the absence of a cold and clammy skin and therefore referred to as warm shock, is due to failure of the vascular smooth muscles to constrict, resulting in vasodilation and poor response to vasopressor drugs.

DEFINITION OF VASOPLEGIA

Vasoplegia is defined as a shock state with difficulty in maintaining mean arterial pressure (MAP) <65 mm Hg with requirement of vasopressors above 0.2 μg/kg/min to 0.5 μg/kg/min of norepinephrine (NE) equivalents and with a cardiac index (CI) >2.2 L/min/m^2.[4]

ETIOLOGY

Vasodilatory shock constitutes >60% of the causes of shock and the causes of vasodilatory shock[4] are not restricted to sepsis alone. Sepsis is the main cause of vasodilatory shock, however any condition in which tissue oxygenation is impaired, such as carbon monoxide poisoning and hypoxic lactic acidosis (nitrogen intoxication) will also lead to vasodilatory shock. Vasodilatory shock is also the final common pathway for long-lasting shock from any cause like hemorrhagic shock after resuscitation and decompensated heart failure with cardiogenic shock.

Spinal cord injury leading to neurogenic shock, postoperative vasoplegia, are important other causes. Systemic inflammatory response syndrome (SIRS) due to condition like acute pancreatitis also leads to vasoplegia. Other conditions such as metformin overdose, cyanide poisoning, mitochondrial disease, and cardiac arrest with pulseless electric activity (PEA) **(Box 1)** are important causes of vasodilatory shock. Hypocalcemia and propofol infusion syndrome are some rare causes of vasodilatory shock. Anaphylaxis, liver failure, and corticosteroid insufficiency are also listed as a probable cause of vasodilatory shock and more commonly encountered in clinical practice; however, the data on the vasodilatation with these causes are limited.[5-8]

PATHOPHYSIOLOGY

Vasodilatory shock is associated with elevated levels of catecholamines and activation of the renin-angiotensin (AT) system, leading to the conclusion that there is failure of smooth muscles contraction leading to hypotension. So, it is not the lack of endogenous catecholamines but the inability of the vascular smooth muscles to respond to the catecholamines that leads to a refractory hypotension. For

BOX 1: Etiology of vasodilatory shock.

1	Sepsis
2	*Tissue hypoxia:* • Hypoxic lactic acidosis • Carbon monoxide poisoning • SIRS due to pancreatitis
3	*Refractory hypotension:* • Hemorrhagic shock • Cardiogenic shock • Cardiopulmonary bypass
4	Lactic acidosis due to metformin toxicity, propofol infusion syndrome
5	Cyanide poisoning, drug overdose with calcium channel blocker, and hydralazine
6	Cardiac arrest with pulseless electrical activity
7	Liver failure, anaphylaxis, and glucocorticoid deficiency-probable causes
8	Spinal cord injury
9	Hypocalcemia
10	Liver failure
11	Anaphylaxis
12	Glucocorticoid deficiency

(SIRS: systemic inflammatory response syndrome)

this failure of response to the vascular smooth muscles, three mechanisms are traditionally proposed:

1. Death of the vascular smooth muscle cells due to inadequate perfusion,
2. Inadequate oxygen extraction by the tissue, and
3. Increased prostaglandin activity.

These mechanisms have little evidence. Recent works have elucidated mechanism of vasoconstriction in vasodilatory shock, and it is proposed that different mechanisms may be active in different etiologies, but a common pathway may be involved in most of the cases.[8,9]

For vasoconstriction to occur, ligands such as NE and AT II bind to and activate receptors on the surface of vascular smooth muscles. Once the neuronal and hormonal ligands bind and activate the receptors on the surface, it results in increased cytosolic concentration of calcium via secondary messengers. The increase in calcium is due to the release of calcium from the internal cytoplasmic stores and entry of extracellular calcium via voltage-gated channels. The increase in calcium in the cytoplasm leads to the binding of calcium to calmodulin and the formation of a calcium-calmodulin complex, which activates a kinase that phosphorylates myosin, the regulatory light chain of muscle contraction **(Fig. 1)**. Phosphorylation of the light chain of myosin leads to activation of myosin adenosine triphosphatase (ATPase) by actin leading to the cycling of myosin cross-bridges along the actin filaments, leading to contraction of the smooth muscle.

The mechanism of vasorelaxation in a vascular smooth muscle involves the activation of a kinase that dephosphorylates the light chain of myosin. The dephosphorylation is mediated by atrial natriuretic peptide (ANP) and nitric oxide (NO) which through the cyclic-guanosine monophosphate (c-GMP) pathway activates myosin phosphatase, which is responsible for the dephosphorylation and thus preventing muscle contraction **(Fig. 1)**.

In addition to the aforementioned mechanism of control of vascular tone, there is growing importance to the role of membrane potential of vascular smooth muscles on the regulation of vascular tone. The modulation of the vascular tone is regulated by the membrane potential

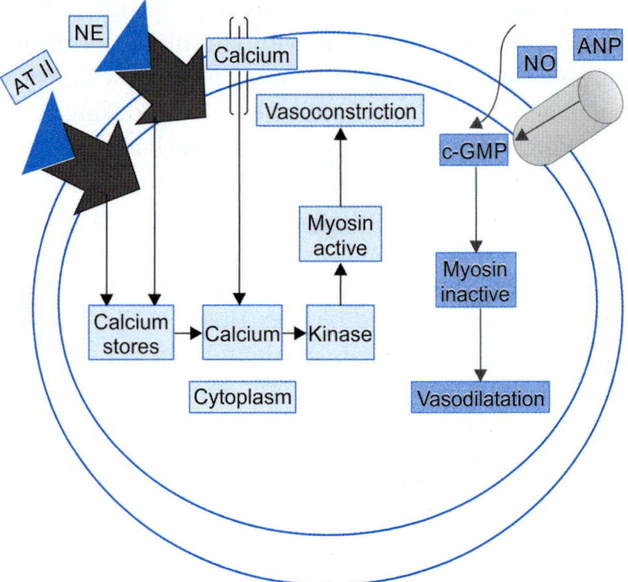

Fig. 1: Mechanism of vasoconstriction and vasodilatation in vascular smooth muscle. Vasoconstriction pathway is shown in black and vasodilation in gray. Influx of calcium is due to second messengers activated by ligands like norepinephrine (NE) and angiotensin II (AT II). Calcium activates myosin kinase which in turn phosphorylates myosin leading to vasoconstriction. Vasodilation occurs due to the action of nitric oxide (NO) and atrial natriuretic peptide (ANP) releasing cyclic-guanosine monophosphate (c-GMP) which activates myosin phosphatase, which dephosphorylates myosin leading to vasoconstriction.

of the vascular smooth muscles. The resting membrane potential of the vascular smooth muscle is about 30–60 mV. Depolarization of the membrane leads to influx of calcium into the cytoplasm through voltage-gated calcium channels leading to vasoconstriction. On the converse, hyperpolarization prevents calcium entry into the cytoplasm and therefore preventing vasoconstriction and causing vasorelaxation **(Fig. 2)**. The sustained hyperpolarization can prevent the action of ligands such as NE and AT from causing vasoconstriction leading to the refractoriness to vasopressors.

Absolute or relative deficiency of endogenous vasoconstrictor hormones (cortisol, AT II) further decreases vasopressor responsiveness. Microcirculatory effect creates low or now flow zone surrounded by zones of profound flow leading to maldistribution of flow despite acceptable hemodynamic parameters.

Over the last two decades, the exact mechanism of smooth muscle failure has been elucidated and three major mechanisms have been proposed to explain the vasodilatory shock.

1. Activation of adenosine triphosphate (ATP) sensitive potassium channels (K_{atp}) on vascular smooth muscles.
2. Increased synthesis of NO.
3. Deficiency of vasopressin.

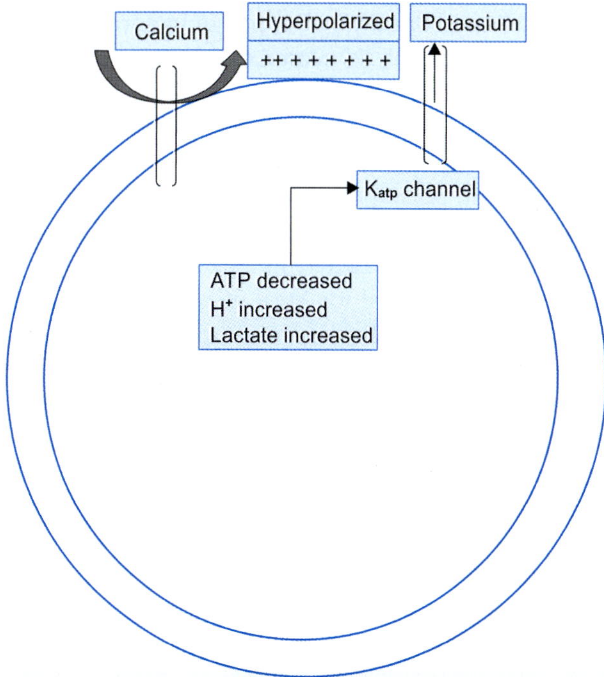

Fig. 2: Control of vascular tone by membrane potential. Depolarization leads to entry of calcium through voltage-gated calcium channels into the vascular smooth muscle cell leading to vasoconstriction. Hyperpolarization of the vascular smooth cell membrane due to movement of potassium out of the cell due to activation of ATP-sensitive potassium channels (K_{atp}) pump which results in closure of calcium channels and prevents vasoconstriction and leads to vasodilation. (ATP: adenosine triphosphate)

Activation of Adenosine Triphosphate-Sensitive Potassium Channels on Vascular Smooth Muscles

The membrane potential of the vascular smooth muscle is maintained by a variety of ion transporters and channels. The potassium channels are the most important in maintaining the membrane potential, and among the four types of potassium channels, the K_{atp} channel is the most studied in its role of maintaining vascular tone. The opening of the K_{atp} channels allows efflux of potassium from the cytosol toward the outside of the cell leading to hyperpolarization and vasodilation. In normal condition K_{atp} channels are closed as evidenced by failure of their inhibitors (e.g., sulfonylurea) to cause vasoconstriction. But in presence of increased cellular metabolism these channels are activated causing vasodilation which can be reversed by sulfonylurea. Activation of these K_{atp} channels leading to their opening and efflux of potassium is by a decreased level of ATP in the cells. The other mechanism of activation of K_{atp} channels are due to increased hydrogen ion concentration and increased lactate concentration inside the vascular smooth muscle cell. The activation of these channels in sepsis, lactic acidosis, and other etiologies leading to intracellular acidosis results in vasodilatory shock. In the late stage of hypovolemic and cardiogenic shock, K_{atp} channels are activated and this results in lowering the expected vascular resistant at this condition. There are roles of other mediators such as atrial natriuretic factor, calcitonin gene related peptide, adenosine, and NO that act on the K_{atp} channels to cause vasodilation.[10]

Increased Synthesis of Nitric Oxide

Plasma concentration of NO is increased in sepsis due to increased expression of nitric oxide synthase (NOS) in vascular smooth muscles and endothelial cells. The *NOS* gene is induced in sepsis due to several inflammatory cytokines released during sepsis. NO causes vasodilatation due to dephosphorylation of myosin due to activation of myosin light chain phosphatase. This is mediated via c-GMP. In addition, NO can activate potassium channels (K_{ca}) leading to hyperpolarization and the refractoriness to vasoconstrictors. NO activates K_{ca} channels by two mechanisms, one is by direct nitrosylation of the channels and second is by a c-GMP-dependent protein kinase. The dysregulated NO metabolism in sepsis also leads to altered microcirculatory flow, decreased bactericidal activity, coagulation modulation, and dysregulated mitochondrial respiration. This in turn leads to a decreased responsiveness to catecholamines, increased blood glucose, decreased calcium, and corticosteroid deficiency.

Deficiency of Vasopressin

Vasopressin has two functions, water conservation and vasoconstriction, these functions depends on concentration. At a concentration of 1–7 pg/mL, vasopressin is involved in regulation of water balance. At concentrations of 10–200 pg/mL, the vasoconstrictor actions of vasopressin are appreciable. Levels of vasopressin are elevated to a vasoconstrictor dose in hemorrhagic shock and sepsis but concentration declines on sustained hypotension for <1 hour. The reason for the decline in vasopressin concentration after prolonged hypotension is unclear but exhaustion of vasopressin stores may be one of the possible explanations.[11] Immunohistochemical analysis of neurohypophysis in dogs subjected to prolonged hypotension reveal a decline in the vasopressin stores pointing to a vasopressin deficiency as a mechanism of vasoplegia. The replacement of vasopressin exogenously at replacement doses leads to a sustained increase in MAP by 25–50 mm Hg. The marked response and increased sensitivity to exogenously administered vasopressin in vasodilatory shock is due to the following reasons:

- Vasopressin receptors on vascular smooth muscle cells are open as their concentration is low.
- Vasopressin response is better in patients who have autonomic failure, which is the case in septic patients who are sedated or are comatose.
- Vasopressin potentiates the effect of NE.
- Vasopressin directly inactivates K_{atp} channels in vascular smooth muscles.
- Vasopressin blunts the increase in c-GMP induced by NO.

Sepsis or tissue hypoxia with lactic acidosis leads to vasodilation due to inappropriate activation of vasodilator mechanism and failure of vasoconstrictor mechanisms, as outlined in **Figure 1**.

MANAGEMENT

Treatment of shock revolves around identification of the etiology of the shock and restoring adequate tissue perfusion with fluids and/or vasopressors and/or inotropes. Vasodilatory shock is the most common type of shock and will require vasopressors to restore vascular tone.

Refractory shock is defined as inadequate response to high-dose vasopressors, i.e., a dose of >0.5 µg/kg/min NE equivalent dose.[4] The NE equivalent doses of the various vasopressors are as illustrated in **Table 1**.

Evaluation of refractory vasodilatory shock entails ruling out contributors such as hypovolemia, pump failure, and obstructive shock. Hemodynamic assessment is required to identify contributors and confirm diagnosis of vasodilatory shock. The purpose of hemodynamic monitoring is to objectively measure the cardiac output and fluid responsiveness. A vasodilatory shock will be evident from a high cardiac output and fluid responsiveness may or may not be present. Cardiac output can be measured directly by Doppler or by surrogates such as pulse contour analysis, central or mixed venous oxygen saturation. Use of pulmonary artery (PA) catheter has got no evidence of benefit. If cardiac output is inadequate, fluid responsiveness can be assessed by tidal volume challenge test, pulse pressure variation (PPV) or stroke volume variation (SVV), or by passive leg rising. Controlled fluid challenge is indicated to optimize the fluid therapy.

The treatment goal for MAP in patients with shock is >65 mm Hg. No vasopressor is superior as compared to each other and the consensus is that the preferred vasopressor is NE. The minimum effective dose of NE is uncertain but doses beyond 0.5 µg/kg/min are generally ineffective in getting the MAP any further. High dose of a single agent leads to toxicity,[12] therefore, use of moderate doses of multiple vasopressors with complementary mechanism is preferred. Dopamine and phenylephrine are weak vasopressors and are not effective in severe or

TABLE 1: Norepinephrine equivalent doses of 0.1 µg/kg/min.

Drug	Dose
Norepinephrine	0.1 µg/kg/min
Epinephrine	0.1 µg/kg/min
Dopamine	15 µg/kg/min
Phenylephrine	1 µg/kg/min
Vasopressin	0.04 U/min

refractory shock; studies have shown that dopamine is associated with an increased rate of cardiac arrhythmias and may worsen outcomes in cardiogenic shock.[13] The choice as an alternative agent is between epinephrine and vasopressin. In case of a low cardiac output situation, epinephrine is preferred, as it has significant β effect. The role of vasopressin as a second-line vasopressor has been evaluated in the vasopressin and septic shock trial (VASST). In this trial, the investigators examined the use of low dose (0.03 U/min) vasopressin or NE added to baseline catecholamine therapy in patients with septic shock and found no difference in mortality.[14] However, there was decreased mortality with vasopressin in the subset of patients with NE dose <15 μg/min. Patients receiving both vasopressin and corticosteroids seem to have the lowest mortality. Subsequent meta-analysis of vasopressin use has thrown up conflicting results as to the benefits of vasopressin. Overall, the evidence is pointing to the safety and efficacy of vasopressin as an adjunct to catecholamines in vasodilatory shock. Higher doses of vasopressin are also safe as evident from the recent study, effect of early vasopressin versus norepinephrine on kidney failure in patients with septic shock (VANISH) study,[15] which compared NE with vasopressin (titrated up to 0.06 U/min) in early septic shock, and there were no significant differences in mortality or adverse events. There is no added advantage of achieving supernormal cardiac output in patients with vasodilation.

Timing of Vasopressors

Traditional approach of initiation of vasopressor in vasodilatory shock is to initiate with a single vasopressor and to titrate the dose according to the goal almost to a toxic level and then introducing a second vasopressor. This approach may not be appropriate for treating a vasodilatory shock since there is coexistent multifactorial pathophysiology involved in vasodilatory shock such as decreased plasma vasopressin level, downregulation of AT receptors, and impaired endogenous catecholamine.[16] Early multimodal balanced vasopressor strategy is probably helpful in treating refractory vasodilation.

Aim for the vasopressor therapy is to push blood into the capillaries and deliver oxygen to tissue early. Delay in vasopressor initiation is associated with increase in organ failure. Every hour of delay leads to 5.3% rise in the risk of death.[17-21] Vasopressor initiation, like antibiotic in septic shock is time bound and the 2018 surviving sepsis guideline, initiation of vasopressor was a part of the 1-hour bundle. However, in the 2021 guideline timing of vasopressor initiation is ambiguous.

The CENSER (Early Use of Norepinephrine in Septic Shock Resuscitation) study[22] which is a prospective single center randomized trial showed early shock reversal with early initiation of NE without any difference in mortality (not powered for mortality). In a recent retrospective study each hour delay in initiation of vasopressin is associated with 12–18% increase in mortality in hospital.

Increased lactate level is the hallmark of poor prognosis in shock and is an independent predictor for early mortality. Hyperlactatemia in shock stem from various mechanisms, e.g., decreased oxygen delivery, inadequate mitochondrial oxygen, anaerobic glycolysis, and poor lactate clearance by liver in presence of acidemia.[23] Increased lactate in patients of shock with vasopressor signifies less survival. Response to vasopressor on lactate gives an insight for vasopressor selection and timing.

The most obvious consequence of the classic stepwise approach of vasopressor is catecholamine burden which causes increased stimulation of peripheral vasculature causing ischemic limbs, splanchnic hypoperfusion as well as incidence of arrhythmia. Increased requirement of NE is associated with increased mortality in PRISM (Preferred Reporting Items for Systematic Reviews) meta-analysis.[24] Catecholamine dose and early reduction is the most robust bedside marker of mortality.

There are emerging biomarkers[25] **(Table 2)** for phenotypic prognostication and to tailor vasopressor

TABLE 2: Biomarkers in vasopressor therapy.

Biomarker	*Vasopressors*	*Clinical association*
ADRβ2	Norepinephrine, epinephrine	Increased organ dysfunction, mortality
AGTRAP	Angiotensin II	Decreased vascular tone, increased shock and mortality
LNPEP	Vasopressin	Vasopressin clearance, shock, and mortality
Angiopoietin-2 level	Vasopressin and analogue	Organ failure, mortality
Renin	Angiotensin II	Hemodynamic response, shock
Vasopressin	Vasopressin	Variable response

(ADRβ2: beta-2 adrenergic receptor; AGTRAP: angiotensin II receptor associated protein; LNPEP: leucyl and cystinyl aminopeptidase)

therapy in vasodilatory shock. The genetic variation of beta-2 adrenergic receptor (ADRβ2) encoding for the β2 receptor is associated with higher NE requirement, greater organ dysfunction. Similarly, variants in *AGTRAP*, the AT II receptor type 1 associated protein is associated with reduced MAP, vasodilation and increased mortality. Defects in LNPEP (leucyl and cystinyl aminopeptidase) or vasopressinase is associated with vasopressin clearance. Elevation of plasma angiopoetin-2 concentration is associated with increased rate of organ failure and mortality. Plasma renin is rapidly rising as a superior predictor of mortality compared to lactate. Renin is stable, and its concentration is not influenced by drugs and renal replacement therapy. The problem is lack of point of care assay and cost.

The more favorable approach may be use of early multimodal so called "broad spectrum" vasopressors followed by extensive use of biomarkers and de-escalation guided by the level of these biomarkers. Where one biomarker stands out as clear signal of benefit of a particular agent. Like if vasopressin levels are found to be disproportionately low probably use of a vasopressin heavy approach would help. High renin level may indicate good response of use of AT II.

Finally, use of noncatecholamine vasoconstricting agents should be given more importance to provide a multimodal approach to resuscitation.

BOX 2: Rescue therapy for vasodilatory shock.

1	Glucocorticoids
2	*Correction of acidosis:* • Intravenous bicarbonate • Tromethamine
3	Renal replacement therapy/extracorporeal membrane oxygenation/extracorporeal blood purification
4	Calcium
5	*Nitric oxide inhibitors:* • Methylene blue • Hydroxycobalamin
6	Vitamin C and thiamine
7	Angiotensin II
8	Selepressin and terlipressin

RESCUE THERAPY FOR REFRACTORY VASODILATORY SHOCK

Several therapies have been studied in refractory vasodilatory shock. They include AT II, selepressin and terlipressin, glucocorticoid therapy, correction of acidosis, renal replacement therapy, NO inhibitors, and calcium and vitamin repletion **(Box 2)**. All these interventions have favorable hemodynamic effect but no effect on mortality.

- *Angiotensin II:* In sepsis there is functional AT converting enzyme and AT II deficiency. The angiotensin II for the treatment of high output shock (ATHOS) trial a pilot study showed human AT II can effectively increase MAP. Subsequently, in a larger ATHOS 3 trial[26] in 74 ICUs, AT II effectively increased blood pressure in vasodilatory shock not responding to high dose of vasopressors. There was no difference in mortality or adverse effects.
- *Selepressin and terlipressin:* Terlipressin reduced NE requirements, and reduced heart rate and a borderline improvement in oxygen consumption index with little influence on mortality.[27] Selepressin has higher vascular selectivity with higher V1 to V2 ratio resulting in fewer side effects compared to vasopressin. Selepressin is associated with equal hemodynamic profile, reduced lung edema, and potential to decrease vascular leakage compared to vasopressin.[28] In the SEPSISACT study,[29] there is no difference in side effect profile compared to placebo.
- *Glucocorticoids:* Glucocorticoid receptors augment vascular α-adrenergic responsiveness and reduce inflammation-mediated vasodilatation. In the vasculature steroid, receptors are present in endothelial smooth muscle which potentiate response to the circulating catecholamine and AT II. In refractory vasodilatory shock, there is also a functional/relative adrenal insufficiency which glucocorticoid replacement replenishes and results in a favorable hemodynamic outcome. In refractory shock, hydrocortisone 200–300 mg/day, irrespective of adrenal function testing, results in decreased vasopressor requirements. The effect on mortality is unclear so far, but less severely ill patients do not seem to have a mortality benefit. The use of hydrocortisone in refractory shock may have a benefit and there is a definite synergism between vasopressin use and hydrocortisone use as a vasopressor.[30]
- *Correction of acidosis:* The accumulation of lactic acid inside the cell is responsible for the activation of the K_{atp} channels and subsequent severe refractoriness to catecholamines and vasoplegia. "Shock begets

shock," the accumulation of lactic acid inside the cell can lead to this vicious cycle of vasoplegia. The vasopressor response to catecholamine is decreased when pH falls below 7.15. Intravenous bicarbonate can reverse acidosis but the increase in MAP is mainly due to the volume expanding effect of hypertonic bicarbonate solution. Intravenous sodium bicarbonate has significant adverse effects mainly related to volume overload, a paradoxical intracellular acidosis, ionized hypocalcemia, and lactic acidosis.[31] Tris-hydroxymethyl-aminomethane (tromethamine), a synthetic nonbicarbonate buffer can be used as an alternative to bicarbonate, however, data regarding its efficacy and safety is lacking.[32]

- *Renal replacement therapy:* Metabolic acidosis associated with acute kidney injury can worsen the vasodilatory shock. Continuous renal replacement therapy can correct the metabolic derangements and improve vasopressor responsiveness. Studies on high volume hemofiltration have shown favorable hemodynamic outcomes but no benefit on mortality. Outcomes are better if renal replacement therapy is initiated soon after onset of shock and initiation of vasopressors.[33]
- *Extracorporeal membrane oxygenation:* Positive experiences in use of both veno-venous extracorporeal membrane oxygenation (VV ECMO) and venoarterial (VA) ECMO is reported. ECMO allows "metabolic rest" which optimize tissue perfusion and reduces dose of vasopressor drugs. Some insights according to recent retrospective study clarified that ECMO appears to achieve bad outcome with distributive shock and high cardiac output but may have a role in early stage of hemodynamic compromise by correcting hypoxemia and acidosis.[34]
- *Extracorporeal blood purification:* These are promising options in severe sepsis with or without acute kidney injury. It involves various techniques such as hemoperfusion/hemoadsorption, high adsorption hemofiltration, high cutoff membrane hemofiltration, plasma exchange, and coupled plasma filtration adsorption.[35] The principle is removal of the inflammatory cytokines and toxins and achieve immune homeostasis which counteracts immune dysregulation. Extracorporeal therapies (ECT) in sepsis are limited with lack of evidence, mainly single center or small trials show therapeutic advantage which are often reversed by larger multicenter trials. The key takeaway message is the fact that the initiation of early therapy in vasodilatory shock can impose maximized benefits. However, timely intervention is critical. Various pharmacokinetic studies on cytokine clearance would be extremely useful to determine the therapy duration. The effect of intervention might vary due to the disease severity. More well-conducted randomized controlled studies with the selection of appropriate patients and endpoints are needed.
- *Calcium:* Calcium is an important element needed for intracellular signaling in vascular smooth muscles and heart muscles. The vasoconstrictor response depends on adequate entry of calcium into the smooth muscle cell and its combination with calmodulin and eventual activation of kinases that phosphorylates myosin leading to coupling of actin myosin cross bridges. A decreased level of calcium is common in critically ill patients due to saponification of necrotic tissue, chelation by citrate in blood products, parathyroid hormone, and vitamin D deficiency. Bolus administration of calcium chloride increases MAP by increasing vascular tone; clinical evidence for this however is lacking and cellular calcium overloading is harmful in sepsis. There is no evidence that calcium administration improves any patient-centered outcomes.
- *Nitric oxide inhibitors:* Nitric oxide overproduction by inducible *nitric oxide synthase* (iNOS) is responsible for the vasodilation and refractory shock in sepsis. NO overproduction also inhibits mitochondrial and organ functioning. Inhibition of NO production by iNOS inhibitors have been studied extensively. The studies reveal no clinical benefit despite vasopressor response and in fact a higher mortality in sepsis due to nonselective iNOS inhibition, leading to the loss of the beneficial effects of NO. Methylene blue is an inhibitor of NOS and soluble guanylate cyclase has been studied in vasoplegic syndromes like cardiopulmonary bypass, with improvement in MAP. A meta-analysis of total 15 studies with 832 patients[36] showed improved hemodynamics, decreased vasopressor requirement, decreased lactate level, and improved survival in patients with vasodilatory shock. It can cause serotonin syndrome by drug-drug interaction since it inhibits mono amine oxidase. Methylene blue also increases pulmonary vascular resistance and can worsen hypoxia. Hydroxycobalamin, a vitamin B_{12} precursor, can reverse NO-mediated vasoplegia and has been

used in cyanide poisoning as a NO scavenger.[37] Its clinical use in refractory shock has not been well studied so far.

- *Vitamin C and thiamine repletion:* Endogenous NE and vasopressin synthesis are governed by enzymes requiring vitamin C as a cofactor. Absolute or relative vitamin C deficiency contributes to shock by decreasing synthesis of endogenous vasopressors. Intravenous high-dose vitamin C can improve hemodynamics.[38] Thiamine is also an essential cofactor in oxidative energy metabolism and lactate metabolism. A recent clinical protocol combining hydrocortisone, vitamin C, and thiamine has shown significant shock reversal and decreased severity of organ failure.[39] A recent randomized controlled study of Vitamin C in sepsis demonstrated higher mortality risk and higher organ dysfunction rates, resulting in abandonment of vitamin C in management of septic shock.[40]

CONCLUSION

Vasodilatory shock is a form of distributive shock characterized by lack of response to catecholamines leading to a refractory shock. Sepsis is a typical example of vasodilatory shock, though other causes which lead to tissue hypoxia also result in a vasodilation. Vasodilatory shock is due to inappropriate activation of vasodilator mechanism and failure of vasoconstrictor mechanism, mediated by three main mechanisms. Activation of K_{atp} channels, increased activity of NO synthase, and decreased vasopressin levels contribute to the vasoplegic state. Management of vasodilatory refractory shock entails cardiac output measurement and objective assessment of fluid responsiveness to rule out secondary contributors to the shock state. Early use of NE coupled with early use of an alternative agent like vasopressin may play an important role in maintaining MAP. Refractory shock may be attenuated by use of rescue therapies, though its effect on mortality needs to be examined in larger trials. AT, like vasopressin, is an alternative vasopressor agent that is in the horizon for treatment of vasodilatory shock.

REFERENCES

1. Cecconi M, De Backer D, Antonelli M, Beale R, Bakker J, Hofer C, et al. Consensus on circulatory shock and hemodynamic monitoring. Task force of the European Society of Intensive Care Medicine. Intensive Care Med. 2014;40(12):1795-815.
2. Vincent JL, De Backer D. Circulatory shock. N Engl J Med. 2013;369(18):1726-34.
3. Weil MH, Shubin H. Proposed reclassification of shock states with special reference to distributive defects. Adv Exp Med Biol. 1971;23(0):13-23.
4. Jentzer JC, Vallabhajosyula S, Khanna AK, Chawla LS, Busse LW, Kashani KB. Management of refractory vasodilatory shock. Chest. 2018;154(2):416-26.
5. Divatia JV, Amin PR, Ramakrishnan N, Kapadia FN, Todi S, Sahu S, et al. Intensive care in India: The Indian intensive care case mix and practice patterns study. Indian J Crit Care Med. 2016;20(4):216-25.
6. Standl T, Annecke T, Cascorbi I, Heller AR, Sabashnikov A, Teske W. The Nomenclature, Definition and Distinction of Types of Shock. Dtsch Arztebl Int. 2018;115(45):757-68.
7. Gabbay U, Carmi D, Birk E, Dagan D, Shatz A, Kidron D. The Sudden Infant Death Syndrome mechanism of death may be a non-septic hyper-dynamic shock. Med Hypotheses. 2019;122:35-40.
8. Landry DW, Oliver JA. The pathogenesis of vasodilatory shock. N Engl J Med. 2001;345(8):588-95.
9. Gkisioti S, Mentzelopous SD. Vasogenic shock physiology. Open Access Emerg Med. 2011;3:1-6.
10. Sohn I, Sheykhzade M, Edvinsson L, Sams A. The effects of CGRP in vascular tissue - Classical vasodilation, shadowed effects and systemic dilemmas. Eur J Pharmacol. 2020;881:173205.
11. Landry DW, Levin HR, Gallant EM, Ashton RC Jr, Seo S, D'Alessandro D, et al. Vasopressin deficiency contributes to the vasodilation of septic shock. Circulation. 1997;95(5):1122-5.
12. Hamzaoui O, Scheeren TWL, Teboul JL. Norepinephrine in septic shock: when and how much? Curr Opin Crit Care. 2017;23(4):342-7.
13. Yamaguchi T, Sumida TS, Nomura S, Satoh M, Higo T, Ito M Y, et al. Cardiac dopamine D1 receptor triggers ventricular arrhythmia in chronic heart failure. Nat Commun. 2020;11(1):4364.
14. Russell JA, Walley KR, Singer J, Gordon AC, Hébert PC, Cooper DJ, et al. Vasopressin versus norepinephrine infusion in patients with septic shock. N Engl J Med. 2008;358(9):877-87.
15. Gordon AC, Mason AJ, Thirunavukkarasu N, Perkins GD, Cecconi M, Cepkova M, et al; VANISH Investigators. Effect of early vasopressin vs norepinephrine on kidney failure in patients with septic shock: The VANISH randomized clinical trial. JAMA. 2016;316(5):509-18.
16. Mayr VD, Dunser MW, Greil V, Jochberger S, Luckner G, Ulmer H, et al. Causes of death and determinants of outcome in critically ill patients. Crit Care. 2006;10(6):R154.
17. Jentzer JC, Coons JC, Link CB, Schmidhofer M. Pharmacotherapy update on the use of vasopressors and inotropes in the intensive care unit. J Cardiovasc Pharmacol Ther. 2015;20(3):249-60.
18. Vincent JL, Moreno R, Takala J, Willatts S, De Mendonça A, Bruining H, et al. The SOFA (Sepsis-related Organ Failure

Assessment) score to describe organ dysfunction/ failure. On behalf of the Working Group on Sepsis-Related Problems of the European Society of Intensive Care Medicine. Intensive Care Med. 1996;22(7):707-10.
19. Dunser MW, Ruokonen E, Pettila V, Ulmer H, Torgersen C, Schmittinger CA, et al. Association of arterial blood pressure and vasopressor load with septic shock mortality: a post hoc analysis of a multicenter trial. Crit Care. 2009;13(6):R181.
20. Dunser MW, Hasibeder WR. Sympathetic overstimulation during critical illness: adverse effects of adrenergic stress. J Intensive Care Med. 2009;24(5):293-316.
21. Schmittinger CA, Torgersen C, Luckner G, Schroder DC, Lorenz I, Dunser MW. Adverse cardiac events during catecholamine vasopressor therapy: a prospective observational study. Intensive Care Med. 2012;38(6):950-8.
22. Permpikul C, Tongyoo S, Viarasilpa T, Trainarongsakul T, Chakorn T, Udompanturak S. Early Use of Norepinephrine in Septic Shock Resuscitation (CENSER). A Randomized Trial. Am J Respir Crit Care Med. 2019;199(9):1097-105.
23. Lee SM, An WS. New clinical criteria for septic shock: serum lactate level as new emerging vital sign. J Thorac Dis. 2016;8(7):1388-90.
24. PRISM Investigators; Rowan KM, Angus DC, Bailey M, Barnato AE, Bellomo R, Canter RR, et al. Early, Goal-Directed Therapy for Septic Shock — a Patient-Level Meta-Analysis. New Engl J of Medicine. 2017;376(23):2223-34.
25. Serano AMN, Alonso JV, Piñero GR, Camacho AR, Benet JS, Vaquero M. Biomarkers in Shock Patients and Their Value as A Prognostic Tool; A Prospective Multi-Center Cohort Study. Bull Emerg Trauma. 2019;7(3):232-9.
26. Khanna A, English SW, Wang XS, Ham K, Tumlin J, Szerlip H, et al. Angiotensin II for the treatment of vasodilatory shock. New Engl J of Med. 2017;377(5):419-30.
27. Huang L, Zhang S, Chang W, Xia F, Liu S, Yang Y, et al. Terlipressin for the treatment of septic shock in adults: a systematic review and meta-analysis. BMC Anesthesiol. 2020;20(1):58.
28. Antonucci E, Giovini M, Agosta S, Sakr Y, Leone M. Selepressin in Septic Shock. Shock. 2022;57(6):172-9.
29. Laterre PF, Berry SM, Blemings A, Carlsen JE, François B, Graves T, et al.; SEPSIS-ACT Investigators. Effect of Selepressin vs Placebo on Ventilator- and Vasopressor-Free Days in Patients With Septic Shock: The SEPSIS-ACT Randomized Clinical Trial. JAMA. 2019;322(15):1476-85.
30. Mirza M, Zafar M, Siddiqui M, Abbas A, Nahas J, Mirza M, et al. Role of steroids in critically-ill sepsis patients: a review article and literature to review. J Community Hosp Intern Med Perspect. 2021;11(6):825-9.
31. Jaber S, Paugam C, Futier E, Lefrant JY, Lasocki S, Lescot T, et al.; BICAR-ICU Study Group. Sodium bicarbonate therapy for patients with severe metabolic acidaemia in the intensive care unit (BICAR-ICU): a multicentre, open-label, randomised controlled, phase 3 trial. Lancet. 2018;392(10141):31-40.
32. Nahas GG, Sutin KM, Fermon C, Streat S, Wiklund L, Wahlander S, et al. Guidelines for the treatment of acidaemia with THAM. Drugs. 1998;55(2):191-224.
33. Tumlin JA, Murugan R, Deane AM, Ostermann M, Busse LW, Ham KR, et al.; Angiotensin II for the Treatment of High-Output Shock 3 (ATHOS-3) Investigators. Outcomes in Patients with Vasodilatory Shock and Renal Replacement Therapy Treated with Intravenous Angiotensin II. Crit Care Med. 2018;46(6):949-57.
34. Mu TS, Becker AM, Clark AJ, Batts SG, Murata LM, Uyehara CFT. ECMO with vasopressor use during early endotoxic shock: Can it improve circulatory support and regional microcirculatory blood flow? PLoS One. 2019;14(10):e0223604.
35. Rimmel T, Kellum JA. Clinical review: Blood purification for sepsis. Crit Care. 2011;15(1):205.
36. Ballarin RS, Lazzarin T, Zornoff L, Azevedo PS, Pereira FWL, Tanni SE, et al. Methylene blue in sepsis and septic shock: a systematic review and meta-analysis. Front Med (Lausanne). 2024;11:1366062.
37. Patel JJ, Willoughby R, Peterson J, Carver T, Zelten J, Markiewicz A, et al. High-Dose IV Hydroxocobalamin (Vitamin B12) in Septic Shock: A Double-Blind, Allocation-Concealed, Placebo-Controlled Single-Center Pilot Randomized Controlled Trial (The Intravenous Hydroxocobalamin in Septic Shock Trial). Chest. 2023;163(2):303-12.
38. Juneja D, Nasa P, Jain R. Current role of high dose vitamin C in sepsis management: A concise review. World J Crit Care Med. 2022;11(6):349-63.
39. Marik PE, Khangoora V, Rivera R, Hooper MH, Catravas J. Hydrocortisone, vitamin C, and thiamine for the treatment of severe sepsis and septic shock: A retrospective before-after study. Chest. 2017;151(6):1229-38.
40. Lamontagne F, Masse MH, Menard J, Sprague S, Pinto R, Heyland DK, et al. Intravenous vitamin C in adults with sepsis in the intensive care unit. N Engl J Med. 2022;386(25):2387-98.

CHAPTER 27

Diagnostic Modality and Hemodynamic Management of Cardiogenic Shock

Ajmer Singh, Yatin Mehta

INTRODUCTION

Cardiogenic shock (CS) is the most severe form of acute heart failure (HF) characterized by low cardiac output (CO) and sustained hypoperfusion despite adequate preload. Despite advances in diagnostic modalities and therapeutic interventions including invasive mechanical support strategies, the overall mortality with CS has plateaued around 40–60%. The incidence of CS has increased from 33.1 per 100,000 person-years in 2007 to 53.7 per 100,000 person-years in 2017.[1] Acute myocardial infarction (AMI) is considered the leading cause of CS. Timely revascularization can potentially reduce the incidence of CS in patients with AMI. The incidence of CS caused by HF is increasing, and this change in the epidemiology of CS is reported by many centers.[2]

DEFINITION AND CLASSIFICATION

The traditional definition of CS includes sustained hypotension [systolic blood pressure (SBP) <90 mm Hg, or mean arterial pressure (MAP) <65 mm Hg for >30 minutes, or requirement for vasoactive medications) with tissue hypoperfusion due to low CO (cardiac index <2.2 L/min/m^2) and pulmonary congestion [pulmonary capillary wedge pressure (PCWP) ≥15 mm Hg or on imaging]. In the absence of hemodynamic data, the diagnosis of CS is made on clinical evidence, and hypotension may not always be present, particularly in patients with severe vasoconstriction. Recent consensus statements have described CS as the presence of hypoperfusion due to ineffective CO with an adequate preload.

The Forrester classification of CS, describing four distinct hemodynamic phenotypes (dry/wet vs. warm/cold), is based on congestion and vascular tone.[3] This also includes left ventricle (LV) predominant vs right ventricle (RV) predominant vs biventricular CS. Clinical findings, echocardiography findings, and pulmonary artery catheter (PAC) derived data are required to define these hemodynamic phenotypes. Another classification based on three different phenotypes, i.e., (1) not congested, (2) cardiorenal, and (3) cardiometabolic has been suggested. A new classification system, the Society for Cardiovascular Angiography and Intervention (SCAI) shock classification system, has come into clinical practice to assess the severity of CS.[4] The prognostic value of this classification has been validated in a wide range of CS cohorts, incorporating AMI-CS, HF-CS, out-of-hospital cardiac arrest (OHCA) survivors, and those receiving venoarterial extracorporeal membrane oxygenation (VA-ECMO). The SCAI shock classification describes five evolutive stages of CS, from A (preshock, i.e., a patient at risk but with no obvious signs of hypoperfusion) to E (extremis, i.e., refractory circulatory collapse) to better define the different levels of CS severity. The *five stages* of the SCAI shock classification are described below.

1. *Class A:* At risk—neither hypotension/tachycardia nor hypoperfusion, but at risk
2. *Class B:* Beginning—hypotension or tachycardia without hypoperfusion
3. *Class C:* Classic—hypoperfusion signs requiring intervention (volume resuscitation, inotropes, vasopressors, and mechanical support) without deterioration after these treatments
4. *Class D:* Deteriorating—similar to category C but getting worse with failure of initial interventions
5. *Class E:* Extremis—refractory circulatory collapse (which is defined by SBP <80 mm Hg or MAP <50 mm Hg under vasoactive drugs; >2 vasoactive drugs or >1 vasoactive drug in association with an intra-aortic balloon pump (IABP); or an admission lactate level of >10 mmol/L), frequently in refractory cardiac arrest.

The predominant pathophysiologic abnormality in CS is diminished CO, which leads to systemic hypoperfusion and diverse cycles of ischemia, inflammation, vasoconstriction, and volume overload, often reaching a pinnacle of multiorgan system failure and death. Patients with CS exhibit a large hemodynamic variability due to the diversity of pathogenic mechanisms, the type of ventricle damage (right, left, or both), systemic inflammation, and associated vascular involvement. A risk score of CS can guide clinical decision making and could improve patient outcomes. The use of invasive hemodynamic monitoring (IHM) has shown lower-in-hospital mortality rate (24.1% vs. 30.6%, p <0.01), and higher use of LV assist device (4.4% vs. 1.3%, p <0.01) and heart transplantation (1.3% vs. 0.7%, p <0.01), compared to the non-IHM group, while there was no difference between the two groups in terms of vascular complications, major bleeding, or the need for renal replacement therapy.[5]

DIAGNOSTIC MODALITIES

It is now clearly established that early recognition, classification, and precise phenotyping of CS via early hemodynamic monitoring improve patient outcomes. The initial assessment should include clinical examination and evaluation of organ dysfunction by echocardiography, invasive arterial pressure, and parameters derived from central venous catheterization. In patients with more severe disease, advanced hemodynamic monitoring with PAC and the use of transpulmonary thermodilution (TPTD) devices is useful to facilitate the right timing of the initiation and weaning from mechanical circulatory support (MCS), and guidance on inotropic treatments, thus helping to reduce mortality.

Initial Evaluation

Clinical examination should consist of continuous monitoring of vital signs, pulse oximetry, BP, heart rate and rhythm, respiratory rate, temperature, and urine output measurement. Signs of hypoperfusion such as mottling, cold and sweaty extremities, dizziness, oliguria (<30 mL/h), and altered mental status should be noted.

Echocardiography

The use of transthoracic echocardiography (TTE) or trans-esophageal echocardiography (TEE) is recommended in patients with CS. TEE should be used when TTE does not provide adequate information. Echocardiography can provide vital information about the etiology of CS. It is helpful for the diagnosis of cardiac tamponade, pulmonary embolism, AMI, LV free wall rupture, ventricular septal rupture, aortic dissection, valvular pathologies such as endocarditis, ruptured chordae, and papillary muscle rupture. Echocardiography can evaluate both the right and left filling pressures, fluid responsiveness, pulmonary artery pressure, and CO. Despite elevated LV pressures seen in most CS patients, hypovolemia can also be present in some cases. The evaluation of right and left heart congestive signs by measurement of inferior vena cava diameter and respiratory variations, mitral E/A and E/é, is important for tailoring therapeutics and determining whether diuretics are needed. In patients with MCS, echocardiography can assist with cannula insertion, monitoring the recovery of cardiac function, timing of weaning, and early diagnosis of complications of MCS therapy.

Invasive Arterial Pressure Monitoring

Non-invasive monitoring tends to overestimate BP in patients with hypotension. Invasive arterial pressure monitoring provides information about SBP, MAP, and diastolic BP which reflects the coronary artery perfusion pressure. Moreover, a low pulse pressure (SBP-diastolic BP) indicates a low stroke volume. Pulse pressure variation (PPV) can predict fluid responsiveness in mechanically ventilated patients. Invasive arterial pressure monitoring also enables titration of inotropes/vasopressors and allows repeated sampling for blood gas analysis and lactate measurement. A lactate value of >2.0 mmol/L is used as a cutoff value for hypoperfusion in CS. A higher lactate value at admission or an increasing trend of lactate defines a deterioration of the condition and is associated with poor prognosis. A lactate value of ≥10 mmol/L at admission is a criterion to diagnose refractory shock.[6] Plasma lactate should be assayed regularly to assess the evolution of shock during treatment every 2 hours in the first 8 hours and then every 8–12 hours thereafter.

Central Venous Catheterization

The routine use of central venous pressure (CVP) monitoring with single-point measurement to predict fluid responsiveness is not recommended. However, the trend of CVP can be helpful to differentiate organ failure related to congestion rather than hypoperfusion, as the right timing of using diuretics to improve organ function following the correction of perfusion is at times ambiguous in CS. A high CVP (>12 mm Hg) in patients with left-sided MCS can help diagnose RV failure and is associated with higher in-hospital mortality rates.[7] Similar to mixed venous saturation (SvO_2), the measurement of central venous saturation ($ScvO_2$) has been advocated for the diagnosis of global tissue hypoxia. In addition, reduced SvO_2 or $ScvO_2$ values along with low BP, low CO, and normal or increased PCWP values despite inotropic/vasopressor support may be helpful in identifying patients who need left-sided MCS. The difference between the CO_2 content of the mixed venous blood and arterial blood [partial venous carbon dioxide tension ($PvCO_2$)-partial pressure of carbon dioxide ($PaCO_2$) or the ΔPCO_2) reflects the balance between its production by tissues and its elimination through the lungs. A ΔPCO_2 of >6 mm Hg suggests that the CO is inadequate to meet the patient's global metabolic demand and should prompt the clinician to increase the CO. ΔPCO_2 remains a valid marker of the adequacy of CO irrespective of the metabolic condition, even if the microcirculation is injured and the oxygen extraction is impaired. In a study by Ospina-Tascón et al., in the early phases of septic shock, ΔPCO_2 could indicate the inadequacy of microvascular blood flow, as increased ΔPCO_2 values were associated with microcirculatory dysfunction, even when SvO_2 was within the normal range.[8]

Pulmonary Artery Catheterization

Right heart catheterization with PAC allows measurements of intracardiac pressures, CO, derived hemodynamic parameters, and SvO_2. The routine use of PACs in critical care medicine has been widely debated over the past few decades, with no survival benefits and increased adverse events with the use of PACs observed in ESCAPE trials. Despite these neutral trials, most recent statements continue to recommend PAC use in CS patients.[9] A recent multicenter review from the Cardiogenic Shock Working Group analyzed outcomes in 1,414 CS patients, stratified by SCAI stage and by the degree of PAC use (complete data, incomplete data, or no PAC data) before initiation of MCS. They found the lowest in-hospital mortality in the complete PAC data group across all SCAI stages.[10] PACs also enable measurement of the cardiac power output (CPO), which is the product of simultaneously measured CO and MAP values (CO × MAP/451) and reflects the cardiac pumping ability. A CPO of ≤0.53 Watts was the strongest predictor of in-hospital mortality in patients with AMI complicated by CS, from the SHOCK registry.[11] PAC also allows the assessment of RV dysfunction using the pulmonary artery pulsatility index (PAPI), which is calculated as the pulmonary artery systolic pressure (PASP); pulmonary artery diastolic pressure (PADP)/right atrial pressure) and reflects components of the right heart system (i.e., the systemic venous system, RV function, and pulmonary circulation). Lower PAPI (<1.5) is associated with worse outcomes, but the cutoff varies with pulmonary vascular resistance. Adopting a standardized team-based approach with a score based on CPO and PAPI to guide clinical decision-making could improve patient outcomes. PAC also allows early identification of patients with significant hemodynamic compromise requiring immediate MCS, before it could cause irreversible end-organ damage. The data derived from a PAC can facilitate early recognition of biventricular shock and timely institution of biventricular support. Monitoring with PAC is helpful in the acute management of patients receiving MCS therapy, as well as in guiding its withdrawal and titrating the pharmacologic therapy of patients with myocardial recovery from CS. In addition, advanced hemodynamic monitoring is useful to assess candidacy for advanced HF therapies, including durable MCS and heart transplantation.

Transpulmonary Thermodilution

Transpulmonary thermodilution methods allow for the assessment of CO by using a central venous and arterial catheter, or by pulse contour analysis. They calculate CO, global end-diastolic volume, and extravascular lung water. TPTD also provides continuous measurement of $ScvO_2$. TPTD devices allow the assessment of indices of cardiac systolic function, which are the cardiac function index (CFI) and the global ejection fraction (GEF). A low CFI is seen in patients with LV systolic dysfunction; however, echocardiography should be done to rule out RV dysfunction. In the absence of RV dysfunction, CFI correlates well with LV ejection fraction.[12] The disadvantages of TPTD methods include intermittent measurement of CO, repeated need for calibration, global end-diastolic volume does not distinguishing between LV and RV, and overestimation of LV systolic function by GEF during ventricular dilation.

MANAGEMENT OF CARDIOGENIC SHOCK

The management of CS includes: (1) Treatment of etiology, e.g., myocardial revascularization for coronary artery disease (CAD), (2) optimization of hemodynamic parameters by improving tissue perfusion and pump function, and (3) prevention and treatment of other organ dysfunction by oxygenation, mechanical ventilation, renal replacement therapy, etc. In patients with refractory CS, early use of MCS should be considered.

Management of Etiology

Emergent myocardial revascularization by percutaneous coronary intervention (PCI) has improved the outcome of patients with AMI-CS. A significant decrease in 6 months (50% vs. 63%, $p = 0.027$) and long-term mortality by early revascularization compared with intensive medical treatment in AMI-CS is emphasized by the SHOCK trial.[13] The European Society of Cardiology (ESC) guidelines have recommended primary PCI as first-line therapy (IB level) for AMI patients presenting with ST-segment elevation.[14] PCI for multivessel CAD or emergent coronary artery bypass grafting in the early stages of CS is not supported by robust evidence. Patients with CS can have arrhythmia and conduction disorders. In such patients, restoration of sinus rhythm, or control of heart rate, can be useful to improve hemodynamic parameters. For hemodynamically unstable ventricular arrhythmia, electrical cardioversion is preferred. For valvular deterioration due to endocarditis complicated by CS, surgery remains the first choice. Transcatheter aortic valve implantation (TAVI) has shown higher 1-year mortality (29.7%) in the CS group compared to the non-CS group (22.6%, $p < 0.01$) in patients with acute decompensated aortic stenosis.[15] For mitral regurgitation, a transcatheter edge-to-edge mitral valve repair in patients ($n = 3{,}249$) with CS was feasible with an excellent device success rate (85.6%) and final mitral regurgitation grade ≤2 + in 88.2% of cases.[16]

Inotropes/Vasopressors

Early use of inotropes is recommended to manage CS patients presenting with hypotension and persistent low CO due to LV systolic dysfunction. Vasopressors are recommended to increase perfusion pressure of vital organs in CS patients with hypotension and normal CO. Most inotropes that act through the cardiomyocyte calcium influx induce tachycardia and can increase myocardial oxygen consumption. Compared to norepinephrine, epinephrine is associated with more arrhythmias, tachycardia, lactic acidosis, and a threefold increase in mortality.[17] Norepinephrine is recommended as the first-line vasopressor in CS. Dobutamine is considered the first-line inotrope to augment myocardial contractility and CO (class IIb). Phosphodiesterase-3 inhibitor, milrinone, and calcium sensitizer, levosimendan, are considered as the second-line inotropes for CS. Levosimendan is particularly useful in CS patients on chronic beta-blocker therapy.

Mechanical Ventilation

Acute respiratory failure is seen in 50–88% of patients with CS, and 80% of them require either noninvasive ventilation (NIV) or invasive mechanical ventilation (IMV). Impaired gas exchange in CS results from interstitial and alveolar fluid accumulation (cardiogenic pulmonary edema), increased RV/LV preload, ventricular systolic and diastolic dysfunction, and inflammatory response. The effect of intermittent positive pressure ventilation (IPPV) on hemodynamics in patients with CS can differ based on the phenotype of RV and LV function. In LV failure, IPPV may improve hemodynamics through a reduction in LV preload and afterload; however, high airway pressures may be deleterious in RV failure by increasing RV preload and afterload, compromising RV performance. Therefore, high-flow nasal cannula oxygen is preferred in conscious patients with RV-predominant CS. CS patients who need IPPV should benefit from early intubation. A recent study by van Diepen et al., has shown that each 1-hour delay in IPPV initiation was associated with higher 30-day mortality [odds ratio (OR), 1.03; 95% confidence interval (CI) 1.00–1.06; $p = 0.03$].[18] Although, ideal oxygenation levels in CS remain undefined, there is enough evidence to suggest that hyperoxemia [arterial oxygen saturation (SaO_2) > 98%] could be deleterious.

Mechanical Circulatory Support

Timely implantation of MCS devices based on invasive hemodynamic data in well-selected patients may improve outcomes. MCS should be considered when immediate hemodynamic stabilization is required despite adequate medical therapy. The MCS devices currently in use include IABP, ventricular assist devices (VAD), and VA-ECMO. The selection of the device depends on the CS phenotype and local expertise. The use of an IABP is not recommended in AMI-CS due to lower efficacy and no evidence of improved outcomes. However, patients with HF-CS may have a more favorable response to IABP as a bridge to definitive therapy. In a recent, large nationwide database in Europe, 20% of AMI-CS patients received an MCS of which 66, 22.7, and 10.5% were Impella, VA-ECMO, or a combination of both devices, respectively.[19] The patients supported with Impella had less adverse events, shorter hospital stays, lower hospital costs, and less in-hospital mortality (61% vs. 67%, $p = 0.001$) compared to VA-ECMO cohorts. Randomized studies such as EURO-SHOCK, ECMO-CS, and ECLS-SHOCK trials have shown mixed results. An ongoing trial ANCHOR (Assessment of ECMO in Acute Myocardial Infarction Cardiogenic Shock) aims to provide further insights. In a large randomized study (ECLS-SHOCK trial) conducted by Thiele and colleagues on patients with AMI complicated by CS, there was no difference in 30-day mortality (the primary endpoint) that occurred in 47.8% of the patients in the ECLS group and in 49.0% of those in the control group.[20] Furthermore, the VA-ECMO group was associated with an increased risk of bleeding and vascular complications. Another issue with the use of VA ECMO is increased LV afterload, which may lead to inadequate unloading of the LV. Combining VA-ECMO with IABP, Impella support, or atrial septostomy could be considered to achieve LV unloading and increased survival. In appropriately selected patients, MCS devices can be used in one of the following ways.

- *Bridge to recovery:* To prevent end-organ damage and to "unload" the heart for "reverse remodeling"
- *Bridge to a decision:* When the decision to implant is unclear
- *Bridge to a destination:* Permanent device in transplant-ineligible patients
- *Bridge to transplant:* Most common indication, allows rehabilitation from severe CS or HF while waiting for the donor.

Lim and colleagues, in a recent state-of-the-art review, have described four therapeutic phases of CS from initial (1) "Rescue" to (2) "optimization," (3) "stabilization" and (4) "de-escalation or exit therapy" (R-O-S-E) to achieve hemodynamic and therapeutic goals.[21] The therapeutic goals vary with the phases of care, which in turn are highly context-dependent. In some cases, the Rescue and Optimization phases may be brief, and the therapeutic goals are easily achieved by the use of inotropes. In more severe cases, the "rescue" phase may necessitate the deployment of VA-ECMO, followed by a prolonged "optimization" phase that includes hemodynamic management such as titration of vasoactive drugs, and escalation of temporary MCS to VA-ECMO. "Stabilization" is characterized by recovery of organ function, diminishing vasoactive drug requirements, and minimizing IHM. In the "de-escalation and exit" therapy, patients are liberated from pharmaco-MCS therapy in the event of sufficient recovery of cardiovascular function.

CONCLUSION

Cardiogenic shock is a life-threatening condition manifesting as a wide spectrum of etiologic, hemodynamic, and phenotyping features. It can rapidly progress into refractory shock and irreversible multiorgan failure. An early recognition, rapid reversal of the underlying cause, and prompt initiation of hemodynamic support may improve patient outcomes and reduce mortality.

REFERENCES

1. Lang CN, Kaier K, Zotzmann V, Stachon P, Pottgiesser T, von Zur Muehlen C, et al. Cardiogenic shock: incidence, survival and mechanical circulatory support usage 2007-2017-insights from a national registry. Clin Res Cardiol. 2021;110(9):1421-30.
2. Ghajar A, Ordonez CP, Philips B, Pinzon PQ, Fleming LM, Motiwala SR, et al. Cardiogenic shock related cardiovascular disease mortality trends in US population: heart failure vs. acute myocardial infarction as contributing causes. Int J Cardiol. 2022;367:45-8.
3. Forrester JS, Diamond G, Chatterjee K, Swan HJ. Medical therapy of acute myocardial infarction by application of hemodynamic subsets (first of two parts). N Engl J Med. 1976;295(24):1356-62.
4. Naidu SS, Baran DA, Jentzer JC, Hollenberg SM, van Diepen S, Basir MB, et al. SCAI SHOCK stage classification expert consensus update: a review and incorporation of validation studies: this statement was endorsed by the American College of Cardiology (ACC), American college of emergency physicians (ACEP), American heart association (AHA), European society of cardiology (ESC) Association for acute cardiovascular care (ACVC), International society for heart and lung transplantation (ISHLT), Society of critical care medicine (SCCM), and Society of Thoracic Surgeons (STS) in December 2021. J Am Coll Cardiol. 2022;79(9):933-46.
5. Tehrani BN, Truesdell AG, Sherwood MW, Desai S, Tran HA, Epps KC, et al. Standardized team-based care for cardiogenic shock. J Am Coll Cardiol. 2019;73(13):1659-69.
6. Jentzer JC, van Diepen S, Barsness GW, Henry TD, Menon V, Rihal CS, et al. Cardiogenic shock classification to predict mortality in the cardiac intensive care unit. J Am Coll Cardiol. 2019;74(17):2117-28.
7. Whitehead EH, Thayer KL, Burkhoff D, Uriel N, Ohman EM, O'Neill W, et al. Central venous pressure and clinical outcomes during left-sided mechanical support for acute myocardial infarction and cardiogenic shock. Front Cardiovasc Med. 2020;7:155.
8. Ospina-Tascón GA, Umaña M, Bermúdez WF, Bautista-Rincón DF, Valencia JD, Madriñán HJ, et al. Can venous-to-arterial carbon dioxide differences reflect microcirculatory alterations in patients with septic shock? Intensive Care Med. 2016;42(2):211-21.

9. Saxena A, Garan AR, Kapur NK, O'Neill WW, Lindenfeld J, Pinney SP, et al. Value of hemodynamic monitoring in patients with cardiogenic shock undergoing mechanical circulatory support. Circulation. 2020;141(14):1184-97.
10. Garan AR, Kanwar M, Thayer KL, Whitehead E, Zweck E, Hernandez-Montfort J, et al. Complete hemodynamic profiling with pulmonary artery catheters in cardiogenic shock is associated with lower in-hospital mortality. JACC Heart Fail. 2020;8(11):903-13.
11. Fincke R, Hochman JS, Lowe AM, Menon V, Slater JN, Webb JG, et al. Cardiac power is the strongest hemodynamic correlate of mortality in cardiogenic shock: a report from the SHOCK trial registry. J Am Coll Cardiol. 2004;44(2):340-48.
12. Perny J, Kimmoun A, Perez P, Levy B. Evaluation of cardiac function index as measured by transpulmonary thermodilution as an indicator of left ventricular ejection fraction in cardiogenic shock. Biomed Res Int. 2014;2014:598029.
13. Hochman JS, Sleeper LA, Webb JG, Sanborn TA, White HD, Talley JD, et al. Early revascularization in acute myocardial infarction complicated by cardiogenic shock. SHOCK Investigators. Should We Emergently Revascularize Occluded Coronaries for Cardiogenic Shock. N Engl J Med. 1999;341(9):625-34.
14. Ibanez B, James S, Agewall S, Antunes MJ, Bucciarelli-Ducci C, et al. 2017 ESC Guidelines for the management of acute myocardial infarction in patients presenting with ST-segment elevation: The Task Force for the management of acute myocardial infarction in patients presenting with ST-segment elevation of the European Society of Cardiology (ESC). Eur Heart J. 2018;39(2):119-77.
15. Goel K, Shah P, Jones BM, Korngold E, Bhardwaj A, Kar B, et al. Outcomes of transcatheter aortic valve replacement in patients with cardiogenic shock. Eur Heart J 2023;44(33):3181-95.
16. Simard T, Vemulapalli S, Jung RG,Vekstein A, Stebbins A, Holmes DR, et al. Transcatheter edge-to-edge mitral valve repair in patients with severe mitral regurgitation and cardiogenic shock. J Am Coll Cardiol. 2022;80(22):2072-84.
17. Levy B, Clere-Jehl R, Legras A, Morichau-Beauchant T, Leone M, Frederique G, et al. Epinephrine versus norepinephrine for cardiogenic shock after acute myocardial infarction. J Am Coll Cardiol. 2018;72(2):173-82.
18. van Diepen S, Hochman JS, Stebbins A, Alviar CL, Alexander JH, Lopes RD. Association between delays in mechanical ventilation initiation and mortality in patients with refractory cardiogenic shock. JAMA Cardiol. 2020;5(8):965-7.
19. Bogerd M, Ten Berg S, Peters EJ, Vlaar APJ, Engström AE, Otterspoor LC, et al. Impella and venoarterial extracorporeal membrane oxygenation in cardiogenic shock complicating acute myocardial infarction. Eur J Heart Fail. 2023;25(11): 2021-31.
20. Thiele H, Zeymer U, Akin I, Behnes M, Rassaf T, Mahabadi AA, et al. Extracorporeal life support in infarct-related cardiogenic shock. N Engl J Med. 2023;389(14): 1286-97.
21. Lim HS, González-Costello J, Belohlavek J, Zweck E, Blumer V, Schrage B, et al. Hemodynamic management of cardiogenic shock in the intensive care unit. J Heart Lung Transplant. 2024;43(7):1059-73.

CHAPTER

Diagnosis and Hemodynamic Management of Obstructive Shock

Armand Mekontso Dessap

INTRODUCTION

Obstructive shock is due to obstruction of the pulmonary circulation [usually by thrombi—severe pulmonary embolism (SPE)] or heart compression [usually by accumulation of fluid, or blood in the pericardial space—cardiac tamponade (CT)].[1] In this review, we will focus on understanding the pathophysiology, presentation, and management of obstructive shock by focusing on CT and SPE. Other causes of obstructive shock, including extrapericardial tamponade (by mediastinal processes, tension pneumothorax, or massive pleural effusion) and intracardiac obstruction (by thrombus or myxoma) will not be discussed here.

EPIDEMIOLOGY

Obstructive shock is relatively rare—2% in a trial involving >1,600 patients with various types of shock.[2] Pericardial effusion may be caused by all categories of diseases, including infectious (e.g., the human immunodeficiency virus infection or tuberculosis), autoimmune, neoplastic, iatrogenic, traumatic, vascular (e.g., ruptured acute myocardial infarction or dissecting aortic aneurysm), and metabolic.[1] SPE represents <5% of all acute pulmonary embolism (PE) but constitutes a medical emergency, associated with a high risk of death (15–50%).[3] There is a wide list of predisposing patient and setting-related factors to PE. Trauma, surgery, oral contraception, infection, and cancer are strong provoking and predisposing factors for PE.[4]

PATHOPHYSIOLOGY

Cardiac tamponade is due to the rise of intrapericardial pressure above intracardiac pressures. This rise is more dependent on the rate of accumulation than on the volume of fluid. Therefore, large effusions may be tolerated if they are progressive while small increases in pericardial volume may produce sudden, critical hemodynamic compromise. SPE induces an abrupt increase in pulmonary vascular resistance, leading to an increase in right ventricular (RV) volume and pressure, which is responsible for a rise in wall tension and myocyte stretch, with RV ischemia.[4] In some patients, right-to-left shunting through a patent foramen ovale occurs as a consequence of an inverted pressure gradient between the right atrium and left atrium and may lead to severe hypoxemia and/or paradoxical embolization and stroke.[5]

Both CT and SPE exacerbate the physiological interdependence of the left and right ventricles.[6] The increase in right ventricle size (especially during spontaneous inspiration) induces a septal shift of the interventricular septum toward the left ventricle, resulting in decreased left ventricle dimension and output.[7]

PRESENTATION

The classical clinical signs of obstructive shock include chest pain and/or dyspnea, tachycardia, hypotension with a narrow pulse pressure (but blood pressure may be preserved in some cases),[8] and venous jugular distension (with increased central venous pressure). The exaggeration of the biventricular interdependence induces the clinical pulsus paradoxus (an inspiratory fall of systolic blood pressure of >10 mm Hg during normal spontaneous breathing), which is an important diagnostic finding in CT.[9] However, it can also be found during SPE and other situations, such as severe acute asthma.[10]

Muffled heart sounds may suggest CT while unilateral leg pain or extremity swelling may suggest deep venous thrombosis associated with PE.

Electrocardiography may show signs of large pericardial effusion in case of CT (with especially low QRS voltage and electrical alternans) and signs of RV strain in case of PE (with inversion of T waves in leads V1–V4, a QR pattern in V1, S1Q3T3 pattern, and incomplete or complete right bundle-branch block).[11]

IMAGING

Echocardiography is the main bedside diagnostic method in case of obstructive shock, with the transthoracic approach being often sufficient. In intubated patients, the transesophageal route may be performed to directly visualize thrombi in the main or right pulmonary arteries in case of SPE[12] or to assess loculated or extrapericardial tamponade that may result in the nonspecific clinical presentation of CT.[6]

During both CT and SPE, the biventricular interdependence typically leads to a paradoxical motion of the interventricular septum, which is usually accompanied by a relaxation impairment of the left ventricle with a diminished stroke volume. Whereas, the RV is often dilated in SPE, it is of normal or reduced size in CT because of cavity compression. In both cases, there is typically an inferior vena cava plethora with blunted respiratory variations.

The other echocardiographic findings in the case of CT are pericardial effusion, heart collapse, and echocardiographic pulsus paradoxus. Pericardial effusion is visualized as an echo-free space between the visceral and parietal pericardium surrounding the heart and is often seen posteriorly, with a "swinging" heart when the effusion is massive. The left pleural effusion (which appears behind the descending aorta on a parasternal long-axis view) and pericardial fat (which is often seen only anteriorly) are the main differential diagnoses.[6] Heart collapse mainly occurs in the right atria (early sign, very sensitive, but poorly specific),[13] and the right ventricle outflow tract (late sign, very specific).[14] The echographic pulsus paradoxus depicts the inspiratory increase of right-sided flows (tricuspid or pulmonary) and the concomitant decrease on the left side (mitral or aortic), which often exceed +25% and –15%, respectively.[15,16]

In the case of SPE, mobile right heart thrombi may be detected by transthoracic or transesophageal echocardiography.[3] A disturbed RV ejection pattern (60–60 sign) or depressed contractility of the RV free wall compared with the RV apex (McConnell sign) have a high positive predictive value for PE.[4] RV function can be assessed at the tricuspid annulus using the time motion mode (tricuspid annular plane systolic excursion) or the tissue Doppler mode (s′ wave). When readily available, computed tomography pulmonary angiography (CTPA) is recommended to confirm PE in patients presenting with obstructive shock and suspected PE. If CTPA is not immediately available or in case of severe hemodynamic instability, bedside transthoracic echocardiography is mandatory to rapidly assess RV overload and potential right cavity thrombi.

MANAGEMENT

The general hemodynamic support for obstructive shock includes cautious fluid loading and catecholamines. Fluid loading improves cardiac index in some patients with SPE or CT, but not in all. Hypotension (systolic blood pressure <100 mm Hg) is a predictor of favorable response during CT.[17] Fluid loading should be used very cautiously (usually 500 mL maximum) during SPE and avoided in case of severe RV dilatation because it may worsen RV overload, ischemia, and left ventricular compression.[18,19] Vasodilators and diuretics are not recommended in the setting of obstructive shock,[1] although the latter have been evaluated in normotensive PE without shock. The comparative effects of catecholamines in obstructive shock are controversial. Norepinephrine seems to be the most indicated to increase blood pressure both in CT[20] and SPE (it restores the coronary perfusion pressure[19] and improves RV performance in this setting[21]). However, dobutamine infusion significantly increases cardiac index while reducing pulmonary vascular resistance during SPE.[22]

The reduction in RV preload and increase in RV afterload induced by mechanical ventilation may decompensate obstructive shock. Intubation should therefore be cautious and high ventilatory pressures avoided.[23]

The specific management of CT involves urgent drainage of the pericardial fluid based on clinical and echocardiographic findings. Real-time echocardiography guidance with microbubbles injection and experienced staff are essential for safe bedside pericardiocentesis.[24] Some etiologies (e.g., type A aortic dissection and ventricular free wall rupture) require surgical drainage when possible.[25] Drainage of an associated large left pleural effusion may also prove useful.[26]

The specific management of SPE includes reperfusion with systemic thrombolytic therapy reperfusion therapy, and anticoagulation by unfractionated heparin.[3] For patients with SPE at high risk of bleeding, alternative options include the use of low-dose thrombolytic therapy, catheter-directed thrombolysis, or surgical embolectomy depending on the local expertise and resources.[3] In the case of refractory obstructive shock secondary to SPE, venoarterial extracorporeal membrane oxygenation should be discussed as a bridge to recovery or pulmonary vascular recanalization.[3]

CONCLUSION

CT and SPE are two emergencies causing obstructive shock, requiring prompt diagnosis and management. Echocardiography is central to diagnosing CT and assessing the consequences of SPE. Pericardial drainage and pulmonary reperfusion are key to the management of CT and SPE, respectively.

REFERENCES

1. Adler Y, Charron P, Imazio M, Badano L, Barón-Esquivias G, Bogaert J, et al. 2015 ESC Guidelines for the diagnosis and management of pericardial diseases: The Task Force for the Diagnosis and Management of Pericardial Diseases of the European Society of Cardiology (ESC) Endorsed by: The European Association for Cardio-Thoracic Surgery (EACTS). Eur Heart J. 2015;36(42):2921-64.
2. Vincent JL, De Backer D. Circulatory shock. N Eng J Med. 2013;369(18):1726-34.
3. Aissaoui N, Konstantinides S, Meyer G. What's new in severe pulmonary embolism? Intensive Care Med. 2019;45(1):75-7.
4. Konstantinides SV, Torbicki A, Agnelli G, Danchin N, Fitzmaurice D, Galiè N, et al. 2014 ESC Guidelines on the diagnosis and management of acute pulmonary embolism. Eur Heart J. 2014;35(43):3033-80.
5. Konstantinides S, Geibel A, Kasper W, Olschewski M, Blümel L, Just H. Patent foramen ovale is an important predictor of adverse outcome in patients with major pulmonary embolism. Circulation. 1998;97(19):1946-51.
6. Mekontso Dessap A, Chew MS. Cardiac tamponade. Intensive Care Med. 2018;44(6):936-9.
7. Hamzaoui O, Monnet X, Teboul JL. Pulsus paradoxus. Eur Respir J. 2013;42(6):1696-705.
8. Argulian E, Herzog E, Halpern DG, Messerli FH. Paradoxical hypertension with cardiac tamponade. Am J Cardiol. 2012;110(7):1066-9.
9. Gauchat HW, Katz LN. Observations on pulsus paradoxus (with special reference to pericardial effusions). Arch Intern Med (Chic). 1924;33(3):350-70.
10. Argulian E, Messerli F. Misconceptions and facts about pericardial effusion and tamponade. Am J Med. 2013;126(10):858-61.
11. Geibel A, Zehender M, Kasper W, Olschewski M, Klima C, Konstantinides SV. Prognostic value of the ECG on admission in patients with acute major pulmonary embolism. Eur Respir J. 2005;25(5):843-8.
12. Meyer G, Vieillard-Baron A, Planquette B. Recent advances in the management of pulmonary embolism: focus on the critically ill patients. Ann Intensive Care. 2016;6(1):19.
13. Gillam LD, Guyer DE, Gibson TC, King ME, Marshall JE, Weyman AE. Hydrodynamic compression of the right atrium: a new echocardiographic sign of cardiac tamponade. Circulation. 1983;68(2):294-301.
14. Armstrong WF, Schilt BF, Helper DJ, Dillon JC, Feigenbaum H. Diastolic collapse of the right ventricle with cardiac tamponade: an echocardiographic study. Circulation. 1982;65(7):1491-6.
15. Appleton CP, Hatle LK, Popp RL. Cardiac tamponade and pericardial effusion: respiratory variation in transvalvular flow velocities studied by Doppler echocardiography. J Am Coll Cardiol. 1988;11(5):1020-30.
16. Leeman DE, Levine MJ, Come PC. Doppler echocardiography in cardiac tamponade: exaggerated respiratory variation in transvalvular blood flow velocity integrals. J Am Coll Cardiol. 1988;11(3):572-8.
17. Sagristà-Sauleda J, Angel J, Sambola A, Permanyer-Miralda G. Hemodynamic effects of volume expansion in patients with cardiac tamponade. Circulation. 2008;117(12):1545-9.
18. Mercat A, Diehl JL, Meyer G, Teboul JL, Sors H. Hemodynamic effects of fluid loading in acute massive pulmonary embolism. Crit Care Med. 1999;27(3):540-4.
19. Ghignone M, Girling L, Prewitt RM. Volume expansion versus norepinephrine in the treatment of a low cardiac output complicating an acute increase in right ventricular afterload in dogs. Anesthesiology. 1984;60(2):132-5.
20. Martins JB, Manuel WJ, Marcus ML, Kerber RE. Comparative effects of catecholamines in cardiac tamponade: experimental and clinical studies. Am J Cardiol. 1980;46(1):59-66.
21. Molloy WD, Lee KY, Girling L, Schick U, Prewitt RM. Treatment of shock in a canine model of pulmonary embolism. Am Rev Respir Dis. 1984;130(5):870-4.
22. Jardin F, Genevray B, Brun-Ney D, Margairaz A. Dobutamine: a hemodynamic evaluation in pulmonary embolism shock. Crit Care Med. 1985;13(12):1009-12.
23. Ho AMH, Graham CA, Ng CSH, Yeung JH, Dion PW, Critchley LA, et al. Timing of tracheal intubation in traumatic cardiac tamponade: A word of caution. Resuscitation. 2009;80(2):272-4.
24. Risti AD, Imazio M, Adler Y, Anastasakis A, Badano LP, Brucato A, et al. Triage strategy for urgent management of cardiac tamponade: a position statement of the European Society of Cardiology Working Group on Myocardial and Pericardial Diseases. Eur Heart J. 2014;35(34):2279-84.
25. Tsang TSM, Enriquez-Sarano M, Freeman WK, Barnes ME, Sinak LJ, Gersh BJ, et al. Consecutive 1127 therapeutic echocardiographically guided pericardiocenteses: clinical profile, practice patterns, and outcomes spanning 21 years. Mayo Clin Proc. 2002;77(5):429-36.
26. Furst B, Liu CJJ, Hansen P, Musuku SR. Concurrent pericardial and pleural effusions: a double jeopardy. J Clin Anesth. 2016;33:341-5.

SECTION

Assessing Cardiac Function

CHAPTER

29 Diastolic Dysfunction in Critically Patients

Rahul Pandit, Prasad Padwal

INTRODUCTION

Diastolic dysfunction or heart failure with preserved ejection fraction (HFpEF) has been recognized since the mid-1990s.[1] The incidence of diastolic dysfunction is known to be between 30 and 70% and of all heart failure (HF) cases admitted to the intensive care unit around 50% are known to be due to diastolic dysfunction.[2] The prognosis of HFpEF is reported to be the same as that of HF with reduced systolic function. It is known that one of the causes of diastolic dysfunction could be coronary artery disease. Therefore, diastolic dysfunction may be present with systolic dysfunction. Thus, a common syndromic hypothesis postulates that diastolic dysfunction is perhaps a precursor of systolic dysfunction and is due to increased interstitial deposition of collagen and modified matricellular proteins.[3] There are many factors that can result in diastolic dysfunction such as ventricular hypertrophy, myocardial fibrosis, infiltrative disease, pericardial constrictive disorders, right ventricular (RV) alterations due to a variety of causes, advanced age, hypoxia, and acidosis. However, with the increased incidence due to better diagnosis, it is now recognized as an important aspect in the treatment and prognosis of a critically ill patient.[3]

PATHOPHYSIOLOGY

Left ventricular (LV) diastole extends from the closure of the aortic valve to the closure of the mitral valve, and its duration, at rest, is usually two-thirds of the cardiac cycle. The LV diastole is typically described in four phases. The first diastolic phase, starting with the closure of the aortic valve up to the opening of the mitral valve, is the isovolumetric relaxation time (IVRT). During this period, the intraventricular pressure decreases rapidly before the ventricular filling begins.[4]

In sinus rhythm, the ventricular filling occurs in three phases. The early or rapid filling phase begins with the opening of the mitral valve due to the reduction of intraventricular pressure below the atrial pressure. During this phase around two-thirds of left atrial (LA) blood volume enters the left ventricle. In the second phase, also called as phase of diastasis or equilibrium phase, the ventricular volume remains constant due to the equalization of the atrioventricular pressure. Finally, the late filling phase, or atrial contraction phase, depends on the increase in atrial pressure due to the atrial contraction. In this phase, the remaining LA blood volume is pushed into the left ventricle due to atrial contraction.[4]

A number of physiological changes occur in ventricular diastole. The fundamental among them are ventricular relaxation, compliance, and atrial contraction.[5] Relaxation of cardiac muscle fibers is an active process that uses energy as adenosine triphosphate (ATP). This energy is required to transfer the cytoplasmic calcium back to the sarcoplasmic reticulum, reactivating the inhibitory effect of the troponin-tropomyosin complex and allowing the dissociation of actin and myosin filaments. Relaxation not only depends on the availability of energy but also on the availability of calcium in the cytoplasm. The effect of the relaxation of the cardiac muscle fibers is a sudden drop in LV pressure. The rate at which pressure decreases during the isovolumetric relaxation period directly reflects the rate of muscle fiber relaxation. This velocity can be measured with invasive techniques and is often defined as the maximum descent velocity (–)dP/dt or the time constant of isovolumetric relaxation (tau).

The relationship between the stretching of the myocardial fiber and stress (force applied by the surface) determines the compliance. It is due to the active relaxation of the sarcomeres and the relative content of elastic and collagen fibers in the connective tissue. These fibers determine the size and the anatomical shape of the left ventricle and configure the matrix that converts the shortening and lengthening of muscle fibers into pressure changes. The force required to stretch the fibers is initially low but increases geometrically as the fibers are stretched. This phenomenon explains that, even in normal subjects, excessive volume overload can result in HF.[5]

Left atrial function depends on its preload, afterload, and contractility. In patients with abnormal ventricular relaxation, atrial preload is increased, leading to a greater atrial ejection volume. This mechanism allows the patient to maintain cardiac output when there is impaired ventricular relaxation. Atrial fibrillation leads to a decrease in cardiac output and the patients may develop congestive symptoms. Atrial contraction is ineffective when ventricular compliance is reduced, as the volume of the atrial ejection passes in a retrograde direction in the absence of valves in pulmonary veins.[6]

The combination of active relaxation and passive myocardial compliance allows the heart to maintain adequate stroke volume and cardiac output with normal filling pressure. In diastolic dysfunction one or both of these properties are altered, and LA pressure needs to be increased to maintain an adequate cardiac output.

DIAGNOSIS OF DIASTOLIC DYSFUNCTION

In the majority of patients clinical signs and symptoms are not able to differentiate between systolic or diastolic HF. Secondly, with a single syndromic hypothesis, both conditions may coexist.

Though cardiac catheterization would be the gold standard in diagnosing diastolic dysfunction, its risk, and the fact that it is an invasive procedure which has made echocardiography a preferred modality of diagnosis.

Two-dimensional Echocardiography

- *LA size and volume:* A LA maximum volume index >34 mL/m^2 supports the presence of elevated LV filling pressures. A normal LA volume is present in the earliest stage of diastolic dysfunction and in case of acute increase of LV pressures.
- *LV and interventricular septum size:*[7] Ventricular hypertrophy is not always present, the absence of hypertrophy does not exclude diastolic dysfunction.[8]
- LV ejection fraction and LV wall motion abnormalities.

Pulse Wave Doppler

Pulse wave (PW) Doppler measures the velocity of intracardiac blood flow generated by the pressure gradient between two chambers and it is expressed in cm/s. Transmitral PW Doppler at the tip of the mitral valve, in sinus rhythm, identifies two waves during LV filling. The first wave (*E*) corresponds to the early diastolic passive filling of the left ventricle. The second wave (*A*) corresponds to the atrial contraction.

Mitral Valve Inflow with Pulse Wave

The mitral inflow signal demonstrates the individual phases of filling as well as displays the contribution of each individual phase in filling. As mitral inflow reflects the pressure difference between the atria and the ventricle, any abnormality of diastolic pressure (as in the presence of diastolic dysfunction) in the chambers will affect the velocity and shape of the Doppler inflow signal. Specifically, diastolic dysfunction alters the relationship between early and late filling (E- and A-wave), how rapidly flow velocity declines in early diastole [E-wave deceleration time (DT)], and how long it takes for filling of the ventricle to start after the ventricle relaxes (length of the IVRT).

Normal Diastolic Function

In preserved diastolic function, blood flows and fills the LV in the early filling phase thus the E-wave is taller than the A-wave, the deceleration time is around 140–200 ms and IVRT is 70–100 mm/s. E/A ratio is between 0.8 and 2 **(Fig. 1)**.

Grade I Diastolic Dysfunction

A stiff ventricle impairs the early filling of the ventricle. Thus, the magnitude of the E-wave will decrease. It will take longer for atrial pressure to be high enough to

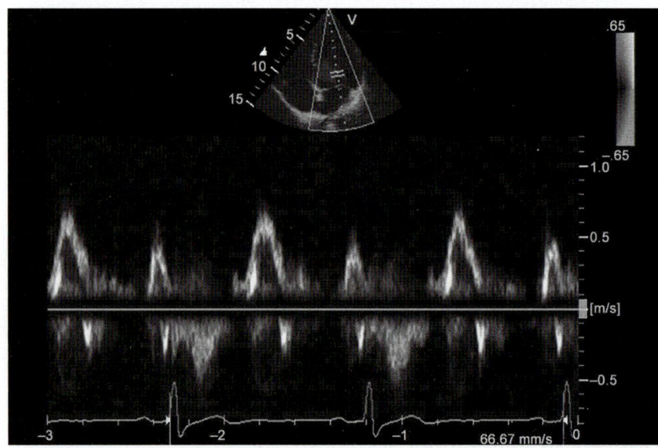

Fig. 1: Normal mitral valve inflow showing E and A waves *(For color version, see Plate 2)*.

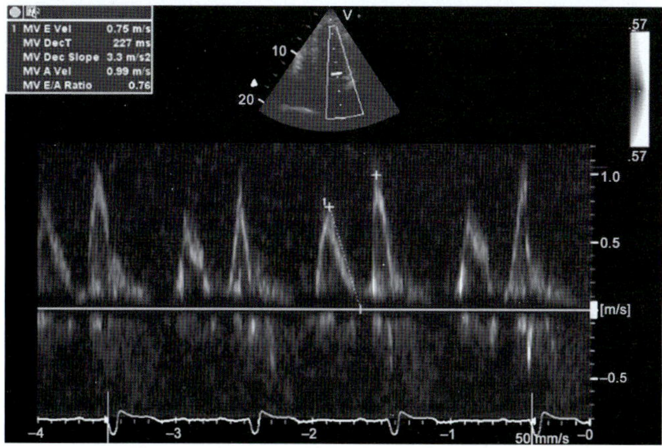

Fig. 2: E and A reversal—grade I dysfunction *(For color version, see Plate 3).*

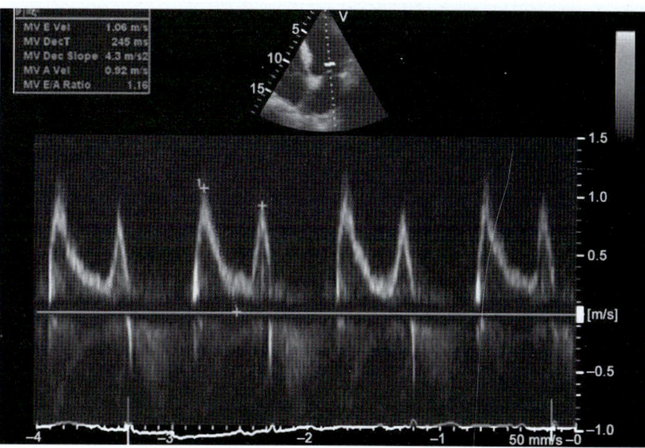

Fig. 3: Pseudonormal pattern grade II dysfunction *(For color version, see Plate 3).*

initiate filling. The IVRT will increase (>100 ms) and the DT will also be prolonged (≥240 ms). As less volume is transported into the left ventricle during early filling, more blood is present at the time of atrial contraction. Therefore, atrial contraction will eject more blood into the left ventricle. The A-wave will be larger than normal and will typically also be larger than the E-wave (E/A ratio ≤0.8) **(Fig. 2)**.

Grade II Diastolic Dysfunction—Pseudonormal

Progressive diastolic dysfunction causes LA pressure to rise. This increases the pressure gradient between the left atrium and the left ventricle and acts as a driving force to fill the ventricle during early diastole. Thus, the size of the E-wave relative to the A-wave will increase, and the E/A ratio will return to the range of 0.8–1.5. DT and IVRT (<90 ms) will also decrease. This will look very similar to that of "normal" diastolic function. This condition is therefore referred to as "pseudonormal." Pseudonormal filling is classified as grade II diastolic dysfunction **(Fig. 3)**.

Several approaches may be used to distinguish between "normal" and "pseudonormal" filling: the most common being the Valsalva maneuver. It unmasks the pseudonormal trace and reverts back to impaired relaxation—grade I dysfunction trace **(Fig. 4)**.

The other approach is to use tissue Doppler imaging at the mitral valve annulus and get the e' and a'. The ratio of E/e' >15 will help unmask pseudonormal dysfunction. Also, the mitral annulus tissue Doppler imaging (TDI) will show a trace-like grade I dysfunction mirror image.

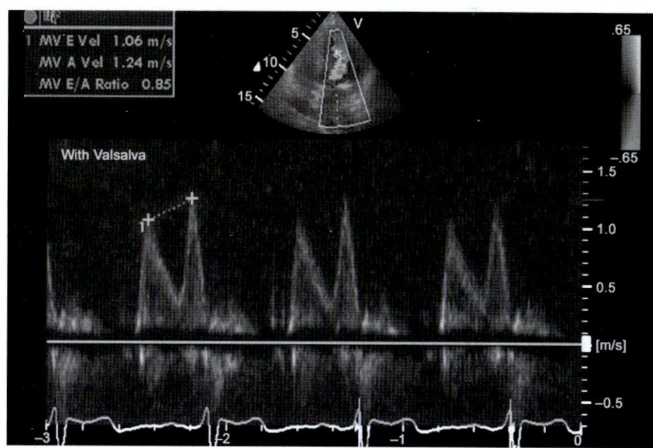

Fig. 4: Unmasking pseudonormal with Valsalva *(For color version, see Plate 3).*

Grade III Diastolic Dysfunction

A further increase in filling pressure will increase the gradient between the left atrium and the left ventricle during early diastole. The E-wave will become even taller and the A-wave shorter. The E/A ratio will be ≥2. In severe forms, the A-wave may be so small as to be nearly invisible and the E/A ratio may reach very high values of 5 or more **(Fig. 5)**.

When filling pressures are high, flow into the ventricle will start early, and filling will terminate quickly. Therefore, typical additional signs of restrictive filling include a short IVRT (≤70 ms) and DT (<140 ms).[8]

Tissue Doppler Imaging of Mitral Valve Annulus

The motion of the mitral valve annulus mirrors systolic as well as diastolic events. During systole, the annulus moves

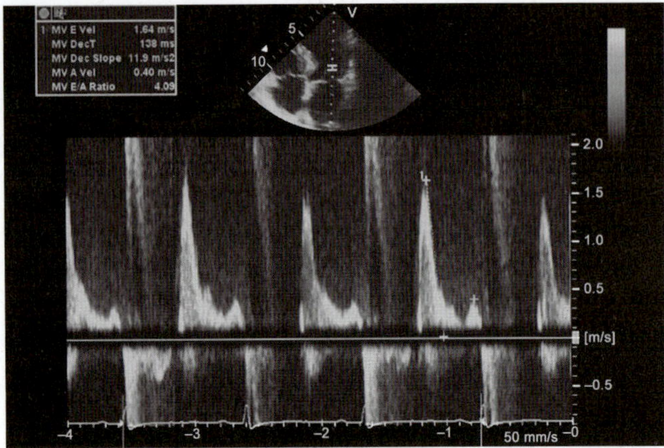

Fig. 5: Grade III diastolic dysfunction *(For color version, see Plate 3).*

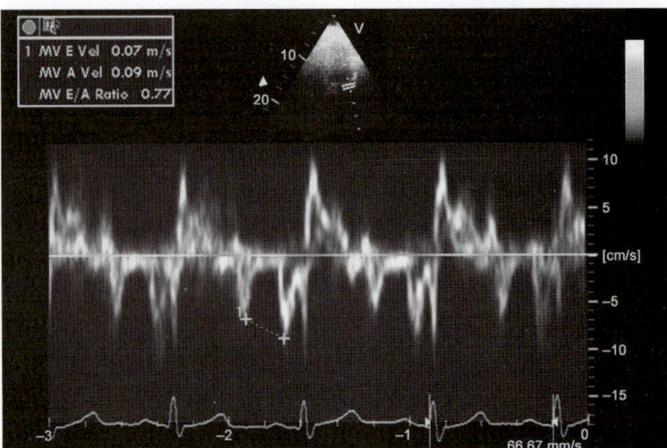

Fig. 6: Abnormal relaxation *(For color version, see Plate 3).*

caudally toward the apex, and during diastole, it moves cranially toward the atrium. The motion of the annulus can be recorded with the help of PW TDI at the medial (septal) as well as the lateral ring (in a four-chamber view).

The tracing of the Doppler wave is a mirror image of negative deflection of diastolic waves same as mitral valve inflow. Except that they are called e' (e prime) and a' (a prime). Together with the mitral valve inflow Doppler, this completes the diagnostics of diastolic dysfunction **(Figs. 6 to 8)**.

A ratio of E/e' helps in understanding the filling pressures and diastolic dysfunction. A ratio >15 correlates with high LV filling pressures and the presence of diastolic dysfunction. A ratio of <8 correlates with normal filling pressures and no diastolic dysfunction. Between 8 and 15 is indeterminate.[8]

By combining all the modalities together one can determine the degree of diastolic dysfunction. A similar assessment can be made using pulmonary valve inflow as well as color Doppler with M-mode. However, there are some indirect signs of diastolic dysfunction that can help point toward diastolic dysfunction such as the presence of LV wall hypertrophy or increased filling pressures as seen by a bulge of interatrial septum toward the right and dilated pulmonary veins.[8]

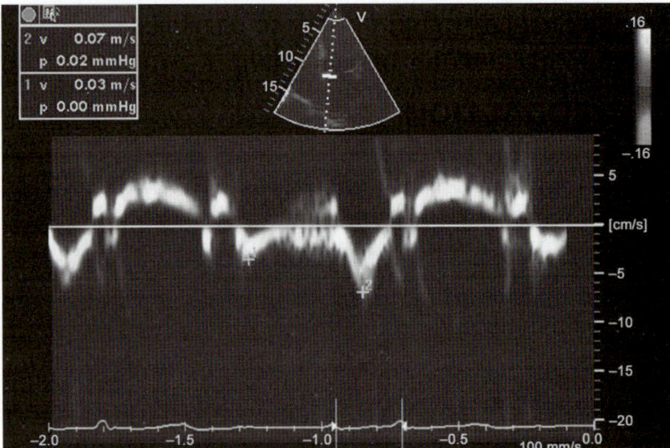

Fig. 7: Pseudonormal *(For color version, see Plate 3).*

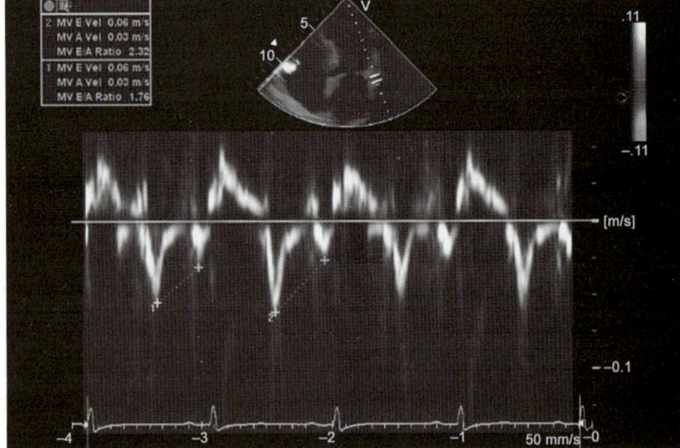

Fig. 8: Restrictive pattern *(For color version, see Plate 4).*

Peak Velocity of Tricuspid Regurgitation Measured by Continuous Doppler

During the development of LV diastolic dysfunction, LV impaired relaxation is transmitted to the right heart chambers, resulting in pulmonary arterial hypertension. Pulmonary arterial pressure significantly increases for each step-up in diastolic dysfunction. Peak velocity of tricuspid regurgitation >2.8 m/s is associated with diastolic dysfunction and elevated LA pressure, once primary lung

Fig. 9: Tricuspid regurgitation *(For color version, see Plate 4).*

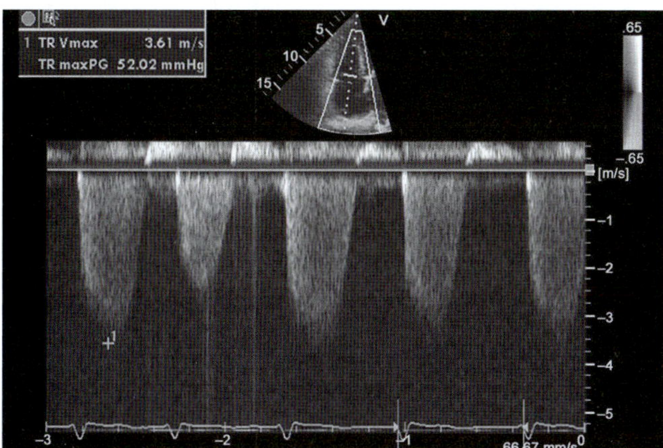

Fig. 10: Tricuspid regurgitation (TR) peak velocity *(For color version, see Plate 4).*

diseases have been ruled out **(Figs. 9 and 10)**. Right atrium pressure must be estimated assessing inferior vena cava size and response to breathing. However, the inferior vena cava size is best correlated only in ventilated patients.

NEW GUIDELINES

The new guidelines recommend taking into account the following four variables when determining whether LV diastolic function is normal or abnormal in the absence of myocardial disease in two-dimensional (2D) echocardiography.

- Annular *e′* velocity (septal *e′* <7 cm/s, lateral *e′* <10 cm/s)
- *E*/*e′* ratio (average >14, septal >15, lateral >13)
- LA maximum volume index >34 mL/m^2
- Peak velocity of tricuspid regurgitation >2.8 m/s.
  The diagnostic criteria are summarized in **Table 1**.

TABLE 1: Grading of left ventricular diastolic dysfunction.

	Normal	*Grade I*	*Grade II*	*Grade III*
Mitral *E*/*A* ratio	≥0.8	≤0.8	>0.8 to <2	>2
Average *E*/*e′* ratio	<10	<10	10–14	>14
Peak TR velocity (m/s)	<2.8	<2.8	>2.8	>2.8
LA volume index	Normal	Normal or increased	Increased	Increased
LV relaxation	Normal	Impaired	Impaired	Impaired
LAP	Normal	Low or normal	Elevated	Elevated

(LA: left atrial; LAP: left atrial pressure; LV: left ventricular; TR: tricuspid regurgitation)

CARDIAC BIOMARKERS

Cardiac biomarkers like brain natriuretic peptide (BNP) and N-terminal proBNP (NT-proBNP) are used for the serologic diagnosis of HF in outpatients, especially in the nonacute setting or when echocardiography is not immediately available.

Natriuretic peptides (BNP and NT-proBNP) are secreted in response to volume overload and increased cardiac wall stretch. In the case of HFpEF BNP levels can be lower or normal compared with patients with systolic HF. In noncritically ill patients, cardiac biomarkers such as BNP and NT-proBNP predict HFpEF more accurately.

Diastolic Dysfunction by Magnetic Resonance Imaging

Different MRI techniques are currently available for the evaluation of diastolic cardiac function, such as cine imaging for global function analysis, phase contrast (PC) imaging for flow analysis, and myocardial tagging for regional function analysis. Simple measurements, such as longitudinal fractional shortening, can be measured quickly and easily by MRI, which has reliably identified echocardiography-evidenced diastolic dysfunction in patients with preserved LV EF.[9]

PRACTICAL APPLICATION OF DIASTOLIC DYSFUNCTION

In the current scenario of intensive care and perioperative period, many studies explain a strong association between diastolic dysfunction and poor outcomes.

Diastolic Dysfunction with Sepsis

In case of sepsis, the patient should undergo an echocardiological examination on priority, which determines dynamic fluid resuscitation status, because, in patients with profound hypovolemia or vasoplegia, the LV diastolic function evaluation parameters show dramatic changes with fluid resuscitation or vasopressors infusion.

Management of patients with diastolic dysfunction includes preload optimization, and maintaining sinus rhythm without tachycardia, whereas in sepsis patients are hypovolemic due to increased permeability with vasoplegia, with tachyarrhythmias (most common is atrial fibrillation).[10,11]

Sepsis management includes controlled fluid resuscitation as a priority, whereas in diastolic dysfunction with rising LV pressures gives a poor window for fluid optimization due to the possibility of pulmonary edema despite fluid responsiveness. This dilemma warrants an understanding of diastolic dysfunction in sepsis before fluid resuscitation.

In sepsis, the well-known fact is increasing levels of cytokines and catecholamines leading to depressed myocardial function.[12,13] E/e′ is considered an independent outcome predictor in sepsis patients.[14] Also e′ <8 cm/s is also an important mortality predictor in malignancy with sepsis.[15] Most popular studies on diastolic dysfunction by Sanfilippo explain higher E/e′ ratio and lower e′ are associated with significant mortality in septic patients.[16]

Left ventricular diastolic dysfunction is not only dependent on preload but also on afterload, which is due to hypertension, vasopressor-induced afterload increase in sepsis, or nonpharmacological rise including increasing intra-abdominal pressures.[17-19] Determination of afterload by echocardiography is a major limitation.

Diastolic dysfunction due to tachycardia is due to reduced LV filling, which is normally compensated by acceleration of LV relaxation, majorly suffered in sepsis.[20-22]

DIASTOLIC DYSFUNCTION IN PERIOPERATIVE MANAGEMENT

Advanced age is the major cause of diastolic dysfunction, it is seen in elderly patients with multiple comorbidities undergoing cardiovascular surgeries. In patients undergoing cardiac surgery, diastolic dysfunction is directly correlated with difficult weaning from cardiopulmonary bypass and higher inotropic needs.[23] Diastolic dysfunction is also related to arrhythmias in the postoperative period, mainly, atrial fibrillation.[24]

Isolated diastolic dysfunction as compared to isolated systolic function is more frequent (43 vs. 8%, respectively) in patients with major vascular surgery. Diastolic dysfunction is also a predictor of postoperative cardiac failure, prolonged hospital stays, and perioperative mortality.[25]

In a study conducted by Arriaza-Cabrera Schulmeyer patients with cardiac comorbidities undergoing noncardiac/nonvascular (abdominal, urological, and orthopedic) surgeries, patients were stratified according to preoperative normal (<8), borderline (8–15), and high (>15) E/e′ ratio. Results suggested that patients with high E/e′ had a higher incidence of perioperative complications such as pulmonary edema, arrhythmias, prolonged ICU and hospital stay, and high mortality than patients with normal E/e.[26]

Preoperative and postoperative diastolic dysfunction evaluation impacts the outcome by identifying stressors affecting diastolic function mainly pain-related tachycardia reducing diastolic time, and volume status.

Diastolic Dysfunction and Weaning

One of the major reasons for weaning failure or prolonged weaning is LV relaxation impairment with a rise in filling pressures. This suggests that 2D echocardiography can be a major tool for the diagnosis and management of weaning failure.

In a study for cardiac dysfunction during weaning from a ventilator, in patients with cardiac output monitoring, weaning-induced pulmonary edema (WiPO) was independent of preload and subsequent SBT responded after diuretic therapy and achieving negative fluid balance. Further, it is observed that fluid balance was equal between patients with WiPO and non-WiPO, but the first group had a significantly higher E/e′ ratio, suggesting diastolic dysfunction.[27] This explains the importance of optimization of diastolic dysfunction in patients with weaning failure.

In a study about postextubation respiratory failure, ultrasound evaluation of cardiac, respiratory, and diaphragmatic components found that detection of lung interstitial water and estimation of LV filling pressure was the most relevant parameters predictive of postextubation respiratory failure. Whereas assessment of systolic function and diaphragmatic excursion were proven as poor predictors of respiratory failure.[28]

Physiologically, relaxation enhancement during exercise blunts the increase in venous return to maintain normal filling pressures.[9] But impaired relaxation can be evident during exercise in patients with mild symptoms of HF due to diastolic dysfunction.[29,30] This is due to weaning being equivalent to cardiopulmonary exercise.[31,32] This pathophysiology explains the increase in filling pressures during weaning failure of cardiac origin, due to poor diastolic reserve due to illness or advanced age.

DIASTOLIC DYSFUNCTION AND ACUTE RESPIRATORY DISTRESS SYNDROME

Acute respiratory distress syndrome (ARDS) is a syndrome with multiple pathophysiological processes at a single moment, where the identification of modifiable factors such as diastolic dysfunction, impacts on recovery from disease. Increased alveolar permeability and edema are the pathophysiology of ARDS, and an increase in edema-promoting forces, such as hydrostatic pressure can worsen pulmonary function leading to poor outcomes.[24] Progressive depression in LV function has the potential to contribute to the development of ARDS in patients with increased alveolar epithelial-capillary endothelial permeability. We need more studies targeting cardiac evaluation in ARDS for assessing cardiac contribution in ARDS. In ARDS, cardiac dysfunction and hydrostatic edema may play a relatively smaller role in development when compared to the high permeability edema that accompanies septic shock.

For ARDS we need to follow the "right ventricle-protective strategy" for ventilation, involving a stricter control of plateau pressures, keeping partial pressure of arterial carbon dioxide ($PaCO_2$) below 60 mm Hg, restricting driving pressures to as low as possible, and definitely proning.[33,34]

MANAGEMENT OF DIASTOLIC DYSFUNCTION

Diastolic dysfunction is difficult to manage pharmacologically and nonpharmacologically. Unfortunately, we do not have studies showing that improving diastolic dysfunction leads to improved prognosis.

Components of correction of hemodynamics in diastolic dysfunction include the following:

- Reduce afterload
- Avoid arrhythmias, mainly tachyarrhythmias
- Use inotropes without negative lusitropism
- Maintaining balanced fluid status
- Maintaining adequate demand–supply balance for LV

In acute clinical conditions, 2D echocardiography-guided fluid management, with dynamic hemodynamic assessment, and adequate use of diuretics, is the mainstay of management. Other pharmacological management includes beta-blockers to ameliorate diastolic dysfunction in HFpEF,[35] beta-blockade to improve LV filling pressures and coronary flow reserve in patients with uncomplicated arterial hypertension.[36] It is observed that in the first large randomized study on beta-blockers in patients with septic shock, esmolol infusions were beneficial and demonstrated decreased requirement of vasopressors due to their negative chronotropic and inotropic effects. Similar studies showed improved LV filling and arterial and ventricular coupling after esmolol infusion in septic patients.[37] Other pharmacological intervention is the use of angiotensin-converting enzyme inhibitors, capable of LV remodeling and improving diastolic function.[38-40] But both medications have demonstrated benefit in chronic conditions as compared to acute settings. Dexmedetomidine (α-2 agonist) and levosimendan are used for improving cardiac function in sepsis but there are no benefits have been demonstrated.[41-43] In acute conditions, diastolic dysfunction grade I is usually easy to manage, but the dominance of the atrial filling ($E < A$) makes them very sensitive to the loss of atrial filling (in arrhythmias like atrial fibrillation) with reduced left ventricular ejection fraction (LVEF). So, prevention and rapid management of arrhythmias is a mainstay in the treatment of grade I.[44]

In the case of diastolic dysfunction grade II, volume assessment is important due to the possibility of developing pulmonary edema as compared to hypovolemia. The LA pressure decreases and patients lose their compensatory mechanism to maintain an LA-to-LV gradient, which can be further worsened by arrhythmias. So, maintaining euvolemia and arrhythmia prevention remains the mainstay of management.

Diastolic dysfunction grade III patients have severe LV filling defects, mainly HFpEF. In case of prolonged QRS, these patients require cardiac resynchronization.[45] Cardiac resynchronization is not possible in acute conditions.[46]

Early diastolic dysfunction related to myocardial ischemia (grade I or II), should be corrected by improving coronary perfusion, pharmacologically or by intervention.[47,48]

CONCLUSION

Diastolic dysfunction is a hidden problem in intensive care patients. Early diagnosis and assessing the severity of dysfunction will help in better management of patients. Echocardiography is the main modality of diagnosis. Early echo will help in guiding fluid and ventilatory management.

REFERENCES

1. European Study Group on Diastolic Heart Failure. How to diagnose diastolic heart failure. European Study Group on Diastolic Heart Failure. Eur Heart J. 1998;19(7):990-1003.
2. Paulus WJ, Tschöpe C, Sanderson JE, Rusconi C, Flachskampf FA, Rademakers FE, et al. How to diagnose diastolic heart failure: a consensus statement on the diagnosis of heart failure with normal left ventricular ejection fraction by the Heart Failure and Echocardiography Associations of the European Society of Cardiology. Eur Heart J. 2007;28(20):2539-50.
3. Owan TE, Hodge DO, Herges RM, Jacobsen SJ, Roger VL, Redfield MM. Trends in prevalence and outcome of heart failure with preserved ejection fraction. N Engl J Med. 2006;355(3):251-9.
4. In: Hall JE (Ed). Guyton and Hall Textbook of Medical Physiology. Philadelphia, PA: Elsevier Health Sciences; 2015.
5. Kitzman DW, Little WC, Brubaker PH, Anderson RT, Hundley WG, Marburger CT, et al. Pathophysiological characterization of isolated diastolic heart failure in comparison to systolic heart failure. JAMA. 2002; 288(17):2144-50.
6. Zile MR, Brutsaert DL. New concepts in diastolic dysfunction and diastolic heart failure: Part II: causal mechanisms and treatment. Circulation. 2002;105(12):1503-8.
7. Nicoara A, Jones-Haywood M. Diastolic heart failure: diagnosis and therapy. Curr Opin Anaesthesiol. 2016;29(1):61-7.
8. Nagueh SF, Smiseth OA, Appleton CP, Byrd BF 3rd, Dokainish H, Edvardsen T, et al. Recommendations for the Evaluation of Left Ventricular Diastolic Function by Echocardiography: An Update from the American Society of Echocardiography and the European Association of Cardiovascular Imaging. Am Soc Echocardiogr. 2016;29(4):277-314.
9. Sanfilippo F, Corredor C, Fletcher N, Tritapepe L, Lorini FL, Arcadipane A, et al. Left ventricular systolic function evaluated by strain echocardiography and relationship with mortality in patients with severe sepsis or septic shock: a systematic review and meta-analysis. Crit Care. 2018;22(1):183.
10. Kuipers S, Klein Klouwenberg PM, Cremer OL. Incidence, risk factors and outcomes of new-onset atrial fibrillation in patients with sepsis: a systematic review. Crit Care. 2014;18(6):688.
11. Vieillard-Baron A, Cecconi M. Understanding cardiac failure in sepsis. Intensive Care Med. 2014;40(10):1560-3.
12. Beesley SJ, Weber G, Sarge T, Nikravan S, Grissom CK, Lanspa MJ, et al. Septic cardiomyopathy. Crit Care Med. 2018;46(4):625-34.
13. Sturgess DJ, Marwick TH, Joyce C, Jenkins C, Jones M, Masci P, et al. Prediction of hospital outcome in septic shock: a prospective comparison of tissue Doppler and cardiac biomarkers. Crit Care. 2010;14(2):R44.
14. Mourad M, Chow-Chine L, Faucher M, Sannini A, Brun JP, de Guibert JM, et al. Early diastolic dysfunction is associated with intensive care unit mortality in cancer patients presenting with septic shock. Br J Anaesth. 2014;112(1):102-9.
15. Sanfilippo F, Corredor C, Arcadipane A, Landesberg G, Vieillard-Baron A, Cecconi M, et al. Tissue Doppler assessment of diastolic function and relationship with mortality in critically ill septic patients: a systematic review and meta-analysis. Br J Anaesth. 2017;119(4):583-94.
16. Krzesinski P, Uzieblo-Zyczkowska B, Gielerak G, Stańczyk A, Kurpaska M, Piotrowicz K. Global longitudinal two-dimensional systolic strain is associated with hemodynamic alterations in arterial hypertension. J Am Soc Hypertens. 2015;9(9):680-9.
17. Ros M, Azevedo ER, Newton GE, Parker JD. Effects of nitroprusside on cardiac norepinephrine spillover and isovolumic left ventricular relaxation in the normal and failing human left ventricle. Can J Cardiol. 2002;18(11):1211-6.
18. Alfonsi P, Vieillard-Baron A, Coggia M, Guignard B, Goeau-Brissonniere O, Jardin F, et al. Cardiac function during intraperitoneal CO_2 insufflation for aortic surgery: a transesophageal echocardiographic study. Anesth Analg. 2006;102(5):1304-10.
19. Janssen PM, Periasamy M. Determinants of frequency dependent contraction and relaxation of mammalian myocardium. J Mol Cell Cardiol. 2007;43(5):523-31.
20. Joulin O, Marechaux S, Hassoun S, Montaigne D, Lancel S, Neviere R. Cardiac force-frequency relationship and frequency-dependent acceleration of relaxation are impaired in LPS-treated rats. Crit Care. 2009;13(1):R14.
21. Ferguson ND, Meade MO, Hallett DC, Stewart TE. High values of the pulmonary artery wedge pressure in patients with acute lung injury and acute respiratory distress syndrome. Intensive Care Med. 2002;28(8):1073-7.
22. Bernard F, Denault A, Babin D, Goyer C, Couture P, Couturier A, et al. Diastolic dysfunction is predictive of difficult weaning from cardiopulmonary bypass. Anesth Analg. 2001;92(2):291-8.
23. Lacalzada J, Jimenez JJ, Iribarren JL, de la Rosa A, Martín-Cabeza M, Izquierdo MM, et al. Early transthoracic

echocardiography after cardiac surgery predicts postoperative atrial fibrillation. Echocardiography. 2016;33(9):1300-8.
24. Matyal R, Hess PE, Subramaniam B, Mitchell J, Panzica PJ, Pomposelli F, et al. Perioperative diastolic dysfunction during vascular surgery and its association with postoperative outcome. J Vasc Surg. 2009;50(1):70-6.
25. Cabrera Schulmeyer MC, Arriaza N. Good prognostic value of the intraoperative tissue Doppler-derived index E/e' after non-cardiac surgery. Minerva Anestesiol. 2012; 78(9):1013-8.
26. Sanfilippo F, Santonocito C, Burgio G, Arcadipane A. The importance of diastolic dysfunction in the development of weaning-induced pulmonary oedema. Crit Care. 2017; 21:29.
27. Silva S, Ait Aissa D, Cocquet P, Hoarau L, Ruiz J, Ferre F, et al. Combined thoracic ultrasound assessment during a successful weaning trial predicts postextubation distress. Anesthesiology. 2017;127(4):666-74.
28. Dusch MN, Thadani SR, Dhillon GS, Hope MD. Diastolic function assessed by cardiac MRI using longitudinal left ventricular fractional shortening. Clin Imaging. 2014;38(5):666-8.
29. Ha JW, Lulic F, Bailey KR, Pellikka PA, Seward JB, Tajik AJ, et al. Effects of treadmill exercise on mitral inflow and annular velocities in healthy adults. Am J Cardiol. 2003;91(1):114-5.
30. Burgess MI, Jenkins C, Sharman JE, Marwick TH. Diastolic stress echocardiography: hemodynamic validation and clinical significance of estimation of ventricular filling pressure with exercise. J Am Coll Cardiol. 2006;47(9):1891-900.
31. Chattopadhyay S, Alamgir MF, Nikitin NP, Rigby AS, Clark AL, Cleland JG. Lack of diastolic reserve in patients with heart failure and normal ejection fraction. Circ Heart Fail. 2010;3(1):35-43.
32. Pinsky MR. Breathing as exercise: the cardiovascular response to weaning from mechanical ventilation. Intensive Care Med. 2000;26(9):1164-6.
33. Cabello B, Thille AW, Roche-Campo F, Brochard L, Gómez FJ, Mancebo J. Physiological comparison of three spontaneous breathing trials in difficult-to-wean patients. Intensive Care Med. 2010;36(7):1171-9.
34. Vieillard-Baron A, Price LC, Matthay MA. Acute cor pulmonale in ARDS. Intensive Care Med. 2013;39(10): 1836-8.
35. Repessé X, Charron C, Vieillard-Baron A. Acute cor pulmonale in ARDS: Rationale for protecting the right ventricle. Chest. 2015;147(1):259-65.
36. Bergstrom A, Andersson B, Edner M, Nylander E, Persson H, Dahlström U. Effect of carvedilol on diastolic function in patients with diastolic heart failure and preserved systolic function. Results of the Swedish Doppler-echocardiographic study (SWEDIC). Eur J Heart Fail. 2004;6(4):453-61.
37. Galderisi M, D'Errico A, Sidiropulos M, Innelli P, de Divitiis O, de Simone G. Nebivolol induces parallel improvement of left ventricular filling pressure and coronary flow reserve in uncomplicated arterial hypertension. J Hypertens. 2009;27(10):2108-15.
38. Morelli A, Singer M, Ranieri VM, D'Egidio A, Mascia L, Orecchioni A, et al. Heart rate reduction with esmolol is associated with improved arterial elastance in patients with septic shock: a prospective observational study. Intensive Care Med. 2016;42(10):1528-34.
39. Siegmund T, Schumm-Draeger PM, Antoni D, Bibra HV. Beneficial effects of ramipril on myocardial diastolic function in patients with type 2 diabetes mellitus, normal LV systolic function and without coronary artery disease: a prospective study using tissue Doppler. Diab Vasc Dis Res. 2007;4(4):358-64.
40. Yalcin F, Aksoy FG, Muderrisoglu H, Sabah I, Garcia MJ, Thomas JD. Treatment of hypertension with perindopril reduces plasma atrial natriuretic peptide levels, left ventricular mass, and improves echocardiographic parameters of diastolic function. Clin Cardiol. 2000;23(6):437-41.
41. Zhang Q, Chen Y, Liu Q, Shan Q. Effects of renin-angiotensin-aldosterone system inhibitors on mortality, hospitalization, and diastolic function in patients with HFpEF. A meta-analysis of 13 randomized controlled trials. Herz. 2016;41(1):76-86.
42. Malik V, Subramanian A, Hote M, Kiran U. Effect of levosimendan on diastolic function in patients undergoing coronary artery bypass grafting: a comparative study. J Cardiovasc Pharmacol. 2015;66(2):141-7.
43. Tarvasmaki T, Lassus J, Varpula M, Sionis A, Sund R, Køber L, Spinar J, et al. Current real-life use of vasopressors and inotropes in cardiogenic shock - adrenaline use is associated with excess organ injury and mortality. Crit Care. 2016;20(1):208.
44. Couture P, Denault AY, Pellerin M, Tardif JC. Milrinone enhances systolic, but not diastolic function during coronary artery bypass grafting surgery. Can J Anaesth. 2007;54(7):509-22.
45. Vieillard-Baron A, Boyd J. Non-antiarrhythmic interventions in new onset and paroxysmal sepsis-related atrial fibrillation. Intensive Care Med. 2018;44(1):94-7.
46. Cleland JG, Daubert JC, Erdmann E, Freemantle N, Gras D, Kappenberger L, et al. The effect of cardiac resynchronization on morbidity and mortality in heart failure. N Engl J Med. 2005;352(15):1539-49.
47. Rinaldi C, Auricchio A, Prinzen F. Left ventricular endocardial pacing for the critically ill. Intensive Care Med. 2018;44(6):915-7.
48. Schwarzl M, Huber S, Maechler H, Steendijk P, Seiler S, Truschnig-Wilders M, et al. Left ventricular diastolic dysfunction during acute myocardial infarction: effect of mild hypothermia. Resuscitation. 2012;83(12):1503-10.

Right Ventricular Failure in the Critically Ill

Srinivas Samavedam, Guruprasad N

INTRODUCTION

The right ventricle (RV) plays a crucial role in the generation of stroke volume (SV). The RV pumps blood into the low-resistance pulmonary circuit, while the left ventricle (LV) pumps blood into the highly resistant systemic circulation. The RV is thin-walled and cannot tolerate any increase in afterload.[1] RV SV is mainly driven by longitudinal shortening with peristaltic bellow-like movement unlike the circumferential thickening of the LV.[2]

VENTRICULAR INTERDEPENDENCE

The LV and RV are enclosed in a stiff envelope, the pericardium. They have similar end-diastolic volumes and there is no free space for acute ventricular dilatation. Thus, when RV end-diastolic volume increases owing to increased RV loading, it can only occur at the expense of the space devoted to the LV, which is prevented from dilating to as large an end-diastolic volume as it would otherwise do given its distending pressure. From a practical point of view this reduced left ventricular end-diastolic volume (LVEDV) is accompanied by decreases in LV diastolic compliance resulting in reduced LV output.

The functions of the RV are:

- To generate adequate pulmonary perfusion pressure for delivery of desaturated mixed venous blood to the alveoli for gas exchange.
- Maintain low systemic venous pressure to prevent organ congestion.[3-5]

Major differences between LV and RV are given in **Table 1** and **Figure 1**.[3-5,6-9]

ACUTE RIGHT HEART SYNDROME

Definition: Sudden deterioration in RV function resulting in failure to deliver adequate blood flow into the pulmonary circulation, finally resulting in systemic hypoperfusion.[10] Acute right heart syndrome (ARHS) is often missed in intensive care units (ICUs) because of the focus being trained on the cardiac output (CO) with SV as its representative. The etiologies of RV dysfunction are given in **Box 1**.

In mechanically ventilated patients, low CO is multifactorial and could be due to:

- Right ventricular systolic dysfunction (due to increased afterload)
- Decreased venous return
- Tricuspid regurgitation
- Ventricular interdependence [dilatation of the RV shifting the interventricular septum (IVS) toward the left and decreasing the LV distensibility and preload]
- Arrhythmias or suboptimal preload.[10]

Clinical Features

Symptoms

- Shortness of breath
- Orthopnea
- Bilateral lower extremity edema
- Epigastric discomfort
- Enlarged tender liver
- Ascites

The clinical features are, however, nonspecific, and difficult to identify in the sedated, critically ill patient.[11]

Signs

- Raised jugular venous pressure
- Gallop rhythm at the left sternal edge
- Systolic murmur of tricuspid regurgitation
- Organomegaly (hepatosplenomegaly)
- Ventricular arrhythmias

TABLE 1: Differences between LV and RV.

	Right ventricle	***Left ventricle***
Morphological structure	Complex, crescentic	Bullet shape; prolate ellipsoid
Structure	Inflow region, infundibulum	No infundibulum mitro-aortic continuity
Shape in cross-section	Semicircular/serpentine shape	Circular
Myocardial characteristics	Thin, heavily trabeculated walls	Thick smooth walls; fine trabeculations
Myocardial architecture	Predominant longitudinal myocyte orientation; angulated intrusion of superficial myocytes right—toward the endocardium myocytes	Predominant radial myocyte orientation in the midlayers; subendocardial myocytes follow hand helix configuration; subepicardial form left-hand helix
Physiological pump conditions	Low-resistance, low-capacitance pump; Peristaltic-like motion from inflow to outflow during ejection, and a bellows-like motion of the free wall towards the septum	High-resistance, high-pressure pump; dominant radial thickening and contraction during ejection
Flow characteristics	No or minimal isovolumic periods; hangout period	Well-defined isovolumic contraction and relaxation; no hangout period
End-diastolic wall thickness	≤3 mm	≤11 mm
End-diastolic volume	49–101 mL/m^2	44–89 mL/m^2
Systolic pressure	25 mm Hg	120 mm Hg
Ejection fraction	40–68%	57–74%
Coronary perfusion	Continuous (Systole and diastole)	Almost exclusively during diastole
Response to disease	Better adaptation to volume overload states, higher compliance than LV	Better adaptation to pressure overload states
Pressure volume loop	Trapezoidal with poorly defined isovolumetric periods—RV pressures rise and ejection continues despite a fall in RV pressure	Rectangular—rapid rise and fall of pressure with ejection

(LV: left ventricle; RV: right ventricle)

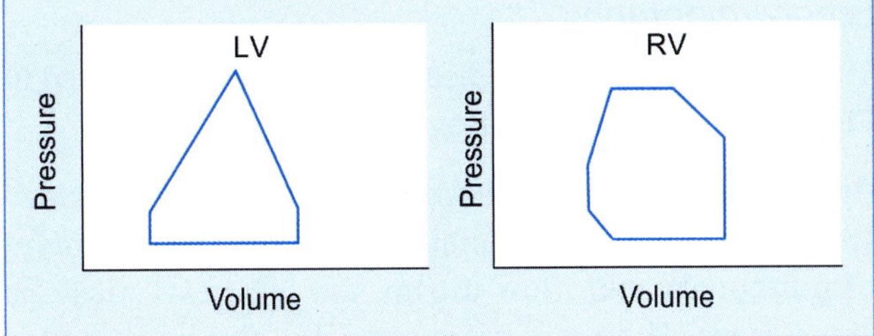

Fig. 1: Pressure volume loops of LV and RV (see text for explanation).
(LV: left ventricle; RV: right ventricle)
Source: Adapted from Kevin LG, et al.[5]

Signs of deep venous thrombosis [in pulmonary thromboembolism (PTE) patients]. If the patient is on the ventilator, the clinical manifestations are:

- Increased oxygen requirements
- Sudden cardiovascular collapse

The various etiologies of ARHS are listed in **Box 1**.

Diagnosis

The diagnosis of RV dysfunction is challenging in a critically ill patient. There are no pathognomonic clinical signs of RV failure.

Chest X-ray

- Enlargement of the main pulmonary artery and regional oligemia are seen in massive pulmonary embolism (PE).
- It helps in differentiating ARHS from atelectasis, pleural effusions, pulmonary edema, and pneumothorax.[19]

Electrocardiography

- Electrocardiography (ECG) is likely to show right-axis deviation, dominant R in V1, dominant S in V5, and P pulmonale suggesting right atrial and ventricular hypertrophy.

BOX 1: Etiologies for ARHS.[6-9,11-16]

RV pressure overload (endothelial dysfunction, vasoconstriction, and mechanical obstruction):
- Massive pulmonary embolism
- Acute respiratory distress syndrome
- Deteriorating chronic pulmonary arterial hypertension
- Postcardiothoracic surgery
- Mechanical ventilation
- Pulmonary valve stenosis
- Hypoventilation state

RV volume overload:
- Pulmonary or tricuspid valve regurgitation
- Left to right shunt due to interatrial defect
- Anomalous pulmonary venous return
- Hyperthyroidism

RV contractile dysfunction:
- RV myocardial infarction
- Relative RV ischemia secondary to RV pressure or volume overload
- Intrinsic myocardial disease, e.g., RV cardiomyopathy, sepsis (cytokine-induced myocardial depression), inflammatory effects of cardiopulmonary bypass, myocarditis
- Pericardial disease, e.g., constrictive pericarditis and tamponade (causing impaired diastolic filling)
- Left ventricular assist device (due to acute unloading of the LV) *LV dysfunction* (by increasing pulmonary venous and pulmonary arterial pressure, myocardial ischemia, LV dilatation leading to restricted RV diastolic function)

Right ventricle and sepsis: Septic cardiomyopathy is defined as the reversible systolic and/or diastolic dysfunction of one or both ventricles. Although RV and LV dysfunction coexist in most patients, multiple studies have reported an incidence of isolated RV dysfunction between 10 and 50%.[17] Apart from the cardiovascular manifestations of LV involvement, refractory vasodilatory shock, myocardial injury, and atrial arrhythmias, sepsis is also characterized by the presence of RV dysfunction.[17] Right ventricle dysfunction in sepsis is multifactorial and is more common in the presence of concomitant acute lung injury, hypoxemia, and hypercapnia.[18]

(ARHS: acute right heart syndrome; LV: left ventricle; RV: right ventricle)

- Right ventricular myocardial infarct as evidenced by elevated ST in V3R and V4R, Q-wave pattern in leads V1–V3, as well as a right-sided Q pattern in leads V3R–V6R.
- Right ventricular strain as evidenced by T inversion in V1–V4, and S1Q3T3.
- Right ventricular dysfunction may manifest with a Qr in V1 (highly associated with troponin leakage and myocardial shear stress).[20]

Central Venous Pressure

- Right ventricular end-diastolic volume (RVEDV) and LVEDV must be measured for assessing the ventricular preload.
- Measuring volume is difficult, so pressures are measured as surrogates assuming constant compliance in all patients.
- Another assumption made is central venous pressure (CVP) = RAP = RVEDP = LAP = LVEDP.
- Right ventricular end-diastolic volume is measured as a surrogate for RVEDP considering that the compliance of RV was normal.
- But if RV compliance is decreased CVP, right ventricular end-diastolic pressure (RVEDP) can be abnormally high despite hypovolemia.
- Central venous pressure can also vary with abnormalities of the intervening valves (tricuspid, pulmonary, and mitral valves).
- So CVP cannot be relied upon in RV failure.[21,22]

Right Heart Catheterization

Acute right heart syndrome is suspected if:
- RA pressure >8–10 mm Hg
- RA pressure to pulmonary capillary wedge pressure ratio ≥0.8 and cardiac index (CI) is low.

In the presence of RV-PA gradient (peak exercise) >25 mm Hg, RV outflow tract obstruction should be excluded by echocardiography.[23,24]

Echocardiography[25–28]

The echocardiographic Indicators of ARHS are depicted in **Figure 2** and are listed in **Box 2**.

Pulsed wave Doppler sampling of the hepatic vein:[24] Hepatic venous flow is analogous to the measurement of pulmonary vein flow during the left heart diastolic assessment. The main components of the hepatic vein waveforms are the systolic wave (S), systolic reversal (Sr), diastolic wave (D), and atrial reversal wave (Ar). The systolic wave predominance over the diastolic wave is normal. When there is RV diastolic dysfunction, the D wave dominates over the S wave (S < D).

RV free wall 2D global longitudinal strain:[29] Many recent studies have demonstrated that RV global longitudinal strain (GLS) assessed by 2D speckle tracking echocardiography correlated well with RV function assessed by cardiac magnetic resonance imaging (CMRI)

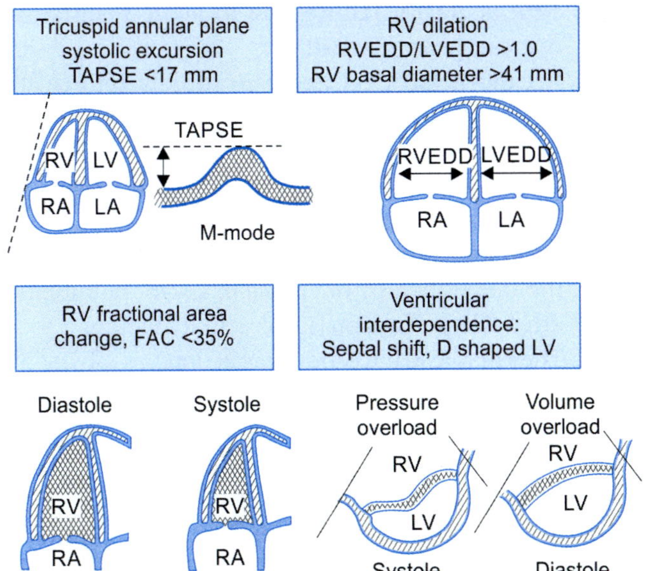

Fig. 2: Indicators of RV strain. (FAC: fractional area change; LA: left atrium; LV: left ventricle; RA: right atrium; RV: right ventricle; RVEDD/LVEDD: right ventricular end-diastolic dimension/left ventricular end-diastolic dimension; TAPSE: tricuspid annular plane systolic excursion)

Source: Harjola VP, Mebazaa A, Čelutkienė J, Bettex D, Bueno H, Chioncel O, et al. Contemporary management of acute right ventricular failure: a statement from the Heart Failure Association and the Working Group on Pulmonary Circulation and Right Ventricular Function of the European Society of Cardiology. Eur J Heart Fail. 2016;18(3):226-41.

which is considered a well-known gold standard for RV assessment. It is done as a postprocessing on software once a good two-dimensional (2D) image is obtained. The machine automatically calculates the GLS and if it is <-23, it suggests decreased RV free wall function.

Arterial Pulse Contour Analysis

A pressure-overloaded RV can show increased pulse pressure variation (PPV) values due to an increase in the RV afterload, and not due to a decrease in RV preload, hence further volume expansion could potentially be harmful.[30,31] When a patient suffers from RV failure or dysfunction, there is reduced ejection of blood when the RV afterload increases during positive pressure ventilation, in the inspiratory phase. Since the infused fluid cannot reach the pulmonary circulation and later the LV, there is no increase in the SV. In other words, if the RV is failing it cannot overcome the increased afterload during inspiration.[32]

BOX 2: Echocardiographic indicators of acute right heart syndrome.

RV systolic dysfunction:
- TAPSE <17 mm
- RV fractional area change <35%
- Tricuspid annular S' < 9 cm/s

RV diastolic dysfunction:
- Lateral tricuspid annular e' velocity <8 cm/s (less load dependent) by tissue pulsed Doppler
- E/A <0.8 by pulsed wave Doppler

Dilated RV chamber:
- Diameter >41 mm at the base
- Diameter >35 mm at the midlevel
- Longitudinal dimension >86 mm
- RVEDD/LVEDD >1.0
- RVEDA/LVEDA >0.6
- Eccentricity index >1 (in PSAX view between the mitral valve and papillary muscles)
- Right ventricle free wall 2D GLS <–0.23

RVOT dilatation: RVOT diameter >27 mm at end-diastole at the level of pulmonary valve

(GLS: global longitudinal strain; LVEDA: left ventricular end-diastolic area; LVEDD: left ventricular end-diastolic diameter; PSAX: parasternal short axis view; RV: right ventricular; RVEDA: right ventricular end-diastolic area; RVEDD: right ventricular end-diastolic diameter; RVOT: right ventricular outflow tract; TAPSE: tricuspid annular plane systolic excursion)

In patients with high PPV and stroke volume variability (SVV), who are nonfluid responders, RV dysfunction should be suspected, and the patient needs further evaluation.

Computed Tomography: Signs Suggestive of Acute Right Heart Syndrome

- Flattening or displacement of the IVS toward the LV (D-shaped LV)
- Reflux of contrast into the inferior vena cava
- Right ventricular diameter (RVD) to left ventricular diameter (LVD) ratio on axial sections >1.0 (RVD axial/LVD axial >1).[33]

Computed tomography pulmonary angiography (CTPA) is being used increasingly as a diagnostic tool in PE, with documented sensitivities of 50–100% and specificities of 81–100%.[31] CTPA has become the preferred diagnostic modality for suspected ARHS due to PE, in hemodynamically stable ICU patients.[33]

In summary, among critically ill patients with clinically suspected ARHS, echocardiography [Transthoracic echocardiogram (TTE) and/or transesophageal echocardiography (TEE)] and right heart catheterization are the preferred diagnostic modalities. If PE is the most likely cause of ARHS, then CTPA is necessary to confirm the diagnosis, provided the patient is suitable for transfer to the radiology suite.

Treatment

Optimization of Right Ventricular Preload

Critically ill patients are:

- Mostly fluid depleted intravascularly due to increased permeability and insensible fluid loss.
- On sedatives which can decrease venous tone and reduce venous return.
- On mechanical ventilation which increases intra-thoracic pressure and reduces RV preload.

Fluid resuscitation in RV failure depends on RV afterload. In the setting of RV myocardial infarction (MI) with normal afterload, fluid resuscitation improves CO. In acute PE with increased RV afterload, fluid resuscitation can cause distension of RV and displacement of IVS toward LV resulting in decreased LV filling. Simultaneously RV distension also increases free wall tension, increased oxygen demand, reduced RV perfusion, and further RV ischemia.[34] Therefore optimization of fluid status in RV failure is difficult.

Optimization of Right Ventricular after Load

In critically ill patients, increased afterload is a common cause of RV failure. Factors that increase pulmonary vascular resistance (PVR) such as hypoxemia, hypercapnia, and acidosis should be corrected immediately. Saturation of peripheral oxygen (SpO_2) needs to be maintained above 92% with a partial pressure of carbon dioxide (pCO_2), pH near-normal values, and ventilator settings to achieve a lung volume near functional residual capacity (FRC).

Pulmonary vasodilators: They act by:

- Decreasing PVR and impedance
- Increasing RV SV and output
- Avoiding systemic hypotension and maintaining coronary perfusion

The examples of pulmonary vasodilators are given here:

- *Inhaled nitric oxide:*
    - It acts by increasing intracellular cyclic guanosine monophosphate (cGMP).
    - It has a rapid onset and short half-life.
    - It improves arterial partial pressure of oxygen (PaO_2)/FiO_2 ratio and CO in ventilated patients with acute RV failure due to acute respiratory distress syndrome (ARDS).[35]
    - It can be an ideal agent to rapidly reduce RV afterload for short-term therapy.
- *Prostacyclin derivatives:*
    - Act by increasing intracellular cyclic adenosine monophosphate (cAMP) levels.
    - Have rapid onset and short half-life and hence, the initial therapy of choice in severe pulmonary arterial hypertension (PAH) with RV failure.
    - They may also have inotropic action.
    - *At present, three prostacyclin derivatives are available:* (1) Epoprostenol, (2) treprostinil, and (3) iloprost.[21,36]
    - All three drugs can be used by inhalational therapy to avoid systemic hypotension.
- *Phosphodiesterase-5 inhibitors:*
    - They inhibit the metabolism of cGMP and potentiate the beneficial effect of nitric oxide.
    - Oral preparations must be used carefully as they cause systemic vasodilation and have a longer half-life.
    - Oral sildenafil and Tadalafil reduce PVR, improve myocardial perfusion, and may improve RV contractility.[37]
    - Intravenous preparation of sildenafil with a shorter half-life is available and can be useful in RV failure in ICU patients on mechanical ventilation.[38]

Other pulmonary vasodilators such as endothelin receptor antagonists (ambrisentan and bosentan) and soluble guanylate cyclase stimulators (riociguat) which are not tried and tested in acute RV failure.

Optimization of Right Ventricular Contractility

Increased RV preload or afterload can lead to RV distension and increase free wall tension and oxygen demand. Simultaneously it causes shifting of IVS toward LV which decreases LV filling and LV output. RV systolic pressure is increased and if there is coexisting chronic pulmonary vascular disease, RV pressure can equalize with LV pressure. The primary goal, therefore, should be to keep systemic blood pressure above RV systolic pressure to prevent shifting of IVS.

Role of Vasopressors

The ideal vasopressor would be the one that increases the systemic vascular resistance and systemic blood pressure without raising PVR and improves RV contractility.

- Norepinephrine principally acts on $\alpha 1$ receptors and causes vasoconstriction with limited $\beta 1$ stimulation and cardiac inotropy.
- Phenylephrine is purely an $\alpha 1$ agonist, causes vasoconstriction, and improves coronary perfusion but it may also increase the PVR.
- Vasopressin at lower doses (0.01–0.03 U/min) causes pulmonary vasodilatation and at higher doses causes pulmonary and systemic vasoconstriction.
- Epinephrine is a mixed α- and β-receptor agonist that causes vasoconstriction and inotropy.

All in all, norepinephrine is the initial agent in hypotensive patients with RV failure.

Inotropes and Inodilators in Acute Right Heart Syndrome

- Dobutamine acts through $\beta 1$ and $\beta 2$ receptors, causes vasodilatation, and improves CO at lower doses. At higher doses, it can cause tachycardia and hypotension.
- Milrinone is a selective phosphodiesterase-III (PDE-III) inhibitor. It slows intracellular cAMP metabolism, causes pulmonary vasodilatation, and improves RV contractility. It is the drug of choice in pulmonary vascular disease with severe PAH and biventricular failure. It is preferred over dobutamine as it has a less chronotropic effect.
- Inotropes can cause tachycardia and should be considered only when there is evidence of inadequate oxygen delivery despite correction of RV preload, RV afterload, and ischemia.
- Levosimendan is a calcium sensitizer. It improves myocardial contractility without increasing cytosolic calcium and oxygen demand. In patients having RV failure with chronic thromboembolic pulmonary hypertension (CTEPH), levosimendan has been shown to improve RV function.[39]

Maintenance of sinus rhythm and heart rate control is important when a patient has an RV failure scenario.

Mechanical Ventilation Strategies

The goals of mechanical ventilation are as follows:

- Adopt lung protective ventilator strategy [low tidal volume, low plateau pressure, and positive end-expiratory pressure (PEEP)].
- Avoid hypoxia, hypercapnia, and high PEEP (10 cmH_2O). RV afterload is determined by PVR, which is affected by the changes in lung volume.

The PVR is high, both at low as well as high lung volumes. At low volumes, PVR is high due to decreased elastic recoil of lung parenchyma leading to extra-alveolar vessel collapse and terminal airway collapse leading to alveolar hypoxia and hypoxic pulmonary vasoconstriction. At high volumes, PVR is high because the stretching of alveolar walls leads to the collapse of alveolar vessels.[40] The total PVR is lowest at FRC, whereas vascular resistance in intra- and extra-alveolar vessels is intermediate. During lung protective strategy in acute RV failure conditions, it is very important to avoid hypercapnia as it can increase PVR and worsen RV function. Hence, in these patients, it is recommended to gradually adopt lung protective ventilation strategies monitoring hypercapnia and RV function.[41] It is important to remember that these patients of acute RV failure on mechanical ventilation may find it difficult to wean off the ventilator, as weaning may worsen (increase) RV afterload due to increasing work of breathing, hypoxemia, or high intrinsic PEEP, which can lead to further RV enlargement. This shifts the IVS toward LV, affecting LV filling and LV output. This can cause pulmonary edema and thus lead to failure in weaning from mechanical ventilation.[32]

MECHANICAL CIRCULATORY SUPPORT

Patients with severe RV failure, not responding to medical treatment, who are hypoxemic and hypercapnic on mechanical ventilation, respond to mechanical circulatory support like extracorporeal membrane oxygenation (ECMO) till the respiratory function improves.[41] Among patients with RV failure due to ARDS, with severe intractable hypercapnic acidosis, where the ventilator therapy is ineffective, extracorporeal carbon dioxide removal devices such as interventional lung assist (Novalung GmbH, Hechingen, Germany), may be useful as they are pumpless and are less invasive than ECMO and ultraprotective lung protection strategy can be instituted.[42] In patients with RV failure due to massive PE, CTEPH, and PAH, venovenous (VV) or venoarterial (VA) ECMO is used successfully as a bridge to pulmonary endarterectomy or lung transplantation.[43,44] Mydin et al. have shown that VA ECMO improves RV function and oxygen delivery in awake spontaneously breathing patients as a bridge to pulmonary endarterectomy.[45] In patients with acute RV failure, due to primary RV pathology and RV dysfunction refractory to medical treatment, mechanical support of RV such as a right ventricular assist device is used as a bridge to recovery or bridge to heart transplant.[46] Recently, pumpless lung assist devices have been developed that connect the PA to the left atrium with low resistance membrane oxygenator and it has been tried in patients with PAH as a bridge to lung transplant. The low resistance circuit offloads the RV and improves LV filling.

CONCLUSION

The right ventricle is a low-resistance, low-capacitance pump; peristaltic-like motion from inflow to outflow during ejection, and a bellows-like motion of the free wall toward the septum. Sudden deterioration in RV function resulting in failure to deliver adequate blood flow into the pulmonary circulation, finally resulting in systemic hypoperfusion is called ARHS. ARDS, PTE, RV infarction, and mechanical ventilation are the common causes of ARHS. CVP and arterial pulse contour analysis are not reliable in RV failure. Echocardiography (TTE and/or TEE) and right heart catheterization are the preferred diagnostic modalities. If PE is the most likely cause of ARHS, then CTPA is necessary to confirm the diagnosis, provided the patient is suitable for transfer to radiology. In RV-MI with normal afterload, fluid resuscitation improves CO. In acute PE with increased RV afterload, fluid resuscitation can cause distension of RV and displacement of IVS toward LV resulting in decreased LV filling, simultaneously RV distension also increases free wall tension, increased oxygen demand, reduced RV perfusion, and further RV ischemia, so be careful during fluid resuscitation. Norepinephrine is the initial agent in hypotensive patients with RV failure. Adopt a lung protective ventilator strategy (low tidal volume, low plateau pressure, and PEEP). Avoid hypoxia, hypercapnia, and high PEEP (10 cmH_2O). Pulmonary vasodilators can be used in severe PAH. Finally, patients with RV failure in shock can be kept on VA-ECMO as a bridge to definitive therapy.

REFERENCES

1. Greyson CR. The right ventricle and pulmonary circulation: basic concepts. Rev Esp Cardiol. 2010;63(1):81-95.
2. Kukulski T, Hübbert L, Arnold M, Wranne B, Hatle L, Sutherland GR. Normal regional right ventricular function and its change with age: a Doppler myocardial imaging study. J Am Soc Echocardiogr. 2000;13(3):194-204.
3. Bleeker GB, Steendijk P, Holman ER, Yu CM, Breithardt OA, Kaandorp TA, et al. Assessing right ventricular function: the role of echocardiography and complementary technologies. Heart. 2006;92(Suppl 1):19-26.
4. Alaverdian A, Cohen R. The right ventricle in critical illness. Open Crit Care Med J. 2010;3:38-42.
5. Kevin LG, Barnard M. Right ventricular failure. Contin Educ Anaesth Crit Care Pain. 2007;7:89-94.
6. Cecconi M, Johnston E, Rhodes A. What role does the right side of the heart play in circulation? Crit Care. 2006;10 (Suppl 3):S5.
7. Haddad F, Hunt SA, Rosenthal DN, Murphy DJ. Right ventricular function in cardiovascular disease, part I: Anatomy, physiology, aging, and functional assessment of the right ventricle. Circulation. 2008;117(11):1436-48.
8. Forrest P. Anaesthesia and right ventricular failure. Anaesth Intensive Care. 2009;37(3):370-85.
9. Giovambattista RD. Hyperthyroidism as a reversible cause of right ventricular overload and congestive heart failure. Cardiovasc Ultrasound. 2008;6:29.
10. Greyson CR. Pathophysiology of right ventricular failure. Crit Care Med. 2008;36(1 Suppl):S57-65.
11. Zochios V, Keeshan A. Pulmonary embolism in the mechanically-ventilated critically ill patient: is it different? JICS. 2013;14(1):36-44.
12. Reis Miranda D, Gommers D, Lachman B. Effect of mechanical ventilation on right ventricular afterload. In: Gullo A (Ed). Anaesthesia, Intensive Care and Emergency Medicine. Trieste: Springer; 2006. pp. 361-6.
13. Lahm T, McCaslin CA, Wozniak TC, Ghumman W, Fadl YY, Obeidat OS, et al. Medical and surgical treatment of acute right ventricular failure. J Am Coll Cardiol. 2010;56(18): 1435-46.
14. Santambrogio L, Bianchi T, Fuardo M, Gazzoli F, Veronesi R, Braschi A, et al. Right ventricular failure after left ventricular assist device insertion: preoperative risk factors. Interact Cardiovasc Thorac Surg. 2006;5(4):379-82.
15. Michael R, Pinsky M. Recent advances in the clinical application of heart-lung interactions. Curr Opin Crit Care. 2002;8(1):26-31.
16. Jardin F, Gueret P, Dubourg O, Farcot JC, Margairaz A, Bourdarias JP. Two-dimensional echocardiographic evaluation of right ventricular size and contractility in acute respiratory failure. Crit Care Med. 1985;13(11):952-6.
17. Vallabhajosyula S, Kumar M, Pandompatam G, Sakhuja A, Kashyap R, Kashani K, et al. Prognostic impact of isolated right ventricular dysfunction in sepsis and septic shock: an 8-year historical cohort study. Ann Intensive Care. 2017;7(1):94.
18. Vieillard-Baron A, Jardin F. Why protect the right ventricle in patients with acute respiratory distress syndrome? Curr Opin Crit Care. 2003;9(1):15-21.
19. Kucher N, Walpoth N, Wustmann K, Noveanu M, Gertsch M. QR in V1—an ECG sign associated with right ventricular strain and adverse clinical outcome in pulmonary embolism. Eur Heart J. 2003;24(12):1113-9.
20. Reems MM, Aumann M. Central venous pressure: principles, measurement, and interpretation. Compend Contin Educ Vet. 2012;34(1):E1.

21. Greyson CR. Right heart failure in the intensive care unit. Curr Opin Crit Care. 2012;18(5):424-31.
22. Matthay MA, Chatterjee K. Bedside catheterization of the pulmonary artery: risks compared with benefits. Ann Intern Med. 1988;109(10):826-34.
23. Goldstein JA, Barzilai B, Rosamond TL, Eisenberg PR, Jaffe AS. Determinants of hemodynamic compromise with severe right ventricular infarction. Circulation. 1990; 82(2):359-68.
24. Rudski LG, Lai WW, Afilalo J, Solomon SD, Louie EK, Schiller MD, et al. Guidelines for the echocardiographic assessment of the right heart in adults: a report from the American Society of Echocardiography endorsed by the European Association of Echocardiography, a registered branch of the European Society of Cardiology, and the Canadian Society of Echocardiography. J Am Soc Echocardiogr. 2010;23(7):685-713;quiz 786-8.
25. Jardin F, Dubourg O, Guéret P, Delorme G, Bourdarias JP. Quantitative two-dimensional echocardiography in massive pulmonary embolism: emphasis on ventricular interdependence and leftward septal displacement. J Am Coll Cardiol. 1987;10(6):1201-6.
26. Hüttemann E. Transoesophageal echocardiography in critical care. Minerva Anestesiol. 2006;72(11):891-913.
27. Wyler von Ballmoos M, Takala J, Roeck M, Porta F, Tueller D, Ganter CC, et al. Pulse-pressure variation and hemodynamic response in patients with elevated pulmonary artery pressure: a clinical study. Crit Care. 2010;14(3):R111.
28. Meluzin J, Spinarova L, Bakala J, Toman J, Krejci J, Hude P, et al. Pulsed Doppler tissue imaging of the velocity of tricuspid annular systolic motion; a new, rapid, and non-invasive method of evaluating right ventricular systolic function. Eur Heart J. 2001;22(4):340-8.
29. Mitchell C, Peter A, Lori A, Canaday B, Finstuen JA, Foster MC, et al. Guidelines for performing a comprehensive transthoracic echocardiographic examination in adults: recommendations from the American Society of Echocardiography. Echocardiography. 2015;32(6):966-74.
30. Daudel F, Tüller D, Krähenbühl S, Jakob SM, Takala J. Pulse pressure variation and volume responsiveness during acutely increased pulmonary artery pressure: an experimental study. Crit Care. 2010;14(3):R122.
31. Kang DK, Thilo C, Schoepf UJ, Barraza JM Jr, Nance JW Jr, Bastarrika G, et al. CT signs of right ventricular dysfunction: prognostic role in acute pulmonary embolism. JACC Cardiovasc Imaging. 2011;4(8):841-9.
32. Gattinoni L, Carlesso E, Langer T. Clinical review: extracorporeal membrane oxygenation. Crit Care. 2011;15(6):243.
33. Ventetuolo CE, Klinger JR. Management of acute right ventricular failure in the intensive care unit. Ann Am Thorac Soc. 2014;11(5):811-22.
34. Price LC, Wort SJ, Finney SJ, Marino PS, Brett SJ. Pulmonary vascular and right ventricular dysfunction in adult critical care: Current and emerging options for management: a systematic literature review. Crit Care. 2010;14(5):R169.
35. Radermacher P, Santak B, Wüst HJ, Tarnow J, Falke KJ. Prostacyclin and right ventricular function in patients with pulmonary hypertension associated with ARDS. Intensive Care Med. 1990;6(4):227-32.
36. Muzaffar S, Shukla N, Angelini GD, Jeremy JY. Inhaled prostacyclin is safe, effective, and affordable in patients with pulmonary hypertension, right-heart dysfunction, and refractory hypoxemia after cardiothoracic surgery. J Thorac Cardiovasc Surg. 2004;128(6):949-50.
37. Vachiery JL, Huez S, Gillies H, Layton G, Hayashi N, Gao X, et al. Safety, tolerability and pharmacokinetics of an intravenous bolus of sildenafil in patients with pulmonary arterial hypertension. Br J Clin Pharmacol. 2011;71(2):289-92.
38. Pitsiou G, Paspala A, Bagalas V, Stanopoulos I. Inhaled iloprost plus levosimendan to decompensate right heart failure due to chronic thromboembolic pulmonary hypertension. Anaesth Intensive Care. 2013;41(4):554-6.
39. Shekerdemian L, Bohn D. Cardiovascular effects of mechanical ventilation. Arch Dis Child. 1999;80(5):475-80.
40. Mekontso Dessap A, Charron C, Devaquet J, Aboab J, Jardin F, Brochard L, et al. Impact of acute hypercapnia and augmented positive end-expiratory pressure on right ventricle function in severe acute respiratory distress syndrome. Intensive Care Med. 2009;35(11):1850-8.
41. Tiruvoipati R, Botha JA, Pilcher D, Bailey M. Carbon dioxide clearance in critical care. Anaesth Intensive Care. 2013;41(2):157-62.
42. Maggio P, Hemmila M, Haft J, Bartlett R. Extracorporeal life support for massive pulmonary embolism. J Trauma. 2007;62(3):570-6.
43. Gregoric ID, Chandra D, Myers TJ, Scheinin SA, Loyalka P, Kar B. Extracorporeal membrane oxygenation as a bridge to emergency heart-lung transplantation in a patient with idiopathic pulmonary arterial hypertension. J Heart Lung Transplant. 2008;27(4):466-8.
44. Mydin M, Berman M, Klein A, Tsui S, Dunning J, Valchanov K, et al. Extracorporeal membrane oxygenation as a bridge to pulmonary endarterectomy. Ann Thorac Surg. 2011;92(5):e101-3.
45. Moazami N, Pasque MK, Moon MR, Herren RL, Bailey MS, Lawton JS, et al. Mechanical support for isolated right ventricular failure in patients after cardiotomy. J Heart Lung Transplant. 2004;23(12):1371-5.
46. Strueber M, Hoeper MM, Fischer S, Cypel M, Warnecke G, Gottlieb J, et al. Bridge to thoracic organ transplantation in patients with pulmonary arterial hypertension using a pumpless lung assist device. Am J Transplant. 2009;9(4):853-7.

SECTION

Supporting the Cardiovascular System

CHAPTER

Fluid Therapy in Shock

Ruchira Wasudeo Khasne, Atul Prabhakar Kulkarni

INTRODUCTION

Shock is defined as a life-threatening, generalized form of acute circulatory failure associated within adequate oxygen utilization by the cells. It is a state of cellular and tissue hypoxia due to reduced oxygen delivery and/or increased oxygen consumption or inadequate oxygen utilization with increased blood lactate levels.[1,2] Quick identification of the condition, and initiation of prompt treatment, i.e., treatment of the cause, fluid therapy, vasopressors, and inotropic agents based on the pathophysiology of shock; plays a pivotal role in improving the outcomes of these patients.

It was more than a half-century ago Max Harry Weil emphasized the role of fluids in shock by gauging objective changes in a patient's clinical condition, such as blood pressure, mental alertness, urine output, peripheral venous filling, and texture of the skin.[3] Intravenous (IV) fluid therapy continues to be one of the first-line therapies to improve patient outcomes when used appropriately. Fluids should be prescribed similarly to any "drug therapy" as both hypovolemia and hypervolemia, are equally harmful.[2] Fluids should be administered as per the phase of acute illness as the hemodynamic status of the patient keeps changing based on the stage of shock. The clinical course of circulatory shock consists of our phases and each phase has different goals of fluid therapy. Two such acronyms describing stages of shock are "ROSE" (Resuscitation, Optimization, Stabilization, and Evacuation),[4] and "SOSD" (Salvage, Optimization, Stabilization, and De-escalation).[1] The concept of fluid stewardship similar to antibiotic stewardship has also been described with the acronym "4 Ds (Four Ds)" (Drug, Dosing, Duration, and De-escalation).[5] All these proposed models point toward a new paradigm in fluid therapy in shock.

PATHOPHYSIOLOGICAL MECHANISMS OF SHOCK[6]

Shock is primarily categorized into four main subtypes: (1) Hypovolemic, (2) cardiogenic, (3) obstructive type, and (4) distributive. At times, the patient may present with a mixed feature with overlapping characteristics. Irrespective of the etiology, the first response of the intensivist when confronted with a patient in shock is to administer an IV fluid bolus. After initially targeting the gross changes in the hemodynamic parameters, the downstream parameters such as lactate and central venous oxygen saturation ($ScvO_2$), can be used to fine-tune the therapy. A detailed discussion about the pathophysiology is beyond the scope of this chapter and can be found in the other chapters in this textbook. We will also not discuss the assessment of fluid responsiveness, as this has been described in detail elsewhere in this book. We will just mention here that the fluid status assessment is based on the "Frank–Starling and Phillip–Marik curves" and the concept of mean systemic filling pressure (Pmsf).[7]

IMPORTANT TERMINOLOGIES IN FLUID THERAPY[4]

- *Resuscitation:* Fluid is administered as a part of the immediate management of life-threatening conditions associated with impaired tissue perfusion.
- *Titration:* Adjustment of type, rate, and amount of fluid based upon context to achieve optimization of tissue perfusion.
- *De-escalation:* Either minimization of fluid administration or mobilization of extravascular fluid to optimize fluid balance.
- *Fluid bolus:* Infusion of a relatively large volume of fluid typically includes the infusion of at least 500 mL over a maximum of 15 minutes to correct absolute or relative fluid deficit rapidly as rescue.[4,8]

- *Fluid challenge:* Standard fluid challenge is when 300–500 mL of fluid is infused over a short period of time (10–15 minutes) to challenge the cardiovascular system and assess the volume response. Inherently it is associated with the risk of fluid overload. Mini-fluid challenge is when a small volume of fluid, (typically 100 mL over 10 minutes) mini-fluid challenge but it requires a very precise measurement of cardiac output (CO).[7]
- *Maintenance fluid therapy:* Fluid administration for the provision of fluids for those who cannot meet their needs by oral route. This should be titrated to patient needs and context and should include the replacement of ongoing losses. In a patient without ongoing losses, this should probably be no >1–2 mL/kg/h.
- *Daily fluid balance:* Daily sum of all intake sand outputs without inclusion of insensible losses. It can be neutral, positive, or negative.
- *Cumulative fluid balance:* The sum total of fluid accumulation over a period of time spent in the intensive care unit (ICU).
- *Fluid accumulation:* It is defined as positive fluid balance with or without associated fluid overload.
- *Fluid overload:* It refers to excess total body water (TBW) content associated with edema formation. This term should be avoided.[9] It is the percentage of fluid accumulation as defined by dividing the cumulative fluid balance in liters by the patient's baseline body weight and multiplying by 100%. A value of 10% as the cutoff value is associated with adverse outcomes.[10]
- *Hypervolemia:* It indicates an excess circulating blood volume where mean systemic circulatory pressure is high, leading to a net fluid loss into the interstitium resulting in edema formation.[9]
- *Hypovolemia:* It refers to a low intravascular blood volume where mean systemic filling pressure is low. There is a net flux of water and electrolytes out of the interstitial and tissue spaces and into the blood stream to support blood volume. But ultimately there is decreased in tissue rigidity and loss of vascular reserve.[9]
- *Testing for fluid responsiveness (FR):* The ideal test for fluid responsiveness will reversibly increase the preload of the heart, and we can assess if there is a significant increase in cardiac output. If this is not possible, the test should predict if the patient will respond to fluid administration by increasing cardiac output, before fluid is administered. The tests based on static indices do not help measure of fluid responsiveness based on static indices such as end-diastolic ventricular volume, area, and diameter LV end-diastolic pressure, and inferior vena cava (IVC) size, which are not very useful, apart from not being reversible. Dynamic indices, i.e., the tests based on heart-lung interaction such as stroke volume variation, pulse pressure variation, aortic blood flow measurement, with velocity time integral (VTI) change, end-expiratory occlusion test (at the end of 0.1 second), tidal volume challenge test, are better for this purpose; however, most of these can only be used in patients who are on controlled mechanical ventilation with a tidal volume >8 mL/kg body weight. Most of these tests also need continuous real-time and accurate measurement of CO.
- *Fluid tolerance:* A degree to which a patient can tolerate the administration of fluids without causation of organ dysfunction.
- *Venous excess ultrasound score (VeXUS):* VeXUS has a promising utility in identifying the end-point of resuscitation, and the onset of fluid congestion and facilitating the initiation of deresuscitation based on a diagnosis of venous congestion by point-of-care ultrasound. Those include the IVC and venous Doppler assessment of the hepatic vein, portal, splenic, interlobar renal, and femoral veins. The degree of congestion is rated in each vein to quantify a VExUS grading and severity is assessed.[11]

IMMEDIATE EVALUATION AND MANAGEMENT

The most common sign of shock is hypotension, though it may not always be the first sign. IV fluids are the mainstay of treatment. IV fluids are useful not only in hypovolemic and septic shock but may be of help in cardiogenic as well as obstructive shock. Identification of the problem, and mechanism of shock with or without mixed pathophysiology is really challenging and is necessary to determine the appropriate treatment strategy. Initial fluid therapy improves microvascular blood flow by increasing preload, stroke volume (SV) and thus the CO. This helps in preserving organ perfusion. Apart from clinical assessment, transthoracic echocardiographic assessment of cardiac function helps to plan further management. A systematic approach to the management of shock can be described by the mnemonic "VIP."[12]

- Ventilation (adequate pulmonary CO_2 and O_2 exchange)

- Infusion (fluids, blood, and electrolyte balance)
- Pumping (restoration of cardiac competence).

A postscript of "PS" has been added to VIP: "P" stands for pharmacological treatment of shock in the form of vasoactive agents, while "S" denotes the specific treatment of the cause. This may include but is not limited to control of bleeding in hypovolemic shock, immediate percutaneous coronary intervention for acute coronary syndromes causing cardiogenic chock, thrombolysis or embolectomy for massive pulmonary embolism leading to obstructive shock, and implementation of sepsis bundle in the form of administration of antibiotics and source control in case of septic shock.

Fluid balance should be meticulously maintained as hypovolemia leads to reduced tissue perfusion, renal failure, anastomotic leaks, risk of cerebrovascular accident (CVA), splanchnic ischemia, and multiorgan failure (MOF). Hypervolemia can cause tissue edema, intra-abdominal hypertension (IAH), respiratory failure, impaired healing, altered mobilization, and MOF.[13] Fluid therapy should be individualized and implemented strategically as per four phases in the treatment of shock, e.g., ROSD/SOSD/ROSE. **Flowchart 1** describes the approach to a patient with hemodynamic compromise. The aim is to restore and maintain intravascular volume at near physiological levels. Simultaneously attempts should be made to find out the cause. Always ask whether intervention is needed by looking for signs of hypoperfusion, worsening hemodynamic parameters, worsening lactates, and skin mottling.

If the answer is NO, watchful waiting with meticulous reassessment is needed.

But if the answer is YES, a multimodal resuscitation strategy is adopted which includes fluid administration,

Flowchart1: Assessment of a patient with hemodynamic compromise.

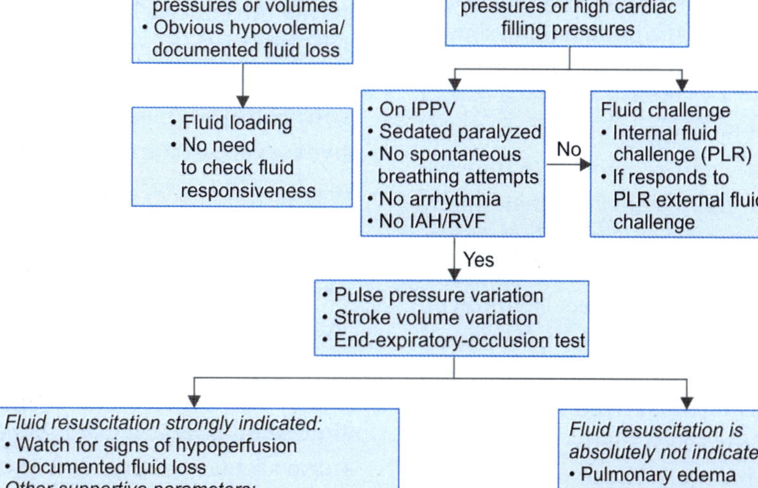

(AKI: acute kidney injury; CVP: central venous pressure; IAH: intra-abdominal hypertension; IPPV: intermittent positive pressure ventilation; MAP: mean arterial pressure; PLR: passive leg raising; RVF: right ventricular failure)

assessment of fluid responsiveness, simultaneous inotropic and/or vasopressor therapy. The patient should be reassessed periodically and after each bolus. Ideally, fluid responsiveness should be looked for before performing volume expansion by tests such as passive leg raising (PLR) test and end-expiratory occlusion test (EEOT).[14]

RATIONAL FOR EARLY FLUID VERSUS EARLY VASOPRESSORS IN SEPTIC SHOCK

Sepsis/septic shock produces a dual metabolic response. There is generalized endothelial injury due to the direct effect of initial cytokines and stress hormones, which leads to the loss of capillary endothelial barrier function called the "ebb phase." It is a hyperdynamic stage characterized by vasodilatation with severe absolute or relative hypovolemia with transcapillary albumin leak resulting in decreased plasma colloid oncotic pressure. This stage has traditionally been treated with large-volume fluid resuscitation for volume expansion. As per Surviving Sepsis Campaign guidelines (SSG), fluid administration at the dose of 30 mL/kg should be given within the first 3 hours.[15] However, the 3-hour duration has been criticized recently, as per the updated Surviving Sepsis Campaign (SSC) bundle which states that fluid administration should begin within the first hour, which is still suboptimal.[10,15]

In fact, giving 500 mL to 1 L of fluid over a short period (definitely <1 hour) should be considered.[13] Thus, fluids should be administered early and generously to improve microcirculation. However, this volume expansion may result in extravascular movement of water, electrolytes, and proteins, leading to organ edema, causing tissue hypoperfusion and hypoxia. This phase is followed by a "flow phase" a balance of equilibrium between proinflammatory and anti-inflammatory reactions and a balance is achieved. It is characterized by increased CO, mobilization of the third space fluids, and diuresis leading to negative fluid balance. Those patients who spontaneously transit from the "ebb phase " to the "flow phase" have a good outcome. For those who fail to enter the "flow phase" spontaneously, deresuscitation becomes complex. In this situation, conservative fluid management and late goal-directed fluid removal (LGFR) should be considered to achieve accumulative negative fluid balance.[10]

Additionally, early use of vasopressors and their combination with smaller amounts of IV fluids in fluid-responsive hypotensive septic shock patients seems to be a safe strategy. It should be preferably implemented in the first hour after diagnosis of septic shock which ultimately reduces the third spacing of fluids and is found to be associated with lower morbidity and mortality in septic patients. Thus, vasopressor therapy should be initiated as soon as possible in patients with septic shock or when the diastolic pressure is <40 mm Hg.[16]

PHASES OF FLUID RESUSCITATION IN SEPTIC SHOCK

Similar to "antibiotic stewardship" in sepsis patients, it is suggested that the time has come to implement "fluid stewardship" in the form of "4 Ds". Thus, the concept of "Four Ds" of fluid therapy, i.e., drug, duration, dosing, and de-escalation has been put forth. It should be implemented in conjunction with fluid strategies "ROSE."[5] "Three hit" model and extended "four hit" model explain the dynamic phases of stages of fluid administration in shock.[7,9]

- *4Ds of fluid therapy:* We must take into account the 4Ds of fluid therapy and these should be modified as per changes in patients' dynamics; to restore microcirculation.[8]
- *Drug:* Fluids are categorized as crystalloids or colloids, terms introduced by Thomas Graham (Professor of Chemistry, University College London, 1836–1855). Various fluids such as crystalloids (saline or buffered salt solutions), and colloids [human albumin, hydroxyethyl starch (HES), dextran, gelatin] are available but uncertainty still exists regarding the safety of different types of fluids. Trials comparing colloids versus crystalloids are as per **Table 1**. It is important to use appropriate fluids considering the risk factors, net fluid balance, risk of capillary leak, source control, and organ function. Choose the fluids correctly as per the patient's clinical condition, e.g., glucose-containing fluid should not be used for resuscitation to correct intravascular volume deficit or acute hypovolemia. The long-standing debate on crystalloids and colloids (appropriate) should now change to "crystalloids alone versus crystalloids plus colloids."[13] Excessive crystalloid infusions can lead to abdominal compartment syndrome (ACS). Whenever large volumes of fluids are needed, the SSG suggests the addition of albumin to crystalloids. Fluid therapy should be initiated promptly to immediately restabilize microcirculation. It should be delivered in an early, "goal-directed manner" and targeted to the physiologic needs of individual patients.

TABLE 1: Trials comparing colloids versus crystalloids.[18-20]

Population	*Outcomes*	*Results*	*Implications*
Hydroxyethyl starch (HES) or saline for fluid resuscitation in Billot L et al. Intensive Care. 2012[18]	• HES group mortality is 18.0% (597 of 3,315 patients) compared to in the saline group it is 17.0% (566 of 3,336) with (relative risk in the HES group, 1.06; 95% CI, 0.96–1.18; $p = 0.26$) • *Need for RRT:* More number of patients in the HES group needed RRT [235 of 3,352 patients (7.0%) in the HES group and 196 of 3,375 (5.8%) in the saline group (relative risk, 1.21; 95% CI, 1.00–1.45; $p = 0.04$)]	90-day mortality, renal failure, renal injury, and need for RRT is high in patients resuscitated with 6% HES (130/0.4) compared to saline	HES causes more harm compared to saline
804 patients with severe sepsis/ septic shock in ICUs (Denmark, Norway, Finland, and Iceland, 2012). Perner A et al. Scandinavian 6S[21]	• *Renal injury:* In HES 34.6% and saline group 38.0% of patients, respectively ($p = 0.005$) • *Renal failure:* In HES 10.4% and saline group 9.2% of patients, respectively ($p = 0.12$). • More adverse events in HES 4.6% in saline group 3.3%, ($p = 0.006$)		HES should not be given to adults with sepsis; HES still linked to adverse outcomes despite the use of a "safer" formulation
	6% HES (130/0.42) to a maximum of 33 mL/kg daily then RL while in ICU until 90 days after enrolment versus RL only. *Composite outcome:* Death or ESRD at 90 days after randomization, need for RRT	HES associated with an increased risk of composite outcome and with an increased proportion of patients requiring RRT	
Meta-analysis of colloids versus crystalloids in critically ill trauma and surgical patients (Qureshi et al. Br J Surg. 2016)[22]	• A systematic review of 59 RCTs with 16,889 patients colloids particularly starches are nephrotoxic, increase the risk of developing AKI, requiring RRT in 9 trials, 11,648 patients; OR 1.35, 1.17–1.57 in patients with sepsis • In 32 trials involving 16,647 patients, colloid for volume replacement does not have any impact on the increase in mortality OR 0.99, 95% CI 0.92–1.06	On subgroup analyses, they demonstrated that pentastarch increases the risk of mortality and the need for RRT primarily. [Mortality (OR 1.47, 1.08–2.02; I2 = 0%). And the need for RRT (OR 1.98,1.35–2.90; I2 = 0%)] whereas the use of tetrastarch is associated with AKI as well as RRT [AKI (OR 1.16, 95% CI 1.01–1.32; I2 = 31%). And the need for RRT (OR 1.27, 1.08–1.50; I2 = 0%)]	These adverse effects are more commonly seen in critically ill patients with sepsis but not in patients with traumatic injuries or as compared to crystalloid, those undergoing nontrauma surgery

(AKI: acute kidney injury; CI: confidence interval; ICU: intensive care unit; RRT: renal replacement therapy; ESRD: end-stage renal disease; OR: odds ratio; RCT: randomized controlled trial; RL: Ringer's lactate; RRT: renal replacement therapy)

Colloids have large molecular weights and they are associated with a modest volume-sparing effect with intravascular expansion ratios of around 1:1.4. One meta-analysis found that in order to meet some targets, a larger volume of crystalloid is required and that the amount required can be reduced by one-third if colloids were given in addition to crystalloids. [Estimated crystalloids/colloids ratio of 1.5 (1.36–1.65)][17] achieve hemodynamic stability faster, stay in circulation longer, with less positive fluid balance, and less amount of edema. However, there is no robust evidence against/for the use of colloids.

Studies such as FIRST (Fluids in Resuscitation of Severe Trauma),[23] BaSES (Basel Starch Evaluation in Sepsis[24] and CRISTAL trials)[21] have not demonstrated any increase in harm with the use of HES compared with crystalloid. CRISTAL suggests the benefits of colloids over crystalloids but the nonblinded nature increases the risk of bias. However, most of the evidence still supports crystalloids.[23] A recent Cochrane review (including 78 trials) concluded that evidence does not support the use of colloids as a resuscitation fluid in terms of mortality in trauma, burns, and postoperative patients. In fact, the use of HES may increase mortality. In addition to that colloids are expensive compared to crystalloids. Thus, its use in ICU is not justified.[21]

Among colloids, HES has been studied the most, and the evidence does not support its use in septic shock. In the CHEST trial[18] tetrastarch, compared to 0.9 NS, was associated with increased acute kidney injury (AKI) and needed for renal replacement therapy (RRT) while in the 6S trial[19] compared to Ringer's acetate, starches led to increased mortality. Evidence suggests that the renal toxicity of starches is related to their storage in tubular cells (osmotic nephrosis) but the data remain controversial. RCTs have confirmed that in patients with septic shock, HES is associated with increased rates of AKI and the need for RRT, and thereby increased mortality in sepsis patients.[25]

Besides that, HES has been shown to be associated with coagulopathy and an increased need for blood transfusions.[26] The renal effect seems to be dose-dependent, but no consensus has been reached as to a safe dose of HES. Thus, there is no indication for the routine use of colloids, except albumin over crystalloids.[27] **Table 1** discusses about trials comparing crystalloids and colloids.[18]

The Food and Drug Administration (FDA) added serious new warnings to HES products but fell short of the European Medicines Agency recommendation. They posted a few recommendations in June 2013 to restrict the use of HES solutions. FDA concluded that "HES solutions should not be used in critically ill adult patients, including patients with sepsis and those admitted to the ICU, and a boxed warning to include the risk of mortality and severe renal injury is warranted." The SSG specifically recommends *not* to use HES in patients with septic shock.

There are additional recommendations from the FDA that emphasize that HES should not be used in critically ill adult patients, including those with sepsis, and those with preexisting renal dysfunction. Additional recommendations from the FDA include:

- Do not use HES solutions in critically ill adult patients, including those with sepsis, and those admitted to the ICU.
- Avoid use in patients with preexisting renal dysfunction.
- Discontinue the use of HES at the first sign of renal injury.
- Need for RRT has been reported up to 90 days after HES administration. Continue to monitor renal function for at least 90 days in all patients.
- Avoid use in patients undergoing open heart surgery in association with cardiopulmonary bypass due to excess bleeding.
- Discontinue use of HES at the first sign of coagulopathy.

Human albumin is a natural colloid, appears safe, has volume expansion effects, and may have beneficial effects in patients with septic shock and those with spontaneous bacterial peritonitis or other bacterial infections. But evidence does not support the benefit of the use of albumin as a resuscitation fluid.[20] Albumin has not been shown to reduce the rate of RRT or improve survival in critically ill patients. Besides that, it is expensive and has a limited shelf life. The results from the SAFE study, a multicenter randomized controlled trial (mRCT) in Australasia (6,997 patients), suggest that fluid resuscitation with either 4% albumin showed that it is safe to use.[28] A more detailed subgroup analysis of patients with septic shock of the SAFE study participants found that albumin did not increase the incidence of renal impairment or other organ failures. Also, there was a trend toward improved outcomes in patients who were given albumin [adjusted odds ratio (OR) for death for albumin versus saline was 0.71 (95% CI: 0.52–0.97; $p = 0.03$)].[28]

The ALBIOS trial in 1,800 patients with sepsis and septic shock, analyzed the efficacy of crystalloid with and without administration of 20% albumin to maintain serum albumin >30 g/L for 28 days or discharge whichever was earlier. In the initial phase, fluids were administered according to early goal-directed therapy. There was no improvement in survival at 28 days in the albumin group. In patients with septic shock, there was a trend toward improved survival at 28 days (RR of death, 0.87; 95% CI 0.77–0.99). The study had several limitations, it did not many enroll patients with early sepsis/septic shock, used a higher concentration of albumin (20% compared to 4% in the SAFE study) and the goal was to maintain serum albumin levels over 30 g/L and not resuscitation.[20] SSC 2021 guidelines suggest that whenever excessive crystalloid administration is required, switching to albumin administration is an alternative.[29]

Not much evidence is available regarding the benefit or harm of gelatins in critically ill patients. Gelatin is a synthetic colloid associated with an increased risk of osmosis nephrosis-induced AKI with gelatin. A systematic review by Thomas-Ruddell and colleagues comparing gelatins with albumin and crystalloids found that the trials included were generally small (10–250 patients), and involved a heterogeneous population, such as those in the perioperative period and (very few) critically ill patients. Many trials lasted for <24 hours. The authors suggested that we should wait before using gelatins till their safety and efficacy are established in clinical practice.[30] The same group of investigators published another systematic review and meta-analysis which included a total of 60 studies comparing gelatins, crystalloids, and other colloids. There was an increased risk of mortality, AKI, need for new RRT, blood transfusion, and anaphylaxis. The authors advised to be cautious in using gelatins till evidence of the safety of gelatins was available.[31]

Dextran solutions have been almost entirely abandoned. However, uncertainty remains regarding the clinical risks and benefits of other colloids from the available evidence.[22]

CRYSTALLOIDS

Evidence suggests that different crystalloid solutions have varying effects on various organ systems. Whether these effects cause deleterious effects such as acid-base disturbance, electrolyte imbalance, coagulation abnormality, renal vasoconstriction, and hepatic dysfunction, and affect outcomes in the critically ill is unclear.[32]

Normal saline (0.9% sodium chloride solution, NS) a chloride-rich solution, is the most commonly used IV fluid. Rapid, high-volume infusion of NS causes hyperchloremic metabolic acidosis, increased risk of AKI, and worsened outcomes in susceptible patients. But firm evidence is lacking.[33]

In a before and after study by Yunos et al. chloride-restrictive strategy was associated with a significant decrease in the incidence of AKI and use of RRT.[34] On extended assessment of the effects of restriction of chloride-rich fluids; the author observed that overall, there is a decrease in the incidence of AKI and RRT requirement in the period in which chloride restrictive strategy was adopted. However, the possibility of the presence of some unidentified confounders or a Hawthorne effect cannot be ruled out which favored chloride-restricted strategy.[35]

The risk of hyperchloremia is reduced with the use of balanced/buffered salt (BSS) solutions in which chloride content is reduced and other cations and anions are added to the solution.[27] Rapid or high-volume infusion of BSS can result in metabolic alkalosis. Because of their hypotonic nature; they are contraindicated in patients with acute brain injury; because of their potential to cause or worsen cerebral edema.

As per a recent international cross-sectional study, BSS are increasingly the preferred fluids of choice for resuscitation.[36] **Table 2** discusses about the details of the trials comparing the crystalloids. The recent RCTs SMART "Isotonic Solutions and Major Adverse Renal Events Trial"[37] and SALT-ED[38] "Saline against Lactated Ringer's or Plasma-Lyte in the Emergency Department" compared buffered crystalloids such as PlasmaLyte A and Ringer's lactate (RL) versus 0.9% NA showed that saline solutions are associated with an increase in major adverse kidney events a composite of death, new RRT, or persistent renal dysfunction. When clinical effects of BSS and saline are compared in noncritically ill patients care mainly outside ICU in the emergency department there is a lower incidence of major adverse kidney events within 30 days with BSS compared to the saline group (4.7% vs. 5.6%; adjusted OR, 0.82; 95% CI: 0.70–0.95; $p = 0.01$).[38] Whereas in critically ill adults these solutions are compared, BSS resulted in a lower rate of the composite outcome of death from any cause, new RRT, or persistent renal dysfunction than the use of saline.[37] The major adverse kidney event (14.3%) with BSS compared with (15.4%) in the saline group [marginal OR, 0.91; 95% confidence interval (CI), 0.84–0.99; conditional OR, 0.90; 95% CI, 0.82–0.99; $p = 0.04$]. In-hospital 30 days mortality was 10.3% in the BSS group and 11.1% in the saline group ($p = 0.06$). The incidence of new RRT is 2.5% with BSS compared to the saline group 2.9% ($p = 0.08$), and the incidence of persistent renal dysfunction is 6.4% with BSS and 6.6% with the saline group respectively ($p = 0.60$). Adverse kidney events are less common with BSS compared to 0.9% NS.

The Balanced Solutions in Intensive Care Study (BaSICS), a multicenter, double-blind, factorial design

TABLE 2: Trials comparing crystalloids.[37,38,41]

Population	*Treatment arms*	*Outcomes*	*Results*	*Implications*
• SMART "Isotonic Solutions and Major Adverse Renal Events Trial" compared • Balanced crystalloids versus saline in critically ill adults.[37] 15,802 adults treated with crystalloid open-label, multiple-cluster crossover randomized single-center trial. N Engl J Med. 2018 (USA)	• RCTs • Buffered crystalloid (Plasma LyteA or RL) versus normal saline	Major adverse kidney events (MAKE, a composite of death, dialysis, or doubling of baseline creatinine concentration) censored at 30 days: MAKE30	Reduced incidence of MAKE30 in a buffered crystalloid group (NNT 99); reduced in-hospital mortality in the buffered crystalloid group ($p = 0.06$)	Adverse kidney events are less common with buffered crystalloids than with saline
• SALT-ED balanced crystalloids versus saline in noncritically ill adults[38] • 13,347 adults treated with crystalloid in a single emergency department, hospitalized outside ICU • Open-label, multiple-cluster cross-over single-center randomized trial. N Eng l J Med. 2018 (USA)	Buffered crystalloid (Plasma LyteA or RL) versus normal saline	Hospital-free days (days alive after discharge before day 28)	No difference in hospital-free days; lower incidence of MAKE30 in the buffered crystalloid group	Adverse kidney events are less common with buffered crystalloids than with saline
• SPLIT trial[41] • Effect of a buffered crystalloid solution versus saline on AKI 2,278 patients admitted to ICUs requiring crystalloid fluid therapy Cluster cross-over trial conducted as pilot study JAMA. 2015 (New Zealand)	Buffered crystalloid (PlasmaLyte 148) versus normal saline	Proportion of patients with AKI (doubling of SCr or baseline SCr 3.96 mg/dL with an increase of 0.5 mg/dL)	No difference in the incidence of AKI cluster	High proportion of elective surgical patients and relatively small volumes of study fluids were used; however, this provides justification for a larger phase III randomized trial in a high-risk population

(RC: Ringer's lactate; NNT: number needed to treat; AKI: acute kidney injury)

RCT conducted in 75 ICUs ($n = 11{,}052$) critically ill patients (48% elective surgery) requiring fluid resuscitation having at least one risk factor for AKI. They were randomized to PlasmaLyte or saline. They observed that contrary to the SMART and SALT-ED trials, Plasma-Lyte did not result in a reduction in 90-day mortality and RRT receipt compared with saline.[39]

Similarly, the Plasma-Lyte 148 versus Saline (PLUS) study,[40] double-blinded RCT was conducted in 53 ICUs in Australia and New Zealand ($n = 5{,}037$) critically ill patients (42% elective surgery). In contrast to previous studies in this study, a larger amount of volume was received (4 L in 6 days), (2.9 L in the BaSICS trial, 2 L in the SPLIT trial, and 1 L in the SMART and SALT-ED trials). They showed the same findings as the BaSICS trial that the administration of a balanced solution did not result in a reduction in 90-day mortality compared with saline.

The SPLIT trial,[41] a cluster RCT, conducted in four New Zealand ICUs, where mainly postoperative patients were included, failed to show any advantage of BSS (Plasmalyte 148®) over NS. However, the amount of fluid infused was <2 L in the entire ICU stay (also <2 days).

Ringer's lactate solution (also called Hartmann's solution) is also not free from criticism. It is hypotonic in nature and should be avoided particularly in patients with neurologic injury. Nonlactate solutions such as Plasmalyte®solution, contain acetate, which may have its own adverse effects. It may cause supraphysiological plasma concentrations of acetate when used as a priming fluid in cardiopulmonary bypass. Even on dialysis, acetate fluid baths may lead to a decrease in myocardial contractility, thus bicarbonate dialysis baths have been preferred for ages. Yet it is still unclear whether such a small amount of acetate present in Plasma-Lyte®

as a resuscitation fluid will also have similar potentially harmful effects. Both 0.9% NS and BSS are feasible choices until some we get some robust evidence.

There is no strong evidence comparing different BSS and the advantage of one BSS over the other. The effects of these nonphysiological concentrations of anions present in BSS are currently unknown.

Dosing: Similar to antibiotics, the pharmacokinetic and pharmacodynamic of fluids and even toxicity profile, e.g., evidence of HES to cause AKI should be considered.

Duration: Fluids should be continued for appropriate duration and preferably should be stopped once shock is resolved and normalization of lactates. Similar to antibiotics, although there is no strong evidence for this, attempts should be made to minimize the duration of fluid therapy. Fluids should not be used to treat low central venous pressure (CVP), or mean arterial pressure (MAP) but to treat shock.

De-escalation: Similar to antibiotic de-escalation (an important component of antibiotic stewardship) fluids should be de-escalated after stabilization with early adequate goal-directed fluid management (EAFM), normalization of lactates, pulse pressure variation (PPV), and CO.

STAGES OF FLUID ADMINISTRATION IN SHOCK

SOSD (Vincent), and a "4 hit model" (Malbrain), should be adopted as strategies of fluid administration, its therapeutic goals, and monitoring which should be adopted as per the time course of phases of septic shock.[1,10] During the first three stages, fluids are administered in the form of resuscitation, maintenance, and then as a replacement however, in the fourth stage, the last stage, fluids need to be actively removed aiming for net negative fluid balance.

A meta-analysis of 3 RCTs comparing early goal-directed therapy (proposed by Rivers et al. in 2000), in sepsis/septic shock with protocolized directed resuscitation to achieve $ScvO_2$ >70%, with usual care found no difference in outcomes. We have to keep in mind that in all three RCTs, the baseline $ScvO_2$ was already >70% in the control group, therefore the intervention was unlikely to improve outcomes.[42]

CLASSIC (Conservative versus Liberal Approach to Fluid Therapy of Septic Shock in Intensive Care) study, a multinational, multicentre RCT aimed to evaluate two fluid management strategies in early septic shock after the initial resuscitation phase. In the restrictive fluid group, fluid boluses were given only if signs of hypoperfusion were present, and in the standard group, fluid therapy was entirely directed by the clinical teams. There was no difference in terms of 90-day mortality, incidence of severe AKI, or days alive without organ support in the two groups. The authors suggested that a restrictive approach is feasible in this patient group.[43]

Salvage or Rescue (Resuscitation Phase) (First Hit) (Table 3)

After an initial inflammatory insult leading to shock, there is a beginning of the "Ebb" phase. This first hit occurs within minutes and is life-threatening. This stage is associated with convective problems of oxygen transport to get into the tissues due to severe hypovolemia and impairment of microcirculation. Fluids should be administered generously to facilitate effective resuscitation in the form of "boluses" whenever there is low MAP, low CO, increased lactate, low left ventricular end-diastolic area index (LVEDAI), low global ejection fraction (GEF)/global end-diastolic volume index (GEDVI), high PPV, and positive PLR or EEOT. Frequent fluid challenges with assessment/re-assessment of ongoing fluid requirements should be the strategy in

TABLE 3: Salvage or rescue phase.

Therapeutic goals	• Assess and treat the cause of instability through rapid assessment by echocardiography • The aim is to keep a positive fluid balance through early goal-directed fluid management (EAFM) to correct the shock
• Hemodynamic targets • Fluid therapy	• *Obtain minimum acceptable BP:* MAP 60–65 mm Hg • Isotonic crystalloid boluses • Fluids should be administered generously in the form of "boluses" • Consider albumin if the patient remains unstable, particularly in sepsis • Consider RBCs, blood products, and tranexamic acid (if obvious bleeding)
Additional treatments	• Start inotrope and/or vasopressor support • Consider damage control surgery if indicated • Retrospective observational studies found that delayed vasopressor initiation was associated with increased mortality in patients with septic shock[44]

this phase. With the aid of hemodynamic monitoring and, the application of dynamic indices of preload responsiveness, fluid administration can be guided, and the need for further fluid infusion should be decided. The clinical parameters such as heart rate, blood pressure, and urine output, for detection of hypovolemia are less sensitive and edema is a late sign of fluid overload.

Optimization Phase (Second Hit) (Table 4)

The main principle of this phase is organ rescue, by optimizing and maintaining tissue perfusion. In this phase, ischemia, reperfusion, and multiorgan dysfunction syndrome (MODS) can occur, which needs to be prevented. This stage can also be associated with "poly compartment syndrome" where two or more anatomical compartments have elevated compartmental pressures. This is a second hit that occurs within hours and is not life-threatening. Here "Ebb phase" turns into a "flow phase" and a risk of fluid overload remains. Hence questions should be asked when to stop fluid infusion and/or when there is any risk with giving further fluids. Thus, a limited amount of fluids should be administered with an ongoing frequent assessment of the patient's fluid status. As fluid accumulation is the biomarker of critical illness at this stage, high GEF/GEDVI, low PPV, negative PLR, positive daily fluid balance, and weight gain should be looked for and further fluids should be avoided. Fluid therapy should be cautiously titrated. Echocardiographic assessment of the degree of filling and cardiac function should be evaluated periodically to monitor the response to treatment. Besides that, the effectiveness of therapy and resolution of shock can be evaluated by serial measurement of blood lactate levels.[45]

TABLE 4: Optimization phase.

Therapeutic goals	• Improved organ perfusion improved alertness peripheral color temperature • Keep neutral fluid balance to maintain tissue perfusion
Hemodynamic targets	• Stage of compensated shock (but at high risk of decompensation) • Mean arterial pressure (MAP) >65 mm Hg • Cardiac index >2.2 L/min/m^2 urine output >0.5 mL/kg/h • Normalization of lactate (usually, <2 mmol/L)
• Fluid therapy • Additional treatments	• Isotonic crystalloid if required • Avoid fluid overload • Conservative use of "fluid challenges" and titrated to maintenance fluids • Ongoing frequent assessment of patient's fluid status • Continue inotrope and/or vasopressor support

Stabilization Phase (Second Hit) (Table 5)

This stage is referred to as the organ support stage or stage of homeostasis to minimize the complications, and it can last for days. This stage is characterized by the absence of shock or impending threat of shock. It focuses mainly on organ support, which may last for some days, where the oxygen transport is affected due to diffusion problems. Thus, fluid therapy should only be used as maintenance therapy and in the presence of normal fluid loss [renal, gastrointestinal (GI)] for replacement therapy. At this stage, fluid accumulation is the biomarker of critical illness. Thus, this stage aims for neutral or negative fluid balance. Various studies have documented that the persistence of positive fluid balance is associated with worsening outcomes. More precisely higher cumulative fluid balance at 72 hours after ICU admission but not during the first 24 hours is independently associated with an increase in the risk of death.[46]

Thus, minimal maintenance of fluids to keep zero or negative fluid balance by late conservative fluid management (LCFM). The hemodynamic targets in this stage are extravascular lung water (EVLWI) <10–12 mL/kg predicted body weight (PBW), pulmonary vascular permeability index (PVPI) <2.5, intra-abdominal pressure (IAP) <15 mm Hg, abdominal perfusion pressure (APP) >55 mm Hg, COP >16–18 mm Hg, and CLI <60. In addition to those biomarkers such as neutrophil gelatinase-associated lipocalin (NGAL), cystatin-C, citrulline, and

TABLE 5: Stabilization phase.

Therapeutic goals	• Similar to the optimization phase • Aim for neutral or negative fluid balance
• Hemodynamic targets • Fluid therapy	• Similar to the optimization phase • No impending threat of shock • Adopt a restrictive fluid strategy approach • Avoid additional fluid or blood products
Additional treatments	• Organ support as needed • Start enteral feeding (unless contraindicated) • Adopt a restrictive approach to oxygen

capillary leak markers such as colloid oncotic pressure (COP), osmolarity (OSM), capillary leak index (CLI), and renal leak index (RLI, i.e., urine albumin over creatinine ratio). RLI and daily cumulative fluid balance should be monitored. If hemodynamics permit fluid removal should be attempted, provided it is not associated with an increased need for vasopressor agents.

Evacuation Phase or Deescalation Stage (Third Hit) (Table 6)

It refers to a stage of global increased permeability syndrome (GIPS). This stage is a stage of organ recovery to mobilizes accumulated fluid and lasts for days to weeks. This stage is managed by restricted fluid administration. Once the patient turns from the second hit to the third hit there is either a recovery or spontaneous flow phase that begins with evacuation of excess of fluids or many of them fail to turn into the flow phase leading to GIPS. GIPS causes worsening of fluid accumulation due to capillary leak which worsens organ dysfunction. Efforts should be made for active fluid removal for days to weeks to support organ recovery by an LGFR strategy (deresuscitation). This stage is identified by increased IAH, EVLWI, high RLI [renal leak index (urine albumin over creatinine ratio)], and worsening of hypoxia. In this stage usually, the patients have recovered from the initial shock. At the bedside, EVLWI can be used as a safety guide to initiate a late conservative fluid management strategy or LGFR. Negative fluid balance is achieved by fluid unloading using either diuresis or fluid removal by ultrafiltration. Diuretics such as loop diuretics and furosemide can be administered if a negative fluid balance is not achieved spontaneously. These are widely used but can lead to hypernatremia if sodium excretion is not adequate and if associated renal dysfunction exists. If the diuretics are not effective, patients may need RRT. Care should be taken that RRT with ultrafiltration does not aggravate hypovolemia as it is difficult to monitor changes in blood volume during RRT.

TABLE 6: Evacuation phase or de-escalation stage.

Therapeutic goals	• Maintenance of parameters achieved during the stabilization phase • Maintain negative fluid balance • Simultaneous reduction of support
• Hemodynamic and other targets • Fluid therapy	• Normalization of parameters • Fluids mainly during food and drug dilution • Obtain negative fluid balance via spontaneous or diuretic-induced diuresis or ultrafiltration
Additional treatments	• Reduce intensity of organ support • Continue enteral feeding • Consider parenteral feeding if enteral goals are not met by day 5, or earlier if preexisting malnutrition

Objective assessment of organ congestion non-invasively by VExUS is an emerging practice. Grades of VExUS are:

- *Grade 0:* No sign of congestion in any organ
- *Grade 1:* Only mild congestive findings (IVC ≥2 cm with normal/mild abnormalities)
- *Grade 2:* Severe findings in only one organ
- *Grade 3:* Severe congestive findings in at least two of three organ systems.

VExUS will not likely provide much information on the need for fluid, it may provide a target for ending fluid administration. It is helpful in identifying patients who are likely to tolerate fluid and also those who are likely to benefit from fluid removal.

Fourth Hit

This stage addresses when to stop unloading fluids. This stage is a stage of organ recovery to mobilize accumulated fluid which lasts for days to weeks. This stage is associated with the risk of hypotension. It mainly focuses on weaning the patient from vasoactive agents and maintaining negative fluid balance by either diuresis or fluid removal by ultrafiltration. We must aim to avoid this stage as it occurs due to iatrogenic cause of excess of fluid removal. At this stage again, convective problems such as hypoperfusion and tissue hypoxia can occur due to hypovolemia which can make the patient hemodynamically unstable. But the cause of hypovolemia is due to fluid removal. Thus, at this stage avoid hypoperfusion and try to maintain a neutral balance to achieve organ support. When a patient shows signs of low APP, decreased hepatic blood flow, low $ScvO_2$, neutral or negative cumulative fluid balance, further fluid removal should be stopped.

FLUID THERAPY TARGETS BASED ON TYPES OF SHOCK AND THERAPEUTIC INTERVENTIONS TO IMPROVE PERFUSION[2]

Fluid therapy should be directed to optimize the hemodynamics by initial fluid resuscitation with early vasopressors to restore tissue perfusion.

Hypovolemic Shock

It is due to internal or external fluid loss, and it is the most common cause of shock in trauma patients. Up to 20% of blood volume loss, the circulatory system works almost normally because of the sympathetic nervous reflexes mediated vasoconstriction. This vasoconstriction mobilizes blood to the central circulation, increasing preload and increasing CO. American College of Surgeons Advanced Trauma Life Support (ATLS) classifies trauma patients based on initial patient presentation and approximate blood loss. The blood loss is categorized into four classes (class I <15%, class II 15–30%, class III 30–40%, and class IV >40%). For class, I and possibly class II, crystalloids are sufficient to optimize patients' hemodynamics.[47] The recently published European guidelines on the management of major bleeding and coagulopathy recommend that fluid therapy using isotonic crystalloid solutions should be initiated in the hypotensive bleeding trauma patient (Grade 1A).[48] Balanced electrolyte solutions are preferred over NS solutions but hypotonic solutions such as RL should be avoided in patients with severe TBI (Grade 1B). The use of colloids should be restricted due to the adverse effects on hemostasis (Grade 1C).

Cardiogenic shock: Cardiogenic shock refers to both new and rapid presentation of acute heart failure or deterioration of known heart failure. It is a complex, heterogeneous clinical syndrome, and a multidisciplinary approach with a high index of suspicion is warranted. Early initiation of specific treatment with urgent revascularization and stabilization of hemodynamics has proven beneficial. Fluid resuscitation strategy is a clinical challenge in the management of cardiogenic shock. It is often difficult to assess the adequacy of resuscitation as it varies over a period of time. No clinical studies have investigated the optimal blood pressure level, and guidelines no longer recommend a target blood pressure, but it should be individualized for all patients.[2] Fluid administration in circulatory shock is mainly based on pathophysiological considerations.[49] Careful fluid challenge of with either 4 mL/kg or 250 mL boluses with repeated ongoing evaluation of further need of fluids to maintain hemodynamics is recommended. In case of hemodynamic instability, start with inotropes in patients with left ventricular dysfunction (provided the MAP is maintained) and with vasopressors in the right ventricular dysfunction with the lowest possible dose and for the shortest possible duration.[49] In right ventricular failure, fluid therapy based on CVP monitoring is crucial. Ventricular interdependence is an important pathophysiological mechanism in right ventricular failure. Even though these patients can be preload dependent, it is important to not overdistend the right ventricle by volume overloading. Volume overload increases wall tension, decreases contractility, aggravates tricuspid regurgitation, increases ventricular interdependence, impairs left ventricular filling, and ultimately reduces systemic CO.

Obstructive Shock

It is less frequent than other types of shock. It is associated with low CO because of low preload, e.g., in pericardial tamponade, tension pneumothorax, or because there is an obstruction to the ventricle efflux, e.g., pulmonary embolism. The mainstay of treatment is directed at the underlying etiology of the obstruction to cardiopulmonary flow. Fluid administration should be attempted in all patients with a critical alteration of tissue perfusion in order to increase preload, even though clinical benefit is unlikely in cases of obstructive shock.

POSITIVE FLUID BALANCE AND OUTCOMES

The association between cumulative positive fluid balance and mortality is seen in various studies.[50,51] It has been clearly established that cumulative positive fluid balance over the ICU stay, is a poor prognostic factor in critically ill patients, particularly in the elderly, with pre-existing cardiac or renal impairment, sepsis, major injury, and burns. It has a tremendous impact on the worsening of organ function **(Table 7)**.[50,51] The pathophysiology of fluid administration causing harm has not been completely understood creating a crucial therapeutic dilemma[52] but positive fluid balance and fluid overload are significantly associated with an increase in days of mechanical ventilation in patients with acute respiratory distress syndrome (ARDS).[53] The kidney, being an encapsulated organ, is also sensitive to the effects of edema and development of fAKI, and the outcome is worsened with positive fluid balance (*hazard ratio:* 1.21; 95% confidence interval: 1.13–1.28; p <0.001). Positive fluid balance is associated with increased mortality in septic shock patients and inpatients with IAH.[54,55] Intransient fluid responders, it has been shown that these effects return to baseline within 90 minutes. Repeated fluid boluses may lead to positive fluid balance and

TABLE 7: Pathophysiologic effects of fluid overload and end-organ damage.[47]

Respiratory system: • Pulmonary edema • Capillary leak • Pleural effusion • Increased EVLW • Impaired gas exchange • Reduced compliance • Increased work of breathing • Difficult weaning	*Renal system:* • Increase renal venous pressure • Increase intracapsular pressure • Renal compartment syndrome • Renal interstitial edema • Reduced renal blood flow • Reduced GFR • Saltwater retention electrolyte disturbance
Central nervous system: • Cerebral edema • Impaired cognition Delirium	*Cardiovascular system:* • Conduction disturbance • Impaired contractility diastolic dysfunction
Gastrointestinal system: • Capillary leak • Gut edema • Mesenteric vein compression intra-abdominal hypertension (IAH) • Polycompartment syndrome • Malabsorption • Ileus	*Hepatic system:* • Hepatic congestion • Hepatic compartment syndrome • Impaired synthetic function • Cholestasis • Reduced cytochrome p450 activity
Others: • Tissue edema • Poor lymphatic drainage • Pressure ulcer • Microcirculatory derangement • Poor wound healing	

(EVLW: extravascular lung water; GFR: glomerular filtration rate)

may carry a risk of long-term adverse effects. Recently, a complex interaction between the heart, abdomen, and kidney which affects body fluid and sodium regulation is identified, known as "cardio-abdominal-renal syndrome(CARS)."[55] In patients who have acute decompensated heart failure and associated elevated IAP have more impaired renal function. Reduction of IAP after tailored medical therapy has been shown to be associated with improvement in renal function. This concept identifies a missing link which explains why some patients with congestive cardiac failure (CCF) have worsening of renal function and need RRT.

Unfortunately, the physiology of fluid resuscitation and the potential adverse effects are incompletely understood. The FEAST trial, a randomized clinical trial in febrile children who received either an NS bolus or an albumin bolus, was compared with those receiving no fluid boluses. This trial was stopped early due to increased mortality in children who were given fluid boluses.[56] Duration of fluid therapy therefore should be as short as possible. Fluid administration should be stopped once a circulatory failure has resolved. It should also be stopped once the patient is no longer preload responsive, or shows signs of fluid accumulation. There has been rising awareness that hidden "fluid creep" from maintenance fluids and drug administration poses a risk of fluid, sodium, and chloride burdens compared to resuscitation fluids.[57]

Different tools are available to assess fluid overload.[58] Clinical signs such as anasarca, pitting edema, body weight, assessment of daily weight, calculating fluid balance and monitoring EVLWI and biomarkers such as β-type natriuretic peptide (BNP), low albumin, low protein levels due to hemodilution, increased urinary albumin, increased urine albumin to creatinine ratio, and increased CRP to albumin ratio have been described. Bedside transthoracic echocardiography to assess filling status, ultrasonography (USG) abdomen to assess bowel edema, lung USG for B-lines, and comet tail artifacts are used to assess fluid overload. EVLWI indicates the development of interstitial edema and its presence is associated with mortality and morbidity. Now fluid overload can be assessed noninvasively by bioelectrical impedance analysis but its role in critically ill patients receiving mechanical ventilation is unclear. It assesses TBW as well as extravascular water (EVW), intravascular water (ICW), ECW/ICW ratio, and volume excess. Dynamics of fluid therapy with adequate initial fluid resuscitation (AIFR) and conservative late fluid management (CLFM) in septic shock with ARDS showed the lowest hospital mortality compared to those who could achieve only AIFR. As per the RIFTS study (Restrictive IV Fluid Trial in Severe Sepsis and Septic Shock), a randomized pilot study published in 2019 involving severe sepsis and septic shock patients, those assigned to a restrictive fluid strategy, that is with ≤60 mL/kg of IV fluid were compared with usual care, observed for first 72 hours. They demonstrated that a restrictive strategy was definitely associated with a reduced amount of IV fluid administered without an increase in mortality, organ failure, or adverse events.[59] Thus, a restrictive strategy does not show any harm and should be explored in larger RCTs.

Rationale of Deresuscitation and Keeping Negative Fluid Balance

Deresuscitation should be considered whenever there is evidence of end-organ damage secondary to fluid overload/positive fluid balance; which manifests in the form of impaired oxygenation, increased capillary leak, and increased abdominal pressure. Till date, there is not a single parameter based on which we can decide about fluid removal.

Deresuscitation can be achieved by either the use of diuretics or the use of RRT. The choice between diuretics and RRT depends on kidney function, urine output, electrolyte abnormalities, diuretic responsiveness, and degree of fluid accumulation.

Intermittent bolus strategy and bolus followed by a continuous infusion of furosemide were compared in a meta-analysis. The authors found that the patients treated with the second strategy had higher urine output but there was no significant difference in mortality or ventilator-free days.[60] Diuretic nonresponsiveness should be assessed. Whenever target urine output is not achieved, diuretics should be not be continued, as in fact, continuation carries a higher risk. Diuretic responsiveness is defined as a furosemide dose equivalent to 1 mg/mL of daily urine output (e.g., 200 mL urine output in response to 200 mg of furosemide at 2 hours is a positive response).

Evidence has shown the clinical advantages and possible mortality benefits of fluid deresuscitation. However, still, there are some unanswered questions and further high-quality multicentric RCTs are needed.

In a systemic review including 47 articles (19,902 patients) and found the following are the observations regarding the negative impact of positive fluid balance.[10]

- *Positive cumulative balance was associated with mortality:* Out of a total of 5,445 patients from 17 studies, 2,609 patients (47.9%) died. They were found to have positive fluid balance by the seventh day of their ICU stay (average cumulative positive fluid balance 4,533.5 + 3,626.7 mL).
- *Restricted fluid regimen was associated with reduced mortality:* 28 studies (15,947 patients) showed improved outcomes with conservative fluid balance [OR 0.42 (95% CI 0.32–0.55)]. In the restrictive fluid regimen group, mortality decreased from 33.2% (2,596 deaths in 7,812 patients) to 24.7% (2,007 deaths in 8,135 patients, $p < 0.0001$).
- *Association of positive fluid balance and development of IAH:* Out of 1,517 patients 597 patients developed IAH (39.4%). They had a positive fluid balance as compared to those without IAH (7,777.9 + 3,803 mL vs. 4,389.3 + 1,996.4 mL). The cumulative positive fluid balance after 1 week of ICU stay was on average 3,388.6 + 2,324.2 mL. World Society of ACS suggested that positive cumulative fluid balance the critically ill patients who had or were at risk of developing IAH/ACS should be avoided after the acute resuscitation has been completed and the inciting issues or source control has been addressed (Grade 2C).[54]
- Therapies of fluid removal to reduce net positive fluid balance are associated with a drop in the incidence of IAH. This systemic review observed that interventions such as either furosemide or RRT may help to reduce IAP. A total fluid removal of 4,876.3 + 4,178.5 mL caused a drop in IAP from 19.3 + 9.1 to 11.5 + 3.9 mm Hg in these patients.
- There is thus abundant evidence to support that protocolized de-escalation/fluid removal is quite feasible, well-tolerated, and is associated with improved outcomes.[61,62]
- Conservative fluid management or deresuscitation in patients with sepsis or ARDS perse has no mortality benefit but there are more ventilator-free days and shorter length of ICU stay. However, well-conducted RCTs are required to confirm these findings in the near future.

Another treatment protocol that has been proposed in order to achieve the negative fluid balance in patients with severe hypoxemia with increased extravascular lung water (EVLW) and IAP is the "PAL treatment protocol". It includes high levels of positive end-expiratory pressure (*P*EEP), hyperoncotic *A*lbumin for small-volume resuscitation, and *L*asix, diuretic for fluid removal or ultrafiltration.[63] In this protocol, the net negative fluid balance can be achieved by an initial 30-minute application of PEEP (which is titrated to counterbalance the effects of increased IAP, 20% albumin) (200 mL boluses over 60 minutes twice on first day and then titrated as her serum albumin levels) and then diuretic (started after the first dose of albumin with initial loading dose of 60 mg followed by infusion of 60 mg/h for first hour and then dose is adjusted between 5 and 20 mg/h as per hemodynamics). This protocol has been found to have beneficial effects in terms of EVLWI, IAP, organ failure, vasopressor therapy, reduction in duration of mechanical ventilation as well as improved mortality. It is important to determine fluid removal targets and fluid removal tolerance. At present, there is no single factor that determines the optimal fluid removal rate. Fluid removal should be stopped once the goal is achieved and/or signs of hypoperfusion occur.

CONCLUSION

Fluids can act as a double-edged sword thus, too much or too little fluid can have a negative impact on patient outcomes. Similar to drugs it should be used with great respect. Right fluids should be used in the right patient at the right time and in the right context considering indications, contraindications, and the possibility of toxicity. We are now in the era of implementation of "fluid stewardship," similar to the use of antibiotics in critically ill patients. It should be adapted to the course of the disease. Clinicians must maintain a heightened awareness about fluid resuscitation strategies such as SOSD, based on the course of the illness. Restrictive fluid administration probably causes a reduction in morbidity and mortality, but larger trials are still needed to confirm this. Crystalloid fluids should be used as first-line therapy in fluid resuscitation. There is no clear benefit of balanced crystalloids over saline to protect kidney function. Among colloids, HES and gelatin should be avoided owing to their unacceptable safety profiles. Albumin offers benefits, particularly in septic shock but there is a weak recommendation supporting its role as an alternative to crystalloids during resuscitation The hemodynamic effects of fluids beyond an initial response are not yet fully understood. Still after the initial resuscitation and correction of hypovolemia, conservative fluid management is safe. All physiological theories on which practice has been based are imprecise. It is quite astonishing that there is no robust outcome data to make fluid resuscitation practices universal all over the world, particularly with regard to indications for fluid boluses, methods of administration, and assessment of response. One must always ask two clinical questions in the presence of hemodynamic compromise: Is any intervention needed? If yes, are fluids likely to be beneficial? We should keep in mind that administration of fluid can cause venous congestion leading to organ dysfunction and it is a real threat. VExUS will not likely provide much information on further need of fluid, it may provide stop points to fluid resuscitation and identify patients who are likely to tolerate and benefit from fluid removal. POCUS may guide fluid resuscitation strategies with better insight in the future.

REFERENCES

1. Vincent J, Backer D De. Circulatory Shock. N Engl J Med. 2013;369(18):1726-34.
2. Cecconi M, Pinsky MR. Consensus on circulatory shock and hemodynamic monitoring. Task force of the European Society of Intensive Care Medicine. Intensive Care Med. 2014;40(12):1795-815.
3. Weil MH, Shubin H, Rosoff RL. Fluid Repletion in Circulatory Shock: Central Venous Pressure and Other Practical Guides. JAMA.1965;192:668-74.
4. Hoste EA, Maitland K, Brudney CS, Mehta R, Vincent JL, Yates D, et al. Four phases of intravenous fluid therapy: a conceptual model. Br J Anaesth. 2014;113(5):740-7.
5. Malbrain MLNG, Van Regenmortel N, Saugel B, et al. Principles of fluid management and stewardship in septic shock: it is time to consider the four D's and the four phases of fluid therapy. Ann Intensive Care. 2018;8(1):66.
6. Weil MH, Shubin H. Proposed reclassification of shock states with special reference to distributive defects. Adv Exp MedBiol.1971;23(0):13-23.
7. Rothe CF. Mean circulatory filling pressure: its meaning and measurement. J Appl Physiol. 1993;74(2):499-509.
8. Malbrain MLNG, Van Regenmortel N, Owczuk R. It is time to consider the four D's of fluid management. Anaesthesiol Intensive Ther. 2015;47:s1-5.
9. Vincent JL, Pinsky MR. We should avoid the term "fluid overload." Crit Care. 2018;22(1):214.
10. Malbrain ML, Marik PE, Witters I, Cordemans C, Kirkpatrick AW, Roberts DJ, et al. Fluid overload, de-resuscitation, and outcomes in critically ill or injured patients: a systematic review with suggestions for clinical practice. Anaesthesiol Intensive Ther. 2014;46(5):361-80.
11. Couture EJ, Gronlykke L, Denault AY. New developments in the understanding of right ventricular function in acute care. Curr Opin Crit Care. 2022;28(3):331-9.
12. Weil H, Shubin H. The "VIP" Approach to the Bedside Management of Shock. JAMA. 1969;207(2):337-40.
13. Vincent JL. Fluid management in the critically ill. Kidney Int. 2019;96(1):52-7.
14. Cavallaro F, Sandroni C, Marano C, La Torre G, Mannocci A, De Waure C, et al. Diagnostic accuracy of passive leg raising for prediction of fluid responsiveness in adults: systematic review and meta-analysis of clinical studies. Intensive Care Med. 2010;36(9):1475-83.
15. Rhodes A, Evans LE, Alhazzani W, Levy MM, Antonelli M, Ferrer R, et al. Surviving Sepsis Campaign: International Guidelines for Management of Sepsis and Septic Shock: 2016. Intensive Care Med. 2017;43(3):304-77.
16. Carlos Sanchez E, Pinsky MR, Sinha S, Mishra RC, Lopa AJ, Chatterjee R. Fluids and Early Vasopressors in the Management of Septic Shock: Do We Have the Right Answers Yet? J Crit Care Med (Targu Mures). 2023;9(3):138-147.
17. Orbegozo Cortés D, Gamarano Barros T, Njimi H, Vincent JL. Crystalloids versus colloids: exploring differences

in fluid requirements by systematic review and meta-regression. Anesth Analg. 2015;120(2):389-402.
18. Myburgh JA, Finfer S, Bellomo R, Billot L, Cass A, Gattas D, et al. Hydroxyethyl starch or saline for fluid resuscitation in intensive care. N Engl J Med. 2012;367(20):1901-11.
19. Perner A, Haase N, Guttormsen AB, Tenhunen J, Klemenzson G, Åneman A, et al. Hydroxyethyl starch 130/0.42 versus Ringer's acetate in severe sepsis. N Engl J Med. 2012;367(2):124-34.
20. Caironi P, Tognoni G, Masson S, Fumagalli R, Pesenti A, Romero M, et al. Albumin replacement in patients with severe sepsis or septic shock. N Engl J Med. 2014;370(15):1412-21.
21. Perel P, Roberts I, Ker K. Colloids versus crystalloids for fluid resuscitation in critically ill patients. Cochrane Database Syst Rev. 2013;(2):CD000567.
22. Qureshi SH, Rizvi SI, Patel NN, Murphy GJ. Meta-analysis of colloids versus crystalloids in critically ill, trauma and surgical patients. Br J Surg. 2016;103(1):14-26.
23. James MF, Michell WL, Joubert IA, Nicol AJ, Navsaria PH, Gillespie RS. Resuscitation with hydroxyethyl starch improves renal function and lactate clearance in penetrating trauma in a randomized controlled study: the FIRST trial (Fluids in Resuscitation of Severe Trauma). Br J Anaesth. 2011;107(5):693-702.
24. ClinicalTrials.gov. (2011). BaSES Trial: Basel Starch Evaluation in Sepsis (BaSES). [online] Available from http://clinicaltrials.gov/ct2/show/NCT00273728 [Last accessed October, 2024].
25. Ostermann M, Liu K, Kashani K. Fluid management in acute kidney injury. Chest. 2019;156(3):594-603.
26. Haase N, Perner A, Hennings LI, Siegemund M, Lauridsen B, Wetterslev M, et al. Hydroxyethyl starch 130/0.38-0.45 versus crystalloid or albumin in patients with sepsis: systematic review with meta-analysis and trial sequential analysis. BMJ. 2013;346:f839.
27. Lira A, Pinsky MR. Choices in fluid type and volume during resuscitation: impact on patient outcomes. Ann Intensive Care. 2014;4:38.
28. SAFE Study Investigators; Finfer S, McEvoy S, Bellomo R, McArthur C, Myburgh J, et al. Impact of albumin compared to saline on organ function and mortality of patients with severe sepsis. Intensive Care Med. 2011;37(1):86-96.
29. Evans L, Rhodes A, Alhazzani W, Antonelli M, Coopersmith CM, French C, et al. Surviving sepsis campaign: international guidelines for management of sepsis and septic shock 2021. Crit Care Med. 2021;49(11):e1063-43.
30. Thomas-Rueddel DO, Vlasakov V, Reinhart K, Jaeschke R, Rueddel H, Hutagalung R, et al. Safety of gelatin for volume resuscitation—a systematic review and meta-analysis. Intensive Care Med. 2012;38(7):1134-42.
31. Moeller C, Fleischmann C, Thomas-Rueddel D, Vlasakov V, Rochwerg B, Theurer P, et al. How safe is gelatin? A systematic review and meta-analysis of gelatin-containing plasma expanders vs crystalloids and albumin. J Crit Care. 2016;35:75-83.
32. Orbegozo Cortés D, Rayo Bonor A, Vincent JL. Isotonic crystalloid solutions: a structured review of the literature. Br J Anaesth. 2014;112(6):968-81.
33. Stenson EK, Cvijanovich NZ, Anas N, Allen GL, Thomas NJ, Bigham MT, et al. Hyperchloremia is associated with complicated course and mortality in pediatric patients with septic shock. Pediatr Crit Care Med. 2018;19(2):155-60.
34. Yunos NM, Bellomo R, Hegarty C, Story D, Ho L, Bailey M. Association between a chloride-liberal vs chloride-restrictive intravenous fluid administration strategy and kidney injuryin critically ill adults. JAMA. 2012;308(15):1566-72.
35. Yunos NM, Bellomo R, Glassford N, Sutcliffe H, Lam Q, Bailey M. Chloride-liberal vs. chloride-restrictive intravenous fluid administration and acute kidney injury: an extended analysis. Intensive Care Med. 2014;41(2):257-64.
36. Hammond NE, Taylor C, Finfer S, Machado FR, An Y, Billot L, et al. Patterns of intravenous fluid resuscitation use in adult intensive care patients between 2007 and 2014: an international cross-sectional study. PLoS One. 2017;12(5):e0176292.
37. Semler MW, Self WH, Wanderer JP, Ehrenfeld JM, Wang L, Byrne DW, et al. Balanced crystalloids versus saline in critically ill adults. N Engl J Med. 2018;378(9):829-39.
38. Self WH, Semler MW, Wanderer JP, Wang L, Byrne DW, Collins SP, et al. Balanced crystalloids versus saline in noncritically ill adults. N Engl J Med. 2018;378:819-28.
39. Zampieri FG, Machado FR, Biondi RS, Freitas FGR, Veiga VC, Figueiredo RC, et al. Effect of intravenous fluid treatment with a balanced solution vs 0.9% saline solution on mortality in critically ill patients: the BaSICS randomized clinical trial. JAMA. 2021;326(9):1-12.
40. Finfer S, Micallef S, Hammond N, Navarra L, Bellomo R, Billot L, et al. Balanced multielectrolyte solution versus saline in critically ill adults. N Engl J Med. 2022;386(9):815-26.
41. Young P, Bailey M, Beasley R, Henderson S, Mackle D, McArthur C, et al. Effect of a buffered crystalloid solution vs saline on acute kidney injury among patients in the intensive care unit: the SPLIT randomized clinical trial. JAMA. 2015;314(16):1701-10.
42. Rowan KM, Angus DC, Bailey M, Barnato AE, Bellomo R, Canter RR, et al. Early, goal-directed therapy for septic shock-a patient-level meta-analysis. N Engl J Med. 2017; 376(23):2223-34.
43. Meyhoff TS, Hjortrup PB, Wetterslev J, Sivapalan P, Laake JH, Cronhjort M, et al. Restriction of intravenous fluid in ICU patients with septic shock. N Engl J Med. 2022;386(26):2459-70.
44. Colon Hidalgo D, Patel J, Masic D, Park D, Rech MA. Delayed vasopressor initiation is associated with increased mortality in patients with septic shock. J Crit Care. 2020;55:145-8.

45. Vincent JL, Quintairos E Silva A, Couto L Jr, Taccone FS. The value of blood lactate kinetics in critically ill patients: a systematic review. Crit Care. 2016;20(1):257.
46. Sakr Y, Rubatto Birri PN, Kotfis K, Nanchal R, Shah B, Kluge S, et al. Higher fluid balance increases the risk of death from sepsis: results from a large international audit. Crit Care Med. 2017;45(3):386-94.
47. American College of Surgeons. ATLS® Student Course Manual, 10th edition. Chicago: American College of Surgeons; 2018.
48. Spahn DR, Bouillon B, Cerny V, Duranteau J, Filipescu D, Hunt BJ, et al. The European guideline on management of major bleeding and coagulopathy following trauma: fifth edition. Crit Care. 2019;23(1):98.
49. Thiele H, Ohman EM, Desch S, Eitel I, de Waha S. Clinical update: management of cardiogenic shock. Eur Heart J. 2015;36(20):1223-30.
50. Hyun DG, Ahn JH, Huh JW, Hong SB, Koh Y, Oh DK, et al. Impact of a cumulative positive fluid balance during the first three ICU days in patients with sepsis: a propensity score-matched cohort study. Ann Intensive Care. 2023;13(1):105.
51. Messmer AS, Zingg C, Muller M, Gerber JL, Schefold JC, Pfortmueller CA. Fluid overload and mortality in adult critical care patients-a systematic review and meta-analysis of observational studies. Crit Care Med. 2020;48(12):1862-70.
52. Acheampong A, Vincent J. A positive fluid balance is an independent prognostic factor in patients with sepsis. Crit Care. 2015;19(1):251.
53. Jozwiak M, Silva S, Persichini R, Anguel N, Osman D, Richard C, et al. Extravascular lung water is an independent prognostic factor in patients with acute respiratory distress syndrome. Crit Care Med. 2013;41(2):472-80.
54. Kirkpatrick AW, Roberts DJ, De Waele J, Jaeschke R, Malbrain ML, De Keulenaer B, et al. Intra-abdominal hypertension and the abdominal compartment syndrome: updated consensus definitions and clinical practice guidelines from the World Society of the Abdominal Compartment Syndrome. Intensive Care Med. 2013;39(7):1190-206.
55. Verbrugge FH, Mullens W, Malbrain M. Worsening Renal Function during Decompensated Heart Failure: The Cardio-abdomino-renal Syndrome. In: Vincent, JL. (eds) Annual Update in Intensive Care and Emergency Medicine 2012. Springer, Berlin, Heidelberg. https://doi.org/10.1007/978-3-642-25716-2_52.
56. Maitland K, Kiguli S, Opoka RO, Engoru C, Olupot-Olupot P, Akech SO, et al. Mortality after fluid bolus in african children with severe infection. N Engl J Med. 2011;364(26):2483-95.
57. Van Regenmortel N, Verbrugghe W, Roelant E, Van den Wyngaert T, Jorens PG. Maintenance fluid therapy and fluid creep impose more significant fluid, sodium, and chloride burdens than resuscitation fluids in critically ill patients: a retrospective study in a tertiary mixed ICU population. Intensive Care Med. 2018;44(4):409-17.
58. O'Connor ME, Prowle JR. Fluid Overload. Crit Care Clin. 2015;31(4):803-21.
59. Corl KA, Prodromou M, Merchant RC,Gareen I, Marks S, Banerjee D, et al. The Restrictive IV Fluid Trial in Severe Sepsis and Septic Shock (RIFTS): A Randomized Pilot Study. Crit Care Med. 2019;47(7):951-9.
60. Ng KT, Yap JLL. Continuous infusion vs. intermittent bolus injection of furosemide in acute decompensated heart failure: systematic review and meta-analysis of randomised controlled trials. Anaesthesia. 2018;73(2):238-47.
61. Silversides JA, McMullan R, Emerson LM, Bradbury I, Bannard-Smith J, Szakmany T, et al. Feasibility of conservative fluid administration and deresuscitation compared with usual care in critical illness: the Role of Active Deresuscitation After Resuscitation-2 (RADAR-2) randomised clinical trial. Intensive Care Med. 2022;48(2):190-200.
62. Bissell BD, Laine ME, Thompson Bastin ML, Flannery AH, Kelly A, Riser J, et al. Impact of protocolized diuresis for de-resuscitation in the intensive care unit. Crit Care. 2020;24(1):70.
63. Cordemans C, De Laet I, Van Regenmortel N, Schoonheydt K, Dits H, Martin G, et al. Aiming for a negative fluid balance in patients with acute lung injury and increased intra-abdominal pressure: a pilot study looking at the effects of PAL-treatment. Ann Intensive Care. 2012;2(suppl 2):S15.

CHAPTER 32 Vasopressors in Critically Ill Patients

Harish MM, Mirza Alamdar Ali Baig, Shivshankar Biradar

INTRODUCTION

Vasopressors are agents that increase vascular tone, thereby enhancing systemic vascular resistance (SVR) and improving end-organ perfusion and tissue oxygenation. These agents are crucial in managing various shock states, patients undergoing major surgeries, or victims of significant trauma. They should be administered via large bore veins, preferably through central veins. This chapter focuses on the various agents, their mechanisms of action, and their application in clinical practice. The commonly used vasopressors have been summarized in **Table 1**.

INDIVIDUAL VASOPRESSOR AGENTS

Epinephrine (Adrenaline)

Epinephrine (adrenaline) is a potent stimulant of both α- and β-adrenergic receptors, with particularly prominent actions on the heart and on vascular and other smooth muscles. It causes blood pressure to rise rapidly to a peak that is proportional to the dose when given via intravenous route. The mechanism of increased blood pressure is via three different pathways: positive inotropic action, positive chronotropic action, and vasoconstriction in many vascular beds—especially in the precapillary resistance vessels of skin, mucosa, and kidney—along with marked constriction of the veins.

The chief vascular action of epinephrine is exerted on the smaller arterioles and precapillary sphincters although veins and large arteries also respond to the drug. Various vascular beds react differently, resulting in substantial redistribution of blood flow. Epinephrine markedly decreases cutaneous blood flow, constricting precapillary vessels and small venules.[1]

Epinephrine also causes an increase in blood sugar levels and increases glycogenolysis in the liver. A transient increase in serum lactate occurs which can confound the management of shock as lactate is used as a marker of tissue hypoperfusion. However, the increase in serum lactate induced by exogenous catecholamines does not appear to be associated with harm and usually returns to baseline values within 12–24 hours.[2] Current randomized evidence showed that continuous intravenous (IV) administration

TABLE 1: List of agents.

Agent	*Dose (max)*	*Receptors*	*Cardiac output*	*MAP*	*SVR*
Epinephrine	1–10 μg/min (up to 20 μg/min)	α1, β1, β2	++	++	+++
Norepinephrine	0.01–0.5 μg/kg/min (up to 1.5 μg/kg/min)	α1, weak β1, β2	+/–	++	+++
Phenylephrine	0.1–0.18 mg/min (up to 9.1 μg/kg/min)	α1	–	++	+++
Dopamine	10–20 μg/kg/min (up to 50 μg/kg/min)	α1*, β1, D1#	++	+	+++
Vasopressin	0.01–0.04 units/min	V1, V2	–	+++	+++
Angiotensin II	20–200 ng/kg/min	AT1	+/–	+++	+++
Selepressin	–	V1a	–	+++	+++
Metaraminol	–	α1	–	++	+++

*High dose
#Low doses
(MAP: mean arterial pressure; SVR: systemic vascular resistance)

of epinephrine as an inotropic/vasopressor agent is not associated with a worse outcome in critically ill patients.[3]

Norepinephrine (Noradrenaline)

Norepinephrine is a sympathomimetic amine derived from tyrosine. It is structurally identical to epinephrine but differs because it lacks a methyl group on its nitrogen atom. This difference makes it primarily agonistic at alpha-1 and beta-1 receptors, with little-to-no beta-2 or alpha-2 activity. At low doses (<2 µg/min), the beta-1 effects may be more pronounced and increase cardiac output. However, in doses higher than 3 µg/min, the alpha-1 effects may predominate. The increased activation of the alpha-1 receptors will result in vasoconstriction and dose-dependent increases in SVR. The ratio of venous to arterial activity is relatively equal.[4,5]

Norepinephrine is predominantly used as a peripheral vasoconstrictor and is approved for blood pressure control in specific acute hypotensive states. It is the first-line agent for treating hypotension in the setting of sepsis that does not respond to fluid resuscitation.[5,6] Norepinephrine generally has more predictable pharmacologic properties than other alpha agonists, and its beta-agonism improves cardiac function relative to pure alpha agonists. This makes norepinephrine a widely used vasoactive agent, particularly in intensive care units to treat hypotension secondary to distributive shock.[7-9]

Pharmacokinetics

After the initiation of intravenous infusion, the steady-state plasma concentration of norepinephrine is attained in 5 minutes. The half-life of norepinephrine is approximately 2.4 minutes. The apparent volume of distribution is 8.8 L, and plasma protein binding is approximately 25%. Norepinephrine crosses the placenta but does not cross the blood–brain barrier. It is metabolized by catechol-O-methyltransferase (COMT) and monoamine oxidase (MAO) in the liver and other tissues, producing metabolites such as normetanephrine and vanillylmandelic acid (VMA). These metabolites are excreted in the urine primarily as sulfate conjugates and, to a lesser extent, as glucuronide conjugates.[9,10]

Administration

Norepinephrine is available as an intravenous solution and should be administered by continuous infusion due to its short half-life. The Food and Drug Administration (FDA) recommends diluting norepinephrine in dextrose-containing solutions before infusion to prevent oxidation and loss of potency. A common infusion technique starts at 8–12 µg/min, titrated to the desired pressure, with an average maintenance dose of 2–4 µg/min. Infusions should ideally be administered through large-bore peripheral intravenous catheters or central venous catheters to reduce the risk of ischemia secondary to extravasation.[11,12]

Adverse Effects

The most common adverse effects of norepinephrine relate to the activation of alpha-1 receptors, resulting in excessive vasoconstriction and decreased end-organ perfusion. Pulmonary vascular resistance may increase, leading to negative sequelae in patients with pulmonary hypertension. Decreased hepatic blood flow can lead to a transient increase in drugs that undergo hepatic metabolism. Reflex bradycardia via the baroreceptor reflex can result in decreased cardiac output despite beta1 agonism.[13,14]

Contraindications and Precautions

Norepinephrine should be avoided in patients with mesenteric or peripheral vascular thrombosis, as vasoconstriction will increase the area of ischemia and infarction. It should also be used cautiously in patients with profound hypoxia or hypercarbia, which can sensitize the myocardium to unstable arrhythmias. Care is necessary when using norepinephrine concomitantly with monoamine oxidase inhibitors or certain antidepressants due to the risk of severe and prolonged hypertension.[15,16]

Monitoring

Blood pressure requires close monitoring whenever vasopressors such as norepinephrine are used. Monitoring should be performed via invasive or noninvasive techniques, with values obtained frequently during initial titration and periodically thereafter. In low doses, titration via cardiac output measurement is preferred. An indwelling arterial catheter (A-line) is recommended for continuous hemodynamic monitoring in critical care settings.[17]

Dopamine

Dopamine, the immediate metabolic precursor of norepinephrine and epinephrine, exhibits dose-dependent effects through different receptors. At low concentrations, dopamine primarily interacts with D1 receptors in the renal, mesenteric, and coronary beds, leading to vasodilation and increased glomerular filtration rate, renal blood flow, and sodium excretion. At moderate concentrations, it exerts positive inotropic effects on the myocardium via β1-adrenergic receptors and induces norepinephrine release, enhancing cardiac effects with minimal impact on diastolic blood pressure. At high concentrations, dopamine activates α1 receptors, causing generalized vasoconstriction.[18,19]

In septic shock management, the 2016 Surviving Sepsis Campaign (SSC) guidelines recommend against using dopamine as a first-line vasopressor, favoring norepinephrine for its superior efficacy and safety profile. Dopamine may be considered in patients with a low risk of tachyarrhythmias and relative bradycardia but is generally avoided due to its arrhythmogenic potential. The Sepsis Occurrence in Acutely Ill Patients (SOAP) study identified dopamine administration as an independent risk factor for intensive care unit (ICU) mortality, and a study by De Backer et al. found a higher incidence of arrhythmias with dopamine compared to norepinephrine.[6]

In acute heart failure, the European Society of Cardiology (ESC) guidelines acknowledge dopamine as a potential inotropic agent, especially in cases of significant hypotension due to its combined inotropic and vasopressor effects.[20] However, caution is advised due to the risk of tachyarrhythmias, and therapy should be individualized based on patient-specific conditions. Dopamine may improve cardiac output and maintain organ perfusion, but other inotropes such as dobutamine and milrinone are also viable options.[20] In pediatric septic shock, a study by Ramaswamy et al. suggested that epinephrine might be more effective than dopamine in resolving fluid-refractory hypotension.

Overall, dopamine's role in critically ill patients is limited by the potential for adverse effects, particularly arrhythmias. Current guidelines favor norepinephrine for septic shock and recommend a cautious, individualized approach to inotropic support in heart failure, considering patient-specific risk factors and clinical response.[19,20]

Phenylephrine

Phenylephrine is a selective α1-adrenergic receptor agonist that increases SVR and blood pressure without significant effects on heart rate or myocardial contractility. It is used to manage hypotension, particularly in patients where tachyarrhythmias are a concern or other vasopressors are contraindicated. The 2016 SSC guidelines recommend norepinephrine as the first-line vasopressor for septic shock, with phenylephrine as a secondary option when norepinephrine and other vasopressors are insufficient or cause adverse effects.[19]

A study during a norepinephrine shortage found that alternative vasopressors, including phenylephrine, did not significantly worsen outcomes in septic shock patients, though norepinephrine remained preferred due to its favorable hemodynamic profile.[11] A randomized controlled trial comparing phenylephrine and norepinephrine for initial hemodynamic support in septic shock showed that while phenylephrine effectively increased blood pressure, it did not improve survival or organ function, highlighting norepinephrine's balanced effects on vascular resistance and cardiac output.[18] Additionally, recent studies indicate that phenylephrine use in septic shock may be associated with higher mortality, particularly in patients with ongoing tachycardia.[21,22] Thus, phenylephrine is generally secondary to norepinephrine in septic shock management, emphasizing individualized patient care based on hemodynamic needs and response to therapy.

Vasopressin

Vasopressin is an endogenous peptide hormone that acts mainly as an antidiuretic hormone by promoting the reabsorption of free water from the collecting tubules. It is a potent vasoconstrictor (V1 receptor-mediated) affecting resistance vessels throughout the circulation. Vasopressin functions through V1 receptors, leading to vasoconstriction, V2 receptors promoting antidiuretic effects, and V3 receptors affecting the central nervous system. Its ability to act on multiple receptors makes it a versatile agent in the management of shock. The drug is particularly beneficial in cases where catecholamines alone do not suffice, providing a multimodal approach to shock management.[23] Despite its potent vasoconstrictor properties, clinical trials like the VASST trial have shown no significant mortality benefit in septic shock, although it remains useful in catecholamine-resistant hypotension.[24]

One of the significant advantages of vasopressin is its role in catecholamine-sparing strategies. By reducing the required doses of catecholamines, vasopressin helps mitigate the adverse effects associated with high doses of catecholamines, such as arrhythmias and excessive vasoconstriction. This strategy is particularly valuable in septic shock, where patients often require high doses of vasopressors to maintain adequate blood pressure.[25] Vasopressin also has potential nephroprotective effects. Studies have suggested that vasopressin can improve renal blood flow and function in patients with septic shock, potentially reducing the incidence of acute kidney injury (AKI). This nephroprotective effect is particularly crucial as AKI is a common and severe complication in critically ill patients. Vasopressin has a short half-life of approximately 10–20 minutes, necessitating continuous infusion to maintain therapeutic levels. It is metabolized by the liver and kidneys, and its clearance can be affected by organ dysfunction commonly seen in critically ill patients. The standard dosing regimen involves an initial infusion rate of 0.01–0.04 units/min, adjusted based on the patient's hemodynamic response.[26] While vasopressin is generally well-tolerated, its potent vasoconstrictive properties can lead to several adverse effects. The most concerning is the risk of ischemia in peripheral tissues, mesenteric circulation, and coronary vessels. Monitoring for signs of tissue ischemia is essential during vasopressin therapy. Other potential side effects include hyponatremia due to its antidiuretic effects and, rarely, hypersensitivity reactions.[27]

The VASST (Vasopressin and Septic Shock Trial) trial is one of the most significant studies evaluating vasopressin's efficacy in septic shock. The trial compared vasopressin to norepinephrine and found no significant difference in mortality rates between the two groups. However, vasopressin did show benefits in catecholamine-resistant patients and helped reduce the norepinephrine dose required to maintain target blood pressure.[24] The VANISH trial also examined the combination of vasopressin and norepinephrine in septic shock and found no significant difference in kidney failure rates but noted a potential reduction in the incidence of atrial fibrillation when using vasopressin[25] **(Fig. 1)**. Further research has explored vasopressin's role in various shock states and its combination with other vasopressors. Studies have highlighted the importance of individualized therapy, considering factors such as the patient's underlying condition, the severity of shock, and the timing of vasopressor initiation.[28]

Combining vasopressin with catecholamines has shown potential benefits, including reducing the incidence of atrial fibrillation and other arrhythmias associated with high-dose catecholamine therapy. A systematic review and meta-analysis by McIntyre et al. demonstrated that vasopressin

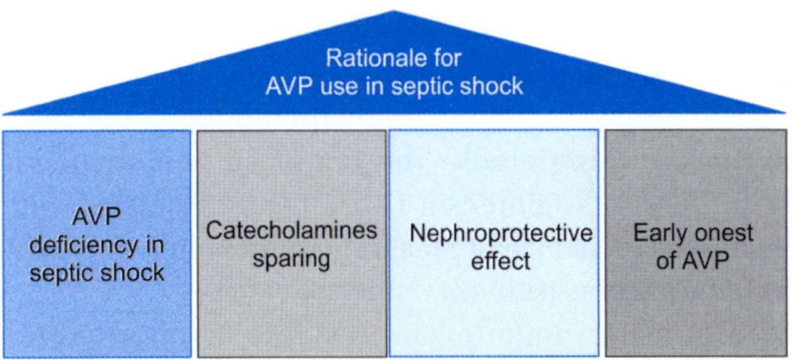

Fig. 1: Rationale for arginine vasopressin (AVP) use in septic shock.
- AVP deficiency present in septic shock.[6]
- As a multimodal strategy for the sparing of catecholamines.
- Its potential nephroprotective effect.
- Early onset of AVP infusion.

when added to catecholamines, was associated with a lower incidence of atrial fibrillation in patients with distributive shock.[27] Vasopressin is a valuable adjunct in the management of vasodilatory shock, particularly in septic shock cases that do not respond adequately to catecholamines alone. Its catecholamine-sparing effects, potential nephroprotective benefits, and efficacy in catecholamine-resistant hypotension make it a crucial component of modern shock management protocols. Early initiation and careful monitoring of vasopressin therapy can optimize outcomes and reduce the adverse effects associated with high-dose vasopressor therapy.

Angiotensin II

Angiotensin II is a powerful vasoconstrictor that plays a crucial role in the body's blood pressure regulation system. It exerts its effects primarily through the angiotensin II type 1 (AT1) receptors, leading to vasoconstriction, increased aldosterone secretion, and sodium and water retention. These mechanisms contribute to its rapid-pressor and slow-pressor responses, as well as promoting vascular and cardiac hypertrophy and remodeling.

The ATHOS-3 trial demonstrated that angiotensin II is effective in increasing blood pressure in vasodilatory shock unresponsive to high doses of conventional vasopressors. This landmark study showed that angiotensin II could significantly improve mean arterial pressure (MAP) in patients with vasodilatory shock who were not adequately responding to standard vasopressors, such as norepinephrine and vasopressin. This makes angiotensin II a potential alternative treatment in refractory vasodilatory shock.[8]

Recent studies and trials have further supported the use of angiotensin II in critically ill patients with vasodilatory shock. A meta-analysis of randomized controlled trials and observational studies indicated that angiotensin II can reduce the need for high dose catecholamines and may improve renal function by promoting better renal perfusion. Additionally, the improved hemodynamic stability with angiotensin II has been associated with decreased incidence of renal replacement therapy (RRT) in some patients with AKI.[29]

Moreover, angiotensin II's role in modulating inflammatory responses has been explored. It has been found to potentially reduce the systemic inflammatory response, which is often elevated in septic shock, thereby contributing to overall hemodynamic stability and improved patient outcomes.[8] This anti-inflammatory effect may be an added benefit in the management of septic shock and other inflammatory states of vasodilatory shock.

However, despite these promising findings, angiotensin II therapy requires careful patient selection and monitoring due to potential adverse effects, such as thromboembolic events and hypernatremia. Continuous monitoring of electrolyte levels and renal function is essential to mitigate these risks.[30]

Terlipressin

Terlipressin, a synthetic analog of vasopressin, has greater selectivity for V1 receptors and a longer half-life. It is effective in managing hepatorenal syndrome and cirrhosis-related septic shock. Treatment with terlipressin and albumin significantly increases creatinine clearance and urine output, with no overt signs of ischemia. Continuous low-dose infusion of terlipressin has been shown to be as effective as norepinephrine in reversing sepsis-induced arterial hypotension while reducing norepinephrine requirements.

Recent trials and studies have reinforced the efficacy of terlipressin in these conditions. The CONFIRM trial demonstrated that terlipressin significantly improves renal function and reduces mortality in patients with hepatorenal syndrome. Additionally, terlipressin has been found to improve hemodynamic stability in patients with cirrhosis and septic shock, making it a valuable therapeutic option in these populations.[31] Another study published in the Journal of Hepatology in 2020 indicated that terlipressin, combined with albumin, could be safely administered with significant improvements in renal function without major adverse effects.[32]

Further research has indicated that terlipressin not only improves systemic hemodynamics but also has beneficial effects on the renal and splanchnic circulations. This multifaceted action makes it particularly useful in managing the complex hemodynamic disturbances seen in hepatorenal syndrome and cirrhosis-related septic shock.[33]

The TERESEP (Terlipressin for Refractory Septic Shock) trial specifically evaluated the use of terlipressin in septic shock and found that terlipressin, when used in conjunction with norepinephrine, improved hemodynamic stability and reduced norepinephrine requirements. This trial also highlighted the potential for terlipressin to reduce the incidence of ischemic complications compared to higher doses of norepinephrine alone.[34]

However, it is important to monitor for potential side effects, such as abdominal cramps, headaches, and ischemic events, especially in patients with underlying cardiovascular disease. Close monitoring and careful patient selection are crucial to optimizing outcomes with terlipressin therapy.[35]

NOVEL AGENTS

Selepressin

A selective vasopressin V1a receptor agonist is designed to avoid the vasoconstrictive side effects associated with nonselective vasopressin analogs. Selepressin acts specifically on V1a receptors, mediating vasoconstriction in vascular smooth muscle without the V2 receptor-mediated antidiuretic effects, which can lead to fluid retention.

The SEPSIS-ACT trial, a multicenter, randomized controlled trial, showed significant reductions in vasopressor load and improved organ function scores in septic shock patients treated with selepressin, highlighting its safety profile.[36] Maier et al. (2022) confirmed these findings, showing that selepressin improved hemodynamic stability and reduced vasopressor requirements, emphasizing its potential to reduce ischemic complications compared to higher doses of norepinephrine alone.[37]

Despite these promising results, further large-scale trials are necessary to confirm the efficacy and safety of selepressin in a broader patient population.

Metaraminol

Metaraminol is an $\alpha 1$-adrenergic agonist that has been re-evaluated for use in critically ill patients, particularly those with septic shock. Recent studies suggest that metaraminol may be beneficial in certain patient populations, providing an alternative when other vasopressors are not suitable. Metaraminol works by stimulating α1-adrenergic receptors, leading to vasoconstriction and an increase in SVR, thereby raising blood pressure. Its utility in septic shock and other critical conditions is still under investigation, but the growing body of evidence supports its role as a supplementary option in vasopressor therapy.[38]

CLINICAL APPLICATION

Septic Shock

Septic shock is a life-threatening condition characterized by decreased end-organ perfusion, potentially progressing to multiorgan dysfunction. Early resuscitation to reduce vasodilation and ensure adequate organ perfusion is paramount. Vasopressors are administered when intravenous fluid resuscitation alone fails to restore blood pressure. Norepinephrine is the first-line agent due to its effectiveness and safety profile, showing fewer adverse effects compared to dopamine and other vasopressors.[5,6]

The SSC[19] is a global initiative aimed at improving the management of sepsis. The campaign was launched in 2002 by the Society of Critical Care Medicine and the European Society of Intensive Care Medicine **(Fig. 2)**. The SSC initially focused on creating guidelines for the treatment of sepsis, which were first published in 2004 and updated in 2008, 2012, 2016, and 2021. These guidelines have become widely accepted as the standard of care for sepsis, to be undertaken as a medical emergency. The SSC guidelines provide evidence-based recommendations for the management of septic shock, including source control, antibiotic therapy, fluid resuscitation, vasopressor therapy, supportive care, and monitoring and follow-up.[19]

The combination of vasopressin with norepinephrine has been explored but shows no significant mortality benefit, although it can be beneficial in catecholamine-resistant cases.[24,25] Vasopressin is particularly beneficial

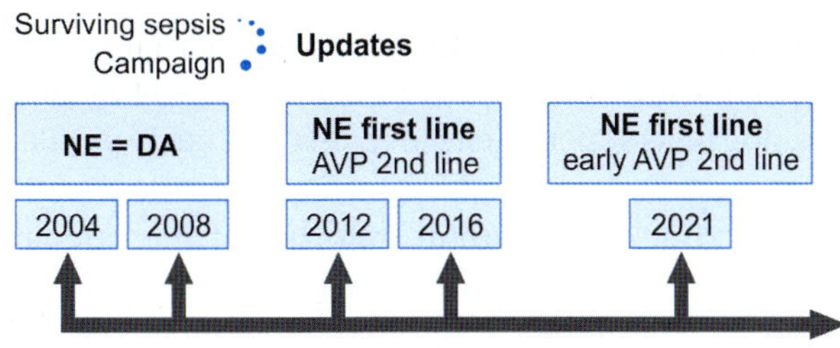

Fig. 2: Surviving Sepsis Campaign updates. (AVP: arginine vasopressin; DA: dopamine; NE: norepinephrine)

in catecholamine-sparing strategies, potentially reducing the adverse effects associated with high doses of catecholamines, such as arrhythmias and excessive vasoconstriction.[23,24]

In refractory cases, angiotensin II has emerged as a potential alternative treatment. The ATHOS-3 (Angiotensin II for the Treatment of High-Output Shock 3) trial demonstrated that angiotensin II could significantly improve MAP in patients with vasodilatory shock who were not adequately responding to standard vasopressors, such as norepinephrine and vasopressin.[8] Additionally, metaraminol has been reevaluated for use in septic shock, providing an alternative when other vasopressors are not suitable.[38]

Phenylephrine can be considered in patients where tachyarrhythmias are a concern or when norepinephrine and other vasopressors are contraindicated. However, studies suggest phenylephrine may be associated with higher mortality rates in septic shock patients, making it a secondary option.[19,18]

Epinephrine may be considered an additional agent when both norepinephrine and vasopressin are insufficient. While epinephrine is a potent vasoconstrictor and inotrope, it can increase serum lactate levels, complicating the assessment of tissue perfusion in septic shock patients.[7]

Dopamine is generally avoided as a first-line vasopressor in septic shock due to its higher incidence of arrhythmias and lack of survival benefit compared to norepinephrine. It may still be considered in select patients with a low risk of tachyarrhythmias and relative bradycardia.[19]

Lastly, terlipressin, used in conjunction with norepinephrine, has shown efficacy in improving hemodynamic stability and reducing norepinephrine requirements in septic shock. The TERESEP trial indicated that terlipressin could reduce the incidence of ischemic complications compared to higher doses of norepinephrine alone.[34]

Vasopressors are administered when intravenous fluid resuscitation alone fails to restore blood pressure. Norepinephrine is the first-line agent due to its effectiveness and safety profile, showing fewer adverse effects compared to dopamine and other vasopressors.[6] The combination of vasopressin with norepinephrine has been explored but shows no significant mortality benefit, although it can be beneficial in catecholamine-resistant cases.[12,14-16]

Cardiac Failure and Cardiogenic Shock

Heart failure and cardiogenic shock are challenging conditions to manage, often requiring inotropes as bridging therapy to stabilize patients until definitive interventions can be performed. Norepinephrine is preferred over dopamine due to a lower incidence of arrhythmias and myocardial ischemia.[6,20] Recent studies have challenged the notion that norepinephrine increases afterload to a detrimental extent in myocardial dysfunction, supporting its use in this context.[8,20]

Dopamine may be considered in patients with a low risk of tachyarrhythmias and relative bradycardia but is generally avoided due to its arrhythmogenic potential. The Sepsis Occurrence in Acutely Ill Patients (SOAP) study identified dopamine administration as an independent risk factor for ICU mortality, and a study by De Backer et al. found a higher incidence of arrhythmias with dopamine compared to norepinephrine.[6]

Cardiac Arrest

Cardiac arrest is a critical emergency where immediate intervention is necessary to prevent death. Vasopressors play a key role in resuscitation efforts. *Epinephrine* is the primary vasopressor used in cardiac arrest. Its potent vasoconstrictive properties increase coronary and cerebral perfusion pressures during cardiopulmonary resuscitation (CPR), improving the likelihood of return of spontaneous circulation (ROSC). Current guidelines recommend administering 1 mg of epinephrine every 3–5 minutes during cardiac arrest, especially in the absence of a shockable rhythm (asystole or pulseless electrical activity).[5]

Duration and Intensity of Treatment

The incidence of septic shock is approximately 31 cases per 100,000 population per year, with mortality ranging from 30 to 60%.[19] Early vasopressor therapy initiation is crucial, with norepinephrine as the preferred first-line agent. The intensity and duration of therapy should be tailored based on the patient's response and prognosis. High-dose vasopressor therapy is associated with high mortality, necessitating careful clinical judgment, and discussions with patient families about prognosis and treatment goals. Studies suggest that when standard high doses of vasopressors fail to normalize blood pressure, further escalation of therapy yields diminishing returns, prompting the need for shared decision-making with the patient's family.[19,20]

Norepinephrine is typically administered as a continuous infusion, titrated to maintain MAP ≥65 mm Hg.[5,6] Vasopressin is often used in conjunction with norepinephrine to reduce the dose of norepinephrine required and to spare catecholamines, administered as a continuous infusion.[24,25] In refractory cases where standard vasopressors are not effective, angiotensin II has emerged as a potential alternative treatment. The ATHOS-3 trial demonstrated that angiotensin II could significantly improve MAP in patients with vasodilatory shock who were not adequately responding to norepinephrine and vasopressin.[8]

Phenylephrine can be used when norepinephrine is contraindicated or in cases of tachyarrhythmias, typically administered as a continuous infusion. However, studies suggest phenylephrine may be associated with higher mortality rates in septic shock patients, making it a secondary option.[19,18] Epinephrine may be used as an additional agent when both norepinephrine and vasopressin are insufficient, administered as a continuous infusion. Although epinephrine is a potent vasoconstrictor and inotrope, it can increase serum lactate levels, complicating the assessment of tissue perfusion in septic shock patients.[7] Dopamine is generally avoided as a first-line vasopressor in septic shock due to its higher incidence of arrhythmias and lack of survival benefit compared to norepinephrine. It may still be considered in select patients, administered as a continuous infusion.[19] Lastly, terlipressin, used in conjunction with norepinephrine, has shown efficacy in improving hemodynamic stability and reducing norepinephrine requirements in septic shock. The TERESEP trial indicated that terlipressin could reduce the incidence of ischemic complications compared to higher doses of norepinephrine alone.[34]

CONCLUSION

Vasopressors are crucial in the management of shock states and other critical conditions in severely ill patients. They function by increasing vascular tone, enhancing SVR, and improving end-organ perfusion and tissue oxygenation. Norepinephrine is the preferred first-line agent for septic shock due to its superior effectiveness and safety profile.

The proper use of vasopressors requires early initiation in septic shock and careful tailoring of the intensity and duration of therapy based on patient response and prognosis. High-dose vasopressor therapy is linked to increased mortality, emphasizing the need for careful monitoring, clinical judgment, and collaboration with patient families regarding treatment goals.

REFERENCES

1. Bearn AG, Billing B, Sherlock S. The effect of adrenaline and noradrenaline on hepatic blood flow and splanchnic carbohydrate metabolism in man. J Physiol. 1951;115(4):430-41.
2. Clutter WE, Bier DM, Shah SD, Cryer PE. Epinephrine plasma metabolic clearance rates and physiologic thresholds for metabolic and hemodynamic actions in man. J Clin Invest. 1980;66(1):94-101.
3. Belletti A, Naggy A, Sartorelli M, Mucchetti M. Effect of Continuous Epinephrine Infusion on Survival in Critically Ill Patients. A Meta-Analysis of Randomized Trials. Critical Care Med. 2020;48(3):398-405.
4. Smith MD, Maani CV. Norepinephrine. In: StatPearls [Internet]. Treasure Island (FL): StatPearls Publishing; 2024.
5. Evans L, et al. Management of septic shock: current guidelines and future perspectives. Crit Care Medi. 2021;49(11):2076-94.
6. De Backer D, Biston P, Devriendt J, Madl C, Chochrad D, Aldecoa C, et al. Comparison of Dopamine and Norepinephrine in the Treatment of Shock. N Engl J Med. 2010;362(9):779-89.
7. Levy B, Clere-Jehl R, Legras A, Morichau-Beauchant T, Leone M, Frederique G, et al. Epinephrine Versus Norepinephrine for Cardiogenic Shock After Acute Myocardial Infarction. J Am Coll Cardiol. 2018;72(2):173-82.
8. Khanna A, English SW, Wang XS, Ham K, Tumlin J, Szerlip H, et al. Angiotensin II for the Treatment of Vasodilatory Shock. N Engl J Med. 2017;377(5):419-30.
9. Russell JA, Walley KR, Singer J, Gordon AC, Hébert PC, Cooper DJ, et al. Vasopressin Versus Norepinephrine Infusion in Patients with Septic Shock. N Engl J Med. 2008;358(9):877-87.
10. Gordon AC, Mason AJ, Thirunavukkarasu N, Perkins GD, Cecconi M, Cepkova M, et al. Effect of Early Vasopressin vs Norepinephrine on Kidney Failure in Patients With Septic Shock: The VANISH Randomized Clinical Trial. JAMA. 2016;316(5):509-18.
11. Vail E, et al. Effect of a norepinephrine shortage on patients with septic shock. Crit Care Med. 2016;45(2):301-9.
12. Chioncel O, et al. European Society of Cardiology Guidelines for the Diagnosis and Treatment of Acute and Chronic Heart Failure. Eur Heart J. 2020;41(2):212-20.
13. McDonagh TA, Metra M, Adamo M, Gardner RS, Baumbach A, Böhm M, et al. 2021 ESC Guidelines for the Diagnosis and Treatment of Acute and Chronic Heart Failure. Eur Heart J. 2021;42(36):3599-726.
14. Bitton S, et al. Norepinephrine use in critical care: A review of indications and current practices. J Intensive Care Medicine. 2022;37(5):517-27.
15. Martin C, Viviand X, Leone M, Thirion X. Effect of Norepinephrine on the Outcome of Septic Shock. Crit Care Med. 2000;28(8):2758-65.
16. Annane D, Vignon P, Renault A, Bollaert PE, Charpentier C, Martin C, et al. Norepinephrine Plus Dobutamine versus Epinephrine Alone for Management of Septic Shock: A Randomised Trial. Lancet. 2007;370(9588):676-84.
17. Myburgh JA, Higgins A, Jovanovska A, Lipman J, Ramakrishnan N, Santamaria J, et al. A Comparison of Epinephrine and Norepinephrine in Critically Ill Patients. Intensive Care Med. 2008;34(12):2226-34.
18. Morelli A, Ertmer C, Rehberg S, Lange M, Orecchioni A, Laderchi A, et al. Phenylephrine versus Norepinephrine for Initial Hemodynamic Support of Patients with Septic Shock: A Randomized, Controlled Trial. Crit Care. 2008;12(6):R143.
19. Rhodes A, Evans LE, Alhazzani W, Levy MM, Antonelli M, Ferrer R, et al. Surviving Sepsis Campaign: International Guidelines for Management of Sepsis and Septic Shock: 2016. Crit Care Med. 2017;45(3):486-552.
20. Hioncel O, et al. European Society of Cardiology Guidelines for the Diagnosis and Treatment of Acute and Chronic Heart Failure. Eur Heart J. 2020;41(2):212-20.
21. Richards E, Lopez MJ, Maani CV. Phenylephrine. In: Treasure Island (FL): StatPearls Publishing; 2024.
22. CIMS Multidisciplinary. (2023). Phenylephrine use ups death risk in septic shock patients. [Online] Available from https://www.mims.com/specialty/topic/phenylephrine-use-ups-death-risk-in-septic-shock-patients [Last accessed October, 2024].
23. García-Álvarez R, Arboleda-Salazar R. Vasopressin in Sepsis and Other Shock States: State of the Art. J Pers Med. 2023;13(11):1548.
24. Russell JA, Lee T, Singer J, Boyd JH, Walley KR; Vasopressin and Septic Shock Trial (VASST) Group. The Septic Shock 3.0 Definition and Trials: A Vasopressin and Septic Shock Trial Experience. Crit Care Med. 2017;45(6):940-8.
25. Ukor IF, Walley KR. Vasopressin in vasodilatory shock. Crit. Care Clin. 2019;35(2):247-61.
26. Sacha GL, Lam SW, Wang L, Duggal A, Reddy AJ, Bauer SR. Association of Catecholamine Dose, Lactate, and Shock Duration at Vasopressin Initiation with Mortality in Patients with Septic Shock. Crit Care Med. 2022;50(4):614-23.
27. McIntyre WF, Um KJ, Alhazzani W, Lengyel AP, Hajjar L, Gordon AC, et al. Association of Vasopressin Plus Catecholamine Vasopressors vs Catecholamines Alone with Atrial Fibrillation in Patients with Distributive Shock: A Systematic Review and Meta-Analysis. JAMA. 2018;319(18):1889-900.
28. Nagendran M, Russell JA, Walley KR, Brett SJ, Perkins GD, Hajjar L, et al. Vasopressin in Septic Shock: An Individual Patient Data Meta-Analysis of Randomised Controlled Trials. Intensive Care Med. 2019;45(6):844-55.
29. Tumlin JA, Murugan R, Deane AM, Ostermann M, Busse LW, Ham KR, et al. Outcomes in Patients with Vasodilatory Shock and Renal Replacement Therapy Treated with Intravenous Angiotensin II. Crit Care Med. 2018;46(6):949-57.
30. Busse LW, McCurdy MT, Ali O, Hall A, Chen H, Ostermann M. Angiotensin II for the treatment of vasodilatory shock:

a clinical review. Pharmacotherapy: The J Hum Pharmacol Drug Therapy. 2019;39(5):576-85.
31. CONFIRM Study Investigators. Terlipressin in Patients with Hepatorenal Syndrome Type 1. N Engl J Med. 2020;382(9): 820-9.
32. Solà E, et al. Terlipressin and Albumin for Type-1 Hepatorenal Syndrome Associated with Acute-on-Chronic Liver Failure: A Cohort Study. J Hepatol. 2020;72(1):42-50.
33. Licata A, et al. Terlipressin for Treatment of Hepatorenal Syndrome: A Review of Current Evidence and Future Perspectives. World J Hepatol. 2021;13(3):294-305.
34. TERESEP Study Investigators. Terlipressin in Septic Shock: A Randomized Controlled Trial. Crit Care Med. 2022;50(7):1016-25.
35. Angeli P, et al. EASL Clinical practice guidelines for the management of patients with decompensated cirrhosis. J Hepatol. 2019;69(2):406-60.
36. SEPSIS-ACT Investigators. Selepressin for Septic Shock: A Multicenter Randomized Controlled Trial. Intensive Care Med. 2021;47(5):569-79.
37. Maier S, et al. Efficacy and safety of selepressin in septic shock patients: a multicenter randomized controlled trial. Crit Care Med. 2022;50(2):182-90.
38. Grauslyte L, Bolding N, Phull M, Jovaisa T. The Use of Metaraminol as a Vasopressor in Critically Unwell Patients: A Narrative Review and a Survey of UK Practice. J Crit Care Med (Targu Mures). 2022;8(3):193-203.

CHAPTER 33

Inotropes in Critically Ill Patients

Natesh Prabu R, Atul Prabhakar Kulkarni

INTRODUCTION

Acute circulatory failure and hypotension are common in intensive care units (ICU). Fluids and vasoactive agents are used to maintain hemodynamic stability. Vasopressors and inotropes are used whenever there is a need to improve vasomotor tone and inotropy of the heart respectively. Most of these vasoactive drugs belong to the catecholamine group and have overlapping actions, i.e., varied combinations of inotropy and vasomotor properties. Almost all vasoactive drugs have both action at the heart (inotropy) and vessel (alter vasomotor tone—either vasoconstriction or vasodilation). There is no pure inotrope, that acts only on the heart and there is no pure vasopressor that acts only on vessels and not on the heart. Improvement in cardiac output may be beneficial in patients having a shock when there is myocardial dysfunction or heart failure. Though it physiologically sounds good to use inotropes in patients with myocardial depression or patients with systolic heart failure with high filling pressures, it has not turned out to be very beneficial.[1] There is always a debate on how to choose a drug, its timing, dosage, etc., as there is no consensus yet.[1] The use of inotropes is seen commonly in critically ill patients with cardiogenic shock (CS) postmyocardial infarction, CS of other etiologies, systolic heart failure, perioperative period, and in patients with sepsis.

EFFECTS OF INOTROPES IN CRITICALLY ILL PATIENTS

Inotropes improve stroke volume by increasing the contractility of the heart. Inotropes also affect systemic and pulmonary vascular resistance. Inotropes are broadly classified into catecholamine (dobutamine) and non-catecholamine [digoxin, phosphodiesterase III inhibitors (PDE-III inhibitors), and levosimendan, omecamtiv mecarbil (OM)] inotropic drugs.[2,3] All noncatecholamine group of inotropes acts by modifying intracellular calcium levels except OM which affects actin-myosin cross bridges. It is a selective small-molecule activator of cardiac myosin.[3]

Inotropes: Classification

Cyclic adenosine monophosphate (cAMP)-dependent inotropes:

- *β-adrenergic receptor agonists:* Dobutamine, dopamine, adrenaline, and isoproterenol
- *PDE-III inhibitors:* Amrinone, milrinone, and enoximone
- *Calcium sensitizers:* Levosimendan
- *Cardiac glycosides:* Digoxin
- *Cardiac myosin activators:* Omecamtiv mecarbil
- *Modulation of sarcoplasmic reticulum Ca^{2+}-ATPase (SERCA2a stimulation):* Istaroxime.
- *Nitroxyl donors:* CXL-1020 (in clinical trials)—has both inotropic and lusitropicic effects.

Action on myocardium: All drugs increase contractility of the heart and may increase myocardial oxygen need (dobutamine > milrinone, levosimendan) except OM. Omecamtiv mecarbil increases the stroke volume by increasing the duration of systole without changing myocardial contraction velocity.[2,3] All other inotropes increase the rate of myocardial contraction and shorten systole duration. Istaroxime by its peculiar action facilitates myocardial diastolic function (lusitropy).[2,4]

Systemic vessels: The majority of inotropes are vasodilators of systemic arteries (inodilators). Dobutamine (β-agonist), levosimendan [adenosine triphosphate (ATP-sensitive potassium channels), and PDE-III inhibitors, all cause vasodilatation leading to hypotension; needing additional vasoconstrictor; to counter the hypotension. All drugs have the potential to cause tachycardia and tachyarrhythmias.

Pulmonary vessels: The majority of drugs cause dilatation of pulmonary vessels and reduce pulmonary arterial and venous resistance. Milrinone and levosimendan cause more pulmonary vasodilation than dobutamine.

Heart rate: Almost all inotropes increase heart rate, and it is not advantageous but rather harmful in patients with myocardial infarction and heart failure. Only digoxin and OM do not increase heart rate, but digoxin may induce bradyarrhythmias and tachyarrhythmias.

Other actions: Levosimendan has additional cardioprotective and pleiotropic (causing multiple effects) properties **(Table 1)**.

These drugs by increasing inotropy and vasodilatation [reduced systemic vascular resistance (SVR)], improve renal blood flow and cause diuresis. Also, the left ventricular diastolic pressure and filling pressure of the heart are reduced. By its properties, the drugs act best in situations with low cardiac output (myocardial failure) and high SVR.

Istaroxime is a novel drug that has a dual action.[4] First is the inhibition of sarcolemmal sodium-potassium ATPase, by which it increases the levels of intracellular Ca^{2+}, thereby enhancing contractility. Another mechanism of action is stimulation of sarcoplasmic reticulum calcium adenosine triphosphatase isoform 2a (SERCA2a). Through this it promotes the reuptake of free Ca^{2+} into the sarcoplasmic reticulum during diastole, improving myocardial diastolic function (lusitropy—rate of myocardial relaxation). The experience with istaroxime is less, further studies will shed light on its use and effects.

Inotropes in Critically Ill: Indications and Clinical Use

Inotropes are used to improve cardiac output in patients with poor cardiac performance. The use of inotropes is not only limited to CS after acute myocardial infarction and heart failure but has also expanded to the perioperative setting, sepsis, bridge-to-heart transplant, and bridge-to-mechanical circulatory devices.[2] A meta-analysis showed beneficial effects with levosimendan in critically ill patients,[5] but the trials included are of poor quality. Inotropes are generally used for short-term, except in cases of advanced heart failure; and have adverse effects such as tachyarrhythmias, myocardial ischemia, and hypotension. Various recommendations are made by different societies regarding the timing and choice of inotropes in patients with heart failure and CS.[6] Inotropes are favored in many situations to maintain tissue perfusion when there is low cardiac output and hypotension or end-organ hypoperfusion. The dynamic nature of shock is also the main factor considered in critically ill patients, which requires frequent titration of drugs. Compared to all inotropic agents, dobutamine has a short half-life and is easily titratable followed by milrinone. Levosimendan has a long half-life, and the effect may last long even after discontinuation of the drug, precluding titration.

So, appropriate use of inotrope is important. Though the evidence is sparse, the need and frequency of using inotropes is increasing; leaving the physician with a challenge in managing such patients.

Cardiogenic Shock

Cardiogenic shock is a state of critical end-organ hypoperfusion due to low cardiac output[7] in patients with primary cardiac dysfunction. When not treated, it progresses to multiorgan failure. Most often CS is caused by ST-segment elevated myocardial infarction with or without mechanical complications.[7] The primary treatment is revascularization and addressing the cause. It is equally important to maintain tissue perfusion by augmenting contractility and perfusion pressure. Norepinephrine is used as a vasopressor of choice and inotropes are commonly used to improve cardiac output. Inotropes initiation is suggested only after revascularization in patients after myocardial infarction, especially in patients with low cardiac output and high systemic vascular resistance.[8] Though dobutamine is recommended as the initial choice,[7] recent studies are favoring non-catecholamine inotropes because of lesser adverse effects, particularly in patients taking β-blockers.[7] Dobutamine causes tachycardia, increased myocardial oxygen need, and hypotension due to its effect on the vessel (β_2 stimulation). In a study that compared epinephrine with combined dobutamine and norepinephrine, the combination was much safer and more effective than epinephrine alone.[9] Another commonly used drug is dopamine. Its usage has reduced due to increased adverse effects and poor outcome[10] and it is not recommended.[7] Interestingly combination of dopamine with dobutamine in patients with CS showed a better increase in mean arterial pressure and pulmonary capillary wedge pressure compared to either drug alone.[11]

Further, there was no growing interest in combination therapy probably due to better properties of newer drugs and more understanding of shock states.

TABLE 1: Inotropes—properties, classification and effects[2,3,6]

Drug	*Classification*	*Mechanism of action*	*Receptors/ site of action*	*Effects*					*Dose*[2,3]	*Half-life*	*Adverse effects*	*Comments*
				Inotropy	*Systolic time*	*Arterial vasodilation*	*Pulmonary vasodilation*	*Heart rate*				
Epinephrine	Catecholamine	Increase intracellular calcium levels	Agonist at $\beta_1 = \beta_2 > \alpha_1$ β effect-at low doses α effect at high doses	↑↑	–	+	+/–	↑↑	0.05–0.5 μ/kg/min	2–3 minutes	Myocardial ischemia, hypertension, ventricular tachyarrhythmias, pulmonary edema, and cerebral hemorrhage	Not commonly used
Dobutamine	Catecholamine	Increase cAMP	$\beta_1 > \beta_2 > \alpha_1$ agonist	↑↑	–	+	+/–	↑↑	2–20 mic/kg/min No bolus	2 minutes	Tachycardia, Arrhythmias, hypotension, myocardial ischemia	Commonly chosen initial choice for cardiogenic shock
Milrinone	PDE-III inhibitors	Increase c-AMP levels by preventing degradation and increase intracellular calcium levels	Bind to PDE-III enzyme at SR	↑	–	++	++	–	0.375–0.75 μ/kg/min 25–75 μ/kg/min over 10–20 minutes (optional)	2.5 hours	Tachyarrhythmias and hypotension	• Low cardiac output postcardiac surgery • Chronic heart failure and acute heart failure • Better efficacy in patients on Beta blocker
Levosimendan	Calcium sensitizers	*Inotropy:* Levosimendan binds and sensitize the cardiac troponin C to calcium. This improves contraction without increasing calcium levels.	Binds to Troponin-C in calcium-dependent manner	↑	–	++	++	–	0.05–0.2 μ/kg/min 12 μ/kg/min over 10 minutes bolus (optional)	1 hour Metabolite OR 1896: 70–80 hours and have another active metabolite	Hypotension, Tachyarrhythmia	• Favored in patients with chronic heart failure and beta-blockade • Evidence is more favoring than other drugs pending large trials

Contd...

Contd...

Drug	Classification	Mechanism of action	Receptors/site of action	Effects					Dose[2,3]	Half-life	Adverse effects	Comments
				Inotropy	Systolic time	Arterial vasodilation	Pulmonary vasodilation	Heart rate				
		Vasodilation: It opens adenosine triphosphate (ATP)-sensitive potassium channels in vascular smooth muscle cells (hyperpolarize and relax) leading to vasodilation	ATP-sensitive potassium channels at the vascular smooth muscle									Has additional cardioprotective and pleiotropic properties
Omecamtiv mecarbil	Cardiac myosin activator	Prolongs the occupancy time of myosin on the actin molecule, increasing the number of myosin molecules bound to actin	Catalytic S1 domain of cardiac myosin	↑	↑	?		↓	Need further studies, oral and IV dose regimens are used in different studies[a]	Elimination half-life is 18.5 hours[a]	Increase cardiac biomarkers, myocardial ischemia	Novel drug, more studies in heart failure patients. Need more studies in critically ill patients
Digoxin	Cardiac glycosides	Increases intracellular calcium levels	Blocks membrane Na-K ATPase	↑	–	?/–		↓	0.125–0.25 mg IV or PO. 0.375–0.5 mg IV or PO daily higher can be tried[b]	36–48 hours	Arrhythmia, gastrointestinal symptoms	In special situations, atrial fibrillation with poor ventricular systolic function with hypotension Narrow therapeutic margin

(ATP: adenosine triphosphate; PDE-III: phosphodiesterase-III enzyme; c-AMP: cyclic adenosine monophosphate; SR: sarcoplasmic reticulum; mic: microgram; +: the effect is present; –: no effect; ?: doubtful or inconclusive effects; PO: per oral; IV: intravenous; ↑: increase; ↓: decrease; +/–: and arrows, the magnitude is relative for comparison and not quantitative)

The comment column is based on common practice, and expert opinion based. Reference VuT 2015[18] and ACCF/AHA 2013[19]

Recent work in cardiogenic shock demonstrates that no single inotrope is superior in overall mortality. Fernando et al. performed a network meta-analysis comparing several inotropes and found no significant differences in mortality outcomes.[12] However, levosimendan has shown promise in several studies.[13] There was no discernible difference in 90-day mortality between milrinone and dobutamine in the SHOCK-MED trial. A recent review showed the potential benefits and use of Levosimendan across various clinical conditions especially cardiogenic shock. The SHOCK-MED trial by Mathew et al. compared milrinone to dobutamine, finding no significant difference in 90-day mortality.[14] It is suggested by experts to tailor inotropes for low cardiac output states and supplement with vasopressors when there is hypotension. Also, there is no preference of any inotrope over the other.[15-17]

Phosphodiesterase-III inhibitors and levosimendan were better in improving cardiac output, left ventricular stroke volume index, and lowering lower pulmonary vascular pressures/resistance and systemic arterial resistance compared to dopamine and dobutamine. In patients with persisting CS refractory to dobutamine, it is better to opt for mechanical circulatory support rather than pharmacological alternatives.[7] Both PDE-III inhibitors and levosimendan had improved myocardial performance and tissue perfusion in such cases, but only levosimendan improved survival.[20] Levosimendan is also a potential option for patients with chronic β-blockade since its action is independent of β-adrenergic receptor stimulation.[7] Though various inotropes are used for improving organ perfusion in CS, none is proven superior. A recent Cochrane review showed a short-term mortality benefit with levosimendan compared to dobutamine which did not remain significant in the long term. However, there is not enough evidence to prove the superiority of one drug over the other. Further larger studies in hemodynamically unstable patients with low cardiac output are required which are correctly planned and executed.[1] So, inotropes in patients with CS are helpful in maintaining hemodynamic stability and tissue perfusion, but the choice depends on clinical profile and physician judgment.

Heart Failure: Acute Decompensated Heart Failure and Chronic Heart Failure

Patients with heart failure present with increasing dyspnea, chest congestion and there may be associated hypotension. In the past inotropic agents were used to improve cardiac performance and patient's symptoms, when patients had acute decompensated heart failure with reduced left ventricular ejection fraction and low cardiac output. Inotropic drugs increase mortality in patients with chronic heart failure when given for the long term.[21,22] The probable explanation could be a chronic increase in intracellular calcium levels; leading to altered gene expression; and malignant ventricular arrhythmias. Later studies focused on short-term use of inotropes in heart failure patients. In the SURVIVE study, levosimendan infusion reduced B-type natriuretic peptide (BNP) levels in patients with acute decompensated heart failure compared to dobutamine infusion.[23] But, it did not reduce all-cause mortality at 180 days. The levosimendan group had more headaches, arrhythmias, hypokalemia, and hypotension. In patients with acute decompensated chronic heart failure, 24-hour levosimendan infusion achieved better hemodynamic improvement at 48 hours compared to dobutamine.[24] The outcome study of SURVIVE patients showed that levosimendan was more effective than dobutamine in those who had a history of congestive cardiac failure and were on β-blockers.[25]

In the RUSSLAN study, levosimendan was given to patients with heart failure complicating acute myocardial infarction in a dose of 0.1–0.4 μg/kg/min, for 6 hours. Patients who received a higher dosage (>0.2 μg) had more hypotension and myocardial ischemia, but the lesser dosage was safer and improved mortality compared to placebo.[26] In the LIDO study, the authors compared levosimendan with dobutamine to study the efficacy and safety of levosimendan in patients with severe low-output heart failure. The primary outcome was an improvement in cardiac output ≥30% and a reduction of pulmonary capillary wedge pressure ≥25%. All patients received an infusion of inotropes for 24 hours and patients who received levosimendan achieved hemodynamic targets more effectively (hemodynamic targets were achieved only in 28% levosimendan group and 15% in dobutamine patients). The study also showed a mortality benefit at 180 days. Further, a few more randomized trials also showed the benefits of adding an inotrope to standard therapy in terms of reduction in symptoms in patients with acute decompensated heart failure.[27] In the REVIVE II study, patients who had dyspnea despite diuretics and left ventricular ejection fraction, ≤35% were randomized to receive levosimendan or placebo infusion. Patients who received levosimendan showed more clinical improvement, less deterioration, and a significant reduction in BNP levels.

Levosimendan may be useful in patients with heart failure to improve symptoms, reduce congestion, and improve perfusion with less increase in myocardial oxygen demand.[28] Compared to dobutamine and placebo levosimendan performed better. Apart from dobutamine, levosimendan, and milrinone, other inotropes have also been tried. The digitalis investigation group (DIG) trial did not show any mortality benefit with digoxin but reduced the rate of hospitalizations. Though the use of digoxin is reduced over the past few years probably due to its adverse effects and no outcome benefits, its use is still not abandoned in patients with heart failure.[29] Digoxin still plays a role in certain patients who have atrial fibrillation with fast ventricular rate and heart failure with reduced ejection fraction when there is a limitation to other therapeutic options.[6] Recently a new drug, OM, is being tried in heart failure patients due to its unique mechanism of action and better safety profile.[30] OM though has less adverse effects and is safe, it is not proven to improve mortality in heart failure patients.[31,32] The studies are emerging and there are no trials done in critically ill patients.

Recent two reviews on levosimendan by Girardis et al.[13] and Mebazaa et al. showed that levosimendan has demonstrated improved hemodynamics in acute heart failure, improved organ perfusion and function. However, there was no discernible advantage in terms of mortality. Bouchez et al. provided expert advice on levosimendan dose and administration in acute and severe heart failure, he showed improved renal function and survival with levosimendan in patients with advanced heart failure.[33] In severe heart failure, intermittent or continuous inotrope therapy may serve as a bridge to recovery, transplantation, or mechanical circulatory support. Arrigo et al. stressed the importance of optimizing medical therapy based on guidelines in addition to inotrope use. In summary, the inotropes are typically prescribed for short-term usage in acute decompensation with signs of hypoperfusion.[34]

Levosimendan is emerging as a potential option for patients with heart failure, but it still needs large studies to prove the benefits.

Sepsis and Septic Shock

Patients with septic shock often have septic cardiomyopathy with reduced left ventricular systolic function.[35] Fluids, vasopressors, and inotropes are the cornerstone to optimize hemodynamic instability. Inotropes are commonly chosen in patients with a low left ventricular systolic function who persistently have low mean arterial pressure and signs of tissue hypoperfusion despite adequate fluid resuscitation and vasopressor therapy. In early goal-directed therapy (GDT) in patients with sepsis, Rivers et al. showed improved survival with targeted hemodynamic resuscitation, but it was challenged recently.[36,37] In early GDT, dobutamine was used in patients with septic shock after fluid resuscitation, vasopressor therapy, and blood transfusion. Surviving sepsis campaign recommends a similar approach in patients with septic shock.[38] The recommendation was only based on physiological improvement in tissue perfusion and not based on randomized trials. In patients with septic shock, inotropes improved cardiac output, in turn improving blood flow and microcirculation. Administration of low-dose dobutamine of 5 μg/kg/min improved capillary flow in septic shock, independent of systemic effects.[39] Another study showed improved capillary perfusion with dobutamine infusion only when there was a low systolic ejection fraction and severe microcirculatory alteration at baseline.[40] Similarly, dobutamine improved microcirculation only in septic shocks patients with low cardiac output with persistent hypoperfusion and not in all patients.[41] Dobutamine infusion does not increase cardiac output in all patients and causes more tachycardia, tachyarrhythmias, increased myocardial oxygen utilization and hypotension necessitating discontinuation of the drug. The beneficial effect of inotropes is confined to only in patients with low left ventricular systolic function and poor tissue perfusion rather than those with normal systolic function.

When the mechanisms of septic myocardial depression are looked into, calcium desensitization is a postulated hypothesis in septic myocardial depression. So, whether calcium sensitization will play a role in managing such patients is an interesting question. This question was answered in a trial where levosimendan, a calcium-sensitizing inotrope, was added to patients who received 48 hours of conventional therapy including 5 μg/kg/min of dobutamine.[42] The group with added levosimendan showed improved systemic and regional hemodynamics in patients with cardiac dysfunction, where only dobutamine was not efficacious. Adding levosimendan is a potential option rather than increasing dobutamine in such cases. Levosimendan also reduced the biomarkers of myocardial injury compared to dobutamine but with no outcome benefits.[43] A recent meta-analysis did not show a mortality benefit with levosimendan compared to dobutamine in septic shock patients[44] necessitating further research. In a recent randomized trial (LeoPARDS) levosimendan infusion for 24 hours in patients with early sepsis was tried aiming at reducing the severity of organ dysfunction. The addition of levosimendan did not improve the severity of organ dysfunction but rather there was a higher incidence of supraventricular arrhythmias.[45] Though many studies have shown the benefits of inotropes in sepsis, it has not translated into improving outcomes[46] and there is no single inotrope that is superior to others.[44]

For septic shock, the Surviving Sepsis Campaign guidelines recommend norepinephrine as the first-choice vasopressor, with vasopressin or epinephrine as second-line agents. Dobutamine is suggested when there is evidence of persistent hypoperfusion despite adequate fluid loading and the use of vasopressor agents.[47]

PERIOPERATIVE PERIOD

Major surgeries cause significant tissue trauma, and exaggerated inflammatory response leading to increased metabolic demand, and tissue oxygen need thus demanding an increase in cardiac output. Low cardiac output and inadequate oxygen delivery may lead to adverse outcomes,[48] especially in patients undergoing cardiac surgeries. Perioperative left ventricular dysfunction is the main contributor to low cardiac output during cardiac surgery. Directing the therapy toward a goal, the GDT has shown beneficial effects in surgical patients.[49] Various combinations of fluids, vasopressors, and inotropes are used to achieve the goal. Inotrope use is more common in cardiac surgical patients during the perioperative period and there is no preference of any one inotrope over others. Though dobutamine is preferred due to the short half-life, easy titration, and less adverse effect pattern, PDE-I and levosimendan are also tried with success. Milrinone and dobutamine were effective in improving systemic hemodynamics in cardiac surgical patients.[50] Also, prophylactic administration of milrinone prevented cardiac deterioration postoperatively and helped to maintain hemodynamic stability.[51] Furthermore, a meta-analysis that focused on patients undergoing cardiac surgery suggested a survival benefit in patients receiving levosimendan compared to placebo.[52] While perioperative inotrope use is prevalent, there is a lack of precise data in the recently reviewed literature. Inotropes are commonly used to treat postcardiotomy shock or vasoplegic syndrome following heart surgery. Levosimendan has been evaluated for potential cardioprotective effects when taken preoperatively in high-risk cardiac surgery patients, according to Mebazaa et al. The emphasis is on tailoring therapy to preoperative cardiac function and kind of surgery.

CONCLUSION

Inotropic therapy improves the hemodynamic status of patients offering short-term benefits. A better understanding of the pathophysiology of shock and its effects as well as the adverse effects of drugs is important to decide on the choice of drugs to achieve the desired therapeutic goal. Routine use of inotropes to improve cardiac output is not favored in patients with heart failure.[44] Inotropes are of benefit in patients with CS after acute myocardial infarction to maintain tissue perfusion, the choice of drug depends on the clinical profile of the patient and the treating physician's preference. Though currently dobutamine is commonly used, levosimendan is safer and beneficial and has been shown to have more survival benefits and faster symptom relief in patients with CS. There is emerging evidence in favor of levosimendan as an inotrope of choice in all patients with low cardiac output state, but at present, the evidence is weak to recommend an individual drug. A combination of different inotropic drugs in smaller doses may be advantageous rather than using high doses of a single drug, but there is no clarity on the drug combinations and choice. The majority of studies were done in noncritically ill populations and the results are extrapolated to critically ill patients. The initiation and choice of inotrope in a given clinical scenario is largely based on the clinical judgment of the physician.

REFERENCES

1. Schumann J, Henrich EC, Strobl H, Prondzinsky R, Weiche S, Thiele H, et al. Inotropic agents and vasodilator strategies for the treatment of cardiogenic shock or low cardiac output syndrome. Cochrane Database Syst Rev. 2018;1(1):CD009669.
2. Overgaard CB, Dzavík V. Inotropes and vasopressors: review of physiology and clinical use in cardiovascular disease. Circulation. 2008;118(10):1047-56.
3. Bistola V, Chioncel O. Inotropes in acute heart failure. Contin Cardiol Educ. 2017;3(3):107-16.
4. Aditya S, Rattan A. Istaroxime: A rising star in acute heart failure. J Pharmacol Pharmacother. 2012;3(4):353-5.
5. Landoni G, Mizzi A, Biondi-Zoccai G, Bignami E, Prati P, Ajello V, et al. Levosimendan reduces mortality in critically ill patients. A meta-analysis of randomized controlled studies. Minerva Anestesiol. 2010;76(4):276-86.

6. Ponikowski P, Voors AA, Anker SD, Bueno H, Cleland JG, Coats AJ, et al. 2016 ESC Guidelines for the diagnosis and treatment of acute and chronic heart failure: The Task Force for the diagnosis and treatment of acute and chronic heart failure of the European Society of Cardiology (ESC). Developed with the special contribution of the Heart Failure Association (HFA) of the ESC. European journal of heart failure. 2016;18(8):891-975.
7. Levy B, Bastien O, Benjelid K, Cariou A, Chouihed T, Combes A, et al. Experts' recommendations for the management of adult patients with cardiogenic shock. Ann Intensive Care. 2015;5(1):1-10.
8. van Diepen S, Katz JN, Albert NM, Henry TD, Jacobs AK, Kapur NK, et al. Contemporary Management of Cardiogenic Shock: A Scientific Statement from the American Heart Association. Circulation. 2017;136(16):e232-e268.
9. Levy B, Perez P, Perny J, Thivilier C, Gerard A. Comparison of norepinephrine-dobutamine to epinephrine for hemodynamics, lactate metabolism, and organ function variables in cardiogenic shock. A prospective, randomized pilot study. Crit Care Med. 2011;39(3):450-5.
10. De Backer D, Biston P, Devriendt J, Madl C, Chochrad D, Aldecoa C, et al. Comparison of dopamine and norepinephrine in the treatment of shock. N Engl J Med. 2010;362(9):779-89.
11. Richard C, Ricome JL, Bottineau G, Bottineau G, Auzepy P. Combined hemodynamic effects of dopamine and dobutamine in cardiogenic shock. Circulation. 1983; 67(3):620-6.
12. Fernando SM, Mathew R, Sadeghirad B, Brodie D, Belley-Côté EP, Thiele H, et al. Inotropes, vasopressors, and mechanical circulatory support for treatment of cardiogenic shock complicating myocardial infarction: a systematic review and network meta-analysis. Can J Anaesth. 2022;69(12):1537-53.
13. Girardis M, Bettex D, Bojan M, Demponeras C, Fruhwald S, Gál J et al. Levosimendan in intensive care and emergency medicine: literature update and expert recommendations for optimal efficacy and safety. J Anesth Analg Crit Care. 2022;2(1):4.
14. Mathew R, Di Santo P, Jung RG, Marbach JA, Hutson J, Simard T, et al. Milrinone as compared with dobutamine in the treatment of cardiogenic shock. N Engl J Med. 2021;385(6):516-25.
15. Bloom JE, Chan W, Kaye DM, Stub D. State of shock: contemporary vasopressor and inotrope use in cardiogenic shock. J Am Heart Assoc. 2023;12(15):e029787.
16. Lepage-Ratte MF, Hibbert B, Mathew R. The role of inotropes in cardiogenic shock: to help, to harm or do nothing at all?Eur Heart J Cardiovasc Pharmacother. 2024;10(2):98-9.
17. Vu T, Ma P, Xiao JJ, Wang YM, Malik FI, Chow AT. Population pharmacokinetic-pharmacodynamic modeling of omecamtiv mecarbil, a cardiac myosin activator, in healthy volunteers and patients with stable heart failure. J Clin Pharmacol. 2015;55(11):1236-47.
18. Yancy CW, Jessup M, Bozkurt B, Butler J, Casey DE Jr, Drazner MH, et al. 2013 ACCF/AHA guideline for the management of heart failure: a report of the American College of Cardiology Foundation/American Heart Association Task Force on Practice Guidelines. J Am Coll Cardiol. 2013;62(16):e147-239.
19. el Allaf D, Cremers S, D'Orio V, Carlier J. Combined haemodynamic effects of low doses of dopamine and dobutamine in patients with acute infarction and cardiac failure. Arch Int Physiol Biochim. 1984;92(4):S49-55.
20. Fuhrmann JT, Schmeisser A, Schulze MR, Wunderlich C, Schoen SP, Rauwolf T, et al. Levosimendan is superior to enoximone in refractory cardiogenic shock complicating acute myocardial infarction. Crit Care Med. 2008;36(8): 2257-66.
21. Felker GM, O'Connor CM. Inotropic therapy for heart failure: an evidence-based approach. Am Heart J. 2001;142(3): 393-401.
22. Packer M, Carver JR, Rodeheffer RJ, Ivanhoe RJ, DiBianco R, Zeldis SM, et al. Effect of oral milrinone on mortality in severe chronic heart failure. The PROMISE Study Research Group. N Engl J Med. 1991;325(21):1468-75.
23. Mebazaa A, Nieminen MS, Packer M, Cohen-Solal A, Kleber FX, Pocock SJ, et al. Levosimendan vs dobutamine for patients with acute decompensated heart failure: the SURVIVE Randomized Trial. JAMA. 2007;297(17):1883-91.
24. Bergh CH, Andersson B, Dahlström U, Forfang K, Kivikko M, Sarapohja T, et al. Intravenous levosimendan vs. dobutamine in acute decompensated heart failure patients on beta-blockers. Eur J Heart Fail. 2010;12(4):404-10.
25. Mebazaa A, Nieminen MS, Filippatos GS, Cleland JG, Salon JE, Thakkar R, et al. Levosimendan vs. dobutamine: outcomes for acute heart failure patients on beta-blockers in SURVIVE. Eur J Heart Fail. 2009;11(3):304-11.
26. Moiseyev VS, Põder P, Andrejevs N, Ruda MY, Golikov AP, Lazebnik LB, et al. Safety and efficacy of a novel calcium sensitizer, levosimendan, in patients with left ventricular failure due to an acute myocardial infarction. A randomized, placebo-controlled, double-blind study (RUSSLAN). Eur Heart J. 2002;23(18):1422-32.
27. Landoni G, Biondi-Zoccai G, Greco M, Greco T, Bignami E, Morelli A, et al. Effects of levosimendan on mortality and hospitalization. A meta-analysis of randomized controlled studies. Crit Care Med. 2012;40(2):634-46.
28. Altenberger J, Gustafsson F, Harjola V. Levosimendan in acute and advanced heart failure: an appraisal of the clinical database and evaluation of its therapeutic applications. J Cardiovasc Pharmacol. 2018;71(3):129-36.
29. Konstantinou DM, Karvounis H, Giannakoulas G. Digoxin in heart failure with a reduced ejection fraction: a risk factor or a risk marker. Cardiology. 2016;134(3):311-9.
30. Kaplinsky E, Mallarkey G. Cardiac myosin activators for heart failure therapy: focus on omecamtiv mecarbil. Drugs Context. 2018;7:212518.

31. Teerlink JR, Felker GM, McMurray JJV, Ponikowski P, Metra M, Filippatos GS, et al. Acute Treatment With Omecamtiv Mecarbil to Increase Contractility in Acute Heart Failure: The ATOMIC-AHF Study. J Am Coll Cardiol. 2016;67(12):1444-55.
32. Papp Z, Agostoni P, Alvarez J, Bettex D, Bouchez S, Brito D et al. Levosimendan Efficacy and Safety: 20 years of SIMDAX in Clinical Use. Card Fail Rev. 2020;6:e19.
33. Bouchez S, Fedele F, Giannakoulas G, Gustafsson F, Harjola VP, Karason K, et al. Levosimendan in acute and advanced heart failure: an expert perspective on posology and therapeutic application. Cardiovasc Drugs Ther. 2018;32(6):617-24.
34. Arrigo M, Jessup M, Mullens W, Reza N, Shah AM, Sliwa K, et al. Acute heart failure. Nat Rev Dis Primers. 2020;6(1):16.
35. Vieillard-Baron A. Septic cardiomyopathy. Ann Intensive Care. 2011;1(1):6.
36. Rivers E, Nguyen B, Havstad S, Ressler J, Muzzin A, Knoblich B, et al. Early goal-directed therapy in the treatment of severe sepsis and septic shock. N Engl J Med. 2001;345(19):1368-77.
37. De Backer, Vincent JL. Early goal-directed therapy: do we have a definitive answer? Intensive Care Med. 2016;42(6):1048-50.
38. Rhodes A, Evans LE, Alhazzani W, Levy MM, Antonelli M, Ferrer R, et al. Surviving Sepsis Campaign: International Guidelines for Management of Sepsis and Septic Shock: 2016. Intensive Care Med. 2017;43(3):304-77.
39. De Backer D, Creteur J, Dubois MJ, Sakr Y, Koch M, Verdant C, et al. The effects of dobutamine on microcirculatory alterations in patients with septic shock are independent of its systemic effects. Crit Care Med. 2006;34:403-8.
40. Enrico C, Kanoore Edul VS, Vazquez AR, Pein MC, Pérez de la Hoz RA, Ince C, et al. Systemic and microcirculatory effects of dobutamine in patients with septic shock. J Crit Care. 2012;27(6):630-8.
41. Hernandez G, Bruhn A, Luengo C, Regueira T, Kattan E, Fuentealba A, et al. Effects of dobutamine on systemic, regional and microcirculatory perfusion parameters in septic shock: a randomized, placebo-controlled, double-blind, crossover study. Intensive Care Med. 2013;39(8):1435-43.
42. Morelli A, Castro S De, Teboul JL, Singer M, Rocco M, Conti G, et al. Effects of levosimendan on systemic and regional hemodynamics in septic myocardial depression. Intensive Care Med. 2005;31(5):638-44.
43. Meng J, Hu M, Lai Z, Ji CL, Xu XJ, Zhang G, et al. Levosimendan Versus Dobutamine in myocardial injury patients with septic shock: a randomized controlled trial. Med Sci Monit. 2016;22:1486-96.
44. Bhattacharjee S, Soni KD, Maitra S, Baidya DK. Levosimendan does not provide mortality benefit over dobutamine in adult patients with septic shock: A meta-analysis of randomized controlled trials. J Clin Anesth. 2017;39:67-72.
45. Santhakumaran S, Mason AJ, Cross M, McAuley DF, Orme RM, Santhakumaran S, et al. Levosimendan for the Prevention of Acute Organ Dysfunction in Sepsis. N Engl J Med. 2016;375(17):1638-48.
46. Wang B, Chen R, Guo X, Zhang W, Hu J, Gong Y, et al. Effects of levosimendan on mortality in patients with septic shock: systematic review with meta-analysis and trial sequential analysis. Oncotarget. 2017;8(9):100524-32.
47. Evans L, Rhodes A, Alhazzani W, Antonelli M, Coopersmith CM, French C, et al. Surviving sepsis campaign: International guidelines for management of sepsis and septic shock 2021. Intensive Care Med. 2021; 47(11):1181-1247.
48. Lobo SM, Rezende E, Knibel MF, Silva NB, Páramo JA, Nácul FE, et al. Early determinants of death due to multiple organ failure after noncardiac surgery in high-risk patients. Anesth Analg. 2011;112(4):877-83.
49. Lobo SM, Mendes CL, Rezende E, Dias FS. Optimizing perioperative hemodynamics: What is new? Curr Opin Crit Care. 2013;19:346-52.
50. Feneck RO, Sherry KM, Withington PS, Oduro-Dominah A; European Milrinone Multicenter Trial Group. Comparison of the hemodynamic effects of milrinone with dobutamine in patients after cardiac surgery. J Cardiothorac Vasc Anesth. 2001;15(3):306-15.
51. Kikura M, Sato S. The efficacy of preemptive Milrinone or Amrinone therapy in patients undergoing coronary artery bypass grafting. Anesth Analg. 2002;94(1):22-30.
52. Greco T, Calabrò MG, Covello RD, Greco M, Pasin L, Morelli A, et al. A Bayesian network meta-analysis on the effect of inodilatory agents on mortality. 2015;114:746-56.

CHAPTER 

Intra-aortic Balloon Pump

Divya Pal, Deepak Govil

INTRODUCTION

After almost six decades since the introduction and first use of intra-aortic balloon pump (IABP) counterpulsation in humans, the evidence regarding the benefits of its use with respect to mortality and morbidity remains conflicting. Despite this, IABP, an internal counterpulsation device, remains the most widely used mechanical circulatory assist device for the failing heart. Different forms of support available for a failing heart include extracorporeal membrane oxygenation (ECMO), internal and external counterpulsation devices, and ventricular assist devices (VADs).

In 1952, Kantrowitz described in animals, the augmentation of coronary flow, by retardation of the arterial pressure pulse.[1] Harken in 1958 suggested the removal of blood via the femoral artery, during systole and replacing it rapidly in diastole, as the treatment for left ventricular (LV) failure.[2] In 1962, Moulopoulos and Kantrowitz developed an experimental prototype of an IABP.[3] In 1968, Kantrowitz reported the use of IABP in two patients with cardiogenic shock (CS) with improvement in urine output, blood pressure (BP), and survival of one of them to discharge.[4] In 1980, the first percutaneous IABP catheter insertion was described by Bergman.[5]

INTRA-AORTIC BALLOON COUNTERPULSATION SYSTEM: THE DEVICE

It is composed of two principal parts:[6]

1. *A mobile console:* It contains a cylinder of gas source that is helium; a valve unit allowing gas delivery; a monitor for acquisition of electrocardiogram (ECG) and arterial BP; and a control unit that develops a trigger signal by processing the ECG and aortic pressure. Both helium and carbon dioxide have been used as the driving gas, but helium has certain advantages over carbon dioxide. It has a lower viscosity, which implies there is little turbulent flow, so the balloon can inflate fast and deflate slowly. Also, it is relatively benign and is absorbed quickly if the balloon ruptures.[7]
2. *A balloon catheter:* It is flexible and has two lumens, one to allow either distal aspiration, flushing, or pressure monitoring and another that permits the periodic delivery and removal of helium gas to the balloon. The balloons are available in capacity between 25 and 50 cc, most commonly 40 cc being used for adults.[6] See **Table 1** for choosing the appropriate size of IABP catheter.

TABLE 1: Approximate size guide for intra-aortic balloon pump catheter.[7]

Height (in cm)	*Size (cc)*
<152	25
152–163	34
164–183	40
>183	50

Principles of Counterpulsation

Intra-aortic counterpulsation attempts to create a balance between myocardial oxygen supply and demand by systolic unloading and diastolic augmentation. This happens by inflation in diastole and balloon deflation in early systole **(Flowcharts 1 and 2) (Figs. 1 and 2)**.[7]

Endocardial Viability Ratio

Endocardial viability ratio (EVR) is the ratio of diastolic pressure time index (DPTI) to tension time index (TTI) **(Fig. 3)**, and is a reflection of the relationship between oxygen (O_2) supply and O_2 consumption of the myocardium, i.e., (EVR = DPTI/TTI).

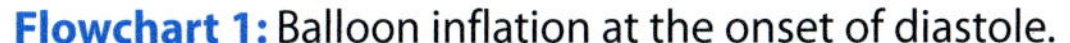

Flowchart 1: Balloon inflation at the onset of diastole.

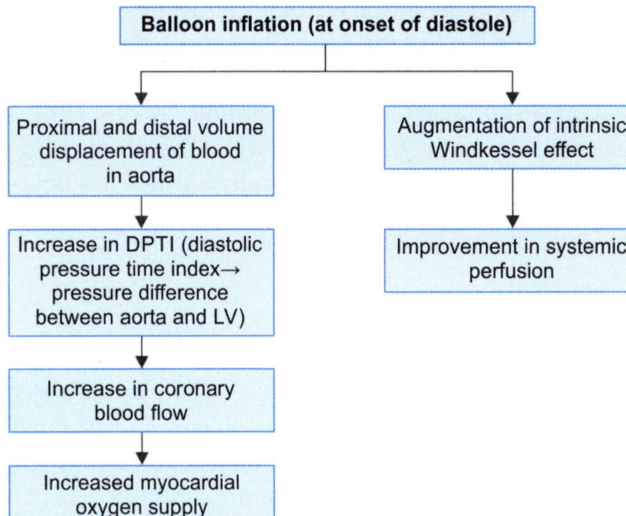

(LV: left ventricular)

Flowchart 2: Balloon deflation in systole.

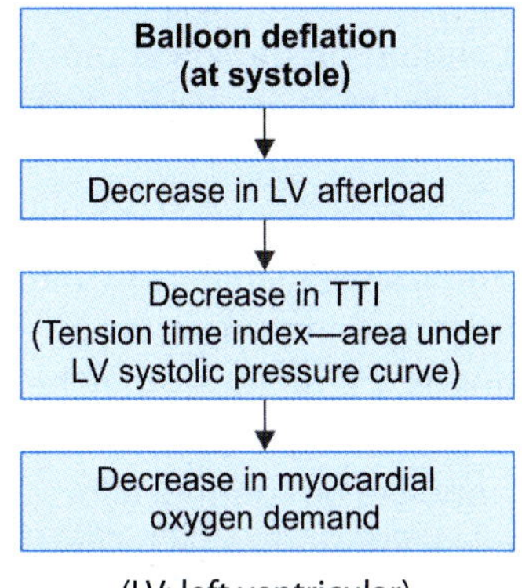

(LV: left ventricular)

Endocardial viability ratio ≥1.0 indicates a normal supply-demand balance while a ratio of <0.7 is indicative of severe myocardial ischemia. IABP by increasing DPTI and decreasing TTI helps in increasing the EVR index, thus improving the demand-supply balance.[8]

Technique of Insertion

The appropriate size of the balloon needs to be selected as per the patient's height **(Table 1)** and the diameter of the balloon should be such that when fully expanded it covers no >80–90% of the diameter of the patient's descending thoracic aorta. The IABP catheter can be inserted percutaneously using a modified Seldinger's technique or by surgical cutdown. A sheathed or a sheathless technique may be used, the latter has been reported to be associated with lesser vascular complications.[9]

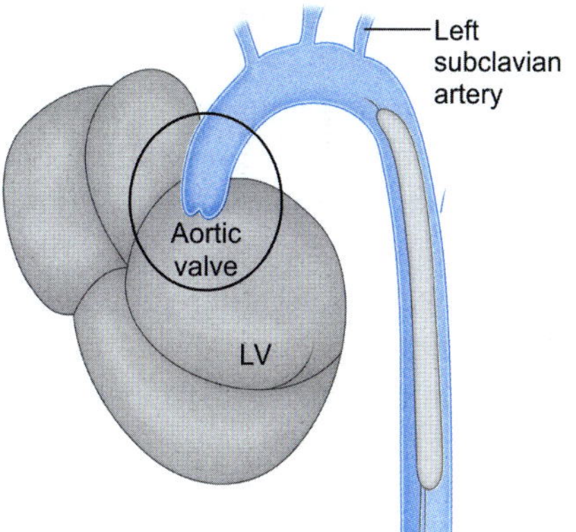

Fig. 1: Balloon inflation in diastole. (LV: left ventricular)
Note: The placement of the balloon in relation to the left subclavian artery in the aorta.

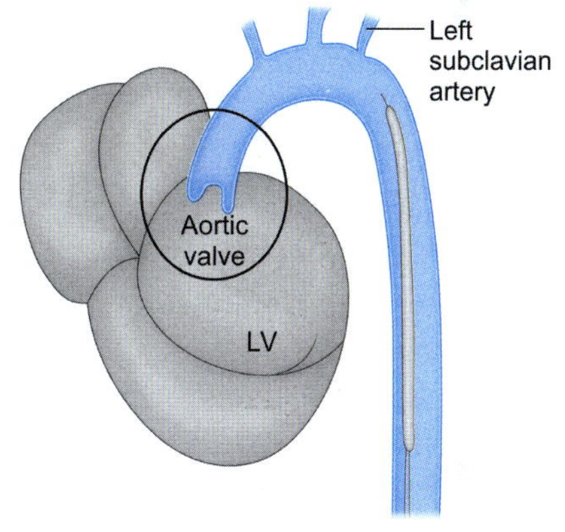

Fig. 2: Balloon deflation in early systole. (LV: left ventricular)
Note: The placement of the balloon in relation to the left subclavian artery in the aorta.

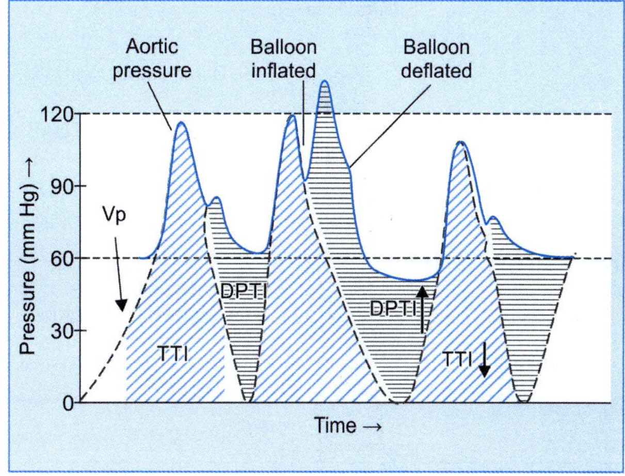

Fig. 3: Effect of intra-aortic balloon pump on diastolic pressure time index and tension time index (TTI).[8]

Most common site of insertion is the femoral artery, others being subclavian, axillary, brachial, or iliac arteries.[7] After informed consent is taken, the patient is positioned supine and site preparation is done using sterile precautions. The balloon is fully collapsed by applying a vacuum using a syringe. After obtaining vascular access, the balloon catheter is advanced over the guidewire through the sheath in the descending thoracic aorta till the estimated distance (measure from sternal angle to umbilicus then to the femoral artery), with its tip placed up to 2–3 cm distal to the origin of left subclavian artery. The position should be such that the proximal end of the balloon is proximal to the origin of renal arteries.[8] Watch for the left radial pulse which may be absent if the balloon is advanced too high. The guidewire is then removed, and the central lumen is connected to the transducer for aortic pressure monitoring. IABP augmentation can be done in 1:1 or 1:2 or 1:3 ratio (trigger ratio—IABP: R wave).

Confirmation of Position

- Look at the morphology of the IABP waveforms **(Fig. 4)**, and the timing of inflation and deflation in 1:2 augmentation.
- The IABP should be positioned such that its distal tip lies 2–3 cm distal to the origin of the left subclavian artery, which can be seen on a chest computerized tomography scan if performed.
- The position can be confirmed on chest X-ray, or fluoroscopy if put under fluoroscopic guidance. On an anteroposterior chest X-ray view, the radiopaque tip lies 1 cm below the top of the aortic arch, at or just above the level of the carina, just above the left main bronchus[10] **(Fig. 5)**.
- Transesophageal echocardiography. A descending aortic short- or long-axis view can be obtained on transesophageal echocardiography and the echo-dense wire within the aortic lumen can be demonstrated as it is advanced into the descending thoracic aorta. After verifying the position of the guidewire, the IABP can be advanced over it.[7]

Monitoring and Patient Care

- Monitor the systolic, diastolic, mean, and diastolic augmented pressures hourly. Regular monitoring of left radial and pedal pulses in the limb that has IAB should also be done. Also, monitor the limb for signs of ischemia.[6,11]
- Watch for urine output, and any signs of bleeding, hematoma, or infection at the insertion site.[6,11]
- The patient should be nursed supine with head end elevation no >30°. The leg with the IAB should be kept straight.[11]
- Do daily chest X-rays, serum electrolytes, blood urea, serum creatinine, coagulation, and hematocrit.[6,11]
- Systemic anticoagulation must be given, particularly if IABP timing is 1:2 or 1:3. It may be reasonable to administer anticoagulation in even 1:1 augmentation, if IABP is planned to be continued for >24 hours, in the absence of any contraindication of anticoagulation.[11,12]

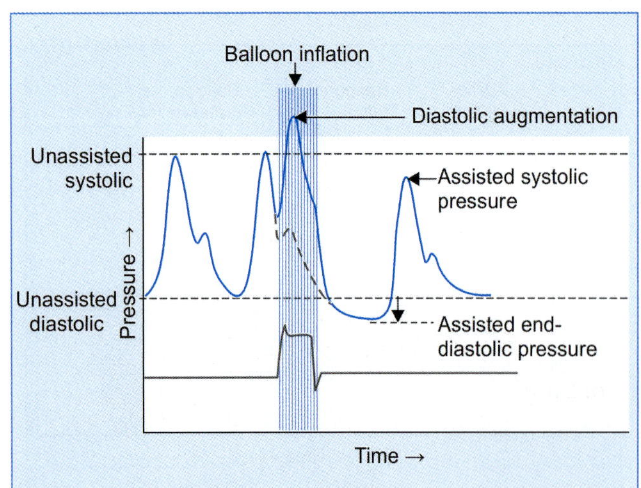

Fig. 4: The normal intra-aortic balloon pump blood pressure waveform.

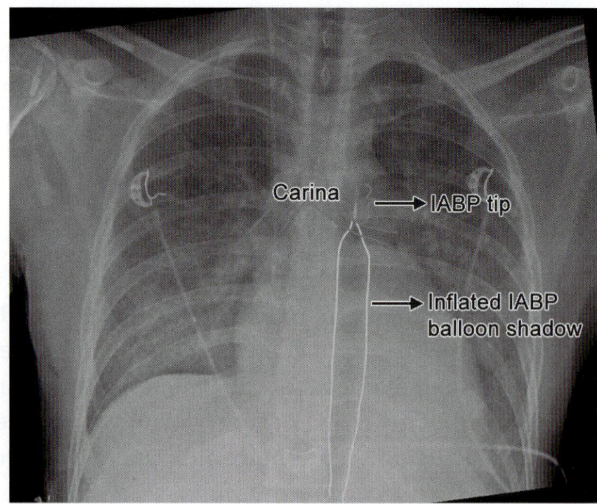

Fig. 5: Position of distal tip of intra-aortic balloon pump (IABP) placed through femoral access *(For color version, see Plate 4)*.

- Any blood or rust-colored flecks in the helium line of the IABP catheter or recurrent gas loss alarm may be suggestive of balloon rupture and should be looked for.[11]

Trigger

It is the way the IABP senses the beginning of the cardiac cycle to correctly time the inflation and deflation of the balloon. Triggering can be achieved by using the following sources:[6,9,12]

- *ECG:* It is the most commonly used trigger. The R wave on ECG is the most reliable trigger, which correlates with the onset of systole and when the deflation of the balloon happens. Inflation of the balloon happens at the beginning of the diastole, which correlates with the midpoint of the T wave **(Fig. 6)**.
- *Pressure:* The systolic upstroke of arterial pressure waveform acts as the trigger signal; this should be used when the ECG signal is lost or distorted.
- *Pacer V/AV*—a trigger mode in ventricular or AV-paced rhythms. Ventricular spike areused as a trigger signal.
- *Pacer A*—a trigger mode in atrial-paced rhythms, the atrial spike is used as a trigger signal.
- *Internal*—the balloon inflation and deflation happen at a preset rate, irrespective of the cardiac activity. Used when the patient is not generating cardiac output or is in cardiac arrest.

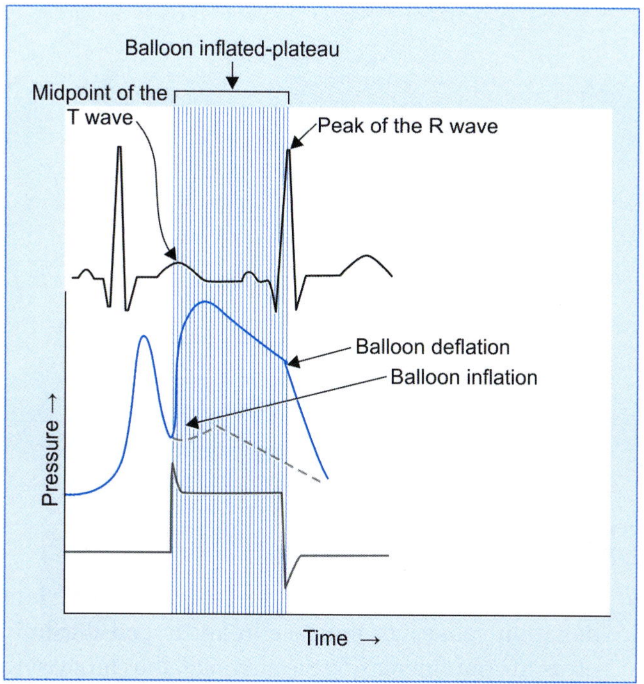

Fig. 6: ECG triggering of intra-aortic balloon pump (IABP).

Hemodynamic Consequences of Intra-aortic Balloon Pump Therapy[6,8,12]

- Reduction in assisted systolic BP (up to 10%), thus, a reduction in afterload.
- Reduction in end-diastolic aortic pressure (up to 30%), thus causing systolic unloading.
- An increase in aortic diastolic pressure (by 30%) and diastolic perfusion pressure gradient, thus increasing the coronary perfusion.
- An increase in CO (up to 30%) and in mean arterial pressure especially in patients with shock due to acute mechanical abnormality, such as mitral regurgitation (MR) and ventricular septal defect (VSD).
- Decrease in preload because of a decrease in LV diastolic volume due to systolic unloading.
- Decrease in calculated peak LV wall stress by around 14% and also decline in the rate of size of LV pressure (dp/dt).

Contraindications for the Use of Intra-aortic Balloon Pump[7,9]

- *Aortic regurgitation:* In the presence of an incompetent aortic valve, the balloon inflation in diastole will increase the LV preload by augmenting the regurgitation.
- *Aortic dissection:* The pulsation of the balloon may increase the blood volume in the false lumen, thus expanding the dissection. Also, it can lead to the dislodgement of any clots forming inside into the systemic circulation.
- *Aortic aneurysm:* The diastolic augmentation would be poor in the presence of aneurysmal dilatation of the aorta as there will be no elastic recoil of the aorta in response to balloon inflation. It may also lead to aortic rupture with a large abdominal aortic aneurysm.
- *Uncontrolled sepsis:* In a septic patient, another invasive device may become a surface to harbor microorganisms. Also, because of vasodilatation in septic shock, the diastolic augmentation would be poor.
- *Severe peripheral vascular disease:* It may lead to worsening of limb ischemia, so it is a relative contraindication of IABP.
- *Contraindication to anticoagulation:* For example, in patients with uncontrolled bleeding, intracranial bleeding, retroperitoneal hematoma, etc., where anticoagulation cannot be given, IABP is a relative contraindication.

TABLE 2: Possible complications associated with intra-aortic balloon pump.

Procedure related	Device related	Vascular	Others
• Local vascular injury—bleeding from insertion site, hematoma • Malpositioning of the balloon—causing cerebral/renal compromise	• Balloon rupture—causing gas embolism • Balloon entrapment • Kinking of the catheter	• Limb ischemia • Aortic dissection • False aneurysm • Peripheral embolization • Compartment syndrome • Cardiac tamponade	• Hemolysis • Thrombocytopenia • Sepsis

Complications

Table 2 shows possible complications associated with IABP.[7,9]

TROUBLESHOOTING

Abnormal Intra-aortic Balloon Pump Waveforms

Early Balloon Inflation (Fig. 7)[7,12]

- *Increased myocardial oxygen demand:* Balloon inflation, while the LV is still contracting leads to increased systemic vascular resistance and increased afterload. Also, there is a backward flow of blood from the aorta into the LV causing an increase in left ventricular end-diastolic volume (LVEDV) and left ventricular end-diastolic pressure (LVEDP), contributing to increased LV stress, aortic regurgitation, and increased O_2 demand.
- *Decreased cardiac output:* Early balloon inflation leads to premature closure of the aortic valve, and premature end of the systole, thus resulting in incomplete emptying of LV and decreased stroke volume (SV).
- *Decreased myocardial oxygen supply:* Due to wasted diastolic augmentation because of early inflation.

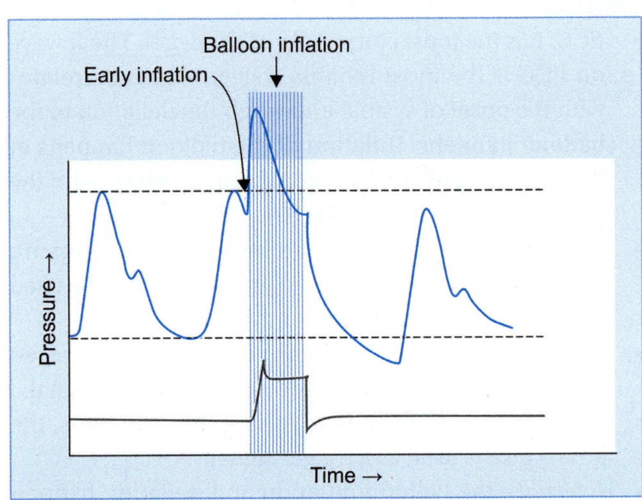

Fig. 7: Early balloon inflation leading to increased afterload.

Late Balloon Inflation (Fig. 8)[7,12]

- Decreased diastolic augmentation leads to decreased coronary perfusion.
- In the IABP waveform there is a loss of sharp "V."

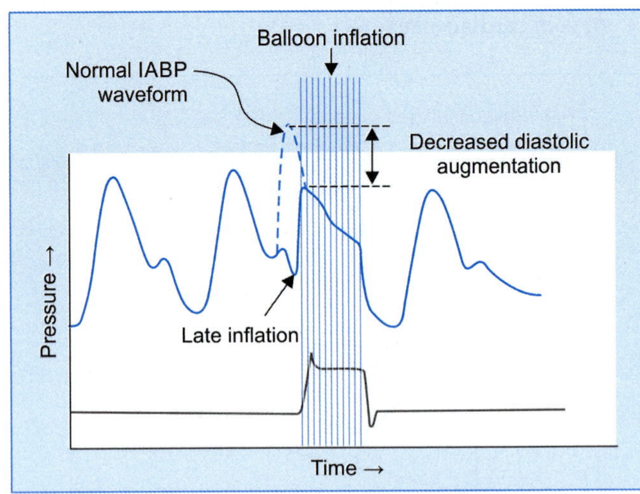

Fig. 8: Late balloon inflation leading to decreased diastolic augmentation. (IABP: intra-aortic balloon pump)

Early Deflation (Fig. 9)[7,12]

- Assisted aortic end-diastolic pressure may be equal to or less than the unassisted aortic end-diastolic pressure, suboptimal afterload reduction, thus leading to failure to decrease the myocardial O_2 demand.
- In the waveform, deflation of IABP is seen as a sharp drop following diastolic augmentation, which may cause suboptimal diastolic augmentation and, thus suboptimal coronary perfusion.

Late Balloon Deflation (Fig. 10)[7,12]

- Increased myocardial oxygen consumption; late deflation causes an increase in aortic end-diastolic pressure, thus increasing the afterload, thus increasing myocardial O_2 consumption.

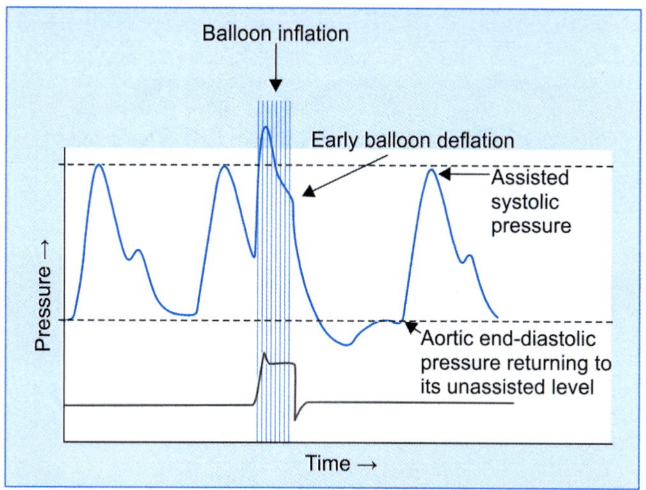

Fig. 9: Early balloon deflation.

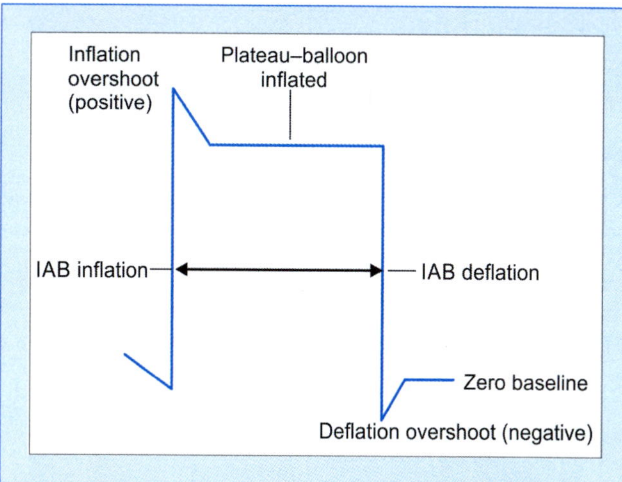

Fig. 11: Normal balloon pressure waveform. (IAB: intra-aortic balloon)

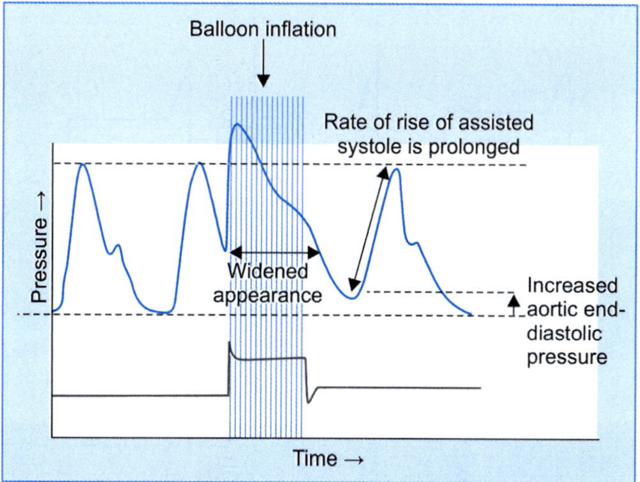

Fig. 10: Late balloon deflation increases afterload.

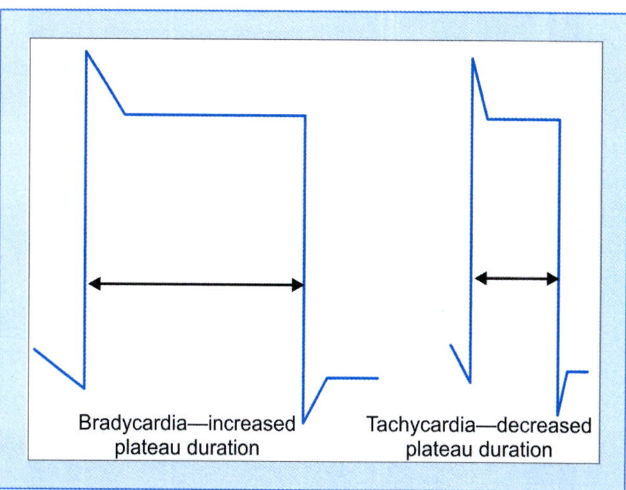

Fig. 12: Effects of bradycardia and tachycardia on plateau duration.

- In the waveform, there is a widening of diastolic augmentation phase, assisted aortic end-diastolic pressure is more as compared to unassisted, and the rate of rise of assisted systole is prolonged.

Balloon Pressure Waveforms-variations[13]

Normal Balloon Pressure Waveform

The width of the waveform corresponds to the duration of balloon inflation during the cardiac cycle. The plateau reflects the pressure within the aorta when the balloon is inflated **(Fig. 11)**.[13]

Bradycardia and Tachycardia

Increased and decreased plateau duration due to respective increased and decreased duration of diastole **(Fig. 12)**.

Arrhythmia

Varying waveform width due to erratic heart rate and diastole duration **(Fig. 13)**.

Hypertension and Hypotension

It can cause an increase and decrease in amplitude, respectively, in the balloon pressure waveform **(Fig. 14)**.

Balloon Catheter Kink or Obstruction

It is leading to the loss of plateau and a rounded pressure waveform. This can also happen if the IAB is too large for the aorta or it is not fully unwrapped or it is malpositioned **(Fig. 15)**.

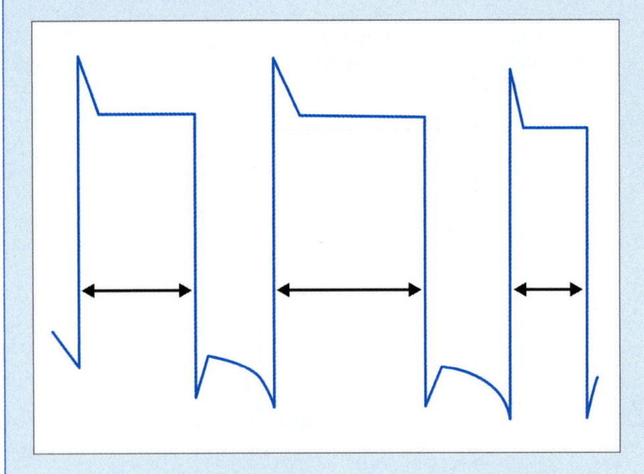

Fig. 13: Arrhythmia leading to varying width.

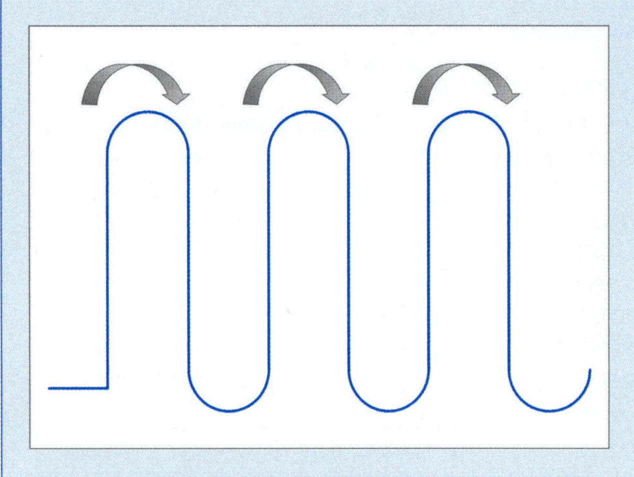

Fig. 15: Loss of plateau leading to rounded waveform.

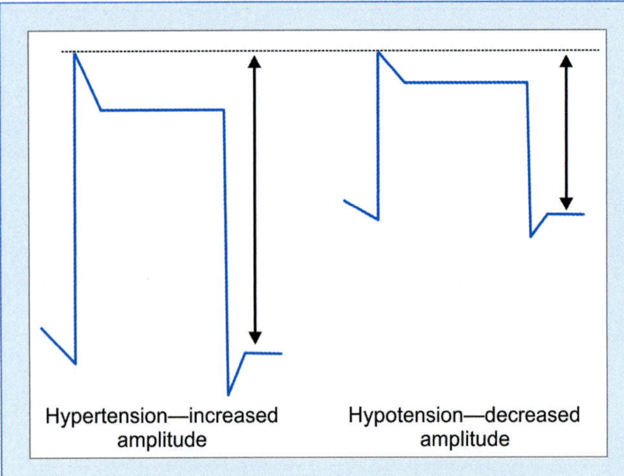

Fig. 14: Blood pressure changes causing effect on amplitude.

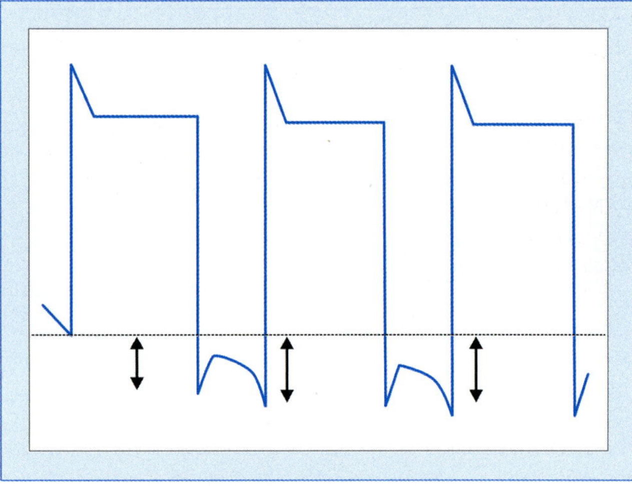

Fig. 16: Balloon gas leak leading to pressure waveform falling below the zero baseline.

Gas Leak

The balloon pressure waveform falls below the baseline **(Fig. 16)**.

Indications of Intra-aortic Balloon Pump Use

Different contexts where there is a possibility of IABP use are discussed below.[14] The guidelines have been summarized in **Table 3**.

- Cardiogenic shock complicating acute myocardial infarction.
- Elective placement of IABP in high-risk percutaneous coronary intervention (PCI).
- CS in nonischemic heart failure/as a bridge to cardiac transplant or LVAD implantation.
- Perioperative IABP in cardiac surgery
- IABP for LV unloading in veno-arterial ECMO (VA-ECMO)

Cardiogenic Shock Complicating Acute Myocardial Infarction

There is pump failure in CS seen as a decrease in SV, increased LVEDV, increased cardiac filling pressure, decreased cardiac contractility, and thus decreased cardiac output (CO) **(Fig. 17)**. IABP helps by causing diastolic augmentation, decreasing LV end diastolic pressure (LVEDP), decreasing afterload, increasing CO, and decreasing myocardial oxygen demand **(Fig. 18)**, as has been discussed before.[15,16]

TABLE 3: Guidelines for the use of IABP in various situations.

Guideline	*Recommendation*	*Class of recommendation, level of evidence*
ISHLT HFSA Guideline on Acute Mechanical Circulatory Support, 2023[21]	Routine IABP use in CS complicating AMI is not recommended	III, A
2021 ACC/AHA/SCAI Guideline for Coronary Artery Revascularization (Hemodynamic Support for Complex PCI)[27]	In selected high-risk patients, elective insertion of an appropriate hemodynamic support device as an adjunct to PCI may be reasonable to prevent hemodynamic compromise during PCI	2b, B-R
2017 ESC STEMI guideline[20]	• Routine IABP use in CS complicating AMI is not recommended • IABP should be considered in patients with hemodynamic instability/ CS due to mechanical complications	III,B IIa, C
2015 SCAI/ACC/HFSA/STS Clinical Expert Consensus Statement on the Use of Mechanical Circulatory Support Devices in Cardiovascular Care[36]	• High-risk PCI [defined as LVEF <20–30% and complex coronary artery disease involving a large territory (sole-remaining vessel, left main, three-vessel disease)] is a suggested indication for consideration of percutaneous MCS (IABP included, though Impella insertion now considered an alternative first-line device) • Peripartum cardiomyopathy is included as a suggested indication for percutaneous mechanical circulatory support (IABP included)	Ungraded Ungraded
2014 ACC/AHA Guideline on Perioperative Cardiovascular Evaluation and Management of Patients Undergoing Noncardiac Surgery[37]	The use of hemodynamic assist devices may be considered when urgent or emergency noncardiac surgery is required in the setting of acute severe cardiac dysfunction (i.e., acute MI and cardiogenic shock) that cannot be corrected before surgery	IIb, C
2014 AHA/ACC Guideline for the Management of Patients With Non-ST-Elevation Acute Coronary Syndromes[38]	Reasonable in the presence of refractory cardiogenic shock following non-ST-elevation myocardial infarction (NSTEMI)	IIa, C
2013 ACCF/AHA Guideline for the Management of ST-Elevation Myocardial Infarction[18]	The use of intra-aortic balloon pump counterpulsation can be useful for patients with cardiogenic shock after STEMI who do not quickly stabilize with pharmacological therapy	IIa, B
2011 ACCF/AHA Guideline for Coronary Artery Bypass Graft Surgery[39]	In the absence of severe, symptomatic aortoiliac occlusive disease or PAD, the insertion of an intra-aortic balloon is reasonable to reduce the mortality rate in CABG patients who are considered to be at high risk (e.g., reoperation, LVEF <30%, or left main CAD)	IIa, B

(ACC: American College of Cardiology; ACCF: American College of Cardiology Foundation; AHA: American Heart Association; ACC: American College of Cardiology; CABG: coronary artery bypass graft; CAD: coronary artery disease; CS: cardiogenic shock; ESC: European Society of Cardiology; HFSA: Heart Failure Society of America; IABP: intra-aortic balloon pump; ISHLT: International Society for Heart and Lung Transplantation; LVEF: left ventricular ejection fraction; MCS: mechanical circulatory support; PAD: peripheral artery disease ; PCI: percutaneous coronary intervention; SCAI: Society for Cardiovascular Angiography and Interventions; STS: Society of Thoracic Surgeons)

Intra-aortic balloon pump which was so widely used earlier, witnessed a progressive down-gradation in recommendation for its use in CS. ACC/AHA ST-elevation MI (STEMI) guidelines in 2013 downgraded the recommendation to IIa(B) from class I(B) (in 2004) in this subgroup of patients.[17,18] Similarly, European Society of Cardiology (ESC) STEMI guidelines in 2012 downgraded the recommendation for IABP use to class IIb from class I(C).[19] Later in 2017 ESC guidelines, the recommendation is against the routine use of IABP in patients with CS (class III). However, class IIa(C) recommendation was given for its use for hemodynamic support in STEMI

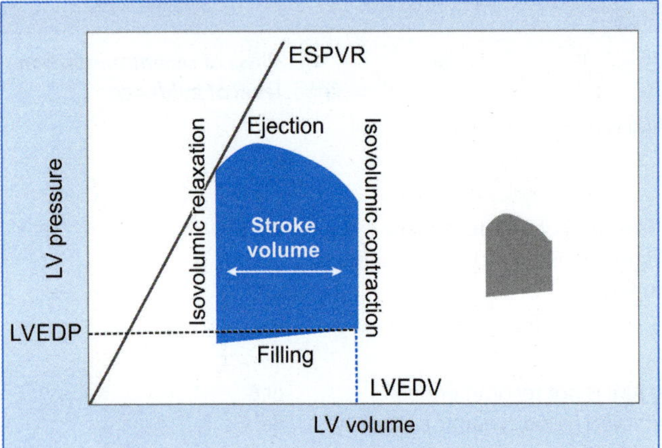

Fig. 17: Pressure-volume loops in normal condition (blue loop) and in CS complicating myocardial infarction (gray loop). In CS, there is decrease in SV (width of loop), increased LVEDV, LVEDP, and decreased cardiac contractility (slope of ESPVR). (CS: cardiogenic shock; ESPVR: end-systolic pressure–volume relationship; LVEDP: left ventricular end-diastolic pressure; LVEDV: left ventricular end-diastolic volume; SV: stroke volume)
Source: Adapted from Lo N, et al.[15]

Fig. 18: Pressure-volume loops in cardiogenic shock and various mechanical ventricular support devices. IABP reduces LVEDP and increases stroke volume. Both Impella and TandemHeart reduce LVEDP. Notably, VA ECMO increases LVEDP, which increases wall stress and myocardial oxygen demand. (CSMI: cardiogenic shock complicating myocardial infarction; IABP: intra-aortic balloon pump; LVEDP: left ventricular end-diastolic pressure; VAECMO: venoarterial extracorporeal membrane oxygenation)
Source: Lo N, et al.[15]

patients with mechanical complications of MI, that is, severe mitral insufficiency or VSD.[20] International Society for Heart and Lung Transplantation (ISHLT)/Heart Failure Society of America (HFSA) guideline on acute mechanical circulatory support, 2023 also recommend against routine IABP use in CS complicating acute myocardial infarction (AMI) (III, A).[21] These recommendations were a result of a lack of improvement in early or late (6 years) outcomes in patients receiving IABP support, observed in the largest trial in this subset, the IABP-SHOCK II trial.[22,23]

Elective Placement of Intra-aortic Balloon Pump During Percutaneous Coronary Intervention in High-risk Group

There have been observational studies that have reported improved outcomes in elective IABP insertion for high-risk PCI. In the BCIS-1 trial, conducted between December 2005 and January 2009, elective IABP insertion was done before PCI in high-risk groups. High risk was defined as severe LV dysfunction with ejection fraction ≤30% and complex multivessel coronary artery disease. They concluded that it did not reduce the incidence of major adverse cardiac and cardiovascular events (MACCE), and did not significantly reduce mortality at 6 months.[24] In the long term mortality data from BCIS-1 trial, the use of IABP was associated with a 34% relative reduction in all-cause mortality at 51 months compared with unsupported PCI.[25] The PROTECT II trial comparing Impella 2.5 with IABP in patients planned for high-risk PCI was terminated early (69% of planned enrolment) in view of futility. There was no significant difference in major adverse events (MAE) at 30 days between the two groups. However, at 90 days, a trend toward decreased incidence of MAE was observed in the Impella 2.5 group.[26] The guidelines suggest the use of an appropriate mechanical circulatory support (MCS) device in selected high-risk patients (e.g., left main or multivessel disease, or disease of the last patent conduit and severe LV dysfunction or CS) as an adjunct to PCI as these devices may provide hemodynamic support in such patients.[27]

Routine IABP placement before reperfusion in acute MI without shock was not found to reduce the infarct size or mortality in the CRISP-AMI trial that randomized 337 patients to IABP or no IABP.[28]

Perioperative Intra-aortic Balloon Pump in Cardiac Surgery

A randomized controlled trial (RCT) by Ranucci et al.[29] has failed to show the benefit of prophylactic IABP in high-risk patients. A meta-analysis by Pilarczyk et al.

(2015) included 9 RCTs with 1,171 patients. It concluded that preoperative IABP in high-risk patients undergoing cardiac surgery is beneficial with regard to mortality, incidence of low cardiac output syndrome (LCOS), and ICU stay.[30] However, it cannot definitely be said whether IABP truly improves outcomes, since the sample size was small in all studies. Also, "high-risk patient" needs to be clearly defined. Further prospective RCTs are needed to give a definitive answer to the question.

Feng Yang et al. concluded that preoperative IABP insertion in acute MI patients without cardiogenic shock undergoing off-pump coronary artery bypass (OPCAB) did not show a 30-day mortality benefit but improved convalescence as shown by shorter postoperative hospital length of stay.[31]

Cardiogenic Shock in Nonischemic Heart Failure/as a Bridge to Cardiac Transplant or Left Ventricular Assist Device Implantation

In a study on 26 patients by Koudoumas D et al., long-term IABP support as a bridge to LVAD implantation was not associated with increased hemorrhagic complication. Long-term preoperative IABP use was defined as IABP placed 3 weeks prior to LVAD implantation.[32] In a randomized trial by den Uil et al., comparing primary IABP versus inotropes for patients with decompensated heart failure (non-ischemic), they observed an increased improvement in organ perfusion in IABP group as measured by mixed-venous oxygen saturation (SvO_2), and also a positive trend in major adverse cardiovascular events and mortality in IABP group. IABP can be placed in decompensated heart failure patients as a bridging modality to decision/bridge/LVAD/transplant.[33]

Left Ventricular Unloading in Venoarterial Extracorporeal Membrane Oxygenation

Venoarterial extracorporeal membrane oxygenation is one of the MCS devices that can be used to support the compromised systemic perfusion in patients with CS, as a bridge to recovery/decision/transplant/VAD. A continuous delivery of blood into the arterial system via the arterial outflow cannula is nonphysiological; and in peripheral VA-ECMO configuration, the delivery is retrograde leading to increased afterload to the LV, which can further lead to decreased SV, stagnation of blood, increased LVEDP, and backward failure causing pulmonary congestion, increased preload and worsening the already injured heart and lungs. Hence, the role of LV unloading.[14,34]

The indications for LV unloading can be categorized into hemodynamic, echocardiographic, and clinical parameters. Increase in pulmonary capillary wedge pressure (PCWP; as a surrogate of LVEDP), lack of pulsatility in the arterial tracing (pulse pressure <15 mm Hg), a distending and hypocontractile LV (LVOT VTI <10 cm), blood stagnation/clot in the LV cavity, persistently closed aortic valve throughout the cardiac cycle, persistent or worsening pulmonary edema, and occurrence of ventricular arrhythmias that are refractory; are among the trigger points for considering LV unloading. Of the various non-invasive and invasive approaches to unload/vent the LV, IABP is a commonly used MCS as an adjunct to VA-ECMO to serve the purpose. Data regarding evidence for the same is limited.[14,34]

In a study by Nishi et al. based on the Japanese Registry of All Cardiac and Vascular Diseases (JROAD), the authors concluded that mortality was significantly less in the VA-ECMO plus IABP group compared from VA-ECMO alone in patients with AMI-CS undergoing primary PCI.[35] There are few ongoing randomized trials [(REVERSE (NCT03431467), ANCHOR (NCT04184635), HERACLES (ISRCTN82431978)] on VA-ECMO with unloading strategies, the results of which might give us a better answer as to which unloading modality should be opted for. In the above sentence, the REVERSE study is "Impella CP with VA-ECMO for Cardiogenic Shock;" ANCHOR is "Assessment of ECMO in Acute Myocardial Infarction Cardiogenic Shock" and HERACLES is "Hemodynamic Effects of Reducing Left Ventricular Afterload With Impella or Intra-aortic Balloon Counterpulsation During Veno-arterial Extracorporeal Membrane Oxygenation in Cardiogenic Shock."

Weaning from Intra-aortic Balloon Pump Support

Weaning from IABP commenced when the patient is hemodynamically stable, and it is evident that its support is no longer required.

Traditionally, two methods of weaning a patient off IABP have been recognized. One is rate-based (RB) weaning, and another is volume-based (VB) weaning.[40] Weaning by ratio is the more commonly used method, especially in high-volume centers. There is large heterogeneity in the method used between the hospitals and countries. There is no published evidence to have convincingly established a difference in clinical outcomes including mortality, need for reinsertion of IABPs, and requirement for inotropic support between RB, VB weaning, and abrupt cessation of IABP support.[41] The only randomized trial by Onorati et al. demonstrated better hemodynamic profiles in the group of patients weaned by VB weaning. They randomized 30 patients to two groups, comparing weaning by the ratio (Group R; 1:2 for 4 hours, followed by 1:3 for an hour, $n = 15$) and progressive volume weaning (Group V; 10% of total volume every hour for 5 hours and then removal; $n = 15$), all in postoperative cardiac surgery patients.[42]

The RB weaning is commenced by decreasing the IABP frequency from 1:1 to 1:2 then 1:3, keeping a watch on the hemodynamics and the clinical state of the patient.

Removal of Intra-aortic Balloon Pump[14]

- Confirm the hemodynamic stability and check the coagulation profile.
- Position the patient supine, put IABP on standby, and then turn it off, and let the balloon deflate.
- Remove the IAB and let the insertion site bleed for 2 seconds to help remove thrombus, if any.
- Sufficient pressure needs to be applied to achieve hemostasis and also allowing distal limb perfusion.

Considerations During Transport with Intra-aortic Balloon Pump

It is imperative to verify the functionality of the equipment. The battery must be fully charged, and wherever possible the console should be connected to power to save battery life. Adaptors compatible with the local facility must be carried along. The helium tank should be filled. The physician and the staff accompanying the patient must be familiar with IABP. A 60 mL syringe and a 3-way stopcock should be carried along in case of need for manual inflation or deflation of the balloon. A thorough neurological and cardiovascular examination, including a distal pulse check, should be performed before transport and after reaching the other facility. In the case of air transport, adjustments need to be made considering the change in atmospheric pressure as the altitude changes. Usually, the IABP machine does the adjustment by itself, for example, in “autofill” mode in the Maquet CS300 system. In case of failure of automatic compensation, a button labeled “pump status” can be pressed, which will lead to an adjustment of the pump as per the altitude.[16]

CONCLUSION

Intra-aortic balloon pumps even though is lacking a strong evidence in their favor, remain popular amongst the MCS devices owing to their ease of insertion, relative affordability, and beneficial effects in terms of hemodynamics improvement. The lack of improvement in outcome in the IABP-SHOCK-II trial may be due to delayed placement of the pump after PCI was done. In high-risk cases, and in patients with pre/impending shock (CS), in the scenario of the nonavailability of other better MCS devices, early IABP implantation may be reasonable.

REFERENCES

1. Kantrowitz A. Experimental augmentation of coronary flow by retardation of the arterial pressure pulse. Surgery. 1953;34(4):678-87.
2. Harken DE. The surgical treatment of acquired valvular disease. Circulation. 1958;18(1):1-6.
3. Moulopoulos SD, Topaz SR, Kolff WJ. Extracorporeal assistance to the circulation and intraaortic balloon pumping. Trans Am Soc Artif Intern Organs. 1962;8:85-9.
4. Kantrowitz A, Tjonneland S, Freed PS, Phillips SJ, Butner AN, Sherman JL Jr. Initial clinical experience with intraaortic balloon pumping in cardiogenic shock. JAMA. 1968;203(2):113-8.
5. Bergman HE, Casarella WJ. Percutaneous intraaortic balloon pumping: initial clinical experience. Ann Thorac Surg. 1980;29(2):153-5.
6. Laham RJ. Intraaortic balloon pump counterpulsation. UpToDate. [online] Available from https:// www.uptodate.com/contents/intraaortic-balloon-pump-counterpulsation [Last accessed October, 2024].
7. Krishna M, Zacharowski K. Principles of intra-aortic balloon pump counterpulsation. Continuing Education in Anaesthesia, Crit Care Pain. 2009;9(1):24-8.
8. Parissis H, Graham V, Lampridis S, Lau M, Hooks G, Mhandu PC. IABP: history-evolution-pathophysiology-indications: what we need to know. J Cardiothorac Surg. 2016;11(1):122.
9. Dedhia JD, KotemaneR NC¸ Ahmed AB. Intra Aortic Balloon Pump (IABP): Past, Present and Future. Ind J Anaesth. 2008;52:387-97.
10. Chaturvedi A, Rotman Y, Hoang T, Jew G, Mandalapu A, Narins C. CT and chest radiography in evaluation of mechanical circulatory support devices for acute heart failure. Insights into Imaging. 2023;14(1):122.
11. Guidelines for Management of the Intra-Aortic Balloon Pump. [Online] Available from https://www.aast.org/Assets/284785ce-1e77-4dae-917f-81bf0ec31720/636075642166370000/a-institutional-guideline-procedure-the-management-of-an-iabp-from-the-university-of-maryland-uploaded-2015-pdf [Last accessed October, 2024].

12. González LS, Chaney MA. Intraaortic Balloon Pump Counterpulsation, Part I: History, Technical Aspects, Physiologic Effects, Contraindications, Medical Applications/Outcomes. Anesth Analg. 2020;131(3):776-91.
13. Bhatt H, Johal GS, Serrao G. Advanced Hemodynamic Support. In: Kini A, Sharma SK (Eds). Practical Manual of Interventional Cardiology. Cham: Springer; 2021.
14. Rossini R, Valente S, Colivicchi F, Baldi C, Caldarola P, Chiappetta D, et al. ANMCO POSITION PAPER: Role of intra-aortic balloon pump in patients with acute advanced heart failure and cardiogenic shock. Eur Heart J Suppl. 2021;23(Suppl C):C204-20.
15. Lo N, Magnus Ohman E. Mechanical Circulatory Support in ST-Elevation Myocardial Infarction. In: Watson TJ, Ong PJL, Tcheng JE (Eds). Primary Angioplasty: A Practical Guide [Internet]. Singapore: Springer; 2018.
16. Gillespie LE, Lane BH, Shaw CR, Gorder K, Grisoli A, Lavallee M, et al. The Intra-aortic Balloon Pump: A Focused Review of Physiology, Transport Logistics, Mechanics, and Complications. J Soc Cardiovasc Angiogr Interv. 2024;3(5):101337.
17. Antman EM, Anbe DT, Armstrong PW, Bates ER, Green LA, Hand M, et al. ACC/AHA guidelines for the management of patients with ST-elevation myocardial infarction—executive summary: a report of the American College of Cardiology/American Heart Association Task Force on Practice Guidelines (Writing Committee to Revise the 1999 Guidelines for the Management of Patients With Acute Myocardial Infarction). Circulation. 2004;110(5):588-636.
18. O'Gara PT, Kushner FG, Ascheim DD, Casey DE Jr, Chung MK, de Lemos JA, et al. 2013 ACCF/AHA guideline for the management of ST-elevation myocardial infarction: executive summary: a report of the American College of Cardiology Foundation/American Heart Association Task Force on Practice Guidelines. 2013;61(4):485-510.
19. Steg PG, James SK, Atar D, Badano LP, Blo m̈strom-Lundqvist C, Borger MA, et al. Task Force on the management of ST-segment elevation acute myocardial infarction of the European Society of Cardiology (ESC). ESC Guidelines for the management of acute myocardial infarction in patients presenting with ST-segment elevation. Eur Heart J. 2012;33(20):2569-619.
20. Ibanez B, James S, Agewall S, Antunes MJ, Bucciarelli-Ducci C, Bueno H, et al. 2017 ESC Guidelines for the management of acute myocardial infarction in patients presenting with ST-segment elevation: The Task Force for the management of acute myocardial infarction in patients presenting with ST-segment elevation of the European Society of Cardiology (ESC). Eur Heart J. 2018;39(2):119-77.
21. Bernhardt AM, Copeland H, Deswal A, Gluck J, Givertz MM; Task Force 1, et al . The International Society for Heart and Lung Transplantation/Heart Failure Society of America Guideline on Acute Mechanical Circulatory Support. J Card Fail. 2023;29(3):304-74. Erratum in: J Card Fail. 2024;30(1):119.
22. Thiele H, Zeymer U, Neumann FJ, Ferenc M, Olbrich HG, Hausleiter J, et al. Intraaortic balloon support for myocardial infarction with cardiogenic shock. N Engl J Med. 2012;367(14):1287-96.
23. Thiele H, Zeymer U, Thelemann N, et al.; On behalf of the IABP-SHOCK II Trial (Intraaortic Balloon Pump in Cardiogenic Shock II) Investigators. Investigators. Intraaortic Balloon Pump in Cardiogenic Shock Complicating Acute Myocardial Infarction: Long-Term 6-Year Outcome of the Randomized IABP-SHOCK II Trial. Circulation. 2019;139:395-403.
24. Perera D, Stables R, Thomas M, Booth J, Pitt M, Blackman D, et al. Elective intra-aortic balloon counterpulsation during high-risk percutaneous coronary intervention: a randomized controlled trial. JAMA. 2010;304(8):867-74.
25. Perera D, Stables R, Clayton T, De Silva K, Lumley M, Clack L, et al. Long-term mortality data from the balloon pump-assisted coronary intervention study (BCIS-1): a randomized, controlled trial of elective balloon counterpulsation during high-risk percutaneous coronary intervention. Circulation. 2013;127(2):207-12.
26. O'Neill WW, Kleiman NS, Moses J, Henriques JP, Dixon S, Massaro J, et al. A prospective, randomized clinical trial of hemodynamic support with Impella 2.5 versus intra-aortic balloon pump in patients undergoing high-risk percutaneous coronary intervention: the PROTECT II study. Circulation. 2012;126(14):1717-27.
27. Lawton JS, Tamis-Holland JE, Bangalore S, Bates ER, Beckie TM, Bischoff JM, et al. 2021 ACC/AHA/SCAI Guideline for Coronary Artery Revascularization: Executive Summary: A Report of the American College of Cardiology/American Heart Association Joint Committee on Clinical Practice Guidelines. Circulation. 2022;145(3):e4-e17. Erratum in: Circulation. 2022;145(11):e771.
28. Patel MR, Smalling RW, Thiele H, Barnhart HX, Zhou Yi, Chandra P, et al. Intra-aortic balloon counterpulsation and infarct size in patients with acute anterior myocardial infarction without shock: the CRISP AMI randomized trial. JAMA. 2011;306(12):1329-37.
29. Ranucci M, Castelvecchio S, Biondi A, Barnhart HX, Zhou Y, Chandra P, et al. A randomized controlled trial of preoperative intra-aortic balloon pump in coronary patients with poor left ventricular function undergoing coronary artery bypass surgery*. Crit Care Med. 2013;41(11):2476-83.
30. Pilarczyk K, Boening A, Jakob H, Langebartels G, Markewitz A, Haake N, et al. Preoperative intra-aortic counterpulsation in high-risk patients undergoing cardiac surgery: a meta-analysis of randomized controlled trials†. Eur J Cardiothorac Surg. 2016;49:5-17.
31. Yang F, Wang L, Hou D, Wang J, Wang X. Preoperative intra-aortic balloon pump inserted in acute myocardial infarction patients without cardiogenic shock undergoing surgical coronary revascularization. Clin Surg. 2020;35(2):145-53.

32. Koudoumas D, Malliaras K, Theodoropoulos S, Kaldara E, Kapelios C, Nanas J. Long-term intra-aortic balloon pump support as bridge to left ventricular assist device implantation. J Card Surg. 2016;31(7):467-71.
33. den Uil CA, Van Mieghem NM, Bastos MB, Jewbali LS, Lenzen MJ, Engstrom AE, et al. Primary intra-aortic balloon support versus inotropes for decompensated heart failure and low output: a randomised trial. Eurointervention. 2019;15(7):586-93.
34. Ezad SM, Ryan M, Donker DW, Pappalardo F, Barrett N, Camporota L, et al. Unloading the Left Ventricle in Venoarterial ECMO: In Whom, When, and How? Circulation. 2023;147(16):1237-50.
35. Nishi T, Ishii M, Tsujita K, Okamoto H, Satoshi K, Nakai M,, et al. Outcomes of Venoarterial Extracorporeal Membrane Oxygenation Plus Intra-Aortic Balloon Pumping for Treatment of Acute Myocardial Infarction Complicated by Cardiogenic Shock. J Am Heart Assoc. 2022;11(7):e023713.
36. Rihal CS, Naidu SS, Givertz MM, Szeto WY, Burke JA, Kapur NK, et al. 2015 SCAI/ACC/HFSA/STS Clinical Expert Consensus Statement on the Use of Percutaneous Mechanical Circulatory Support Devices in Cardiovascular Care: Endorsed by the American Heart Assocation, the Cardiological Society of India, and Sociedad Latino Americana de Cardiologia Intervencion; Affirmation of Value by the Canadian Association of Interventional Cardiology-Association Canadienne de Cardiologie d'intervention. J Am Coll Cardiol. 2015;65(19):e7-26.
37. Fleisher LA, Fleischmann KE, Auerbach AD, Barnason SA, Beckman JA, Bozkurt B, et al. 2014 ACC/AHA guideline on perioperative cardiovascular evaluation and management of patients undergoing noncardiac surgery: a report of the American College of Cardiology/American Heart Association Task Force on practice guidelines. J Am Coll Cardiol. 2014;64(22):e77-137.
38. Amsterdam EA, Wenger NK, Brindis RG, Casey DE Jr, Ganiats TG, Holmes DR Jr, et al. 2014 AHA/ACC Guideline for the Management of Patients with Non-ST-Elevation Acute Coronary Syndromes: a report of the American College of Cardiology/American Heart Association Task Force on Practice Guidelines. J Am Coll Cardiol. 2014;64(24):e139-228.
39. Hillis LD, Smith PK, Anderson JL, Bittl JA, Bridges CR, Byrne JG, et al. 2011 ACCF/AHA guideline for coronary artery bypass graft surgery: executive summary: a report of the American College of Cardiology Foundation/American Heart Association Task Force on Practice Guidelines. Circulation. 2011;124(23):2610-42.
40. Gelsomino S, Lozekoot PWJ, Lorusso R, de Jong MJ, Parise O, Matteucci F, et al. The Optimal Weaning Strategy for Intraaortic Balloon Counterpulsation: Volume-Based Versus Rate-Based Approach in an Animal Model. Ann Thorac Surg. 2016;101(4):1485-93.
41. Rogersa L, Cochraneb E, Blundellb D, Zakkar M. What is the optimum method of weaning intra-aortic balloon pumps? Interac Cardiovasc Thorac Surg. 2016;23(2):310-3.
42. Onorati F, Santini F, Amoncelli E, Campanella F, Chiominto B, Faggian G, et al. How should I wean my next intra-aortic balloon pump? Differences between progressive volume weaning and rate weaning. J Thorac Cardiovasc Surg. 2013;145(5):1214-21.

CHAPTER

Left Ventricular Assist Devices in the Management of Acute Cardiogenic Shock

Suresh Rao KG, Rahul Pandit, Muralikrishna T

INTRODUCTION

Cardiogenic shock (CS) is a state of low or ineffective cardiac output, primarily due to a cardiac dysfunction, resulting in end organ hypoperfusion. The definitions of CS are derived from studies which have looked at patients with acute coronary syndrome (ACS).[1] There is a poor understanding of CS in patients who have underlying congestive cardiac failure, often also termed as population which is often not considered in ACS. CS can be secondary to both ischemic and nonischemic causes. Whatever the underlying cause is, it is an acute emergency and should be treated as early as possible. The main goal of treatment in CS is to establish the normal vital organ perfusion as soon as possible, because the mortality is very high, if not treated early.[1]

DEFINITION AND DIAGNOSTIC CRITERIA

Criteria for diagnosis of CS are divided in clinical and hemodynamic. Clinical criteria include a systolic blood pressure of ≤90 mm Hg for ≥30 minutes or need of support to maintain systolic blood pressure ≤90 mm Hg and urine output ≤30 mL/h or cool extremities. Hemodynamic criteria include a depressed cardiac index (≤2.2 L/min/m^2 of body surface area) and an elevated pulmonary-capillary wedge pressure (>15 mm Hg).[1,2] The European Society of Cardiology also considers acidosis, increased lactate levels, and elevated creatinine levels, as laboratory criteria.[3,4] The usual line of management is treating the underlying cause for the shock, inotropes, inodilators, diuretics, drugs to control the rate, and rhythm. Refractory cardiogenic shock (RCS) is defined as cardiac and circulatory failure, resulting in organ hypoperfusion unresponsive to conventional medical therapies.

MECHANICAL CIRCULATORY SUPPORT

Delay in effective treatment despite conventional medical therapies of CS leads to increase in mortality and morbidity. In patients with refractory CS, mechanical circulatory support (MCS) has shown to help, at times to act as a bridge to recovery, and in some cases, mechanical support acts as destination therapy. Intra-aortic balloon pump (IABP) is an easily available bed-side mechanical circulatory device, which can be instituted in a short time. IABP is timed to inflate and deflate in concert with cardiac cycle; thus, a diastolic inflation increases coronary perfusion, and a systolic deflation results in reduction of left ventricular after load. Before 2012, American and European guidelines supported IABP use for CS with a Class I recommendation. The IABP-SHOCK II trial, which enrolled patients with myocardial infarction (MI)-associated CS, found no differences in the primary end point of 30-day mortality, prespecified secondary end points, or 1-year outcomes between those with and those without IABP support.[5] These results led to the IABP being downgraded to a Class IIIA recommendation for routine use in CS in the most recent European revascularization and non–ST-segment–elevation ACS guidelines.[6] The other options of MCS include extracorporeal membrane oxygenator (ECMO) and ventricular assist device (VAD) often differentiated into left ventricular assist device (LVAD), right ventricular assist device (RVAD), and if both ventricles are supported then Biventricular assist device (BiVAD).

Advantages and Disadvantages of Extracorporeal Membrane Oxygenator versus Ventricular Assist Device (Figs. 1A and B)

Extracorporeal membrane oxygenator is one of the preferred ways of MCS. ECMO as an option of MCS has the following advantages and limitations.

Advantages

- Easy to institute and can be done on the bedside.
- Can be done by percutaneous method.

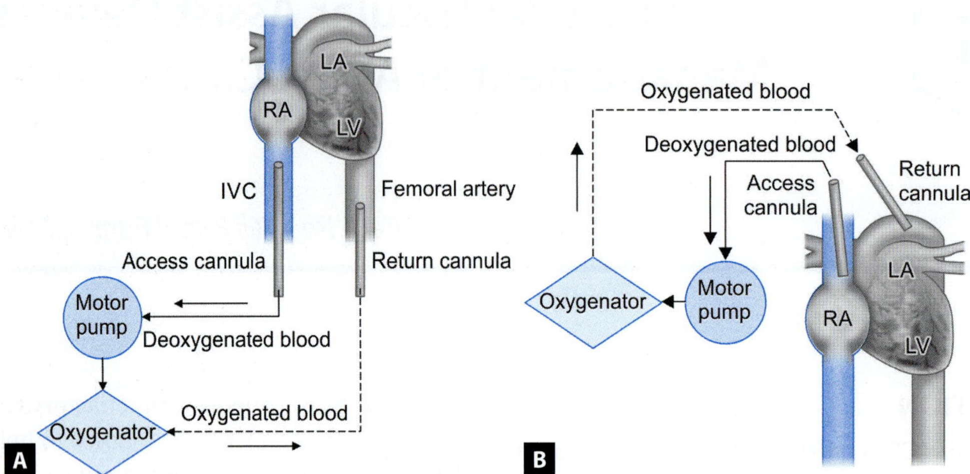

Figs. 1A and B: Two different configurations of venoarterial extracorporeal membrane oxygenation (VA-ECMO): (A) Peripheral and (B) Central VA-ECMO. (IVC: inferior vena cava; LA: left atrium; LV: left ventricle; RA: right atrium)

Source: Adapted from Ng GW, Yuen HJ, Sin KC, Leung AK, Yeung KA, Lai KY. Clinical use of venoarterial extracorporeal membrane oxygenation. Hong Kong Med J. 2017;23(3):282-90.

- Needs less time to establish the support.
- Can be instituted by intensivist or surgeon.
- Biventricular support (predominantly right ventricular support).
- Supports both heart and lungs.
- Can be instituted through peripheral vascular access (without opening the chest).

Limitations

- In peripheral ECMO, afterload to left ventricle (LV) is increased, thereby affecting left ventricular recovery.
- Bleeding complications due to need for anticoagulation.
- Can be used as a support only for few weeks.
- Need to maintain higher activated clotting time (ACT) since it has oxygenator in the circuit.
- Vascular complications and decreased distal limb perfusion.

In comparison to ECMO, VAD has the following advantages and limitations.

Disadvantages

- Ventricular assist device decompresses the ventricle, thereby increasing the chances of its recovery.
- Can be used as a long-term support.
- Patient can be mobilized on VAD.
- Needs lesser anticoagulation than ECMO (as there is no oxygenator).

Limitations

- Supports only LV, needs BiVAD if the patient is having severe right ventricular dysfunction.
- Does not support the lungs (however oxygenator can be connected in a LVAD circuit if required, and complexity increases).
- Takes time to establish the support.
- Cannot be done bedside in the intensive care unit (ICU).

VENTRICULAR ASSIST DEVICES

There are two types of VAD, temporary, one meant for short-term support and destination LVADs meant for long-term support. In CS, temporary VADs are used. The following are the different types of LVAD available for support in acute CS:

- Impella® (Abiomed, Inc. Headquarters USA)
- Tandem heart
- CentriMag

Impella (Figs. 2 and 3)

Impella is a minimally invasive catheter-based cardiac assist device. It is a percutaneous ventricular assist device (PVAD) with continuous, nonpulsatile axial flow pump. It is inserted through the femoral artery; the tip of the device crosses the aortic valve and is positioned in the LV. It drains blood from the tip which is positioned in the LV

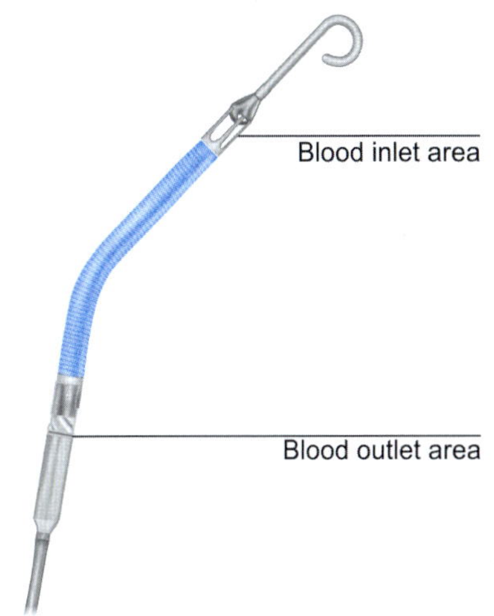

Fig. 2: Impella 2.5® (Abiomed, Danvers, MA, USA) device.

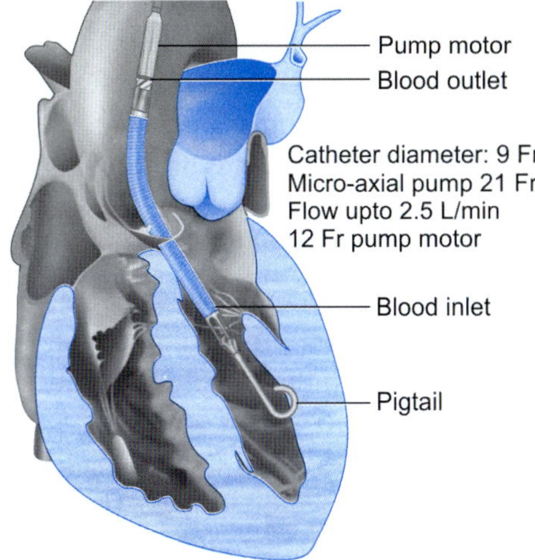

Fig. 3: Impella 2.5® (Abiomed, Danvers, MA), USA device in situ.

and delivers to the ascending aorta. Impella does not need electrocardiogram (ECG) or arterial waveform as a trigger, so it will work even if there is a cardiac arrest. There are four types of Impella devices. The Impella 2.5 and Impella CP devices are inserted percutaneously and provide cardiac output from 2.5 to 4.0 L/min.[7] Impella 5.0 can deliver flows up to 5 L/min, it requires a larger sheath, and it is inserted by surgical cutdown of femoral artery. Impella RP supports the right ventricle (RV); it is inserted through the femoral vein, it drains the blood from the inlet area which is positioned in the inferior vena cava and delivers blood through the outlet area near the tip in the pulmonary artery. Impella 2.5 and Impella CP are approved for temporary

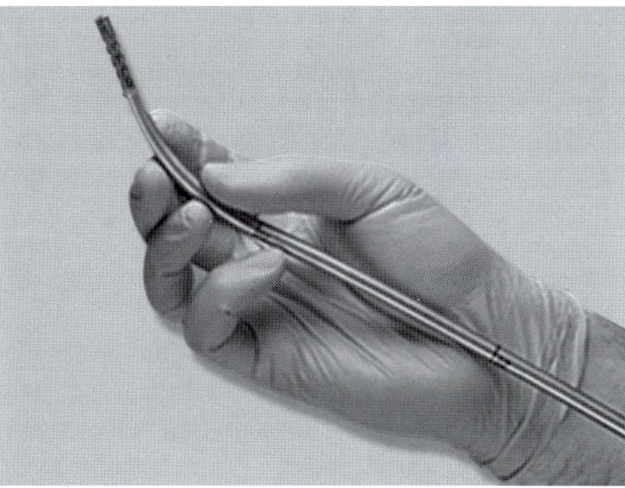

Fig. 4: TandemHeart kit component, Protek Solo transseptal cannula: The curved distal tip enables placement in the left atrium (LA) and has 14 side holes for draining blood from LA *(For color version, see Plate 4)*.

ventricular support for up to 4 days, and Impella 5.0 is approved for support up to 14 days. The main advantage is ease of insertion and the ability to establish a circulatory support in a short time. It reduces the ventricular workload and provides the necessary circulatory support, thereby providing a window for recovery of heart or to plan further interventions. It is contraindicated in patients having left ventricular mural thrombus, moderate-to-severe aortic regurgitation, mechanical aortic valve, severe aortic stenosis, and peripheral artery disease. The main complications with Impella are device migration, device thrombosis, hemolysis, bleeding, arrhythmias, limb ischemia, tamponade, injury to aortic, mitral valves, and stroke.

Tandem Heart (LivaNova)

Tandem heart (LivaNova) is a temporary circulatory support device that can be inserted percutaneously.[8] It is inserted through the femoral venous access. The cannula tip is positioned in the left atrium (LA) through a transseptal puncture **(Fig. 4)**. It drains blood from the LA, thereby decompressing the LV. The blood is returned through an outflow cannula placed through the femoral artery approach and is positioned in the iliac or femoral artery. The advantages with the tandem heart are: It can be inserted percutaneously, can be done in catheterization laboratory, decompresses the LV, and supports flows up to 4 L/min **(Fig. 5)**. The tandem heart cannot be used in

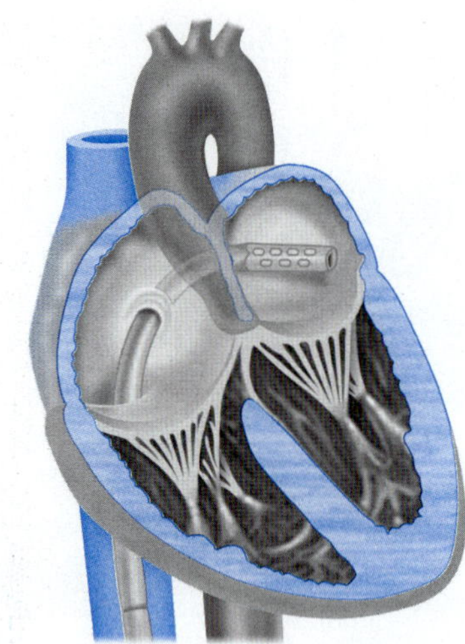

Fig. 5: Protek Solo transseptal cannula in situ: It bypasses the left ventricle, taking up its work and allows it to rest.

cases where transseptal puncture cannot be performed. A modified version of tandem heart can be used to support the RV.

CentriMag™ Circulatory Support System (Abbot Cardiovascular)

CentriMag[9] is a paracorporeal type of VAD. It has a continuous, nonpulsatile centrifugal flow pump that provides flows. The cannula has to be inserted surgically. The inflow cannula is in LV or in the LA, and the outflow is usually to the ascending aorta or a major artery. This pump can provide flow equivalent to that of cardiac output. A different version of this pump PediMag can be used to support the circulation in the pediatric patients with CS. The advantages with this VAD are that it provides full support, can be used for long-term support, patients can be mobilized while they are on this VAD, coagulation and bleeding related complications are less when compared to ECMO, we can add an oxygenator in the circuit, and it can be used as an RVAD if required. The main limitations are: the pump has to be inserted by surgical technique, and it cannot be done at the bedside in ICU or in catheterization laboratory.

Acceptable Indications for Ventricular Assist Devices

Cardiogenic shock can be secondary to multiple causes such as:

- Acute coronary syndrome
- Decompensation of a patient with cardiomyopathy
- Postcardiac surgery
- Postpartum cardiomyopathy
- Myocarditis
- Arrhythmias
- Severe valvular heart diseases

The point at which the MCS has to be considered needs to be decided on the clinical basis, and continuous close monitoring of these patients in CS is essential as this will help in taking appropriate decisions at the right time. If the patient is clinically improving with medical management as manifested by adequate tissue perfusion, decreasing lactates, good urine output then the option of mechanical support can be delayed. However, if the patient is not clinically improving or rapidly deteriorating (arrhythmias or severe hypotension) MCS should be established as early as possible. Decision-making at appropriate time has impact on outcomes of mortality and morbidity. MCS should be established before end organ damage happens. INTERMACS (Interagency Registry for Mechanically Assisted Circulatory Support) criteria help us in guiding on this. For patients who are in INTERMACS level 1, MCS has to be established as soon as possible and the options here are ECMO and percutaneous devices **(Table 2)**.[10]

Assessment for Left Ventricular Assist Device

Ventricular assist device should be considered in patients with refractory CS. Before proceeding, we should assess the patient in detail, to decide whether that particular patient can undergo LVAD or not, and which LVAD should be considered. The assessment should include a detailed clinical examination, echocardiography, assessment of other systems (renal, hepatic, neurological, and pulmonary), and any associated problems (infection and coagulopathies).

The following are the situations in which an LVAD is considered a contraindication or it should not be done. These should be actively looked into, before deciding to proceed with LVAD support.

- Right ventricular dysfunction (unless it is secondary to left heart failure)
- Irreversible neurological dysfunction
- Coexisting severe terminal comorbidity (irreversible) (renal, pulmonary, liver disease, or advanced malignancy)
- Active bleeding or contraindication for anticoagulation
- *Anatomical factors*: Ventricular septal rupture, cannulation site issues, or body surface area for which suitable VAD is not available

TABLE 1: Different types of left ventricular assist devices (LVAD).

Therapy	*Inflow*	*Outflow*	*Mechanism*
VV-ECMO	Right atrium	Right ventricle	• No RV or LV support • Improves oxygenation • Increase in RV load
VA-ECMO	Right atrium	Ileo-femoral	• Supports RV • Improves oxygenation • Increases load to LV
pLVAD	Left ventricle	Aorta	• Supports and offloads LV • Increases RV load
pRVAD	IVC	PA	RV support and decrease RV load
BiPella	IVC	PA	• Supports and offloads RV and LV • No improvement in oxygenation
	LV	AO	
ECPella	RA	IF	Antegrade and retrograde flow
	LV	AO	

(AO: aorta; IVC: inferior vena cava; PA: pulmonary artery; pLVAD: percutaneous left ventricular assist device; pRVAD: percutaneous right ventricular assist device; VA-ECMO: venoarterial extracorporeal membrane oxygenation; VV-ECMO: venovenous extracorporeal membrane oxygenation)

TABLE 2: INTERMACS (Interagency Registry for Mechanically Assisted Circulatory Support) criteria for mechanical circulatory support (MCS).

INTERMACS level	*Clinical picture*	*Time for mechanical support*	*Options of MCS*
1	Critical cardiogenic shock	Immediately	ECMO, percutaneous devices, and CentriMag
2	Sliding on inotropes	Within days	ECMO and LVAD
3	Stable on inotropes	Within weeks	LVAD
4	Requires intermittent inotropic support		LVAD
5	NYHA Class 4 symptoms, stable at rest		
6	NYHA Class 3 symptoms, fatigue after few minutes of activity, exertion limited		
7	NYHA Class 3 symptoms		

(ECMO: extracorporeal membrane oxygenator; LVAD: left ventricular assist device; NYHA: New York Heart Association)

- Chance of recovery of native heart function is not there and no clear plan for further management options such as destination LVAD or transplant.

The following things should be looked in the echocardiography in a patient for LVAD:

- Detailed assessment of left heart function to ascertain the cause for shock
- Detailed study of right ventricular function to determine if there is any dysfunction
- Presence of any atrial septal defect (ASD), patent foramen ovale (PFO), and ventricular septal defect (VSD)
- Aortic regurgitation, aortic stenosis, and mitral stenosis (in presence of any of these lesions, the surgical plan may be altered to suit the condition)
- Presence of any intracardiac clot or mass
- Status of the cannulation sites (to look for any thrombus, atheromas)

The assessment of right heart should include a clinical examination, interpretation of hemodynamic parameters [central venous pressure (CVP), pulmonary arterial pressure (PAP), pulmonary artery occlusion pressure (PAOP), mean arterial pressure (MAP), systemic vascular resistance (SVR), pulmonary vascular resistance (PVR), and right ventricular stroke work index (RVSWI)]. If possible, a right heart hemodynamic study should be done to get an idea about the function.

Echocardiography Assessment

A detailed echocardiography study is mandatory.[11] The assessment should include left ventricular chamber dimensions, systolic function assessment, diastolic function assessment. Left atrial volume and pressure should be measured. Mitral annulus dimensions, tethering of mitral valve leaflets, are secondary to the geometric changes of LV and papillary muscles. Quantification of mitral regurgitation, assessment of aortic valve area, quantification of aortic regurgitation, and stenosis should be made.

The right heart assessment should include sizes of right atrium (RA) and RV, position of the interventricular septum, fractional area change of RV, tricuspid annular plane systolic excursion (TAPSE), color Doppler assessment of the flow, tissue Doppler indices of right heart function, and assessment of RV mechanics. If the clinical situation demands, there may be a need to evaluate further with a coronary angiogram. The decision whether the right ventricular function is suitable for LVAD placement should be taken after taking into account all of the above parameters. Further risk stratification for the chance of right ventricular dysfunction in the postoperative period will help us in optimizing the patient better and plan with strategies to manage the right ventricular dysfunction.

In the presence of a PFO or ASD or VSD, we have to ensure that the lesion has to be addressed along with the insertion of LVAD or else patient will have persistent desaturation post-LVAD due to right to left shunt. In the presence of valvular heart diseases, the option of the LVAD and the approach has to be changed accordingly. Presence of severe aortic regurgitation or severe aortic stenosis is a contraindication for Impella. Severe aortic regurgitation has to be addressed before putting the patient on CentriMag. In case of severe mitral stenosis, the inflow cannula for CentriMag has to be placed in the LA.

Postoperative Care of Left Ventricular Assist Device Patient

Postoperative care of these patients includes the standard care of all cardiac surgical patients plus care specifically guided at LVAD. The invasive hemodynamic monitoring includes parameters such as MAP, CVP, PAP, cardiac output, SVR, and PVR. The choice of inotropes/inodilators/vasoactive drugs is based on the above values, keeping a target of adequate cardiac index with MAP >70 mm Hg and CVP <14 mm Hg. There can be changes in the values of the hemodynamic parameters in the immediate postoperative period because of multiple reasons, so these values should be serially monitored at regular intervals, and the inotropes/inodilators/vasoactive medications should be titrated accordingly. Echocardiographic guidance is essential in management of these patients; hence, echo should be done at regular intervals and during trouble shooting of these patients. Right ventricular function, interventricular septal position, LVAD cannula position, volume status, and pericardial collection should be assessed on echo regularly. The target is to have a good right ventricular function and interventricular septum deviated toward right side.

The interface of the LVAD monitor is unique to each device. The intensivist should be aware of the parameters on display, knobology and alarms of the monitor. Typically almost all the LVAD monitors display the pump speed in revolutions per minute (RPM) and flow. The target is to have an adequate cardiac index without very high RPM. If there is graphical or waveform display, it will indicate the flow and filling characters at that point of time. Reading these waveforms or graphical display, we can assess whether the volume status of the patient is adequate or not. Abnormal waveforms require further interrogation that requires looking into clinical parameters and echo to diagnose the underlying problem (hypovolemia, RV dysfunction, cannula malposition, thrombosis, and tamponade). We may have to adjust the RPM and flows according to the clinical situation. It takes few days for the immediate postoperative fluctuations to settle and to identify the final RPM and flows, till then these parameters should be watched continuously.

ANTICOAGULATION MANAGEMENT

In the postprocedure period, anticoagulation is vital in this group of patients. Usually a continuous infusion of unfractionated heparin is started postprocedure once the hemostasis is secured and this is continued in the postoperative period. It is monitored by serially monitoring activated partial thromboplastin time (aPTT) levels. The consensus guidelines recommend an aPTT of 60–80 seconds, which is around 2–3 times the baseline.[12] There is a possibility that these patients may have coagulopathy secondary to multiple causes, anticoagulation in these patients should be titrated to the specific individual patient based on the clinical scenario. Since aPTT reflects the function of heparin on intrinsic pathway of the coagulation cascade, whereas the anti-factor Xa (anti-Xa) assay measures the heparin impact on antithrombin, it is now increasingly recommended that in LVAD patients aPTT may not accurately reflect the anticoagulation and hence anti Xa should be measured for anticoagulation.[13]

Since the blood circulates outside the body in the paracorporeal VADs such as CentriMag, there is a risk of developing hypothermia (more so in pediatric patients); hence all precautions to prevent temperature loss should be taken. Apart from these, the regular postoperative care, similar to any critical cardiac surgical patient, has to be given to these patients. Ventilatory support is continued, and patient is weaned and extubated when he is deemed fit. Preprocedure left ventricular dysfunction induced pulmonary edema is common in these patients; this should be addressed before extubation. Other supportive therapies such as fluid balance management, nutrition management, infection control and treatment, physiotherapy, and rehabilitation play an important role in the postoperative recovery.

COMMON COMPLICATIONS IN THE POSTOPERATIVE PERIOD

The following are the common complications for these patients in the postoperative period:

- *Right ventricular dysfunction:* RV dysfunction is a common complication post-LVAD. It can be primary RV dysfunction or secondary to pulmonary hypertension, cardiac tamponade, and pulmonary causes such as collapse, pulmonary edema. RV dysfunction can lead to shifting of the interventricular septum toward left side, thereby leading to change in geometry of RV, collapse of LV, and no flow through the LVAD; this is called suction event. It is identified by high CVP, low MAP, and low LVAD flows. Echocardiography aids in both diagnosis and management of these cases. If not treated, RV dysfunction is a cause of mortality and morbidity in these patients. The standard line of management includes inotropes, inodilators, diuretics, optimizing the lung function, and antipulmonary hypertension measures (nitric oxide and sildenafil).[14] Continuous renal replacement therapy (CRRT) may help in fluid removal and decongesting the RV. Further high LVAD flows can cause RV dysfunction; temporarily decreasing the flows can help in improvement of RV function. If the medical management cannot optimize the right ventricular failure, then the option of MCS has to be considered. ECMO and RVAD are the available options for supporting the RV, the choice has to be decided depending on the clinical situation.
- *Pulmonary hypertension:* This can be due to a high PVR or due to lung conditions such as pulmonary edema, collapse of lung, etc. This can lead to secondary right ventricular failure. Appropriate management includes optimizing the ventilatory management, sedation, nitric oxide, inodilators, phosphodiesterase inhibitors, endothelin receptor antagonists, diuretics, and optimizing the lung function.
- *Coagulation abnormalities:* These patients can have coagulation abnormalities due to multiple reasons, preoperative cardiac failure, congested liver, antiplatelets in ACSs, and consumptive coagulopathy due to shock. This can result in blood loss, increased transfusions, and risk of tamponade. Point-of-care tests will help in guiding the treatment. Lactate dehydrogenase (LDH) levels should be serially monitored in these patients; persistently elevated levels with an increasing trend should raise a suspicion of thrombus in the circuit and hemolysis.
- *Hemolysis:* This can happen due to blood flowing through a narrow orifice at high speeds. This is a known complication of percutaneous assist devices. This can also happen if inadequate anticoagulation leads to thrombus formation in the cannula. The underlying cause has to be identified and rectified. Adequate hydration is required to prevent renal injury.
- *Equipment-related issues:* Cannula dislodgement, cannula malposition, and equipment malfunction.
- *Vascular complications:* Groin vessels are used in percutaneous VADs; there is always a risk of vascular compromise in the lower limb. Further patients can have hematoma, vessel injury, stenosis, and pseudoaneurysm.
- *Renal and liver dysfunction:* These patients can have renal and liver dysfunctions due to their preoperative CS. These organ dysfunctions can be temporary if the MCS is established at the earliest. A variety of postoperative factors such as drugs, hemodynamic instability, bleeding, transfusions, and sepsis can lead to further derangement of renal and liver functions. In cases where medical management is not sufficient,

then organ support with renal replacement therapy has to be considered.

- *Infection:* Because of their preoperative status, prolonged stay in hospital, stay in ICU, requirement of transfusions increases the risk of infections in these patients. Appropriate antibiotic therapy guided by the culture sensitivity reports will help in treating the infections.

HOW LONG CAN A PATIENT BE TREATED WITH MECHANICAL CIRCULATORY SUPPORT?

The duration for which the circulation can be supported by these temporary LVADs is limited. According to the regulatory body approval, Impella can be used for up to 2 weeks and tandem heart can be used for up to few days; however, there are instances where the support is extended beyond the recommended duration. Compared to the percutaneous devices, CentriMag support can be used for up to few months, and patient can be mobilized with a CentriMag support in place. These devices are used as bridges for recovery, transplant, high-risk procedure, bridge, destination LVAD, or decision-making. A clear-cut plan for further course of action should be chalked out; patient should be regularly assessed to look for signs of recovery. If the clinical parameters and echo show signs of recovery, then the LVAD support should be gradually weaned. Anticoagulation should be carefully titrated during the weaning period as there is a higher risk for clot formation due to lower flows. Once the LVAD flows are lowest and patient is tolerating well, the LVAD support can be taken off followed by surgical repair of the vascular access. If there are no signs of recovery of the native heart function, then the patient's candidacy for *transplant or destination LVAD has to be evaluated.*

CONCLUSION

Cardiogenic shock refractory to medical management has high mortality and morbidity. MCS can help in salvaging these patients. ECMO is easy to institute and can be done bedside. Percutaneous VADs have the advantage of rapid initiation of support and can be used for few days. CentriMag has to be inserted surgically and can be continued for months. All these strategies essentially serve as bridge therapies for recovery or for further management. Patient selection, timing of initiation, close monitoring, and having a clear plan about the patient management help in having good outcomes.

TRIALS

The PROTECT II trial was designed to compare outcome in over 600 symptomatic patients with complex three-vessel or unprotected left main coronary artery disease and severely depressed left ventricular function [EF <35%] randomly assigned to and Impella [2.5] or an IABP. The trial was stopped for futility at 69% of planned enrollment. There was no significant difference in the primary endpoint of major adverse event at 30 days.[15]

Intravascular microaxial LVAD and IABP have also been compared with acute MI and cardiogenic shock.[16-17]

These studies have found no mortality advantage to microaxial LVAD and a higher rate of bleeding.

In a 2020 propensity-matched, registry-based retrospective cohort study of over 28,000 patients with acute MI and CS in the American College or Cardiology's National Cardiovascular Data Registry, 1680 propensity-matched pairs were identified.[16] The rate of in-hospital death or bleeding at 30 days was higher with intravascular microaxial LVAD (45.0% vs. 34.1%; absolute risk difference, 10.9 percentage points, 95% CI: 7.6–14.2 and 31.3% vs. 16.0%; absolute risk difference, 15.4 percentage points, 95% CI: 12.5–18.2, respectively).

These data are limited by small numbers or unmeasured confounding. Larger randomized trials in this population are needed.

REFERENCES

1. Hochman JS, Sleeper LA, Webb JG, Sanborn TA, White HD, Talley JD, et al. Early revascularization in acute myocardial infarction complicated by cardiogenic shock. SHOCK Investigators. Should We Emergently Revascularize Occluded Coronaries for cardiogenic shock. N Engl J Med. 1999;341:625-34.
2. Thiele H, Zeymer U, Neumann FJ, Ferenc M, Olbrich HG, Hausleiter J, et al. IABP-SHOCK II Trial Investigators. Intraaortic balloon support for myocardial infarction with cardiogenic shock. N Engl J Med. 2012;367:1287-96.
3. Ponikowski P, Voors AA, Anker SD, Bueno H, Cleland JGF, Coats AJS, et al. 2016 ESC guidelines for the diagnosis and treatment of acute and chronic heart failure: The Task Force for the diagnosis and treatment of acute and chronic heart failure of the European Society of Cardiology (ESC) Developed with the special contribution of the Heart Failure Association (HFA) of the ESC. Eur Heart J. 2016;37:2129-200.
4. Combes A, Leprince P, Luyt CE, Bonnet N, Trouillet JL, Léger P, et al. Outcomes and long-term quality-of-life of patients supported by extracorporeal membrane oxygenation for refractory cardiogenic shock. Crit Care Med. 2008;36:1404-11.

5. Thiele H, Zeymer U, Neumann FJ, Ferenc M, Olbrich HG, Hausleiter J, et al. Intraaortic Balloon Pump in Cardiogenic Shock II (IABP-SHOCK II) trial investigators. Intra-aortic balloon counterpulsation in acute myocardial infarction complicated by cardiogenic shock (IABP-SHOCK II): final 12 month results of a randomised, open-label trial. Lancet. 2013;382:1638-45.
6. Windecker S, Kolh P, Alfonso F, Collet J-P, Cremer J, Falk V, et al. 2014 ESC/EACTS Guidelines on myocardial revascularization: The Task Force on Myocardial Revascularization of the European Society of Cardiology (ESC) and the European Association for Cardio-Thoracic Surgery (EACTS) Developed with the special contribution of the European Association of Percutaneous Cardiovascular Interventions (EAPCI). Eur Heart J. 2014;35:2541-619.
7. O'Neill WW, Schreiber T, Wohns DH, Rihal C, Naidu SS, Civitello AB, et al. The current use of Impella 2.5 in acute myocardial infarction complicated by cardiogenic shock: results from the USpella Registry. J Interv Cardiol. 2014;27:1-11.
8. Kar B, Adkins LE, Civitello AB, Loyalka P, Palanichamy N, Gemmato CJ, et al. Clinical experience with the TandemHeart percutaneous ventricular assist device. Texas Heart Inst J. 2006;33:111-5.
9. Aziz TA, Singh G, Popjes E, Stephenson E, Mulvey S, Pae W, et al. Initial experience with CentriMag extracorporeal membrane oxygenation for support of critically ill patients with refractory cardiogenic shock. J Heart Lung Transplant. 2010;29:66-71.
10. Stewart GC, Kittleson MM, Patel PC, Cowger JA, Patel CB, Mountis MM, et al. INTERMACS (Interagency Registry for Mechanically Assisted Circulatory Support) Profiling Identifies Ambulatory Patients at High Risk on Medical Therapy After Hospitalizations for Heart Failure. Circ Heart Fail. 2016;9:(11):e003032.
11. Mended LA, Picard MH, Sleeper LA, Thompson CR, Jacobs AK, White HD, et al. Cardiogenic shock: predication of outcomes based on right and left ventricular size and function at presentation. Coron Artery Dis. 2005;16:209-15.
12. Feldman D, Pamboukian SV, Teuteberg JJ, Birks E, Lietz K, Moore SA, et al. The 2013 International Society For Heart And Lung Transplantation Guidelines for mechanical circulatory support: executive summary. J Heart Lung Transplant. 2013;32:157-87.
13. Vandiver JW, Vondracek TG. Antifactor Xa levels versus activated partial thromboplastin time for monitoring unfractionated heparin. Pharmacotherapy. 2012;32:546-58.
14. Lahm T, McCaslin CA, Wozniak TC, Ghumman W, Fadl YY, Obeidat OS, et al. Medical and surgical treatment of acute right ventricular failure. J Am Coll Cardiol. 2010;56:1435-46.
15. O'Neill WW, Kleiman NS, Moses J, Henriques JP, Dixon S, Massaro J, et al. A prospective, randomized clinical trial of hemodynamic support with Impella 2.5 versus intra-aortic balloon pump in patients undergoing high-risk percutaneous coronary intervention: the PROTECT II study. Circulation. 2012;126:1717-27.
16. Dhruva SS, Ross JS, Mortazavi BJ, Hurley NC, Krumholz HM, Curtis JP, et al. Association of Use of an Intravascular Microaxial Left Ventricular Assist Device vs Intra-aortic Balloon Pump With In-Hospital Mortality and Major Bleeding Among Patients With Acute Myocardial Infarction Complicated by Cardiogenic Shock. JAMA 2020; 323:734-45.
17. Ouweneel DM, Eriksen E, Sjauw KD, van Dongen IM, Hirsch A, Packer EJS, et al. Percutaneous Mechanical Circulatory Support Versus Intra-Aortic Balloon Pump in Cardiogenic Shock After Acute Myocardial Infarction. J Am Coll Cardiol. 2017;69:278-87.

Extracorporeal Cardiovascular Support: Extracorporeal Cardiopulmonary Resuscitation

Jitendra Choudhary, Rahul Pandit

INTRODUCTION

Extracorporeal membrane oxygenation (ECMO) is a modification of the conventional cardiopulmonary bypass technique. It is performed by using intrathoracic or extrathoracic cannulation to support patients with cardiac or respiratory failure who are not responsive to conventional therapeutic interventions. "Extracorporeal life support (ECLS)" was the term proposed by Zwischenberger and Bartlett to describe prolonged but temporary cardiopulmonary support using mechanical devices.[1] ECMO nomenclature generally covers modalities that can be used for pulmonary support involving extracorporeal oxygenation and carbon dioxide (CO_2) removal, and ECLS is a term used for both cardiac and pulmonary supports, but these terminologies are used interchangeably.

TYPES OF EXTRACORPOREAL MEMBRANE OXYGENATION

Extracorporeal membrane oxygenation is an invasive technique where blood is drawn out from the venous system, oxygenated via an oxygenator, and then returned to the patient. Depending on where oxygenated blood is returned, ECMO has two basic types: Venovenous (VV) ECMO and venoarterial (VA) ECMO.

1. VV ECMO is used in respiratory failure patients and provides gas exchange support when standard ventilatory treatment fails.
2. VA ECMO provides circulatory as well as pulmonary support whenever heart and/or lung failure is present which is intractable to inotropes, intra-aortic balloon counterpulsation, and ventilation.
3. Venopulmonary artery (VPa) ECMO is a third type of ECMO that is used to provide right heart support ± gas exchange support in conjunction with a left-ventricular assist device (LVAD).

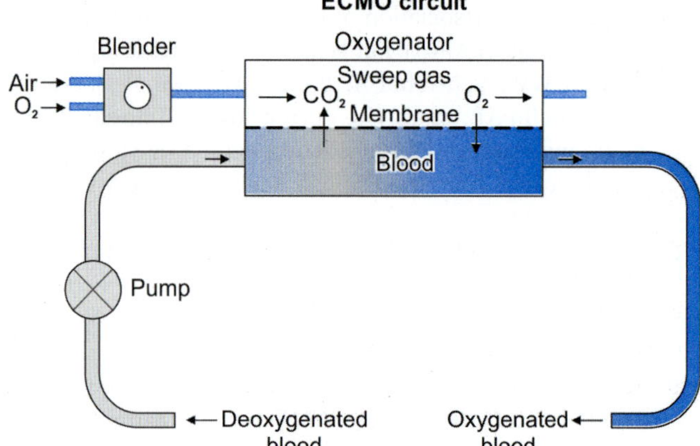

Fig. 1: Basic extracorporeal membrane oxygenation (ECMO) circuit.

The ECMO circuit consists of a large bore drainage cannula inserted into a large vein; a blood pump (capable of providing circulatory support); an oxygenator (that facilitates the exchange of oxygen and CO_2); a heater-cooler (to maintain the blood temperature at an acceptable level); and a large bore return cannula that is either inserted into a large vein (in the case of VV ECMO) or a large artery (in the case of VA ECMO) or the pulmonary artery (PA) (in the case of VPa ECMO).[2-4] **Figure 1** shows the basic ECMO circuit.

Venovenous Extracorporeal Membrane Oxygenation

Venovenous ECMO is used for lung failure intractable to usual mechanical ventilation. It only provides gas exchange support and helps in decreasing mechanical ventilation dramatically, and eases lungs into recovery, without any cardiac support. The effects of VV ECMO on patient arterial O_2 and CO_2 are as follows:

- *CO_2:* CO_2 removal by the ECMO circuit is related to sweeping gas flow across the oxygenator. Greater sweep gas flow via an oxygenator will clear more CO_2.
- *O_2:* During VV ECMO, if one presumes native lungs are not contributing to gas exchange and there is minimal recirculation in ECMO, final arterial O_2 is decided by association among ECMO pump flow and the patient's cardiac output. If ECMO pump flow persists to be low with respect to the patient's cardiac output, arterial O_2 will be low. Locker et al. (2003) indicated that providing ECMO pump flow equivalent to approximately 66% of cardiac output is essential to attain patient saturation >90%.[5]

In summary, if there is a major discrepancy between the ECMO blood flow and the total cardiac output, the PaO_2 will drop. This can be rectified by:

- Increasing the blood pump flow by inserting an additional drainage cannula to allow increased blood flow and decrease recirculation and improve arterial saturation.[6]
- Decreasing the patient's cardiac output by measures such as sedation, neuromuscular blockade, administration of negative chronotropic medications such as dexmedetomidine and β-blockers, and by consideration of cooling.

In VV ECMO, oxygen-deprived blood is drained from femoral vessels, and oxygen-rich blood is reinfused through the right internal jugular vein. In adults, the most common central veins cannulated are femoral veins. However, if a second venous cannula is needed to increase the flow, it is often inserted via the internal jugular vein.

The largest trial till date comparing ECMO versus conventional treatment is the CESAR (Conventional Ventilatory Support vs extracorporeal. Membrane oxygenation for Severe Adult Respiratory Failure) trial, which randomized 180 patients to receive VVECMO versus conventional treatment. ECMO group had better survival. However, there were significant differences in care received in both the groups (more lung protective ventilation and steroids used in ECMO groups) and nearly 25% of patients in the ECMO group did not actually receive ECMO. So, the mortality difference in both the groups was more because of better care at the high-volume center than because of ECMO itself.[4] The recent EOLIA (ECMO to Rescue Lung Injury in Severe ARDS) trial compared the efficacy of VV ECMO for severe ARDS, which found no mortality difference in patients randomized to ECMO versus conventional ventilation. The majority of patients in the control arm received prone ventilation but 28% of patients from the control group migrated to the ECMO arm and received ECMO as rescue therapy. Thus, data suggest a possible clinical benefit from ECMO over standard care, especially if used early rather than late.[7]

Indications

Common indications:

- Acute lung (graft) failure following transplantation
- Severe pneumonia, in particular, legionella pneumonia
- Status asthmaticus
- Severe acute refractory distress syndrome (ARDS) refractory to conventional ventilation and prone ventilation

Possible indications:

- Alveolar proteinosis to facilitate whole lung lavage
- Smoke inhalation
- Pulmonary contusion
- Bridge to lung transplantation

Venoarterial Extracorporeal Membrane Oxygenation

Venoarterial ECMO is used to support both cardiac as well as respiratory failures whenever traditional treatment modalities fail. VA ECMO can be used at low flow rates as partial assistance to native cardiac output, or at high flow rates which replaces almost the entire native cardiac output.[7]

The VA ECMO may be applied via central or peripheral cannulation. With central cannulation, blood is drawn out from the right atrium and returned to the ascending aorta. In peripheral ECMO, blood is drawn from the proximal great veins (via a femoral or jugular vein) using either surgical cut-down or modified Seldinger technique. The oxygenated blood is returned to the aorta by cannulating the carotid, axillary, or femoral artery. In the case of peripheral VA ECMO, the remaining native cardiac output passes through the patient's lungs.[6] In case the lungs are significantly affected, or mechanical ventilation is not adequate, the blood passing through the lungs remains substantially hypoxic. This hypoxic blood after entering systemic circulation is preferentially delivered to upper body circulation. This causes differential circulation between the upper body and lower body. This is called "Harlequin syndrome." To find out about differential hypoxia, saturation and pulse pressure at the right radial artery should be monitored.[8,9]

Indications

Common indications:

- *Primary graft failure:* After heart/heart-lung transplantation
- Nonischemic cardiogenic shock, including acute fulminant myocarditis and acute decompensated dilated cardiomyopathy
- Ischemic cardiogenic shock[10]
- Cardiopulmonary arrest with potentially reversible or treatable cause of cardiac arrest, especially in young patients
- Cardiomyopathy as a "bridge" to longer-term ventricular assist device
- *Postcardiotomy shock:* Unable to wean safely from cardiopulmonary bypass using conventional supports
- Drug overdose with profound cardiac depression
- Sepsis with profound cardiac depression
- Pulmonary embolism
- Severe anaphylaxis
- Cardiac or major vessel trauma
- Massive hemoptysis/pulmonary hemorrhage
- Pulmonary trauma

Venopulmonary Artery Extracorporeal Membrane Oxygenation

Venopulmonary artery ECMO, is used to support the right heart with or without gas exchange support with an LVAD. Blood is drained via a peripherally inserted venous cannula and returned into PA. ECMO pump flow is set to deliver less flow than cardiac output to avoid overwhelming the left ventricle. Fresh gas flow is adjusted to provide normal partial pressure of carbon dioxide in arterial blood ($PaCO_2$). Oxygenation parameters are usually high whilst the ECMO circuit delivers most of the oxygenated blood.

Indications

Common indications: Right heart failure following insertion of LVAD.

Possible indications: Respiratory failure following insertion of LVAD (or a combination of right heart and lung failure).

HEMODYNAMICS ON EXTRACORPOREAL MEMBRANE OXYGENATION

Venoarterial Extracorporeal Membrane Oxygenation

On ECMO, blood flow is nonpulsatile and has a very narrow pulse pressure (which reflects the perfusion pressure). Blood flow during ECMO is usually maintained at around 80% of calculated total blood flow and acceptable pulse pressure is between 10 and 15 mm Hg.

During partial VA ECMO support, the coronary artery blood flow is being derived from native left ventricular (LV) flow, which may be desaturated because of the return from the bronchial flows. Also, LV afterload is increased with the arterial cannula positioning into a right brachiocephalic artery, leading to increased metabolic demand. Thereby, in this scenario, failing LV may not be rested on partial VA ECMO. The heart is exposed to elevated preload, afterload, and increased wall tension; this results in increased oxygen consumption and hypoxic coronary circulation. Thus, higher ECMO flow may be required to decompress LV completely. Factors that increase oxygenation in VA ECMO are increased hemoglobin, increased flow, increased mixed venous oxygen saturation, and decreased shunt flow. After initiation of ECMO, in the first 72 hours, the peak and mean blood flow velocities decline by 30–50% and then revert to baseline. Ventricular stroke volumes for right and left ventricles are virtually similar and differ inversely with pump flow rate. Total aortic flow, which is the sum of pump flow and ventricular cardiac output, remains the same with either an increase or a decrease in pump flow.

Venovenous Extracorporeal Membrane Oxygenation

The VV ECMO does not provide circulation support and thus has no effects on hemodynamics, as blood withdrawn from the right atrium (RA) is returned back into the RA. In VV ECMO, the mixed venous oxygen saturation is high.

The oxygenation is blood flow dependent, and more blood must pass through the oxygenator to achieve a good degree of oxygenation. With VV ECMO, increased oxygen flows to the PA, the increased blood flow increases pulmonary vascular resistance and increases RV afterload which may lead to right ventricular myocardial stunning.

The VV ECMO systems may actually recirculate previously oxygenated blood depending on the placement of the inflow and outflow catheters. Factors which affect recirculation are:

- *Pump flow:* Recirculation increases linearly (from negative suction) with increasing pump flow.
- *Catheter position and cardiac output:* Increased CO, decreased recirculation (better forward flow).

ANTICOAGULATION MANAGEMENT

The goal of anticoagulation for ECMO is to achieve perfect equilibrium between platelet attenuation and thrombin activation to avert life-threatening thrombosis and also prevent excessive bleeding. The most commonly used anticoagulation is heparin. The activated clotting time (ACT) may be used to titrate heparin in the first 24 hours and is measured 2 hourly until established and stable, and then 6 hourly after the first day. Activated partial thromboplastin time (APTT) is preferred but there may be delays in obtaining results so may only be available for 6 hourly. The usual target for the ACT is 180–200 seconds.

Following the first day, APTT-guided heparin therapy is continued. The target range for the nonbleeding patient is 50–75 seconds.

The hemoglobin target should be 10–12 g/dL; this helps in maximizing oxygen delivery.

An albumin target of approximately 4.0 g/dL is important to ensure plasma volume is maintained.

Drug sequestration and altered volume of distribution of various drugs are very common on ECMO, so therapeutic drug level monitoring should be done especially for antimicrobials, vancomycin, opioids, and voriconazole.

VENTILATION STRATEGY FOR ECMO[11] VENOVENOUS EXTRACORPOREAL MEMBRANE OXYGENATION

The aim is to implement a "lung rest strategy" to prevent barotrauma and volutrauma [peak inspiratory pressure (PIP) <35 cmH_2O, plateau pressure (P_{Plat}) <30 cmH_2O, tidal volume (TV) <6 mL/kg ideal body weight (IBW), rate ~6 breaths/min, and positive end-expiratory pressure (PEEP) 10–15 cmH_2O].

The aim is to prevent hypoxemia by maintaining suitable oxygenation (e.g., PaO_2 of >60 mm Hg and saturation of >88% may be adequate for some individuals). The fraction of inspired oxygen (FiO_2) is between 0.4 and 1.0 (aim for 0.5 when possible). Oxygenator function needs to be confirmed and make sure that there is no recirculation through the ECMO circuit [on preoxygenator arterial blood gases (ABG) if preoxygenator saturation >75% and PO_2 >45 mm Hg suggest recirculation].

Generally, once lung pathology reversal is adequate (increasing TVs, during recruitment maneuvers improves compliance), a transition from lung rest strategies toward efforts to ventilate lung tissue should be done. It can occur between day 7 and day 21, or earlier.

Venoarterial Extracorporeal Membrane Oxygenation

The aim of ventilation is to provide sufficient aeration, maintain normal functional residual capacity (FRC), and to prevent atelectasis. (Usual settings include: FiO_2 0.5, rate 6–12 beats/min, TV 6–9 mL/kg IBW and best PEEP).

Aim for Normal Partial Pressure of Carbon Dioxide in Arterial Blood

Avoid overventilating the lungs, as when flow through the cardiopulmonary system is minimal, there will not be any gas exchange from native lungs even when ventilatory settings are of normal lungs.

COMPLICATIONS

Extracorporeal membrane oxygenation-related complications are as follows:[12-16]

- *Vascular complications:* These are the leading cause of mortality in ECMO patients. These include limb ischemia, vascular injury (dissection, pseudoaneurysm, and retroperitoneal hematoma), and late vascular complications such as vascular stenosis.
- *Bleeding complications:* The most common site of bleeding is from the cannula insertion site and other surgical sites. Bleeding can also occur from the airway and gastrointestinal (GI) tract. Intracranial bleeding is the most dreaded complication and can be rapidly fatal. Etiology for bleeding can be overanticoagulation, coagulopathy, platelet dysfunction or thrombocytopenia, and acquired von Willebrand syndrome.
- *Neurological complications:* Neurological damage can include seizure, stroke, intracranial hemorrhage, ischemic encephalopathy, and brain death. Paraplegia and spinal cord infarction are very rare complications of ECMO.

- *Technical complications:* These are a mechanical failure, an acute clot in the pump head, and device-related coagulopathy.
- Infection

HEMODIALYSIS ON EXTRACORPOREAL MEMBRANE OXYGENATION

Many patients requiring extracorporeal support are at high risk of developing acute kidney injury requiring renal replacement therapy. Continuous renal replacement therapy (CRRT) is the preferred modality of renal replacement therapy.

Indications

- Persistent metabolic acidosis (pH <7.1), despite intravenous sodium bicarbonate, especially when the metabolic derangements are unlikely to improve due to the severity of the cardiopulmonary failure.
- Persistent severe hyperkalemia or rapidly increasing levels despite antikalemic measures.
- Fluid overload not responding to diuretics.
- Uremic symptoms/signs like altered sensorium, convulsions, and pericardial rub.

Technical Aspects of Combining Extracorporeal Membrane Oxygenation and Continuous Renal Replacement Therapy

Continuous renal replacement therapy can be combined with ECMO either through independent venous access or a CRRT device can be included in the ECMO circuit. The advantages of including CRRT into the ECMO circuit are: (1) No need for separate vascular access; (2) No need for separate anticoagulation; (3) Better control of ultrafiltration and fluid balance. Also, Studies have shown longer hemofilter life of with this method than when CRRT was performed through an independent venous access.[12,17]

The CRRT machine can be linked to the ECMO circuit's venous section before the pump. This setup allows the blood to be propelled from the ECMO system into the CRRT machine. Following the cleansing process, the purified blood is then reintroduced into the ECMO circuit upstream of the ECMO pump. This integration facilitates the simultaneous support of both cardiac and renal functions. Dialyzed blood from CRRT is returned to the ECMO circuit before the oxygenator. This helps to trap air or clots before returning to the patient and also avoids venous admixture due to shunt.

WEANING THE PATIENT FROM EXTRACORPOREAL MEMBRANE OXYGENATION

The decision to wean ECMO is made by the medical team. The principles of VA ECMO weaning are as follows:

- Assessment of native heart function must be done by reducing ECMO circuit flows with appropriate changes in ventilator and oxygenator gas flow settings. ECMO pump flows should not be <1 L/min. Flows <1 L/min may be associated with precipitate quick clotting of the ECMO circuit.
- Transthoracic echocardiography and continuous cardiac output monitoring with PA catheter may be helpful in weaning from ECMO. Transesophageal echocardiography may help in assessing cardiac function.

The principles of VV ECMO weaning: When a weaning trial is given, the turn of the oxygenator fresh gas flow and a mechanical ventilator are increased. It is not necessary to reduce ECMO blood pump flow rates during this process since ECMO pump flow is generally set throughout to run at the lowest flow that provides adequate support (NB: ECMO pump flow is never <1 L/min due to the increased risk of circuit clotting).[3,7,18]

Extracorporeal Cardiopulmonary Resuscitation

Extracorporeal cardiopulmonary resuscitation (ECPR) means rapid deployment of VA ECMO during cardiac arrest to provide cardiac support when there is no return of circulation with conventional CPR. ECPR is not just ECMO applied in a CPR setting. Two important trademarks of these scenarios are an abrupt presentation of cardiac arrest patients, whether in hospital or out of hospital cardiac arrest, and other is uncertainty about its cause.

American Heart Association (AHA) guidelines state that ECPR should be considered in patients with easily reversible events. In out-of-hospital cardiac arrest and the majority of in-hospital cardiac arrest, the cause may not be readily known. In view of these uncertainties, one may decide about cannulation and ECPR in two ways:

1. By application of various scores used to predict mortality such as SAVE score, Acute Physiology and Chronic Health Evaluation (APACHE) II score, ENCOURAGE score, and HOPE survival probability score.[19-21]

2. By strict application of various prognostic criteria in CPR studies such as witnessed arrest, bystander CPR, shockable rhythm, and good quality CPR.[22]

But realistically none of these parameters are very reliable when the decision has to be made within a few minutes available to the ECMO team members. Many a time, contraindications such as aortic disease can be identified only after cannulation. Thus, the best strategy is in patients in whom the arrest is witnessed, and the duration of no-flow before resuscitation efforts is less than 5 minutes, one should begin the process of decision-making within 10 minutes of beginning resuscitative measures and the decision should be made by 15 minutes. The goal of initiation of support should be 30 minutes and not >60 minutes from the onset of resuscitation. Also, ECPR is now the treatment of choice for deep hypothermic arrest, usually refractory to conventional CPR.[23-25]

Extracorporeal Life Support Organization (ELSO) registry has reported a cumulative survival of 29–44% in patients receiving ECPR.[29-30] Also, studies comparing ECPR with conventional CPR have shown better survival in ECPR groups and but evidence to support better 6-month neurological outcomes in ECPR patients is lacking.[26,29,30] Deep hypothermic arrest managed with ECPR appears to have a better prognosis.[27]

Rationale for Extracorporeal Cardiopulmonary Resuscitation

Several factors such as initial rhythm (shockable vs. nonshockable), time to initiate cardiac compression and adequacy of compression, time to defibrillation in case of shockable rhythm, and time to return of spontaneous circulation are important determinants of outcome after cardiac arrest.

The institution of ECMO may help in the mitigation of some of these factors. ECMO helps in providing an immediate and certain return of circulation, thus providing adequate perfusion. This also improves myocardial perfusion, which may allow success at defibrillation in shockable rhythm and improvement in myocardial function.[28]

The ECMO also helps in the rapid establishment of hypothermia in the postcardiac arrest resuscitation phase and better outcomes.

Immediate full ECMO support in the postoperative period is essential to improve and maintain adequate peripheral perfusion and helps in reducing oxygen debt. Richardson et al. have shown that ECMO flow has gradually increased from 3.0 L/min in 2002 to 3.6 L/min in 2014. Regulation of ECMO flow is a delicate balance between maintaining higher flow to restore systemic circulation and causing LV distention, stasis, and pulmonary edema because of higher flow. Though, recent studies have not shown 6 months of better neurological outcomes compared to standard CPR, but ECPR has definitely shown survival benefits for out-of-hospital cardiac arrest (OHCA).

Weaning of ECMO should be undertaken when cardiorespiratory recovery has occurred.

CONCLUSION

ECPR provides a valuable option in critical care and resuscitation, extending the limits of conventional life-saving measures. As healthcare systems gain more experience and data, ECPR may become an increasingly integral part of advanced cardiovascular support, offering hope for survival in otherwise fatal cardiac events.

REFERENCES

1. Bartlett RH, Gazzaniga AB, Jefferies MR, Huxtable RF, Haiduc NJ, Fong SW. Extracorporeal membrane oxygenation (ECMO) cardiopulmonary support in infancy. Trans Am Soc Artif Intern Organs. 1976;22:80-93.
2. Chauhan S, Subin S. Extracorporeal membrane oxygenation, an anesthesiologist's perspective: physiology and principles. Part 1. Ann Card Anaesth. 2011;14(3): 218-29.
3. Chauhan S, Subin S. Extracorporeal membrane oxygenation—an anaesthesiologist's perspective—Part II: clinical and technical consideration. Ann Card Anaesth. 2012;15(1):69-82.
4. Peek G, Clemens F, Elbourne D, Firmin R, Hardy P, Hibbert C, et al. CESAR: conventional ventilatory support vs extracorporeal membrane oxygenation for severe adult respiratory failure. BMC Health Serv Res. 2006;6:163.
5. Locker GJ, Losert H, Schellongowski P, Thalhammer F, Knapp S, Laczika KF, et al. Bedside exclusion of clinically significant recirculation volume during venovenous ECMO using conventional blood gas analyses. J Clin Anes. 2003;15(6):441-5.
6. Extracorporeal Life Support Organization (ELSO) General Guidelines for all ECLS Cases. (2017). [online] Available from https://www.elso.org/Portals/0/ELSO%20Guidelines%20General%20All%20ECLS%20Version%201_4.pdf [Last accessed October, 2024].
7. Combes A, Hajage D, Capellier G, Demoule A, Lavoué S, Guervilly C, et al. Extracorporeal membrane oxygenation

for severe acute respiratory distress syndrome. NEJM. 2018;378(21):1965-75.

8. Rao P, Khalpey Z, Smith R, Burkhoff D, Kociol RD. Venoarterial extracorporeal membrane oxygenation for cardiogenic shock and cardiac arrest. Circ Heart Fail. 2018;11(9):e004905.
9. Ensminger SL, Puehler T, Benzinger M, Morshuis M, Kizner L, Gummert J. The role of extracorporeal mechanical assists (ECLS et al.) App Cardiopulmonary Pathophysiol. 2012;16(2):192-201.
10. Guglin M, Burchettl A. VA-ECMO in cardiogenic shock in adults: indications and outcomes. VAD J. 2016;2(8):1-22.
11. Schmidt M, Pellegrino V, Combes A, Scheinkestel C, Cooper DJ, Hodgson C. Mechanical ventilation during extracorporeal membrane oxygenation. Crit Care. 2014;18(1):203.
12. Cheng R, Hachamovitch R, Kittleson M, Patel J, Arabia F, Moriguchi J, et al. Complications of extracorporeal membrane oxygenation for treatment of cardiogenic shock and cardiac arrest: a meta-analysis of 1,866 adult patients. Ann Thorac Surg. 2014;97(2):610-6.
13. Nasr DM, Rabinstein AA. Neurologic complications of extracorporeal membrane oxygenation. J Clin Neurol. 2015;11(4):383-9.
14. Samadi B, Nguyen D, Rudham S, Barnett Y. Spinal cord infarct during concomitant circulatory support with intra-aortic balloon pump and veno-arterial extracorporeal membrane oxygenation. Crit Care Med. 2016;44(2): e101-5.
15. Mateen FJ, Muralidharan R, Shinohara RT, Parisi JE, Schears GJ, Wijdicks EFM. Neurological injury in adults treated with extracorporeal membrane oxygenation. Arch Neurol. 2011;68(12):1543-9.
16. Lo Coco, Lorusso R, Raffa GM, Malvindi PG, Pilato M, Martucci G, et al. Clinical complications during veno-arterial extracorporeal membrane oxigenation in post-cardiotomy and non post-cardiotomy shock: still the achille's heel. J Thorac Dis. 2018;10(12):6993-7004.
17. Symons JM, McMahon MW, Karamlou T, Parrish AR, McMullan DM. Continuous renal replacement therapy with an automated monitor is superior to a free-flow system during extracorporeal life support. Pediatr Crit Care Med. 2013;14(9):e404-8.
18. Lafçı G, Budak A, Yener A, Cicek OF. Use of extracorporeal membrane oxygenation in adults. Heart, Lung Circ. 2014; 23(1):10-23.
19. Schmidt M, Burrell A, Roberts L, Bailey M, Sheldrake J, Rycus PT, et al. Predicting survival after ECMO for refractory cardiogenic shock: The survival after veno-arterial-ECMO (SAVE)-score. Eur Heart J. 2015;36(33):2246-56.
20. Kim KI, Lee HS, Kim HS, Ha SO, Lee WY, Park SJ, et al. The pre-ECMO simplified acute physiology score II as a predictor for mortality in patients with initiation ECMO support at the emergency department for acute circulatory and/or respiratory failure: a retrospective study. Scand J Trauma Resusc Emerg Med. 2015;23:59.
21. Muller G, Flecher E, Lebreton G, Luyt CE, Trouillet JL, Nicolas Bréchot, et al. The ENCOURAGE mortality risk score and analysis of long-term outcomes after VA-ECMO for acute myocardial infarction with cardiogenic shock. Intensive Care Med. 2016;42(3):370-8.
22. Debaty G, Babaz V, Durand M, Gaide-Chevronnay L, Fournel E, Blancher M, et al. Prognostic factors for extracorporeal cardiopulmonary resuscitation recipients following out-of-hospital refractory cardiac arrest. A systematic review and meta-analysis. Resuscitation. 2017;112:1-10.
23. Arora A, Amin A, Tsangaris A. Extracorporeal membrane oxygenation for cardiogenic shock: National trends in the United States 2008-2012. J Heart Lung Transplant. 2018;37(4):S48.
24. Conrad SA. Extracorporeal cardiopulmonary resuscitation. Egypt J Crit Care Med. 2016;4:11-5.
25. Nakashima T, Noguchi T, Tahara Y, Nishimura K, Ogata S, Yasuda S, et al. Patients With Refractory Out-of-Cardiac Arrest and Sustained Ventricular Fibrillation as Candidates for Extracorporeal Cardiopulmonary Resuscitation—Prospective Multi-Center Observational Study. Circulation. 2019;83(5):1011-8.
26. Ryu J, Chung C, Cho Y, Sung K, Jeon K, Suh GY, et al. Neurologic outcomes in patients who undergo extracorporeal cardiopulmonary resuscitation. Ann Thorac Surg. 2019; 108(3):749-55.
27. Sawamoto K, Bird SB, Katayama Y, Maekawa K, Uemura S, Tanno K, et al. Outcome from severe accidental hypothermia with cardiac arrest resuscitated with extracorporeal cardiopulmonary resuscitation. Am J Emerg Med. 2014;32(4):320-4.
28. Pappalardo F, Montisci A. What is extracorporeal cardiopulmonary resuscitation? J Thorac Dis. 2017;9(6): 1415-9.
29. Yannopoulos D, Bartos J, Raveendran G, Walser E, Connett J, Murray TA, et al. Advanced reperfusion strategies for patients with out-of-hospital cardiac arrest and refractory ventricular fibrillation (ARREST): a phase 2, single centre, open-label, randomised controlled trial. Lancet. 2020;396(10265):1807-16.
30. Belohlavek J, Smalcova J, Rob D, Franek O, Smid O, Pokorna M, et al. Effect of Intra-arrest Transport, Extracorporeal Cardiopulmonary Resuscitation, and Immediate Invasive Assessment and Treatment on Functional Neurologic Outcome in Refractory Out-of-Hospital Cardiac Arrest: A Randomized Clinical Trial. JAMA. 2022;327(8):737-47.

CHAPTER

37 Hypotension and its Prediction: An Update

TWL Scheeren

INTRODUCTION

Critically ill patients frequently develop hypotension at some time point during their stay in the intensive care unit (ICU). However, it is a relatively late symptom of a compromised cardiovascular state of hemodynamic instability. The development of hypotension not only forces the attending clinician to treat it and to establish an individual "tolerable threshold" of hypotension, but also to assess and monitor the potential mechanisms causing hypotension as a prerequisite for the appropriate treatment, and finally to evaluate the effects of these potential treatment modalities.

In the current era, complex algorithms that use machine learning tools for interpreting the many (continuous) input signals from hemodynamic monitors like pulse wave analysis, provide a prediction of ensuing hemodynamic events, such as hypotension, even before it develops. This chapter focuses on recent developments in the context of predicting hypotension in critically ill patients using machine learning algorithms.

Hypotension is a widespread problem that occurs frequently in the perioperative setting and in the ICU. Maintaining arterial blood pressure (ABP) at a constant and adequate level is well-regulated in healthy individuals by multiple factors, which include a combination of metabolic, (para)sympathetic, and endocrine factors. Maintaining ABP ultimately aims to provide an optimal perfusion *inflow* pressure for various organs.

The development of hypotension during critical illness represents an imbalance between the three cardinal features of cardiocirculatory physiology: Preload, afterload, and cardiac contractility. In patients with a distributive septic shock, for instance, both afterload and preload will likely be reduced, which in combination with septic cardiomyopathy may contribute to the development of hemodynamic instability resulting in hypotension. Intrinsically, derangements in cardiocirculatory balance are very common in critically ill patients, and so is the incidence of hemodynamic instability or hypotension in these patients. As organ perfusion is highly dependent on inflow pressure—and thus on ABP—hypotension may lead to organ dysfunction due to insufficient supply of oxygen and other nutrients. While both the heart, brain, and kidneys adjust their vascular tone to maintain organ blood flow independent of ABP (autoregulation)—at least within certain limits—these organs are at particular, increased risk of dysfunction in case ABP exceeds these limits. Other organs (e.g., splanchnic) may even be endangered at relatively "normal" ABP levels.

Currently, hemodynamic instability including hypotension is managed by the combined administration of fluids, vasopressors, and inotropes, depending on the underlying pathophysiology and the "goals" that are defined.

In recent years, multiple studies have investigated the relationship between hypotension and outcomes in critically ill patients.[1,2] In a large retrospective study in 8,782 adult patients with sepsis, the association between the time-weighted average (TWA), which equals the product of the magnitude and cumulative duration of hypotension for different thresholds and in-hospital mortality, acute kidney injury, and myocardial injury was assessed.[3] The authors found that for every increase in a unit of TWA-MAP <65 mm Hg, the odds of in-hospital mortality increased by 11.4%, while the odds of AKI and myocardial injury increased by 7.0 and 4.5%, respectively. A previous study in 274 septic patients found comparable results concerning mortality but found a higher cut-off value (i.e., a MAP of 75 mm Hg) for the association with acute kidney injury and the need for renal replacement therapy.[4] The impact of postoperative hypotension at various absolute hemodynamic thresholds (≤75, ≤65, and ≤55 mm Hg) on outcomes in the ICU following noncardiac surgery has been assessed in a multicenter retrospective cohort study including 3,185 patients.[5] Postoperative hypotension in the ICU was associated with an increased risk of 30-day major adverse cardiac or cerebrovascular events at MAP ≤65 mm Hg [hazard ratio (HR) 1.52; 98.4% confidence interval (CI) 1.17–1.96] and ≤55 mm Hg (HR: 2.02, 98.4% CI: 1.50–2.72). Mean arterial pressures (MAP) of ≤65 mm Hg and ≤55 mm Hg were also associated with higher 30-day mortality [MAP ≤65 mm Hg, (HR 1.56, 98.4% CI 1.22–2.00); MAP ≤55 mm Hg, (HR 1.97, 98.4% CI 1.48–2.60)] and 90-day mortality [MAP ≤65 mm Hg, (HR: 1.49, 98.4% CI: 1.20–1.87); MAP ≤55 mm Hg, (HR: 1.78, 98.4% CI 1.38–2.31)]. Furthermore, the authors found an association between postoperative hypotension with MAP ≤55 mm Hg and acute kidney injury (HR: 1.68, 98.4% CI 1.02–2.77).

In a different patient population, the relationship between the lowest MAP and a composite of myocardial injury and mortality was assessed in a recent retrospective study of 2,833 postoperative ICU patients after non-cardiac surgery.[6] Here, the authors found a strong association between this composite endpoint and the lowest daily MAP when comparing the lowest quartile of lowest MAP (<78 mm Hg) with patients with MAP at 87 mm Hg. In addition, the authors found this association to be dependent on the amount of intraoperative hypotension (IOH) the patient was exposed to.

In a slightly different context, but of relevance to the critical care physician, is the perioperative setting. Here, the association between IOH and postoperative outcome has been well established.[7-10] Multiple studies have shown that both the severity of hypotension (e.g., MAP <65 mm Hg vs. MAP <55 mm Hg) and the duration of IOH contribute to the development of either acute kidney injury[11,12] or myocardial injury,[13-15] as well as increased 30-day mortality.[16,17] Even for a MAP threshold of 65 mm Hg, maintaining MAP below this value intraoperatively for >13 minutes was associated with an odds ratio (OR) of 1.34 (1.06–1.68) for myocardial injury and 1.20 (1.02–1.40) for acute kidney injury (AKI), while OR's further increase for prolonged hypotension [>28 minutes; OR = 1.60 (1.28– 2.01) and 1.35 (1.14–1.58), respectively].[13]

The studies above led to the recommendations that—on a population base—maintaining MAP ≥65 mm Hg is associated with reduced morbidity and mortality.[10,18] However, clear evidence is lacking to a certain extent, especially for defining the "optimal" MAP threshold for guiding therapy in the individual patient. Official recommendations, e.g., from the Surviving Sepsis Guidelines (level 1B evidence, strong recommendation, moderate evidence), define a target MAP value ≥65 mm Hg as the threshold/target for resuscitation in the initial phase of septic shock.[19] On the other hand, several studies could not demonstrate a beneficial effect of striving for even higher MAP values, both in ICU patients[20-22] and after noncardiac surgery.[23,24] Nevertheless, in individual patients, e.g., those with chronic hypertension, maintaining higher MAP values may be beneficial.[20]

THE SOLUTION: MACHINE LEARNING-BASED ALGORITHMS

It may be clear that once hypotension has developed in the individual patient, it is suggestive of hemodynamic instability and a substantially impaired cardiocirculatory state, and it forces the clinician to react or, more precisely, resuscitate the patient. As pointed out previously, the development of hypotension is usually not an early clinical sign, but happens secondarily to a substantially jeopardized cardiocirculatory state, after failure or exhaustion of several compensatory mechanisms.[25] Therefore, it represents a state in which the perfusion of vital organs is already severely threatened, and the development of multiorgan failure will or has already ensued. Treatment, however, currently only starts after recognition of hypotension (with some delay), whereas, from a physiological point of view, it might be better to recognize the development of hypotension *before* it ensues, and thus prevent these hypotensive events (with potential benefits to patient outcome).

Predicting the evolution of hypotension before it ensues requires the recognition of the initial phase of hemodynamic deterioration, which might be subtle and influenced by other factors, e.g., pain-causing tachycardia or tachypnea. The complexity of correctly interpreting clinical signs in critically ill patients was illustrated recently in a large cohort, where it was shown that clinical examination alone fails to recognize shock, as reflected by a decreased cardiac index.[26]

The use of machine-learning tools may prove beneficial in predicting hemodynamic events.[27] Artificial intelligence (AI) in medicine is used to develop clinical decision support systems in acute and critical care environments to support clinicians, not replace them at the bedside.[28] More specifically, large datasets are analyzed to develop prediction models or algorithms. AI-based solutions can transform healthcare delivery, improving patient outcomes, and enhancing the clinician-patient relationship.[29]

The arterial pressure waveform is the gold standard for monitoring ABP. While it provides the clinician with information on the absolute values of ABP, it also gives a visual impression of the generated pulse wave. Using automated algorithms, additional information such as pulse pressure variation, stroke volume, cardiac output, and stroke volume variation can be derived, which is already available to the attending clinician. Nevertheless, as many features of the cardiac cycle are represented by the complex curves of the arterial pressure waveform, subtle and not visible to the human eye, additional information could be provided by using artificial intelligence about other features of the circulation, such as cardiac contractility, arterial tone, and aortic compliance. If these complex, high-frequency data are input into machine-learning algorithms and combined with ABP as output, it is possible to develop prediction models for hypotension.

Such an algorithm has recently become commercially available and is incorporated in the HemoSphere clinical monitoring platform from Edwards Lifesciences (Irvine, CA, USA). The Acumen "hypotension prediction index" (HPI) represents a unitless index value ranging from 0 to 100. The higher the HPI value, the higher the likelihood of impending hypotension—defined as a decrease in MAP <65 mm Hg for at least one minute—within the following 5–15 minutes. In case HPI exceeds 85, it provides the clinician a warning sign, aimed to help in preemptively taking appropriate measures to prevent hypotension. The underlying algorithm divides the arterial pressure waveform into five distinct phases. It identifies associated physiologic components of the waveform (e.g., pulse pressure, the duration of systolic rise) and measures of the waveform morphology.[30] The HPI algorithm uses a multidimensional space of 23 hemodynamic combinatorial features of the arterial pressure waveform for the prediction of hypotension, based on data from a retrospective cohort (internal validation; *n* = 1,334 ICU/OR patients with 25,461 hypotension episodes). The underlying processes captured are complex alterations in compensatory mechanisms related primarily to preload, afterload, and contractility. Subsequently, the algorithm was externally validated by prospective data from 204 OR patients, with 1,923 episodes of hypotension. For hypotension occurring within 10 minutes, the sensitivity and specificity of the HPI were 89 and 90%, respectively, which was still 88 and 87% 15 minutes before the onset of hypotension. Based on discussions on the validity of the validation method, a reevaluation of the algorithm using different methods has been performed on a large dataset of 4,152,124 measurements obtained from 2,022 patients from previously reported studies.[31] This study confirmed the high utility of the HPI index to predict future hypotensive events.

The use of HPI software in combination with a treatment protocol has been shown to reduce the severity and duration of hypotension in perioperative and critically ill patients in >20 randomized controlled trials (RCTs) and cohort studies, summarized in recent meta-analyses.[32,33] These studies demonstrated a strong predictive performance of the HPI algorithm [area under the receiver operating characteristic curve (AUROC) = 0.89], and showed a significant reduction in hypotension duration, the TWA of MAP <65 mm Hg, and the area under the MAP <65 mm Hg threshold in the patient groups where HPI was used.

Moreover, it has been shown that the HPI software and an associated warning of impending hypotension as displayed on a bedside screen can change the behavior of the clinician and convert the treatment of hypotension from reactive to proactive.[34] As such, an HPI-derived warning for ensuing hypotension can buy time for evaluating the specific reason behind the impeding hypotensive event as a prerequisite for taking appropriate measures.

The decision support regarding the underlying cause of the hypotensive event may change our clinical practice from reactive to proactive and from unspecific to root-cause-specific blood pressure management. Yet, the impact on outcome in terms of major morbidity and mortality warrants further research, particularly in critically ill patients.

CONCLUSION

Critically ill patients frequently develop hypotension at sometime point during their stay in the intensive care unit (ICU). However, it is a relatively late symptom of a compromised cardiovascular state of hemodynamic instability. The development of hypotension not only forces the attending clinician to treat it and to establish an individual "tolerable threshold" of hypotension, but also to assess and monitor the potential mechanisms causing hypotension as a prerequisite for the appropriate treatment, and finally to evaluate the effects of these potential treatment modalities.

In the current era, complex algorithms that use machine learning tools for interpreting the many (continuous) input signals from hemodynamic monitors such as pulse wave analysis, provide a *prediction* of ensuing hemodynamic events, such as hypotension, even before it develops.

REFERENCES

1. Vincent JL, Nielsen ND, Shapiro NI, Gerbasi ME, Grossman A, Doroff R, et al. Mean arterial pressure and mortality in patients with distributive shock: a retrospective analysis of the MIMIC-III database. Ann Intensive Care. 2018;8(1):107.
2. Schuurmans J, van Rossem BTB, Rellum SR, Tol JTM, Kurucz VC, van Mourik N, et al. Hypotension during intensive care stay and mortality and morbidity: a systematic review and meta-analysis. Intensive Care Med. 2024;50(4):516-25.
3. Maheshwari K, Nathanson BH, Munson SH, Khangulov V, Stevens M, Badani H, et al. The relationship between ICU hypotension and in-hospital mortality and morbidity in septic patients. Intensive Care Med. 2018;44(6):857-67.
4. Dünser MW, Takala J, Ulmer H, Mayr VD, Luckner G, Jochberger S, et al. Arterial blood pressure during early sepsis and outcome. Intensive Care Med. 2009;35(7): 1225-33.
5. Smischney NJ, Shaw AD, Stapelfeldt WH, Boero IJ, Chen Q, Stevens M, et al. Postoperative hypotension in patients discharged to the intensive care unit after non-cardiac surgery is associated with adverse clinical outcomes. Crit Care. 2020;24(1):682.
6. Khanna AK, Maheshwari K, Mao G, Liu L, Perez-Protto SE, Chodavarapu P, et al. Association Between Mean Arterial Pressure and Acute Kidney Injury and a Composite of Myocardial Injury and Mortality in Postoperative Critically Ill Patients: A Retrospective Cohort Analysis. Crit Care Med. 2019;47(7):910-7.
7. Wesselink EM, Kappen TH, Torn HM, Slooter AJC, van Klei WA. Intraoperative hypotension and the risk of postoperative adverse outcomes: a systematic review. Br J Anaesth. 2018;121(4):706-21.
8. Wijnberge M, Schenk J, Bulle E, Vlaar AP, Maheshwari K, Hollmann MW, et al. Association of intraoperative hypotension with postoperative morbidity and mortality: systematic review and meta-analysis. BJS Open. 2021; 5(1):zraa018.
9. Gregory A, Stapelfeldt WH, Khanna AK, Smischney NJ, Boero IJ, Chen Q, et al. Intraoperative Hypotension Is Associated With Adverse Clinical Outcomes After Noncardiac Surgery. Anesth Analg. 2021;132(6): 1654-65.
10. Scott MJ, APSF Hemodynamic Instability Writing Group. Perioperative Patients With Hemodynamic Instability: Consensus Recommendations of the Anesthesia Patient Safety Foundation. Anesth Analg. 2024;138(4):713-24.
11. Mathis MR, Naik BI, Freundlich RE, Shanks AM, Heung M, Kim M, et al. Preoperative Risk and the Association between Hypotension and Postoperative Acute Kidney Injury. Anesthesiology. 2020;132(3):461-75.
12. Shaw AD, Khanna AK, Smischney NJ, Shenoy AV, Boero IJ, Bershad M, et al. Intraoperative hypotension is associated with persistent acute kidney disease after noncardiac surgery: a multicentre cohort study. Br J Anaesth. 2022; 129(1):13-21.
13. Salmasi V, Maheshwari K, Yang D, Mascha EJ, Singh A, Sessler DI, et al. Relationship between Intraoperative Hypotension, Defined by Either Reduction from Baseline or Absolute Thresholds, and Acute Kidney and Myocardial Injury after Noncardiac Surgery: A Retrospective Cohort Analysis. Anesthesiology. 2017;126(1):47-65.
14. van Lier F, Wesdorp F, Liem VGB, Potters JW, Grune F, Boersma H, et al. Association between postoperative mean arterial blood pressure and myocardial injury after noncardiac surgery. Br J Anaesth. 2018;120(1):77-83.
15. Sessler DI, Meyhoff CS, Zimmerman NM, Mao G, Leslie K, Vasquez SM, et al. Period-dependent Associations between Hypotension during and for Four Days after Noncardiac Surgery and a Composite of Myocardial Infarction and Death: A Substudy of the POISE-2 Trial. Anesthesiology. 2018;128(2):317-27.
16. Mascha EJ, Yang D, Weiss S, Sessler DI. Intraoperative Mean Arterial Pressure Variability and 30-day Mortality in Patients Having Noncardiac Surgery. Anesthesiology. 2015;123(1):79-91.
17. Barboi C, Stapelfeldt WH. Mortality following noncardiac surgery assessed by the Saint Louis University Score (SLUScore) for hypotension: a retrospective observational cohort study. Br J Anaesth. 2024;133(1):33-41.
18. Sessler DI, Bloomstone JA, Aronson S, Berry C, Gan TJ, Kellum JA, et al. Perioperative Quality Initiative consensus statement on intraoperative blood pressure, risk and outcomes for elective surgery. Br J Anaesth. 2019;122(5):563-74.
19. Evans L, Rhodes A, Alhazzani W, Antonelli M, Coopersmith CM, French C, et al. Surviving sepsis campaign: international guidelines for management of sepsis and septic shock 2021. Intensive Care Med. 2021; 47(11):1181-247.
20. Asfar P, Meziani F, Hamel JF, Grelon F, Megarbane B, Anguel N, et al. High versus low blood-pressure target in patients with septic shock. N Engl J Med. 2014;370(17): 1583-93.
21. D'Amico F, Pruna A, Putowski Z, Dormio S, Ajello S, Scandroglio AM, et al. Low Versus High Blood Pressure Targets in Critically Ill and Surgical Patients: A Systematic

Review and Meta-Analysis of Randomized Controlled Trials. Crit Care Med. 2024;52(9):1427-38.
22. Kotani Y, D'Andria Ursoleo J, Murru CP, Landoni G. Blood Pressure Management for Hypotensive Patients in Intensive Care and Perioperative Cardiovascular Settings. J Cardiothorac Vasc Anesth. 2024;38(9):2089-99.
23. Wanner PM, Wulff DU, Djurdjevic M, Korte W, Schnider TW, Filipovic M. Targeting Higher Intraoperative Blood Pressures Does Not Reduce Adverse Cardiovascular Events Following Noncardiac Surgery. J Am Coll Cardiol. 2021;78(18):1753-64.
24. Marcucci M, Painter TW, Conen D, Lomivorotov V, Sessler DI, Chan MTV, et al. Hypotension-Avoidance Versus Hypertension-Avoidance Strategies in Noncardiac Surgery: An International Randomized Controlled Trial. Ann Intern Med. 2023;176(5):605-14.
25. Pinsky MR. Complexity modeling: identify instability early. Crit Care Med. 2010;38(10 Suppl):S649-55.
26. Hiemstra B, Koster G, Wiersema R, Hummel YM, van der Harst P, Snieder H, et al. The diagnostic accuracy of clinical examination for estimating cardiac index in critically ill patients: the Simple Intensive Care Studies-I. Intensive Care Med. 2019;45(2):190-200.
27. Michard F, Pinsky MR, Vincent JL. Intensive care medicine in 2050: NEWS for hemodynamic monitoring. Intensive Care Med. 2017;43(3):440-2.
28. Pinsky MR, Bedoya A, Bihorac A, Celi L, Churpek M, Economou-Zavlanos NJ, et al. Use of artificial intelligence in critical care: opportunities and obstacles. Crit Care. 2024;28(1):113.
29. Cecconi M, Greco M, Shickel B, Vincent JL, Bihorac A. Artificial intelligence in acute medicine: a call to action. Crit Care. 2024;28(1):258.
30. Hatib F, Jian Z, Buddi S, Lee C, Settels J, Sibert K, et al. Machine-learning Algorithm to Predict Hypotension Based on High-fidelity Arterial Pressure Waveform Analysis. Anesthesiology. 2018;129(4):663-74.
31. Davies SJ, Sessler DI, Jian Z, Fleming NW, Mythen M, Maheshwari K, et al. Comparison of differences in cohort (forward) and case control (backward) methodologic approaches for validation of the Hypotension Prediction Index. Anesthesiology. 2024;141(3):443-52.
32. Mohammadi I, Firouzabadi SR, Hosseinpour M, Akhlaghpasand M, Hajikarimloo B, Tavanaei R, et al. Predictive ability of hypotension prediction index and machine learning methods in intraoperative hypotension: a systematic review and meta-analysis. J Transl Med. 2024; 22(1):725.
33. Pilakouta Depaskouale MA, Archonta SA, Katsaros DM, Paidakakos NA, Dimakopoulou AN, Matsota PK. Beyond the debut: unpacking six years of Hypotension Prediction Index software in intraoperative hypotension prevention—a systematic review and meta-analysis. J Clin Monit Comput. 2024.
34. de Keijzer IN, Vos JJ, Yates D, Reynolds C, Moore S, Lawton RJ, et al. Impact of clinicians' behavior, an educational intervention with mandated blood pressure and the hypotension prediction index software on intraoperative hypotension: a mixed methods study. J Clin Monit Comput. 2024;38(2):325-35.

SECTION

Ultrasonography and Echocardiography in the Critically Ill

CHAPTER 38

Basic Physics of Ultrasonography and Doppler Imaging

Bindiya Salunke, Amol Trimbakrao Kothekar, Vijaya Prakash Patil

INTRODUCTION

Ultrasonographic (US) technology has been used for several decades in imaging the human body. Point-of-care ultrasound (POCUS), which includes both ultrasonography and Doppler imaging, has become an essential component of patient care in critical care, anesthesia, and emergency medicine. It is used for evaluating hemodynamic function, securing vascular access, and performing peripheral nerve blocks.

Ultrasonographic technology is non-invasive, safe, and provides real-time imaging, making it invaluable across various medical fields. Therefore, a thorough understanding of the physical principles underlying ultrasound is crucial for generating high-quality images and providing accurate diagnostic information. This chapter covers the basic physics of ultrasonography and Doppler imaging, including the generation, propagation, and interaction of ultrasound waves with tissues.

BASIC PRINCIPLES OF ULTRASONOGRAPHY

Sound is a mechanical vibration transmitted by pressure waves through an elastic medium (it does not travel in a vacuum). Ultrasound refers to the portion of the sound spectrum with frequencies higher than what humans can hear, typically >20,000 cycles per second (20 kHz).

The diagnostic utility of ultrasound is enhanced by the following characteristics:

- *Directional and focused:* Ultrasound can be directed as a beam and focused.
- *Reflection and refraction:* Ultrasound follows the laws of reflection (where the incident ray, reflected ray, and the normal to the surface lie in the same plane) and refraction (where the incident ray, refracted ray, and the normal to the interface lie in the same plane) as it passes through a medium.

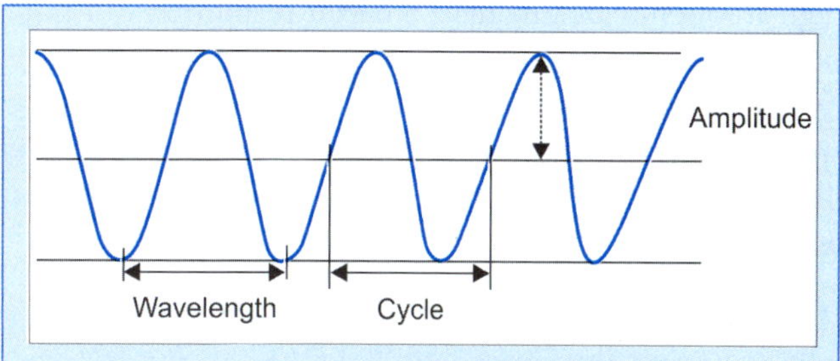

Fig. 1: Diagrammatic representation of an ultrasound wave. An actual ultrasound wave is a longitudinal wave.

- *Detection of small targets:* Even relatively small targets can reflect ultrasound, allowing for their detection and characterization.

Major disadvantages of ultrasound include its poor transmission through gaseous media (such as air or lung tissue) and its rapid attenuation.

As ultrasound waves propagate through a medium, pressure changes of vibrating molecules are transferred mechanically to neighboring molecules, producing longitudinal waves with alternating areas of compression and rarefaction. The ultrasound wave is often graphically represented as a sine wave **(Fig. 1)** with peaks (areas of compression) and troughs (areas of rarefaction).

BASIC TERMS

The sum of one compression and one rarefaction constitutes *one cycle of an ultrasound wave*. The time required to complete one cycle is called *the period, measured in microseconds.* The period of an ultrasound wave is determined by the source and cannot be altered by the sonographer.

Wavelength is the distance between two similar points along an ultrasound wave. In soft tissue, the wavelength of diagnostic ultrasound ranges from 0.15 to 1.5 mm. Wavelength determines resolution (ability to distinguish two adjacent structures as different structures). Shorter wavelengths allow for higher resolution, enabling the detection of smaller targets. *Frequency* is the inverse of the period and is defined by the number of wavelengths per unit of time, measured in Hertz (Hz). Similar to period, and wavelength, frequency is also determined by the source and cannot be changed. Clinical ultrasound frequencies range from 1 to 20 MHz (1 MHz = 1,000,000 Hz). Frequency is a major factor, which determines the depth of ultrasound beam penetration. Low-frequency beams penetrate deeper but have a lower resolution; whereas, high-frequency beams have a better resolution but poor penetration.

The velocity of ultrasound or propagation speed is the speed of movement of sound through a given medium. It is the product of the wavelength and frequency of ultrasound waves.

$$\text{Velocity (v)} = \text{Frequency (f)} \times \text{Wavelength} (\lambda)$$

Velocity depends on the medium's density and stiffness. It is directly proportional to stiffness and inversely to density. Thus, different media propagate sound at different speeds. The velocity of ultrasound within human soft tissues is approximately 1,540 m/s **(Table 1)**.

Amplitude refers to the strength of the ultrasound wave and is defined as the difference between the peak value and the average value of the waveform. It is depicted as the height of the sine wave above and below the baseline and is measured in decibels (dB). Amplitude can be adjusted by the sonographer.

The *power* of ultrasound is the rate of energy transfer measured in Watts. It is determined by the sound source and decreases as the beam propagates through the body.

The intensity of the ultrasound beam is the power per unit cross-sectional area, measured in watts/cm^2. Intensity also decreases as the ultrasound propagates through tissue.

TABLE 1: Velocity of sound through different media.[1]

Medium	Velocity (m/s)
Air	330
Fat	1,450
Water	1,480
Soft tissue	1,540
Kidney	1,560
Muscle	1,580
Bone	4,080

INTERACTION BETWEEN ULTRASOUND AND TISSUE

Attenuation: Attenuation refers to the reduction in ultrasound energy as the wave propagates through a medium **(Fig. 2)**. It measures the rate at which the intensity of the ultrasound beam diminishes (waves decay) as it travels through any medium. Attenuation consists of three main components: (1) Absorption, (2) scattering, and (3) reflection.

Absorption is the conversion of ultrasound energy into heat as it interacts with tissue. Scattering occurs when ultrasound waves interact with irregular or small structures, causing the waves to disperse in different directions. Reflection happens when ultrasound waves bounce back from interfaces between tissues of different densities.

Attenuation increases with the depth and frequency of the transmitted beam. In soft tissue, attenuation of ultrasound wave occurs between 0.5 and 1.0 dB/cm/MHz, for example, if we are using a 3 MHz probe, for each cm depth there will be a loss of 3–6 dB taking into account the round trip of ultrasound waves from probe to tissue and back to probe.[1] The higher the frequency of the ultrasound wave, the better is the resolution but it has higher attenuation of the ultrasound beam, therefore ultrasound penetration will be poor, and deeper structures will not be visualized clearly. Conversely, low-frequency probes will have good penetration but poor resolution.

Acoustic impedance is the product of the velocity of sound in a particular medium (measured in meters per second) and the density of the medium (measured

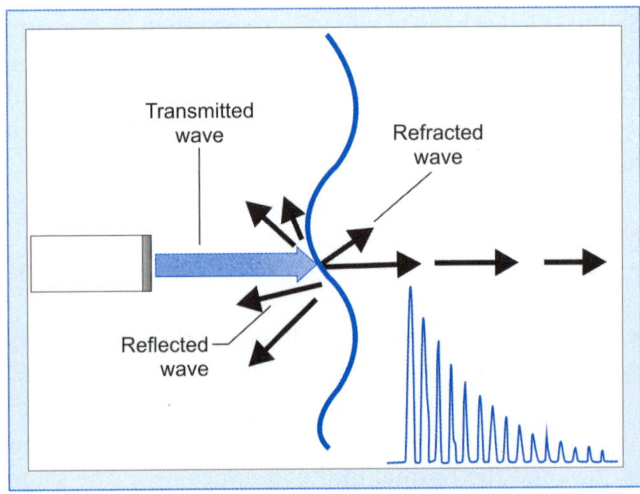

Fig. 2: Attenuation of ultrasound wave.

TABLE 2: Acoustic impedance of different materials.[2]

Material	Acoustic impedance (Rayls)
Air	400
Fat	1,380,000
Water	1,430,000
Soft tissue	1,630,000
Bone	7,800,000

in kilograms per cubic meter). The unit of acoustic impedance is Rayls (or Rayleigh).

1 Rayls = 1 kg/m^2/s acoustic impedance helps in understanding the amount of ultrasound wave that is reflected, refracted, or transmitted when it encounters the boundary between two different media. Acoustic impedance varies significantly across different materials **(Table 2)**. Acoustic impedance mismatch between two mediums is the deciding factor of the amount of reflection, refraction, and transmission of sound when it travels from one medium to another. Because air has such low impedance relative to soft tissue, using an acoustic coupling gel is necessary during ultrasound procedures. The gel helps eliminate air between the transducer and the skin, reducing reflection and allowing efficient transmission of ultrasound waves into the body. If the gel is not used, >99% of the ultrasound energy will be reflected at the air-tissue interface, leading to a poor image.

INTERACTION BETWEEN ULTRASOUND AND TISSUES

The interaction between ultrasound and tissues is determined by the on acoustic impedances of different tissues, and the relative size of the target compared to the wavelength and frequency of the ultrasound beam.

- *Reflection of ultrasound* ***(Fig. 3)****:* When ultrasound waves hit a smooth surface, they undergo specular reflection, similar to how light reflects according to the laws of optics. In this case, the angle of incidence equals the angle of reflection. Larger targets (relative to the wavelength of the ultrasound beam) produce specular echoes.
- *Refraction* ***(Fig. 3)****:* Refraction occurs when the ultrasound beam crosses the boundary between two media with different acoustic impedances at an angle that is not 90°. This change in direction is similar to light bending when it moves between materials, such as air and water. Refraction can lead to artifacts in imaging, as the ultrasound beam's path is altered.

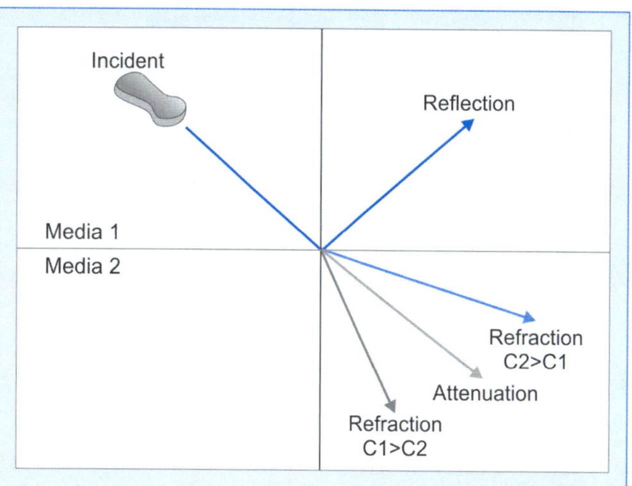

Fig. 3: Reflection, refraction, and attenuation of ultrasound waves. C1 and C2 are the speed of sound in materials 1 and 2 respectively. The angle of refraction depends on the difference between C1 and C2.

- *Absorption:* As the ultrasound wave travels through tissue, some of its mechanical energy is converted into heat energy. This process reduces the amplitude (or intensity) of the wave as it penetrates deeper into the tissue. The higher the frequency of the ultrasound wave, the greater the absorption, leading to more rapid attenuation of the beam. This is why higher-frequency ultrasound waves, although better for resolution, have less penetration.
- *Scattered reflection:* These are scattered echoes reflected in multiple directions from smaller targets. These scattered reflections allow imaging of tissues and surfaces that are not perpendicular to the beam. Each of these interactions—reflection, scattering, refraction, and absorption—affects the quality of the ultrasound image and the accuracy of the diagnostic information obtained.

GENERATING ULTRASOUND AND IMAGE PRODUCTION

The piezoelectric transducer is the most critical component of an ultrasound machine, enabling both the generation and reception of ultrasound waves. The transducer contains piezoelectric crystals, which possess the unique ability to convert electrical energy into mechanical energy (ultrasound waves) and vice versa.

- *Generation of ultrasound:* When *alternating current* is applied across the electrodes coupled with the piezoelectric crystals, these crystals *vibrate* and change

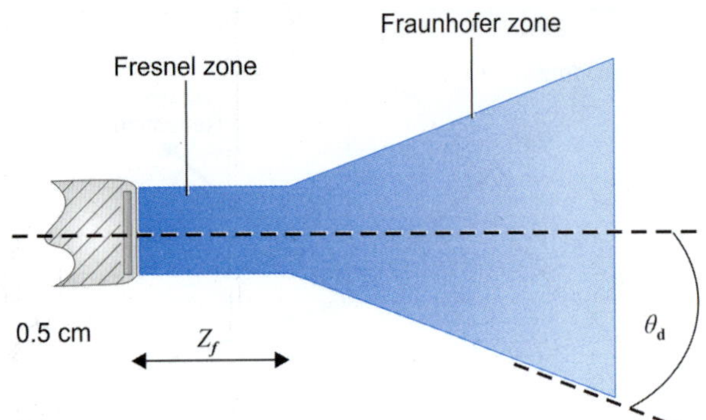

Fig. 4: Fresnel zone (near field) and Fraunhofer zone (far field). Z_f is the length of the near zone. θ_d is the angle of the cone-shaped Fraunhofer zone.

their shape. This vibration generates the ultrasound waves that are transmitted into the tissue.

- *Reception of echoes:* When the *returning echoes* from the tissue apply pressure on the transducer, the piezoelectric crystals *vibrate again*, converting this mechanical energy back into *electrical signals*. These electrical signals are then processed, amplified, and converted into an ultrasound image.

This dual function of the transducer, as both a *sound transmitter* and *receiver*, is the basis of ultrasound imaging. The returning echoes provide information about the structure and composition of tissues, which is then processed into real-time images.

Dampening material is an important component of the transducer. It reduces the ringing response of the piezoelectric material and absorbs backward and laterally transmitted ultrasound waves.

The ultrasound transducer can direct or focus the beam as it leaves the transducer. This creates a proximal cylindrical-shaped beam known as the near field or Fresnel zone **(Fig. 4)**. As this beam propagates, it further diverges and becomes a cone-shaped or Fraunhofer zone. This is the reason why the structures within a near field are better visualized. The length of a near zone (Z_f) is calculated by the square of the radius of the transducer divided by the wavelength of the ultrasound wave ($l = r^2/\lambda$).

TRANSMITTING ULTRASOUND ENERGY

When a brief alternating current is applied intermittently to the piezoelectric crystals, they generate a burst/pulse of ultrasound waves that are emitted from the transducer at fixed intervals. The time interval between the two consecutive pulses is known as the dead time, during which the transducer receives signals from returning echoes. To visualize deeper structures, it is necessary to increase the dead time. The number of ultrasound pulses emitted by the transducer over a designated period of time is known as pulse repetition frequency (PRF).

Gain compensates for attenuation by amplifying returning echoes. Time-gain compensation (TGC) is a technique used to selectively amplify echoes from deeper structures to achieve uniform brightness in the image **(Figs. 5A and B)**. Normally, ultrasound beams reflecting from deeper structures would have less energy compared to those from superficial structures due to attenuation. The primary purpose of this is to enhance the far echoes while suppressing near echoes, thereby improving image quality without introducing artifacts.

SCANNING MODES

- *A-mode (amplitude mode):* This mode scans in one dimension and thus it is used primarily for measuring distances. It is most commonly utilized in ophthalmology to measure eye dimensions.
- *B-mode (brightness mode):* In this mode, a linear array of transducers scans a plane through the tissue creating a series of reflected echoes. This produces a two-dimensional (2D) black-and-white image of the planes through which the ultrasound beam passes.
- *M-mode (motion mode):* This mode provides a time-motion display of the ultrasound wave along a chosen line, known as the M-line. The M-line is insonified repeatedly at a high sampling rate to examine the movement of a structure (e.g., a heart valve) over time.

Choice of an ideal probe: The choice of a USG probe varies based on wavelength, frequency, and penetration resolution. Low-frequency ultrasound provides greater penetration but lower resolution, making it useful for visualizing deeper structures. Commonly used low-frequency probes include the curvilinear (abdominal) probe and the phased array (echocardiography) probe. High-frequency ultrasound, on the other hand, offers excellent resolution but poor penetration, making it ideal for imaging superficial structures. The linear (vascular) probe and the hockey-stick transducer are the most commonly used high-frequency probes. Intermediate frequencies are seen in probes, such as the microconvex, endocavitary, and pediatric echocardiography probes.

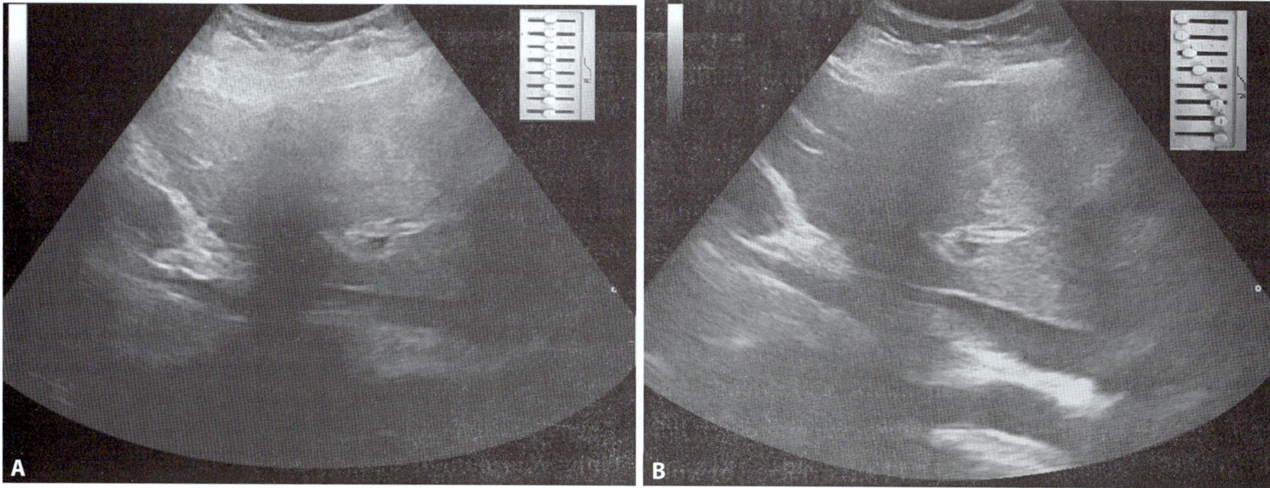

Figs. 5A and B: Time gain compensation (TGC). (A) Target at greater depth is poorly visualized; (B) Target at greater depth is clearly visualized.

ULTRASOUND ARTIFACTS

Ultrasound artifacts are common and can interfere with image interpretation. Understanding, recognizing, and minimizing these artifacts is crucial for accurate ultrasound imaging and optimal patient care. Ultrasound imaging relies on several key assumptions, but in clinical sonography, these assumptions are often not fully maintained leading to artifacts. The key assumptions are as follows:

- *Signal path:* Signal sent from ultrasound probe and returning echo travel in a straight line.
- *Ultrasound beam origin:* The echoes detected by the probe have originated from the rectangular main ultrasound beam.
- *One echo per reflector:* There is one echo per reflector
- *Depth relation:* The depth of an object is directly related to the time it takes for an ultrasound pulse to return to the transducer as an echo.
- *Constant speed of sound:* The speed of sound in human tissue is assumed to be constant at 1,540 m/s.
- *Uniform attenuation:* Acoustic energy in an ultrasound field is uniformly attenuated.

Artifacts Associated with Ultrasound Beam Characteristics

One of the assumptions in ultrasound image processing is that the echoes detected originate from within the main ultrasound beam. However, not all the energy generated by the transducer remains within the central beam. Some energy propagates radially, creating side lobes, and this phenomenon is known as the *edge effect*. Side lobes are multiple beams of low-amplitude ultrasound energy that emanate radially from of the piezoelectric crystals, projecting outward from the main beam axis. As a result, if a strong reflector is located outside of the main ultrasound beam, it may generate echoes that are falsely detected by the transducer as having originated from within the main beam.

Artifacts Associated with Multiple Echoes

Another assumption in ultrasound image processing is that an echo returns to the transducer after a single reflection, and the depth of an object is directly related to the time it takes for the returning echo to reach the transducer. However, when two parallel, highly reflective surfaces are present, the echoes generated from a primary ultrasound beam may repeatedly reflect back and forth between the surfaces before returning to the transducer. This results in multiple echoes being displayed. The echo that returns to the transducer after a single reflection will be displayed at the correct depth, but the subsequent echoes, which take longer to return will be placed at increasing distances from the transducer. This is visualized in imaging as multiple, equally spaced linear reflections, a phenomenon known as reverberation artifact. Comet tail artifact **(Fig. 6)** is a form of reverberation.

Ring-down artifact appears similar to comet tail artifact but occurs due to a completely different mechanism. This artifact is seen in the presence of gas bubbles. Whenever

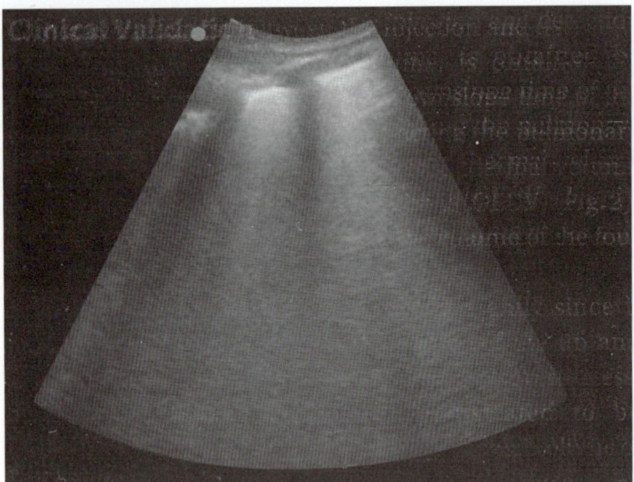

Fig. 6: Comet tail artifact.

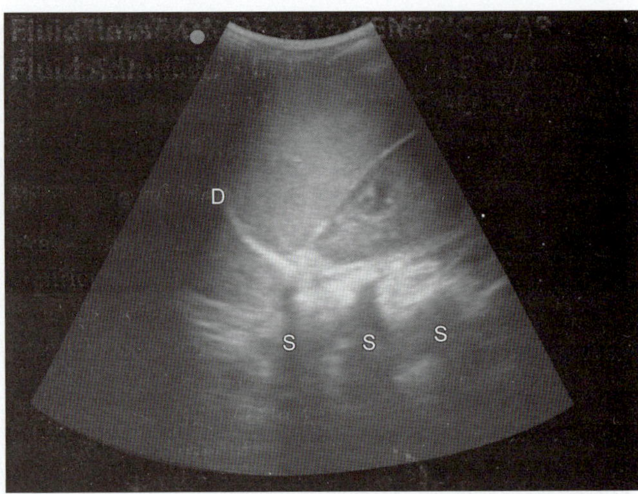

Fig. 7: Mirror image artifact. Note the discontinuation of the spine (S) below the diaphragm (D).

transmitted ultrasound energy causes resonant vibrations within fluid trapped between a tetrahedron of air bubbles, it produces a continuous sound wave that is transmitted back to the transducer. A line or series of parallel bands extending posteriorly from the gas collection are observed. This artifact is commonly seen in the bowel in the presence of gas and liquid.

Mirror image artifacts are most commonly encountered at the level of the diaphragm, where the pleura-air interface acts as a strong reflector **(Fig. 7)**. In this situation, the primary ultrasound beam encounters a highly reflective interface, resulting in an initially reflected echo. This echo then strikes the backside of a structure and then is reflected back toward the reflective surface before finally reaching the transducer. This phenomenon results in the display of a duplicated structure, equidistant from but deeper than the strongly reflective interface. This artifact can resemble lung consolidation due to the virtual reflection of the liver. In this situation continuation of spine shadows above the diaphragm (the thoracic spine sign or spine sign) suggests consolidation, pleural effusion, or hemothorax. In contrast, its absence is suggestive of mirror image artifacts.

Artifacts Associated with Velocity Errors

Another assumption in ultrasound image processing is that an ultrasound beam travels at a constant speed through human tissue. However, when sound passes through tissue with lower density, such as the area of focal fat, its speed decreases, causing the returning echo to take a longer time to reach the transducer.

The image processor, assuming the time of the echo's round trip is solely related to distance, will inaccurately display the structure deeper than it actually is. This phenomenon is known as the *speed displacement artifact*.

Additionally, refraction of sound waves will occur when they travel from one media to another with different densities. Here also ultrasound processor assumes that sound travels only in a straight line and thus it will misinterpret the returning echoes to be originating from the side rather than its original location. The best example of this is false visualization of duplication of the aorta when viewed in the midline at the rectus muscle junction.

Artifacts Associated with Attenuation Errors

Another assumption in ultrasound image processing is that acoustic energy within the ultrasound field is uniformly attenuated. However, when an ultrasound beam encounters a focal area that attenuates the sound to a greater or lesser extent than the surrounding tissue, then the amplitude of the beam distal to that area will be either weaker or stronger compared to its surrounding image. For instance, when the ultrasound beam encounters a structure with a high attenuation coefficient, such as a bladder stone, the echoes returning from beyond this structure will appear as a hypoechoic band, a phenomenon known as acoustic shadowing. Conversely, when an ultrasound beam passes through a weakly attenuating focal region like a fluid-filled structure, the amplitude of the beam beyond this structure will be greater than in the surrounding field at the same depth. This causes the area to appear falsely more echogenic than it should and is known as acoustic enhancement.

Doppler Ultrasound Imaging

The Doppler effect was first described by Austrian physicist Christian Doppler in 1842. He observed that when a sound source is stationary, the frequency of sound remains constant. However, if the source moves toward the listener, its pitch or frequency increases, and if it moves away from the listener, the frequency decreases.

In medical ultrasound, the Doppler effect is utilized to assess the direction and speed of blood flow through the heart and blood vessels. Where B-mode ultrasound provides structural information about tissues, Doppler imaging offers functional insights, particularly regarding blood flow dynamics.

Types of Doppler Ultrasound

- Pulse wave Doppler (PWD)
- Continuous wave Doppler (CWD)
- Color flow imaging
- Tissue Doppler imaging
- Duplex scanning

Pulse wave Doppler: In PWD, similar to B-mode ultrasound, the transducer emits short ultrasound pulses at intervals to allow time for receiving reflected echoes. The returning echoes are then analyzed at these fixed and brief intervals. By adjusting the timing between transmission and reception, specific points along the transmitted beam can be sampled, providing good depth acuity. However, a major drawback of PWD is that at higher velocities it generates inaccurate measurements due to an artifact known as *aliasing*.

What is aliasing?

Aliasing occurs when a sampling rate (number of pulses transmitted by Doppler transducer per second) is slower than the event rate, resulting in uncertainty about the direction and velocity of the signal **(Fig. 8A)**. *Continuous wave Doppler can be employed to overcome this issue.*[3]

Continuous wave Doppler: In CWD, there is continuous transmission and reception of ultrasound waves. This is achieved by using separate, dedicated transducers for transmitting and receiving the Doppler signals. The primary advantage of continuous wave Doppler is that aliasing does not occur, allowing for accurate measurements of very high velocities **(Fig. 8B)**. However, the major disadvantage of CWD is its inability to indicate the exact depth of the displayed velocity. CWD is particularly useful for measuring high-velocity jets, such as tricuspid regurgitation and stenotic lesions.

Tissue Doppler imaging: This technique is designed to record the movement of tissue rather than blood flow. The Doppler settings are adjusted to detect a lower range of tissue velocities.

Duplex scanning: This Doppler mode combines B-mode imaging with Doppler waveform analysis. It is predominantly used for evaluating for deep vein thrombosis, and venous insufficiency, as well as cerebrovascular, mesenteric, renal, and aortoiliac diseases.

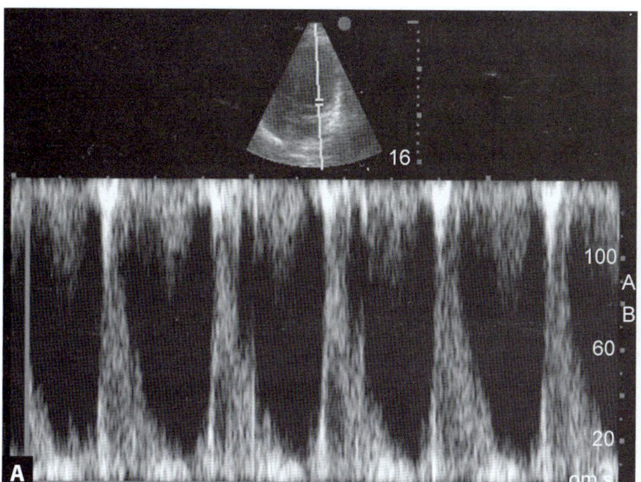

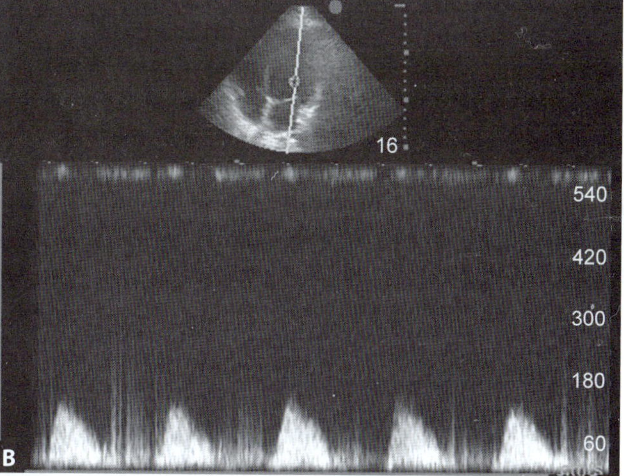

Figs. 8A and B: (A) Aliasing with pulse wave Doppler; (B) Disappearance of aliasing with continuous wave Doppler.

Color flow imaging: This technique of visually detects motion or blood flow by integrating a color map that is incorporated into a standard B-mode image. Based on the pulsed wave Doppler principle, it allows for the visualization of blood vessels and their flow characteristics, as well as the surrounding tissue. Color flow imaging is primarily used to assess the direction and general velocity of blood flow across the heart valves during echocardiography.

Doppler Imaging-related Artifacts

Spectral Broadening Artifact

This artifact occurs due to an increased range of flow velocities within the sample volume and is commonly observed in vessels downstream of a stenosis, indicating turbulent flow. However, it may also appear in normal-caliber vessels if the sampling area is too wide or positioned too close to the vessel wall **(Fig. 9A)**. To mitigate this, the Doppler sample volume gate should be set to approximately two-thirds of the vessel's width and centered within the vessel, which helps eliminate slow velocities near the vessel wall **(Fig. 9B)**.

Blooming Artifact

This artifact occurs when the Doppler gain is set too high, causing the amplification of signals beyond the vessel walls. As a result, the color extends outside the true boundaries of the blood vessels, creating the illusion that the vessels are larger than their actual size **(Fig. 10A)**. Adjusting the Doppler gain setting to optimum can lead to the disappearance of blooming artifact **(Fig. 10B)**.

Biosafety of Ultrasound

Clinical applications of ultrasound are showing a rising trend, and it is used in every branch of medicine. Ultrasound is mechanical energy that propagates longitudinally and has the potential to react with biological systems.

Thermal Effects

As an ultrasound beam travels through tissues, it generates frictional forces that produce heat. The rate of heat generation depends on several factors, including the characteristics of ultrasound like pulse repetition frequency, pulse length, duration of ultrasound exposure, transducer frequency, zoom function, etc. Tissue characteristics such as tissue perfusion, thermal conduction, and anatomical configuration also influence heat generation, etc. Animal studies indicate that fetal tissues are particularly susceptible to thermal effects during organogenesis.

Mechanical Effects

Besides thermal effects, ultrasound can cause mechanical effects in the form of a cavitational phenomenon that involves the expansion and collapse of gas bubbles in tissues. The generation of shear forces by these bubble implosions can lead to cell lysis and free radical formation. Animal experiments have demonstrated lung, kidney, and other organ injuries due to the mechanical effects of ultrasound.

Most of these studies are in animal models. Human studies done in obstetric diagnostic settings have till now

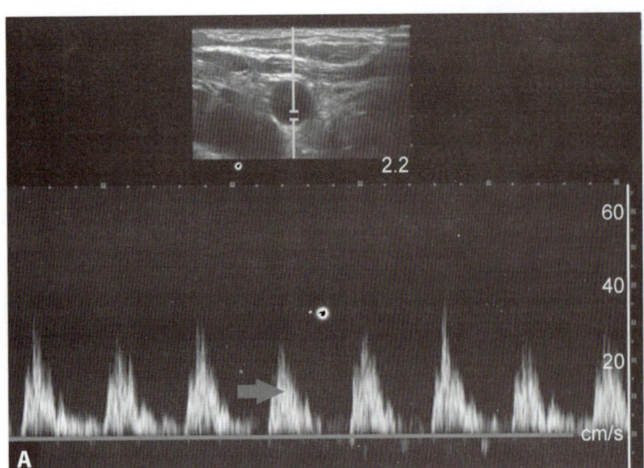

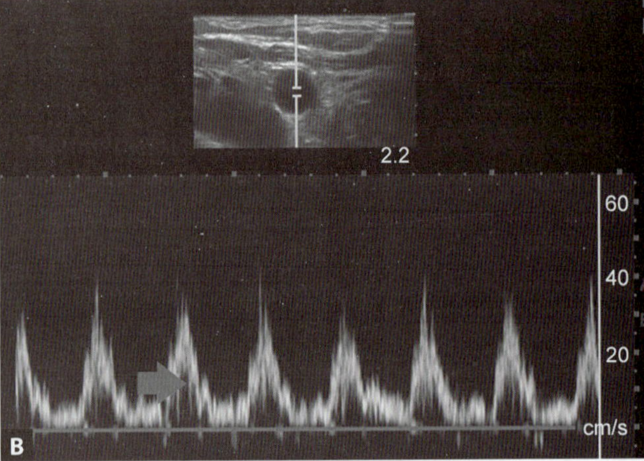

Figs. 9A and B: (A) Incorrect sample gate causing spectral broadening artifact; (B) Correct sample gate with no spectral broadening artifact *(For color version, see Plate 5)*.

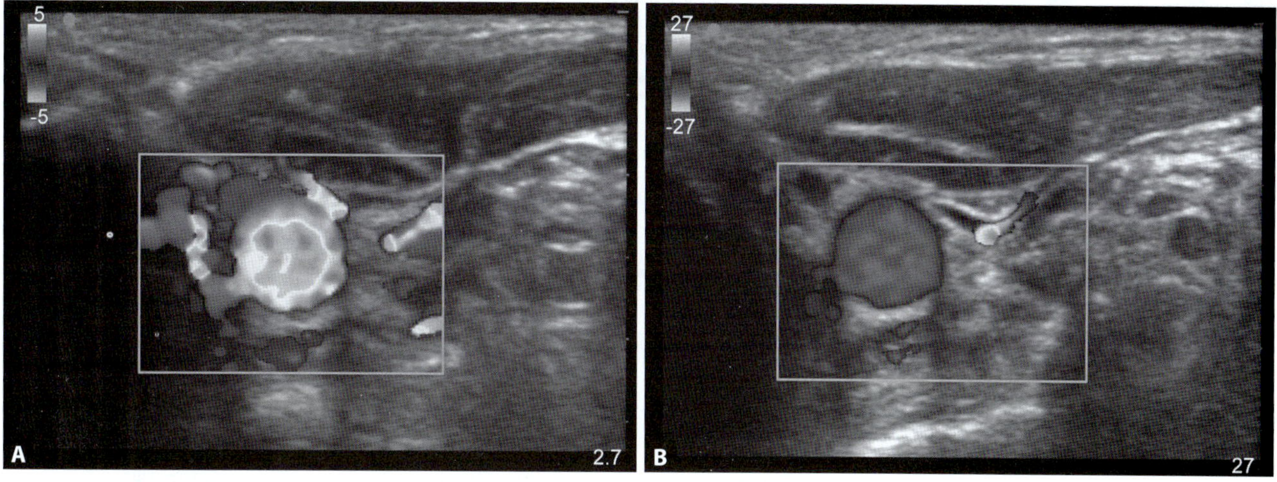

Figs. 10A and B: (A) Excessively high Doppler gain causing blooming artifact; (B) Optimal Doppler gain setting causing disappearance of blooming artifact *(For color version, see Plate 5)*.

shown reassuring results and have failed to show a causal relationship between diagnostic ultrasound and adverse effects.[4,5] These risk potentials, although theoretical, should guide us to use ultrasound with prudence.

CONCLUSION

Ultrasound imaging employs high-frequency sound waves to create internal images, with properties such as frequency and wavelength significantly impacting image resolution and depth. Artifacts are unintended distortions in the images and include reverberation (multiple echoes), shadowing (dark areas behind dense objects), enhancement (increased brightness in fluid areas), and mirror images (duplications near reflective surfaces). Recognizing these artifacts is crucial for accurate interpretation.

A solid understanding of the physics underlying ultrasonography and Doppler imaging is essential for effectively utilizing these modalities in clinical practice. Mastering these principles enables clinicians to enhance image quality, interpret results accurately, and minimize diagnostic errors caused by artifacts. Today, ultrasonography and Doppler imaging are integral components of high-quality, evidence-based patient care, evolving beyond mere diagnostic tools to become essential elements in comprehensive medical assessments.

REFERENCES

1. Armstrong WF, Ryan T. Physics and instrumentation. In: Feigenbaum's Echocardiography, 7th edition. Philadelphia: Lippincott Williams & Wilkins; 2010. pp. 9-37.
2. Taylor PM. Ultrasound for anaesthetists. Curr Anaes Crit Care. 2003;14:237-49.
3. Sohn D, Chai I, Lee DJ, Kim HC, Oh BH, Lee MM, et al. Assessment of mitral annulus velocity by Doppler tissue imaging in the evaluation of left ventricular diastolic function. J Am Coll Cardiol. 1997;30(2):474-80.
4. Salvesen KA, Vatten LJ, Eik-Nes SH, Hugdah K, Bakketeig LS. Routine ultrasonography in utero and subsequent handedness and neurological development. BMJ. 1993;307(6897):159-64.
5. Newnham JP, Doherty DA, Kendall GE, Zubrick SR, Landau LL, Stanley FJ. Effects of repeated prenatal ultrasound examinations on childhood outcome up to 8 years of age: follow-up of a randomised controlled trial. Lancet. 2004;364(9450):2038-44.

CHAPTER

Utility of Echocardiography and Ultrasound in a Patient with Shock

Ian Seppelt

INTRODUCTION

Shock is defined as "acute circulatory failure associated with inadequate oxygen utilization by the cells".[1] Many different types of "shock" are described, but all ultimately lead to a failure of cellular oxygen usage, whether because of a failure in organ perfusion (a failure of oxygen delivery) or a failure of cellular utilization of available oxygen (cytotoxic shock). Traditionally shock has been considered in terms of hypovolemic shock, cardiogenic shock, obstructive shock (either preventing venous return to the heart or preventing forward flow of blood from the heart), and distributive shock where paradoxically cardiac output (CO) can increase while tissue oxygen utilization fails. The most common cause of distributive shock is severe sepsis (or "septic shock").[2]

Treatments for shock are based on fluid volume replacement, drugs to alter vascular tone or myocardial function, relief of mechanical obstruction to blood flow, and source control and antibiotic treatment for sepsis. There are ongoing debates, and an increasing amount of high-quality evidence, to address the questions of which fluid, how much fluid, and which vasoactive drugs to use. There is comparatively much less evidence about what can be done at the level of the microcirculation and at cellular level.

In the 21st century, bedside ultrasound, and especially echocardiography, is an essential element of both the diagnosis of the cause of shock and exclusion of other possible causes, and the ongoing reevaluation of the response to treatment.[3] Ultrasound is an essential component of emergency diagnostic algorithms, discussed elsewhere in this book. Increasingly ultrasound is being utilized as a hemodynamic monitor.[4] Basic (level 1) echocardiography is now considered essential for all trainees in intensive care medicine, in collaboration with experts (level 2) and referral intensive care units (ICUs) (level 3).[5] Bedside echocardiography is mandatory for any patient who is not rapidly responding to the primary treatment to find out the most likely diagnosis.

ECHOCARDIOGRAPHY FOR DIAGNOSIS OF THE CAUSE OF SHOCK

Initial assessment is a focused ultrasound, using one of the published Rapid Assessment by Cardiac Echocardiography (RACE) algorithms.[6] This is not looking for subtle findings, but rather to rapidly identify, or exclude, causes of shock, which require urgent treatment. A rapid assessment should answer the following:

- Is the heart working?
- Is the heart really empty or really full?
- Is there an acute valve rupture?
- Is there a pericardial effusion with signs of tamponade?
- Is there lung sliding, or could there be a tension pneumothorax?

These questions are deliberately framed in terms of obvious abnormalities, which should be urgently treated, before a more comprehensive echocardiographic examination can be undertaken.

Hypovolemia

The assessment of intravascular volume is one of the most difficult tasks in critical care medicine, and one most open to debate. There is clear recognition that static measures such as central venous pressure (CVP) or pulmonary artery occlusion pressure (PAOP) bear no relationship at all to a patient's intravascular volume or cardiac preload [left ventricular end-diastolic volume (LVEDV)].[7] There is a better relationship with dynamic measures of fluid responsiveness including change of CO, pulse pressure variation (PPV), and response to passive leg raise (PLR), while recognizing the fact that a patient can be demonstrated to be fluid responsive still does not mean that the patient requires fluid to be given.

At the extremes, hypovolemia is confirmed by a hyperdynamic collapsing left ventricle (the "kissing" sign), whereas fixed bowing of the atrial septum into the right atrium throughout the cardiac cycle confirms elevated left atrial (LA) pressures, and that further fluid is unlikely to be beneficial. Neither of these signs is absolute and must still be taken in context but is generally helpful when seen. Other indices such as left ventricular end-diastolic area (LVEDA) are useful in anesthetized patients with intraoperative transesophageal echocardiography (TOE) but are difficult to translate into the intensive care environment.

Inferior vena cava (IVC) and superior vena cava (SVC) diameter and variation throughout the respiratory cycle have been recommended as reasonable guides to intravascular volume, recognizing the effect measurement errors (such as off-axis Doppler) can have on the conclusions and the difference between spontaneous ventilation and positive pressure ventilation. In particular, the IVC diameter needs to be measured at the same point between 0.5 and 3 cm from the caval-right atrial junction in the subcostal view, and the sonographer must take care to obtain a good longitudinal view parallel to the IVC, and then tilt the probe to ensure that the maximum diameter is being measured. Inexperienced operators have confused the aorta for the IVC, leading to spurious conclusions, and the IVC moves inferiorly during inspiration so it is possible to be measuring two different segments of the vessel during inspiration and expiration on M-mode.

In a spontaneously breathing patient, an IVC diameter (D) of <21 mm that collapses >50% with a "sniff" indicates a normal right atrial pressure (RAP) of 3 mm Hg, whereas an IVC diameter >21 mm which collapses <50% indicates an RAP of >15 mm Hg. This can be further quantified as a collapsibility index (CI) = $(D_{max} - D_{min})/D_{max} \times 100\%$ or distensibility index (DI) $(D_{max} - D_{min})/D_{min} \times 100\%$.[8] Such techniques have been trialed in the emergency department and in trauma patients, where IVC dilatation has been used as an endpoint for volume replacement.[9]

For a spontaneously breathing, shocked patient, the IVC diameter has been used as a predictor of fluid responsiveness. If the IVC diameter is <10 mm then fluid is appropriate, if >20 mm then fluid is unlikely to be appropriate, and if between 10 and 20 mm and >50% collapsing then a trial of fluid is reasonable, with frequent reassessment of the clinical results after fluid administration. In nonbreathing patients on positive pressure ventilation, the DI has been used to predict fluid responsiveness with a threshold of 18% between responders and nonresponders, with 90% sensitivity and specificity.[10] An alternative approach in ventilated patients is to use a TOE probe to examine the SVC, where collapse of >36% during inspiration can distinguish between fluid responders and nonresponders with a sensitivity of 90% and specificity of 100%.[11]

Regardless of what is being measured, passive (or snapshot) measurements are usually unhelpful, particularly in the most difficult "intermediate" group of patients where the problem is not entirely obvious, and dynamic assessments of volume responsiveness are much more likely to lead to appropriate treatment. Different techniques have been utilized to assess either the change in stroke volume (SV) and therefore CO, or PPV.

The best validated technique is the PLR, which is effectively a "reversible transfusion", designed to assess the hemodynamic consequences of a fluid bolus before one is actually given.[12] SV is measured using pulsed-wave Doppler with sample volume at the level of the aortic annulus, such that the product of the velocity time integral (VTI) and cross-sectional area (CSA) = SV, and CO = SV × heart rate.[13,14] Having assessed a baseline CO, the legs are elevated and after a period of equilibration, the CO measurement is repeated. An increase in CO of >15% during the PLR is predictive of fluid responsiveness, although some researchers have suggested 12% or even 10% may be a reasonable cut point. False positive responses to PLR may be seen in the context of increased intra-abdominal pressure, and the technique is both operator and patient dependent (see Chapter 6 for detailed discussion on PLR).

Cardiogenic Shock

Cardiogenic shock likewise can be difficult to define but refers to an inadequate CO due to intrinsic cardiac dysfunction. Overall mortality from cardiogenic shock is high, and echocardiography is essential, both to define the severity of the ventricular dysfunction and to exclude specific mechanical causes of cardiogenic shock such as mitral valve (papillary muscle) rupture. While most literature relates to cardiogenic shock due to underlying myocardial ischemia, in intensive care, other things including toxins, sepsis, and catecholamines (takotsubo syndrome) can all lead to cardiogenic shock.

A basic assessment of biventricular function is part of rapid bedside (RACE) examination and should identify a severe global LV dysfunction, significant segmental wall motion abnormalities, and significant valve pathology. Obvious abnormalities can be identified by visual inspection. The VTI in the left ventricular outflow tract is a useful single measure that can be rapidly obtained as a surrogate for the SV, with VTI >20 cm normal and >18 cm evidence of adequate SV.[15] Left ventricular ejection fraction (LVEF) is the traditional way to assess LV systolic function, and a variety of techniques have been described to estimate LVEF from echo-derived indices. The most accepted is Simpson's biplane method, but this can be technically difficult in some patients and requires skill and experience to perform accurately.

Left ventricular systolic function cannot be assessed in isolation, and in critical illness, loading conditions (preload and afterload) and the use of inotropic drugs can all influence interpretation of LV systolic function. Where there is some mitral regurgitation dP/dt (integral of pressure with respect to time) can be estimated, which in normal LV systolic function is >1,200 mm Hg/sec and <800 mm Hg/sec is markedly abnormal. Newer techniques such as strain rate imaging and speckle tracking are currently under investigation in critically ill patients.[16,17]

Aside from acute myocardial ischemia and myocardial infarction, cardiogenic shock can be caused by acute valve lesions, peri-infarction rupture of a papillary muscle, causing severe mitral regurgitation, acute aortic regurgitation (which can be associated with an aortic dissection), and peri-infarction ventricular septal defects. Acute right ventricular (RV) failure is pathophysiologically distinct but can also be considered under the general category of cardiogenic shock. A transthoracic echocardiogram is the investigation of choice to identify or exclude a cardiac cause of shock with positive predictive value 97% and negative predictive value 100%.[18]

Obstructive Shock

A focused rapid echocardiogram (RACE) specifically looks for mechanical (obstructive) causes of shock, including acute pulmonary embolus (PE), pericardial effusion with tamponade, and tension pneumothorax, and dynamic causes of left ventricular outflow tract obstruction (LVOTO) can also be considered under the category of obstructive shock.

While it is unusual to see an actual PE on ultrasound (though occasionally a saddle embolus can be seen with good images of the pulmonary trunk, and a "clot in transit" is sometimes seen within the right heart chambers), there are characteristic changes of acute cor pulmonale, which are not diagnostic of, but are consistent with, massive PE, whereas a normal echocardiogram can at least exclude PE as a cause of shock, though not exclude a hemodynamically insignificant PE. Diagnostic criteria include dilated right heart chambers (RV/LA area ratio >0.6), impairment in right heart contraction [tricuspid annulus plane systolic excursion (TAPSE) <16 mm], elevated pulmonary artery pressures [assessed using the tricuspid regurgitation (TR) jet or pulmonary acceleration time], with paradoxical septal motion and a D-shaped left ventricle on short axis, and decreased CO associated with reduced left heart filling. Some consider the McConnell sign (good apical but poor free wall contraction) diagnostic of PE, but it can also be seen in RV infarction and can be difficult at times to assess.[19]

Pericardial tamponade is seen when the intrapericardial pressure exceeds the RV end-diastolic pressure, causing obstructive shock. Ultimately tamponade is a clinical diagnosis, not an echocardiographic one, but there are many associated signs. Pericardial effusion is generally easy to identify, though must be distinguished from pericardial fat and from pleural effusion (and a pericardial effusion >20 mm must lead to the question whether it is not actually pleural fluid that is being seen). The echo findings supportive of tamponade are right atrial wall systolic collapse for more than one-third of the cardiac cycle, RV diastolic collapse (best assessed on M-mode), and a dilated IVC.[20]

Ultrasound guidance should be considered mandatory for urgent or elective pericardiocentesis. Traditional landmark-based approaches (such as subxyphoid aiming at the tip of the ipsilateral scapula) frequently lead to misdirection of the needle and increase the chances of RV puncture. Using ultrasound it is possible to plan the best approach, looking for the most obvious target through the chest wall, and also confirm intrapericardial placement of the catheter by the injection of blood or agitated saline through the catheter, with appearance of the bubbles in the pericardial space on ultrasound. A medial-to-lateral approach from a parasternal entry point is recommended, which directs the needle away from the pericardium, rather than a steeper approach, which directs the needle toward the pericardium.[21]

Dynamic LVOTO is classically associated with hypertrophic cardiomyopathy where asymmetric septal hypertrophy and systolic anterior motion of the anterior mitral leaflet obstruct CO during systole. LVOTO can be seen in critical illness in the absence of LV hypertrophy, however, particularly in older patients with hypovolemia, tachycardia, and high doses of inotropes. Characteristic findings are turbulent flow in the LVOT on color flow Doppler, and high velocities associated with obstruction on continuous wave Doppler. The characteristic "dagger-shaped" LVOT flow is often seen on a spectral Doppler tracing. Treatment involves fluid resuscitation, control of tachycardia to restore normal diastolic coronary blood flow, and minimizing inotrope dosage.

Finally, tension pneumothorax is another cause of obstructive shock when high intrathoracic pressures prevent venous return to the heart. An extension to the RACE examination is lung ultrasound looking for evidence of a normal lung pattern (which excludes a pneumothorax), lung sliding or a lung point (suggestive of simple pneumothorax), or a complete absence of normal lung pattern which in the context of a shocked patient is supportive evidence of the clinical diagnosis of tension pneumothorax.[22]

Distributive Shock

In distributive shock (septic shock but also anaphylaxis, neurogenic shock, acute hypoadrenalism, and other rarer causes of shock), the echocardiogram may be normal or hyperdynamic, which is reassuring as a means of excluding other possible diagnoses and focusing attention on the cause. Sepsis can, of course, also be associated with cardiogenic shock (septic cardiomyopathy) and at times with takotsubo syndrome (apical ballooning and akinesia associated with good basal contraction) or LVOTO. Importantly, the myocardial dysfunction associated with sepsis is usually reversible and resolves over several days. If coronary angiography is performed, the coronary arteries are usually normal.

CONCLUSION

Ultrasound is an essential component of the evaluation of every shocked patient who is not rapidly responding to treatment of the most likely diagnosis. A simple bedside examination (RACE) can confirm both life-threatening diagnoses, such as causes of obstructive shock, diagnose cardiogenic shock, or reassure clinicians that the heart is not the problem, and diagnostic and therapeutic efforts should be directed elsewhere.

While a straightforward RACE examination is an essential skill for every intensivist, it must always be followed up with a comprehensive examination by someone skilled in critical care ultrasound. There are multiple possible pitfalls for the novice. Accurate SV assessment is essential, the PLR has to be done properly, RV dysfunction must be assessed systematically, and it is important not to miss LVOTO.[23] It is recommended that all focused examinations be stored for subsequent offline evaluation, education, and quality assurance. With the ready availability of high-capacity digital storage, ultrasound images are essential components of the medical record and will also assume medicolegal importance in the future. While it is accepted that critical care echo is a first-line modality for the evaluation of shock, increasingly it will also be used as a monitor of therapeutic response, and novel techniques under investigation will both simplify assessment and make it more accurate.[24]

REFERENCES

1. Cecconi M, De Backer D, Antonelli M, Beale R, Bakker J, Hofer C, et al. Consensus on circulatory shock and hemodynamic monitoring. Task force of the European Society of Intensive Care Medicine. Intensive Care Med. 2014;40:1795-815.
2. Vincent JL, De Backer D. Circulatory shock. N Engl J Med. 2013;369:1726-34.
3. McLean AS. Echocardiography in shock management. Crit Care. 2016;20:275.
4. McGee WT, Raghunathan K, Adler AC. Utility of functional hemodynamics and echocardiography to aid diagnosis and management of shock. Shock. 2015;44:535-41.
5. Cholley B. International expert statement on training standards for critical care ultrasonography. Intensive Care Med. 2011;37:1077-83.
6. McLean AS, Huang SH. Critical Care Ultrasound Manual, 1st edition. Churchill Livingstone, Australia: Elsevier; 2012.
7. Marik PE, Cavallazzi R. Does the central venous pressure predict fluid responsiveness? An updated meta-analysis and a plea for some common sense. Crit Care Med. 2013;41:1774-81.
8. Rudski LG, Lai WW, Afilalo J, Hua L, Handschumacher MD, Chandrasekaran K, et al. Guidelines for the echocardiographic assessment of the right heart in adults: a report from the American Society of Echocardiography. J Am Soc Echocardiogr. 2010;23:685-713.
9. Yanagawa Y, Sakamoto T, Okado Y. Hypovolemic shock evaluated by sonographic measurement of the inferior vena cava during resuscitation in trauma patients. J Trauma. 2007;63:1245-8.
10. Barbier C, Loubières Y, Schmit C, Hayon J, Ricôme JL, Jardin F, et al. Respiratory changes in inferior cava diameter

are helpful in predicting fluid responsiveness in ventilated septic patients. Intensive Care Med. 2004;30:1740-6.
11. Vieillard-Baron A, Chergui K, Rabiller A, Peyrouset O, Page B, Beauchet A, et al. Superior vena cava collapsibility as a gauge of volume status in ventilated septic patients. Intensive Care Med. 2004;30:1734-9.
12. Monnet X, Rienzo M, Osman D, Anguel N, Richard C, Pinsky MR, et al. Passive leg raising predicts fluid responsiveness in the critically ill. Crit Care Med. 2006; 34:1402-7.
13. McLean AS, Needham A, Stewart D, Parkin R. Estimation of cardiac output by noninvasive echocardiographic techniques in the critically ill subject. Anaesth Intensive Care. 1997;25:250-4.
14. Mercado P, Maizel J, Beyls C, Titeca-Beauport D, Joris M, Kontar L, et al. Transthoracic echocardiography: an accurate and precise method for estimating cardiac output in the critically ill patient. Crit Care. 2017;21:136.
15. Dalen H, Thorstensen A, Vattan LJ, Aase SA, Stoylen A. Reference values and distribution of conventional echocardiography Doppler measures and longitudinal tissue Doppler velocities in a population free from cardiovascular disease. Circ Cardiovasc Imaging. 2010; 3:614-22.
16. Vignon P, Huang SJ. Global longitudinal strain in septic cardiomyopathy: The hidden part of the iceberg? Intensive Care Med. 2015;41:1851-3.
17. Orde SR, Pulido JN, Masaki M, Gillespie S, Spoon JN, Kane GC, et al. Outcome prediction in sepsis: Speckle tracking echocardiography based assessment of myocardial function. Crit Care. 2014;18:R149.
18. Joseph MX, Disney PJ, Da Costa R, Hutchison SJ. Transthoracic echocardiography to identify or exclude cardiac cause of shock. Chest. 2004;126:1592-7.
19. Torbicki A. Echocardiography diagnosis of pulmonary embolism: A rise and fall of McConnell sign. Eur J Echocardiogr. 2005;6:2-3.
20. Ristić AD, Imazio M, Adler Y, Anastasakis A, Badano LP, Brucato A, et al. Triage strategy for urgent management of cardiac tamponade: a position statement of the European Society of Cardiology Working Group on Myocardial and Pericardial Disease. Eur Heart J. 2014;35:2279-84.
21. Osman A, Chuan TW, Ab Rahman J, Via G, Tavazzi G. Ultrasound-guided pericardiocentesis: a novel parasternal approach. Eur J Emerg Med. 2018;25:322-7.
22. Rudas M, Orde S, Yang Y, Nalos M. Reporting focused lung ultrasound studies in critical care. Recommendations from the College of Intensive Care Medicine Ultrasound Special Interest Group. Australas J Ultrasound Med. 2019;22:217-24.
23. Orde S, Slama M, Hilton A, Yastrebov K, McLean A. Pearls and pitfalls in comprehensive critical care echocardiography. Crit Care. 2017;21:279.
24. Vignon P. What is new in critical care echocardiography? Crit Care. 2018;22:40.

CHAPTER 40

Transthoracic Echocardiography in the Critically Ill

Ashish Kumar Srivastava, Shrikanth Srinivasan

INTRODUCTION

Transthoracic echocardiography (TTE), done by intensivist on the bedside, is a problem-based, goal-directed modality that is dictated by the patient's symptoms. It attempts to provide answers to a clinically relevant problem. TTE has tremendous scope in the intensive care setting. It can give an insight to cardiovascular pathophysiology and mitigates diagnostic uncertainty at bedside. It should be used as a basic screening tool for rapid assessment of circulation in hemodynamically unstable patient and is a valuable adjunct to clinical examination.

This chapter will review some fundamental aspects of TTE. These include basic echo window acquisition skills, principle of Doppler, left ventricular systolic function assessment, identification of regional wall abnormalities, measurement of stroke volume (SV), assessment of right-sided heart function, identification of preload responsiveness, and identifying pericardial effusion and tamponade pathophysiology.

Intensivist uses TTE for qualitative or semiquantitative assessment with pattern—recognition and in-context interpretation. Self-explanatory pictures are found throughout the text and are a key element of this chapter. A basic knowledge of cardiac anatomy, probe manipulation, and orientation is required for acquiring good TTE windows.

BASIC CARDIAC ANATOMY FOR ECHOCARDIOGRAPHY

The heart is obliquely placed in the chest cavity with the apex toward the left. The right ventricle and part of left ventricle form the anterior part of the heart; hence on 2D TTE, the ventricles are seen on the top of the screen, and the atria are seen to be located deeper (**Fig. 1**: Basic cardiac anatomy for echocardiography).

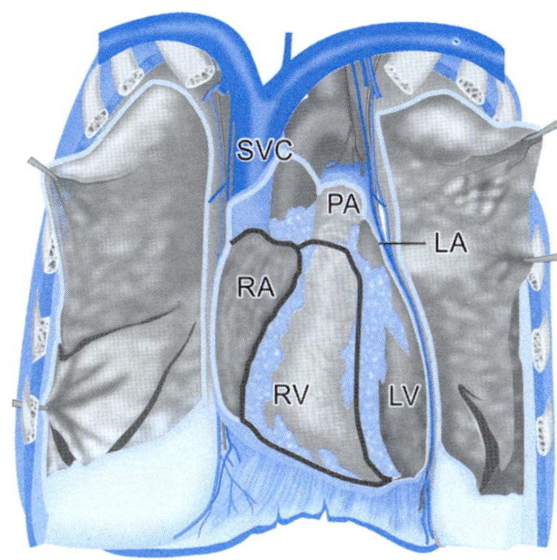

Fig. 1: Anatomy of heart. (LA: left atrium; LV: left ventricle; PA: pulmonary artery; RA: right atrium; RV: right ventricle; SVC: superior vena cava)

Probe Selection

The phased array probe is used for TTE. It has a smaller footprint (scan head), which allows it to be placed between the ribs to scan the heart.

This probe is called the phased array probe because the piezoelectric crystals generating the ultrasound waves fire in phases to get a constantly updated image of a rapidly moving structure (heart) **(Fig. 2)**.

Probe Manipulation

Probe manipulations refer to several ergonomic movements done while moving the cardiac probe in order to access a good cardiac window; these movements are: Sliding, rocking, rotation, and tilting.

Sliding

It refers to moving the probe in its long axis of the probe across the body to find the best echocardiographic window **(Fig. 3)**.

Rocking

Rocking is manipulating the transducer in its long axis, toward or away from the indicator. It allows focusing the area of interest or enhancing the field of view in one direction or the other, i.e., cephalic/caudal or right/left **(Fig. 4)**.

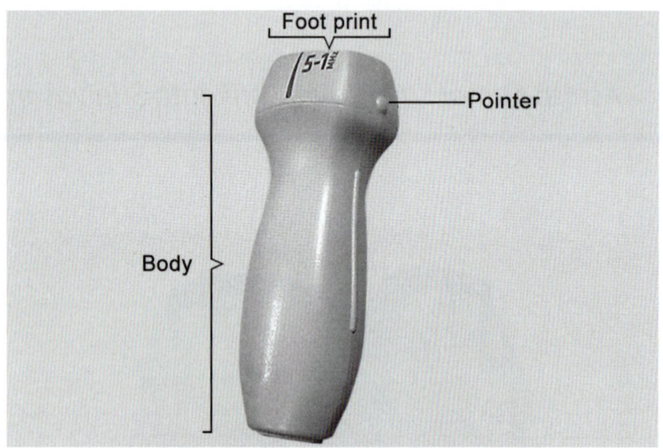

Fig. 2: Cardiac or phased array probe (1–5 MHz).

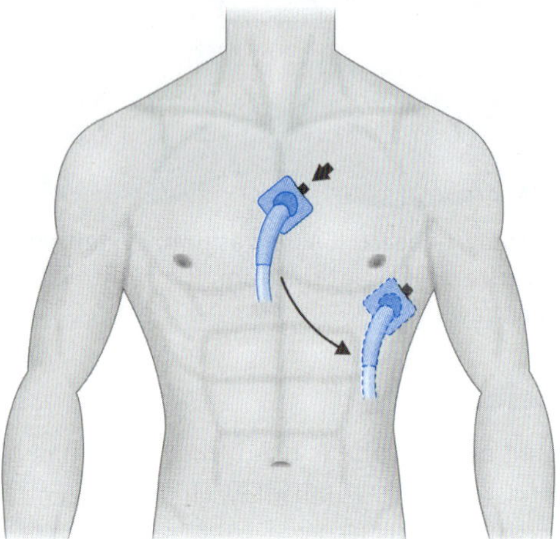

Fig. 3: Sliding probe in its long axis from the parasternal to apical view.

Rotation: It is moving the probe in a clockwise or counter-clockwise direction **(Fig. 5)**.

Tilting

Tilting motion of the probe is perpendicular to rocking motion. The tilting motion allows visualization from cephalic to caudal or right to left depending on the orientation of the probe **(Fig. 6)**.

STANDARD VIEWS ATTAINED DURING TRANSTHORACIC ECHOCARDIOGRAPHY

The heart enclosed in a bony rib cage; in order to visualize the various chambers of the heart, several well-defined acoustic windows are identified, which allow the examiner to view specific parts of the heart and assess its function and pathology **(Fig. 7)**.

These acoustic windows are:

- *Parasternal window:*
  - Parasternal long-axis (PLAX) view
  - *Parasternal short-axis (PSAX) view:*
    - PSAX base view
    - PSAX mid-papillary view
    - PSAX apical view
- *Apical view:*
  - Apical four-chamber view
  - Apical five-chamber view
- *Subcostal view:*
  - Subcostal four-chamber view
  - Subcostal inferior vena cava (IVC) view
- Suprasternal view

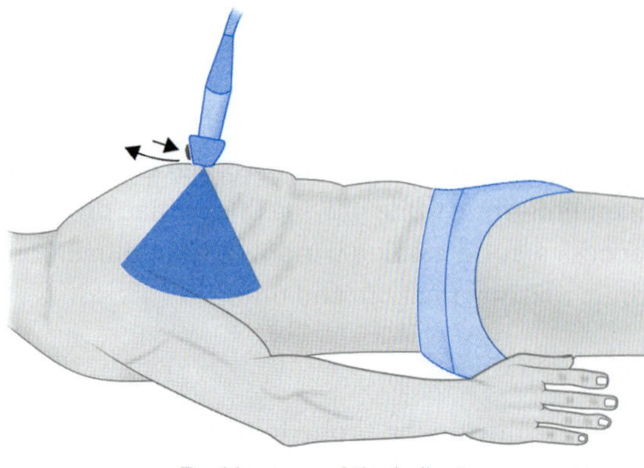

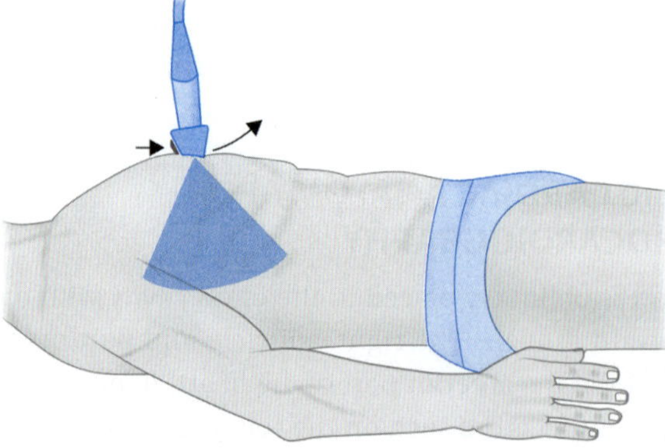

Fig. 4: Rocking motion is done in the long axis of the probe along a fixed point.

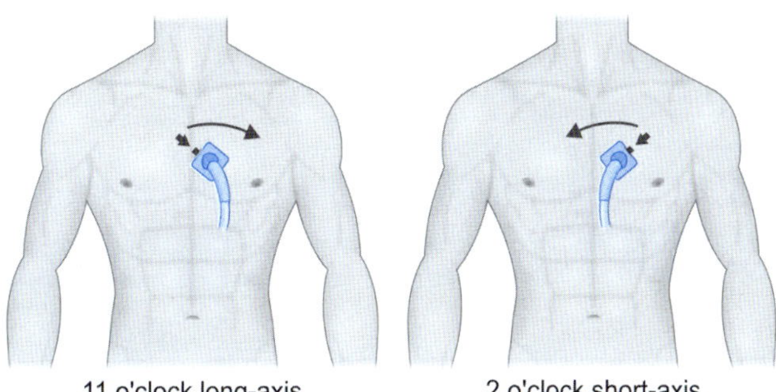

Fig. 5: In parasternal views, rotating the probe from 11 o'clock to 2 o'clock changes the window from long- to short-axis view.

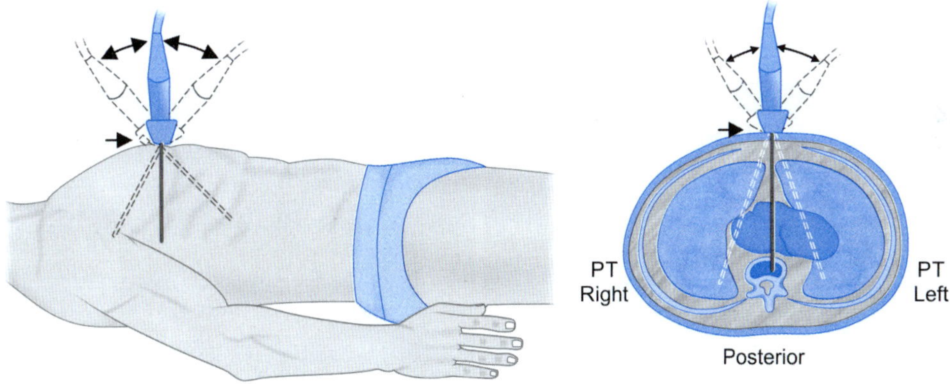

Fig. 6: Base to apex of heart can be visualized by tilting the probe in parasternal short-axis view.

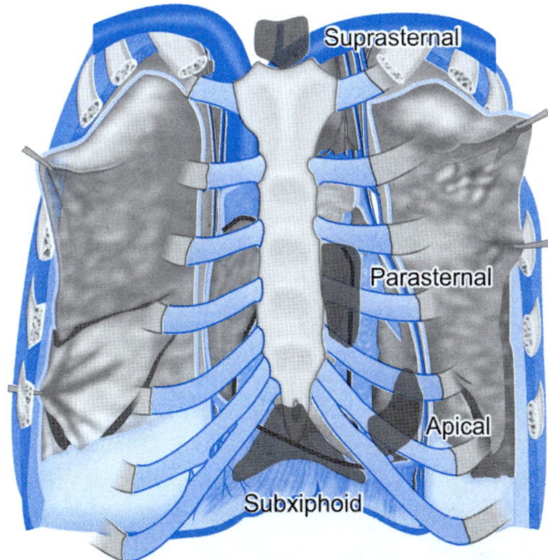

Fig. 7: Cardiac windows.

Parasternal Long-axis View

Transducer position: Left sternal edge; second to fourth intercostal space. Marker dot direction: points toward right shoulder **(Figs. 8A to D)**. The PLAX view is commonly the first view obtained in an echo examination and is useful for:

- Assessing contractility
- Visually calculating ejection fraction (EF) in M-mode
- Detecting regional wall motion abnormalities
- Measuring LV outflow tract diameter for cardiac output studies.

Parasternal Short-axis View

Transducer position: Probe in third or fourth intercostal space, left of sternum; probe indicator to the left shoulder, at 2 o'clock position **(Figs. 9A and B)**. This view is further divided into four parts based on which area of the heart the cross-section (short-axis) view is being taken:

1. Papillary muscle view (mid-PAP)
2. The mitral valve (MV) level view
3. LV apex view
4. Base view

Parasternal Mid-papillary Short Axis

This view is used to assess the fluid status and EF by the *eyeballing* method **(Figs. 10A and B)**.

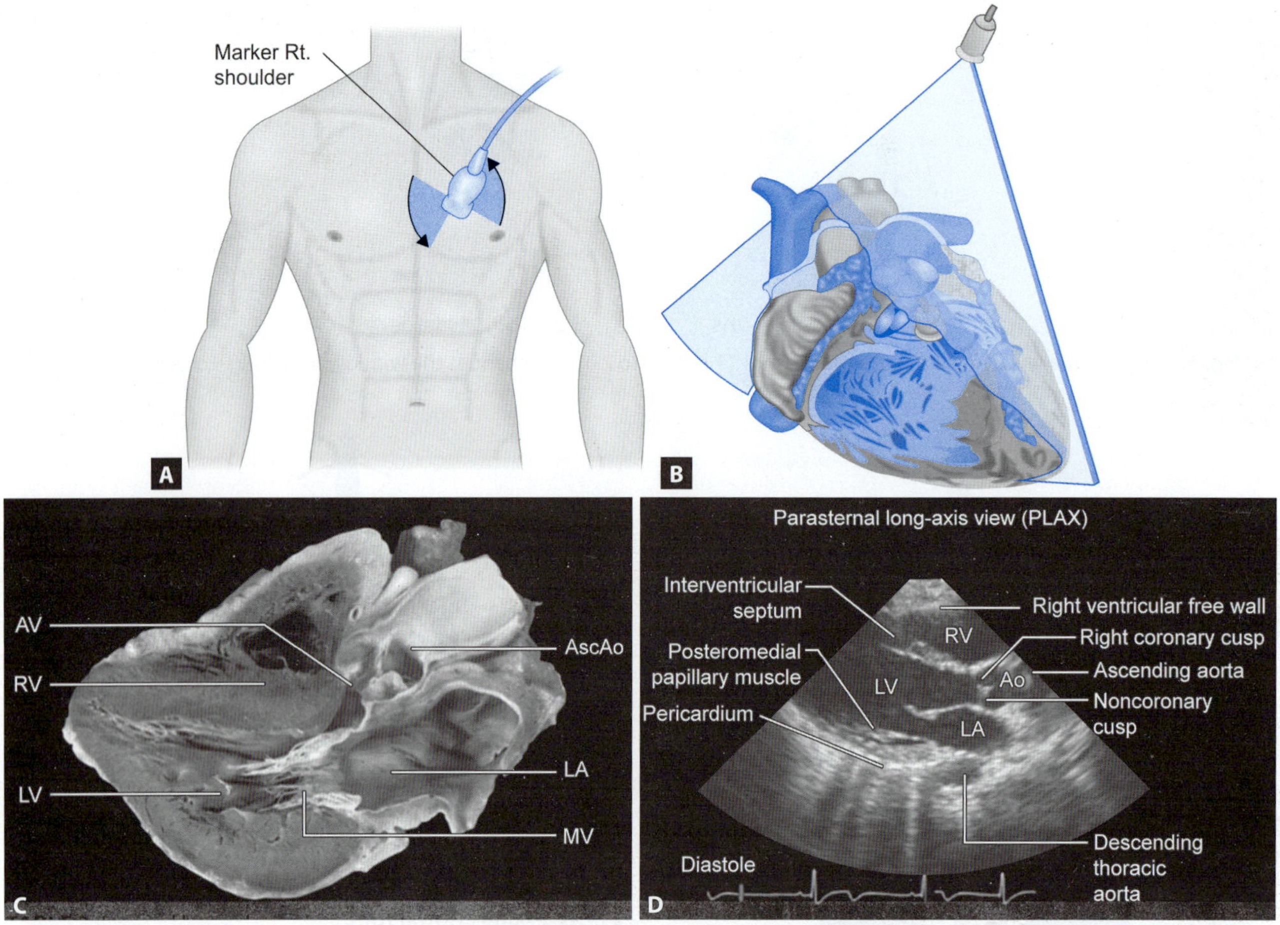

Figs. 8A to D: Parasternal long-axis (PLAX) view. (Ao or AscAo: ascending aorta; AV: aortic valve; LA: left atrium; LV: left ventricle; MV: mitral valve; RA: right atrium; Rt: right; RV: right ventricle) *(For color version, see Plate 5)*

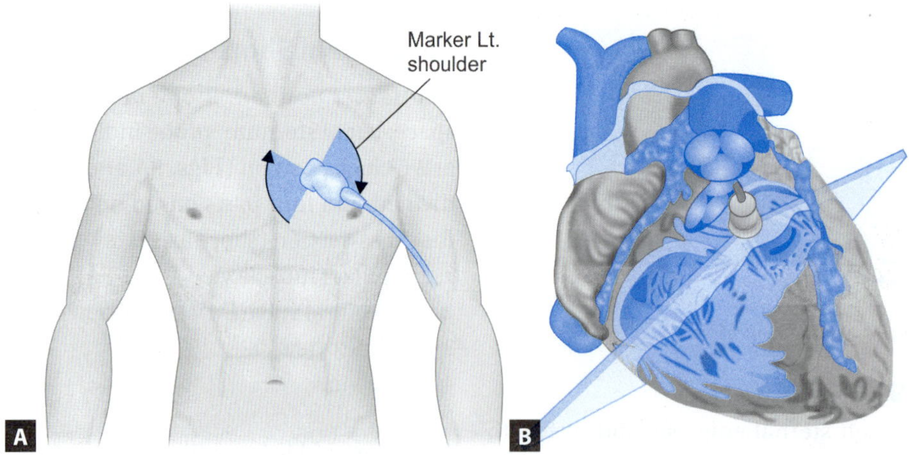

Figs. 9A and B: Parasternal short-axis (PSAX) view. (Lt: left)

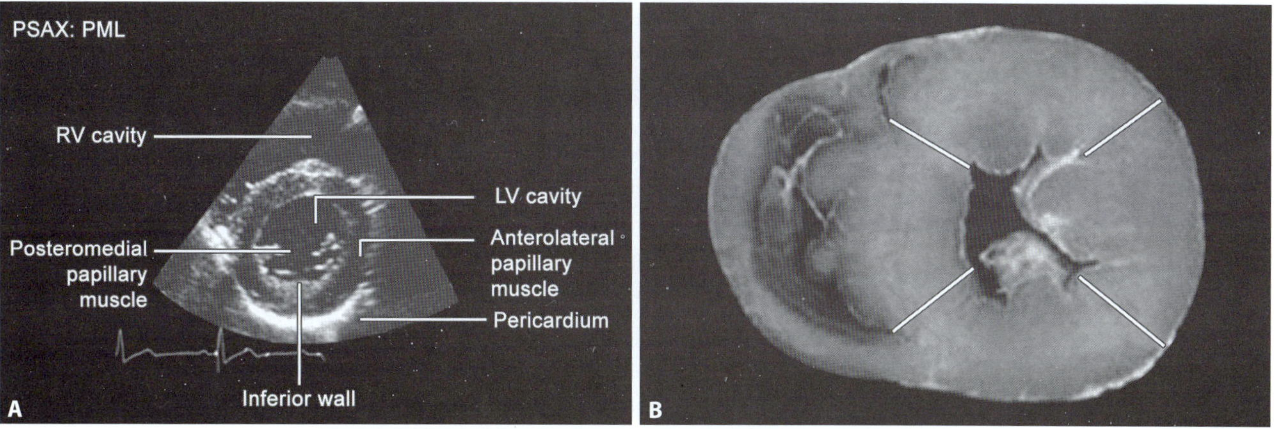

Figs. 10A and B: Parasternal mid-papillary short-axis view. (LV: left ventricle; RV: right ventricle)

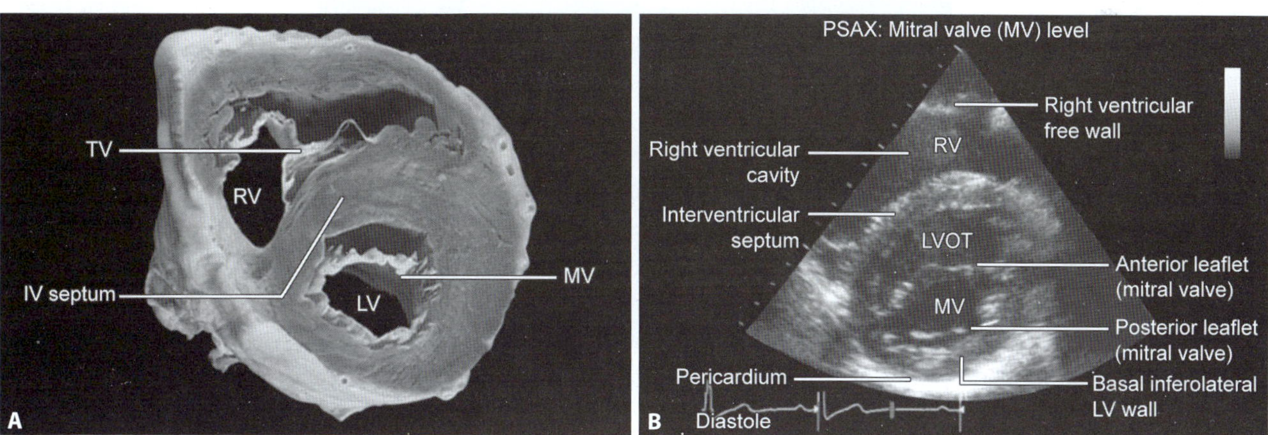

Figs. 11A and B: Parasternal short-axis mitral valve view. (IV septum: interventricular septum; LV: left ventricle; MV: mitral valve; RV: right ventricle; TV: tricuspid valve) *(For color version, see Plate 5)*

Examine the myocardial segments and wall motion:

- Anterior
- Septal
- Inferior
- Posterior/lateral

Mitral Valve Level—Parasternal Short-axis View

From the position of the papillary muscles, by tilting the transducer upward toward the right shoulder, a view of the MV can be obtained **(Figs. 11A and B)**.

- Note the *fish mouth*
- Examine MV function
- Note any severe stenosis
- Examine the wall segments

Parasternal Base Short Axis

From the position of the MV, angling the transducer upward with the footprint toward the right shoulder, a view of the aortic valve and the right ventricular outflow tract can be obtained **(Figs. 12A to C)**.

Ultrasonographic findings:

- Examine aortic valve and pulmonary valve function and note any severe stenosis.
- Note the Mercedes-Benz sign representing the aortic valve.
- Examine the aortic valve, right ventricular outflow tract, and the pulmonary valve.
- Use color flow Doppler (CFD) to examine for any pulmonary insufficiency, which can help in the measurement of the pulmonary artery pressure (PAP) by Doppler method.
- Examine the main pulmonary artery for regurgitation.
- Examine the right and left pulmonary artery.
- May be able to detect a large pulmonary embolus.

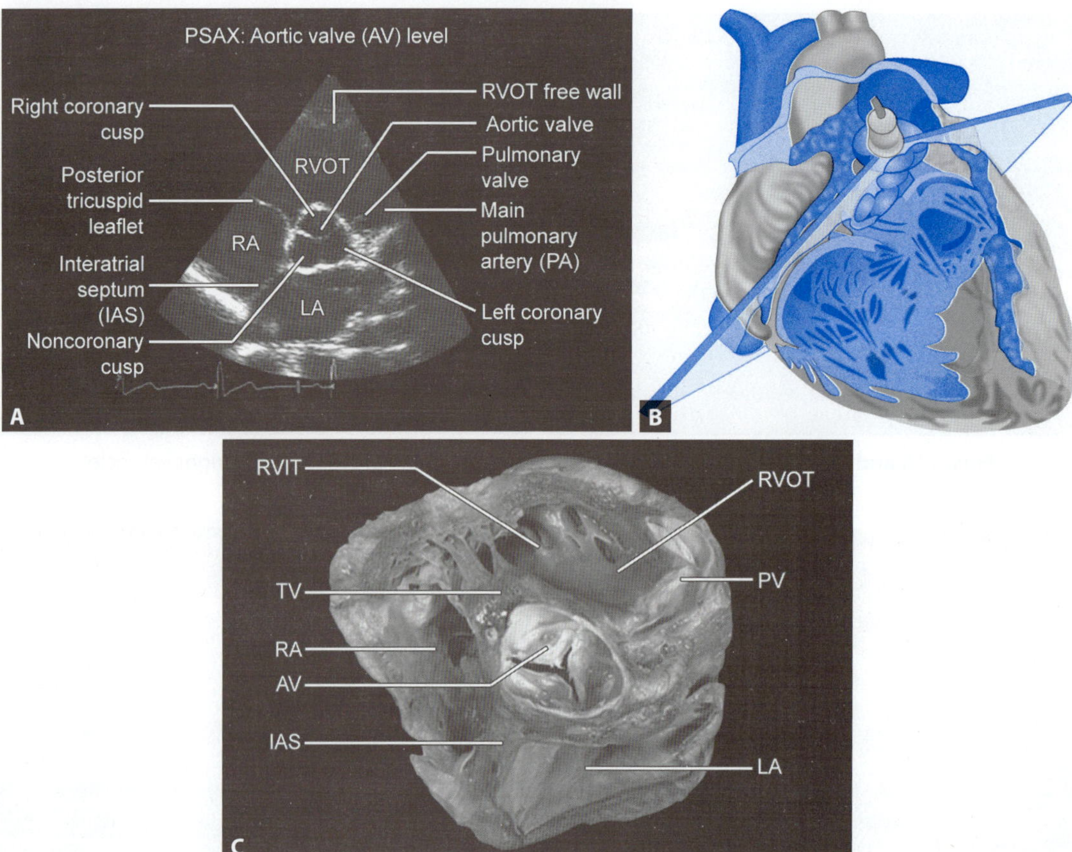

Figs. 12A to C: Parasternal short-axis base view. (AV: aortic valve; LA: left atrium; LV: left ventricle; MV: mitral valve; PV: pulmonary valve; RA: right atrium; RV: right ventricle; RVIT: right ventricular inflow tract; RVOT: right ventricular outflow tract; IAS: interatrial septum; TV: tricuspid valve) *(For color version, see Plate 6)*

Parasternal Apical Short-axis View

Tilting the probe downward from the mid-papillary view—left ventricle cavity (papillary muscle), apex can be visualized.

Here, the transducer is tilted downward with the footprint pointing toward the left thigh to obtain a short axis image at the apical level **(Figs. 13A to C)**.

- To evaluate the myocardial segments and note any apical hypokinesis
- *Assess:* Contractility
- *Look for:* Regional wall motion abnormality

Apical Four-chamber View (Fig. 14)

- Keep probe at the apex of heart, usually along the point of maximum impulse, fifth intercostal space.
- Probe pointer to the left.
- Aim toward right shoulder to get the apical four-chamber view.
- Measure and compare dimensions of right and left ventricles.
- The width from myocardial inner wall to septal inner wall of the right ventricle is about half of the left ventricle during both systole and diastole.
- Examine the overall cardiac contractility.
- Note any wall motion abnormality in different segments: Lateral, apical, and septal.
- Can be used to estimate the EF of left ventricle.
- Can be used to evaluate the RV function.
- Use CFD to examine the MV and tricuspid valve (TV) function and detect any significant flow abnormality.
- Note any significant MV, TV stenosis, or regurgitation.

Apical Five-chamber View

Tilting the transducer upward at the apex to open up the left ventricular outflow tract (LVOT) and aortic valve (the fifth chamber) **(Fig. 15)**:

- Using color flow and pulse wave Doppler (PWD) to calculate the SV as well as any significant regurgitation.

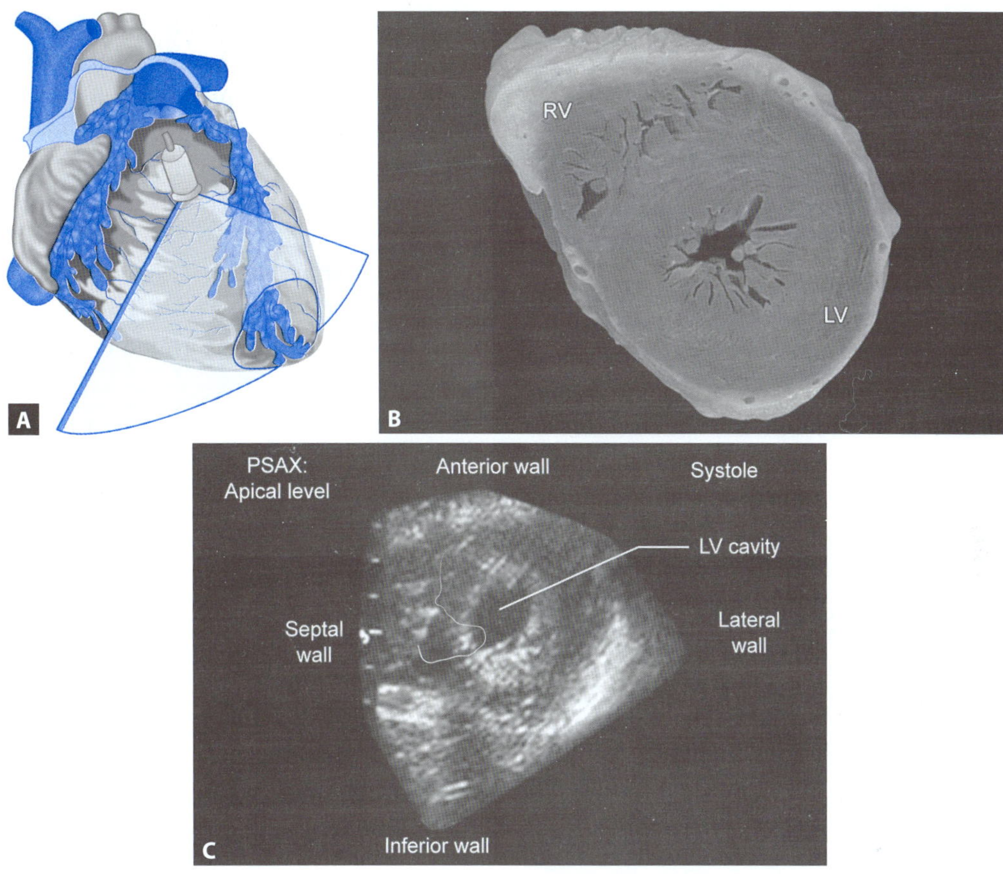

Figs. 13A to C: Parasternal short-axis apex view *(For color version, see Plate 6)*.

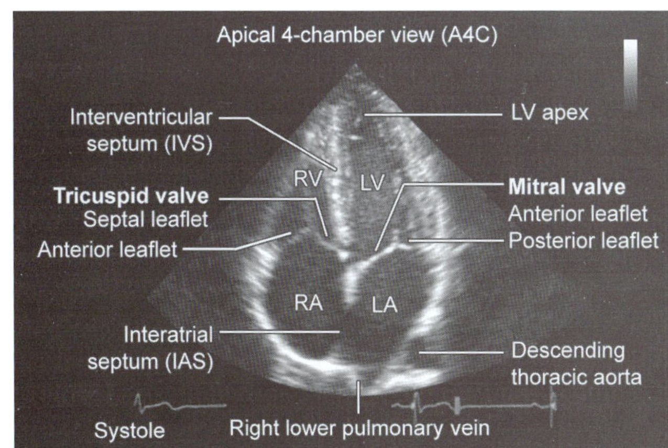

Fig. 14: Apical four-chamber view. (LA: left atrium; LV: left ventricle; RA: right atrium; RV: right ventricle)

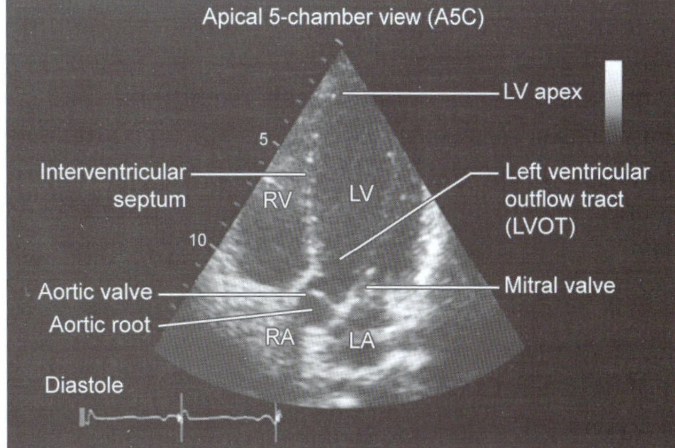

Fig. 15: Apical five-chamber view. (LA: left atrium; LV: left ventricle; RA: right atrium; RV: right ventricle) *(For color version, see Plate 6)*

Subcostal/Subxiphoid—Four-chamber View

Below the xiphoid process, the footprint pointing toward the left shoulder; the marker is at about 3 o'clock position **(Fig. 16)**.

- Evaluate the function of all chambers.
- Note any wall motion abnormality.
  This is a good view to detect any pericardial effusion.

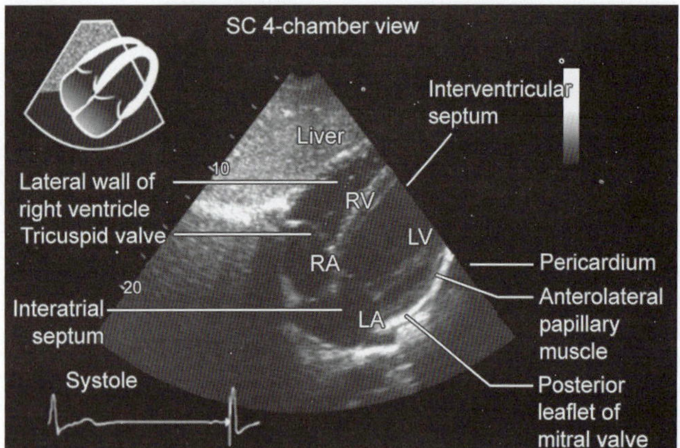

Fig. 16: Subxiphoid four-chamber view. (LA: left atrium; LV: left ventricle; RA: right atrium; RV: right ventricle)

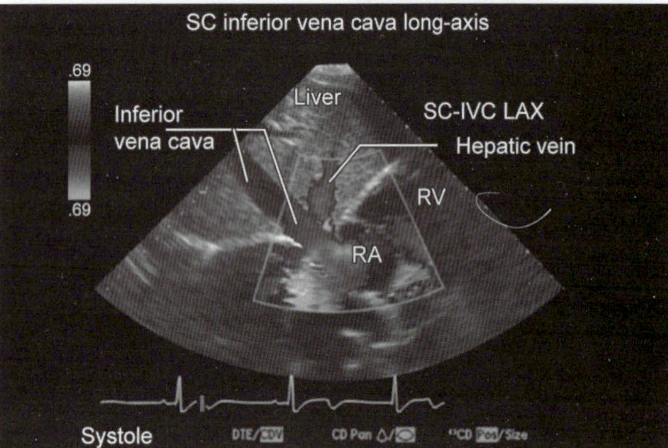

Fig. 17: Subcostal inferior vena cava view. (RA: right atrium; RV: right ventricle).

Subcostal Inferior Vena Cava View (Fig. 17)

- Subxiphoid view
- Probe marker toward head/cranium
- Right of the midline

BASIC PRINCIPLES OF DOPPLER

The fundamental basics of Doppler effect are present in our daily life and experienced by all of us. Suppose a car is honking and coming toward you and crossing. The horn pitch is louder (higher frequency) when it is coming toward you compared to when it has crossed and moved away from you. This implies that the intensity of sound depends on relative motion of source and receiver. In TTE, the source of sound wave is transducer and the reflecting surface is RBCs or myocardium, which is moving relative to one another. Therefore, frequency of returning sound wave will differ with the one which was transmitted from transducer. This change in frequency of the transmitted wave and the reflected wave is used in Doppler equation to estimate the velocity of the reflector.

The change of frequency (Doppler Shift, Fd) is directly proportional to ratio of velocity of blood (V), original frequency (Fo), and inversely proportional to speed of sound (C).

Doppler shift (Fd) = V/C × Fo Velocity of blood
= Fd × C/Fo

Further refining this formula to calculate velocity of blood:

$$V = Fd \times C/2Fo \times \cos\theta$$

We have to multiply the original frequency (Fo) by 2 because the change in frequency happens twice, during the ultrasound insonation and also once it is reflected back. Cos theta is used for correcting the angle between the insonated wave and the blood flow. Therefore, the sonographer must ensure to align the axis of interrogation as parallel to blood flow as possible.

The clinical application of this Doppler shift principle is assessment of intracardiac pressure using simplified Bernoulli equation.

$$\text{Pressure gradient (delta P)} = 4 \times V^2$$

Various modalities of Doppler applied are: PWD, CFD, and continuous wave Doppler (CWD).

Pulsed Wave Doppler

The underlying principle of PWD is that the ultrasound waves are transmitted in pulses and waits for reflected ultrasound after every pulse. Therefore, the sampling rate is limited as there is time delay in receiving back the reflected waves. It cannot be applied for assessing high velocities.

Color Flow Doppler

Color flow Doppler is a version of PWD, in which we have a visual display of blood flow, in form of color-coded map. By convention, the blood flow toward the transducer is coded in shades of red while flow away from transducer is coded in shades of blue. The turbulence created by high velocity gives a mosaic pattern.

Continuous Wave Doppler

Continuous wave Doppler modality transmits and receives the ultrasound waves continuously, allowing measurement of high velocity blood flow. But it is unable to precisely localize high velocity at a specific point along the width of ultrasound beam. This Doppler modality is used for detection of high-velocity signals that occurs with stenotic or regurgitant valvular lesion.

MEASUREMENT OF STROKE VOLUME

The cardiac SV may be accurately measured with echocardiography.[1] Multiplication of SV by heart rate equals the cardiac output.

Measurement Technique

In PLAX view, we can measure diameter of the LVOT **(Fig. 18)**, immediately below the hinge point of the aortic valve leaflets. The LVOT area (cm^2) is calculated from the diameter measured using the formula:

$$\text{LVOT area } (cm^2) = (\text{LVOT diameter}/2)^2 \times 3.14.$$

Next, acquire the apical five-chamber view and place the PWD sample volume in the LVOT to measure the systolic velocity envelope of blood flow in the LVOT. Integration of the resulting velocity-time envelope gives the velocity time integral (VTI), which is the distance in centimeters that blood has moved over the course of systole through the LVOT. The SV is then calculated as follows:

$$\text{SV (mL)} = \text{LVOT area } cm^2 \times \text{VTI (cm)}$$

Normal values of VTI range between 18 and 22 cm, and LVOT diameter ranges between 1.8 and 2.2 cm.

Practical Problems with Measurement of Stroke Volume

Incorrect measurement of LVOT diameter will be squared when calculating the area. Ideally measure the LVOT dimension in mid-systole with maximal separation of aortic leaflets. Best method is to zoom in on the LVOT to achieve good visualization of aortic root. It needs acquiring PLAX view with clear endomyocardial borders and caliper orientation, which is 90° to the walls of LVOT.

Determination of the VTI is subject to problems-related to Doppler measurement. The site of the measurement is important.[2] The PWD sample volume is placed just proximal to aortic valve. VTI recording must show a smooth velocity curve and well-defined peak. When measuring VTI, the Doppler wave should be in line with the flow of blood through the LVOT. Any angle between the Doppler wave and LVOT can result in underestimation of VTI, and therefore SV.

Since the LVOT area is constant, changes in VTI represent changes in SV, even if exact VTI is not calculated with each cardiac cycle. Changes in VTI that occur during ventilator cycle may be used to determine preload sensitivity, as these changes reflect changes in SV.

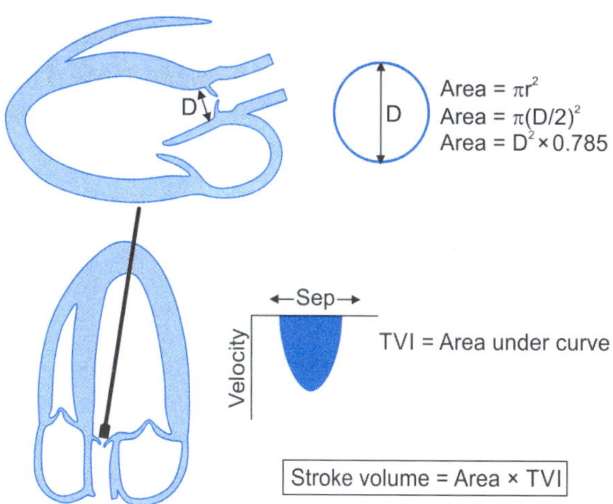

The amount of blood going through the LVOT is given by the VTI (velocity time integral) of the flow, obtained by tracing the signal's envelope:

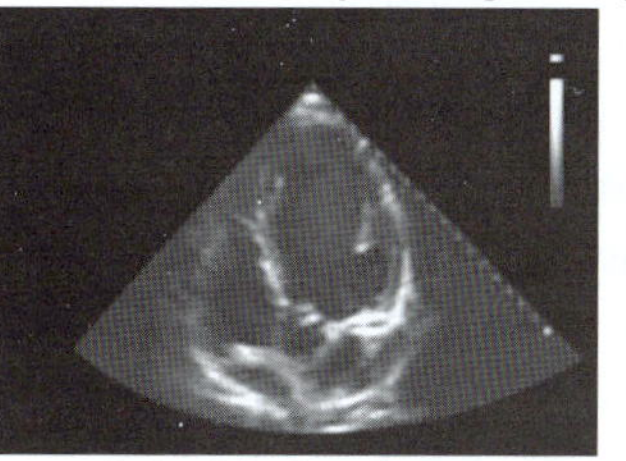

Apical 5 chamber

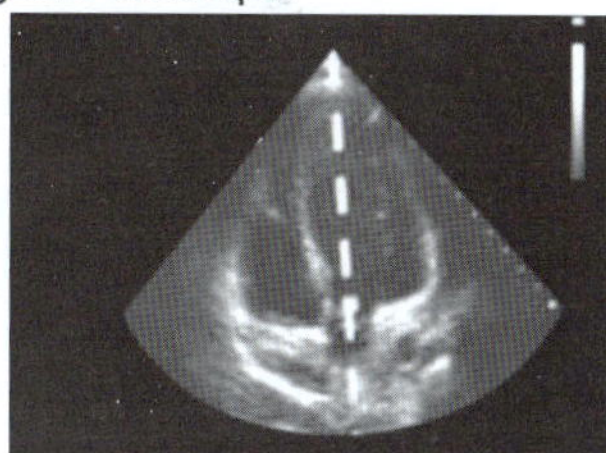

Pulsed Doppler (PW) sample in LVOT +++ Doppler beam MUST be alighed with the LV outflow +++

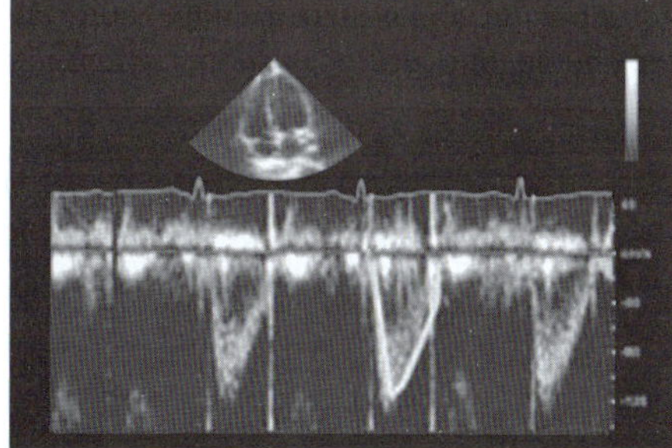

Trace envelope of LVOT flow → VTI of LVOT

Fig. 18: Calculation of left ventricular outflow tract (LVOT), velocity time integral (VTI), and stroke volume (SV).

ASSESSMENT OF LEFT VENTRICULAR FUNCTION AND REGIONAL WALL MOTION ABNORMALITY

Measurement Technique

With the qualitative approach, the intensivist can eyeball overall LV function. The contractile function of the left ventricle in the standard TTE windows thus can be eyeballed. In the PSS view, assessment of LV function is done at level of the papillary muscles. The nomenclatures commonly used are normal, mildly reduced, moderately reduced, severely reduced, and hyperdynamic LV function. Quantitative estimation of LV function uses Simpson method, where the end-systolic and end-diastolic areas of the left ventricle are measured in the apical four-chamber and apical two-chamber views to calculate an EF. Because of time limits and technical problems in obtaining the requisite high-quality images, in critically ill patients, it is not much useful to intensivist. Assessment of LV function is useful for categorizing shock state in intensive care unit (ICU).

ASSESSMENT OF SEGMENTAL WALL FUNCTION OF LEFT VENTRICLE

Standard segmental wall anatomy includes 17 segments.[3] Wall motion and thickening for each myocardial segment is graded as normal, hypokinetic, akinetic, or dyskinetic.

Akinesia means lack of movement or contraction of a region of the heart muscle. Dyskinesia means abnormal movement—instead of shortening and contracting in systole, that segment of myocardium bulges out in systole. Hypokinesia means reduced movement or contraction of a segment of the heart muscle. For quantitative assessment, wall thickening of <50% or wall excursion of <5 mm defines abnormal segmental contractility.

Wall motion abnormalities at the segmental level may be identified qualitatively by visual examination of the 2D-Echo image set in multiple standardized views. The coronary distribution of these segments is illustrated in **Figure 19**.

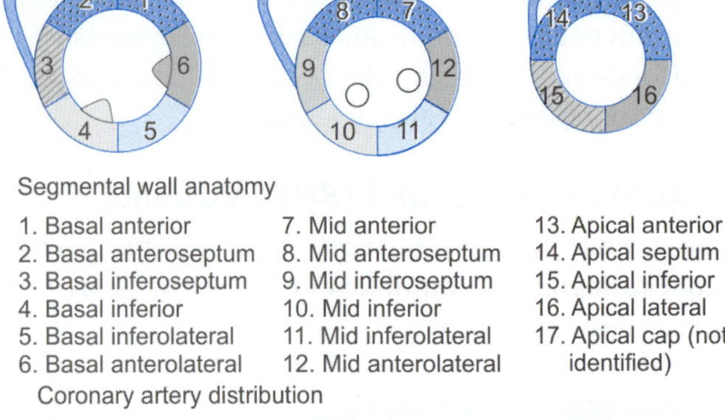

Fig. 19: Coronary segments on 2D ECHO. (Cx: circumflex artery; LAD: left anterior descending artery; RCA: right coronary artery)

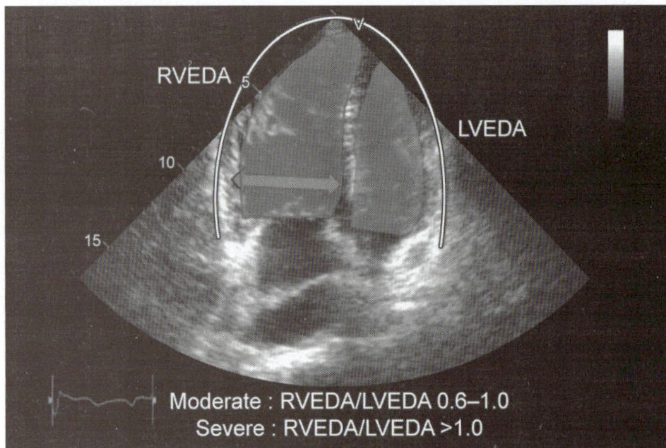

Fig. 20: RV/LV ratio. (LV: left ventricle; LVEDA: left ventricular end-diastolic area; RV: right ventricle; RVEDA: right ventricular end-diastolic area) *(For color version, see Plate 6)*

ASSESSMENT OF RIGHT VENTRICULAR FUNCTION

The American Society of Echocardiography has recommended multiple measurements that may be used to evaluate RV function.[4]

- *RV size and thickness:* RV size is best seen in the apical four-chamber or subcostal views, with direct comparison with the LV size. Normal RV size is 60% of LV size at end diastole. An end-diastolic RV cavity size between 60–100% and >100% of end-diastolic cavity size of the left ventricle indicates moderate or severe RV enlargement, respectively **(Fig. 20)**.

  The thickness of the RV free wall in the PLAX views identifies the patient with chronic elevation of RV afterload. The normal RV free wall thickness is <4 mm and is abnormal if it is more than 5 mm.
- *Septal kinetics:* Volume or pressure overload of the right ventricle results in paradoxical motion of the septum. This is seen as movement of the septum toward the left ventricle during ventricular contraction. The use of

M-mode helps in extensive analysis of septal kinetics and is useful in identifying patterns consistent with RV dysfunction.[5] The M-mode sampling line is placed through the septum in PLAX view **(Figs. 21A to C)**.

- *RV systolic function:* The degree of longitudinal systolic movement of the tricuspid annulus correlates with overall RV systolic function. To measure the tricuspid annular plane systolic excursion (TAPSE), an M-mode sampling line is placed through the tricuspid lateral annulus in the apical four-chamber (AP4) view **(Fig. 22)**. Normal TAPSE is >17 mm; measurements below this value indicate reduced RV systolic function.[6]
- *Pulmonary artery systolic pressure (PASP):* The CWD echocardiography sampling line is placed along the main axis of the tricuspid regurgitation (TR) jet to measure the blood flow velocity of the regurgitant jet. With the use of the modified Bernoulli equation, the pressure gradient across the valve is calculated. Once the pressure gradient is known, adding the right atrial pressure (RAP) to this gradient yields an estimate of the PASP. The RAP may be measured directly if a central venous catheter is in place or estimated from the size and respiratory variation of the IVC **(Fig. 23)**.[7]

PRELOAD RESPONSIVENESS ASSESSMENT

An important use of SV measurement and its surrogate LVOT VTI is assessment of preload responsiveness.

Measurement Technique

The Doppler echocardiography sample volume is placed in the LVOT using the five-chamber view. The LVOT VTI is measured serially while the ventilator is cycling. Instead of the VTI, the peak velocity of the systolic velocity envelope may be used because it is easier to measure.[8] Measurement of the change in the VTI or peak velocity of the VTI envelope is sufficient as a surrogate for change of SV. An increase of VTI or velocity of >12% during passive inflation with the ventilator is indicative of preload sensitivity.[9]

The major limitation of using variation in the VTI to identify preload responsiveness is that it requires the patient to be on a mechanical ventilator and making no respiratory effort. In addition, the degree of variation of SV depends on the tidal volume. When making the measurement, the patient should be receiving 8 mL/kg tidal volume, and serial measurements should be made at the same tidal volume.[10]

An arrhythmia invalidates the measurement.

PASSIVE LEG RAISING

The change in SV after passive leg raising has been validated as a means of assessing preload responsiveness.[11,12] This method is also useful in patients with spontaneous respiratory effort. The patient is placed in a supine, semi-recumbent position with the torso at 45°. The LVOT VTI is measured from the five-chamber view.

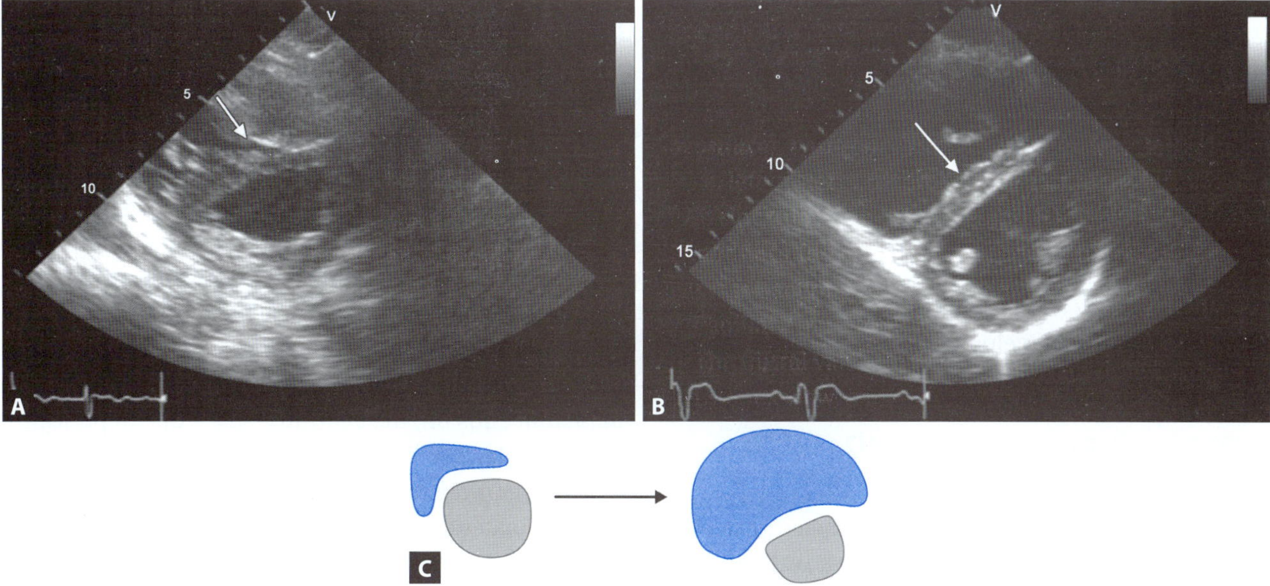

Figs. 21A to C: Interventricular septal motion: Flattened septum ["D" shape of left ventricle (LV)].

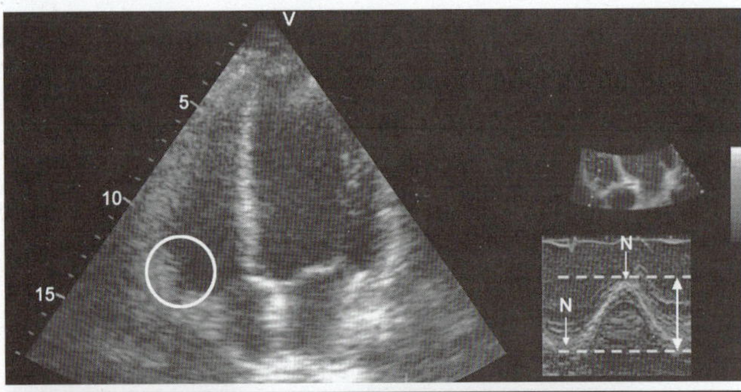

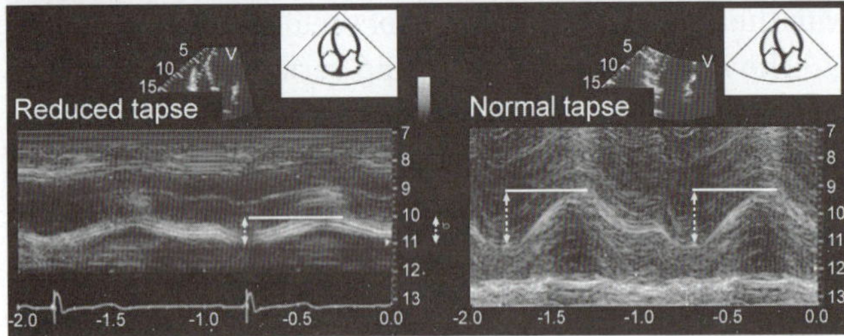

Fig. 22: RV systolic function (TAPSE). (RV: right ventricle; TAPSE: tricuspid annular plane systolic excursion) *(For color version, see Plate 6)*

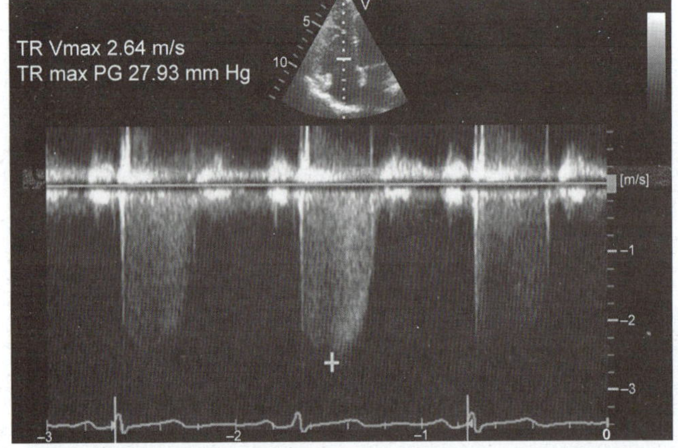

Fig. 23: Tricuspid regurgitation (TR) tracing for pulmonary artery systolic pressure (PASP) *(For color version, see Plate 6)*.

The patient position is then changed so that the torso is at 0° with the legs elevated to 45°. One minute after leg raising, the LVOT VTI is measured again. A >12% increase of LVOT VTI or peak velocity is predictive of preload responsiveness.

PERICARDIAL EFFUSION AND TAMPONADE PHYSIOLOGY

Pericardial effusion creates an echo-free space posteriorly between the left ventricular posterior wall and the pericardium as well as anteriorly between the right ventricular free wall and the anterior chest wall. Posterior accumulation of fluid precedes collection in the anterior space **(Fig. 24)**.

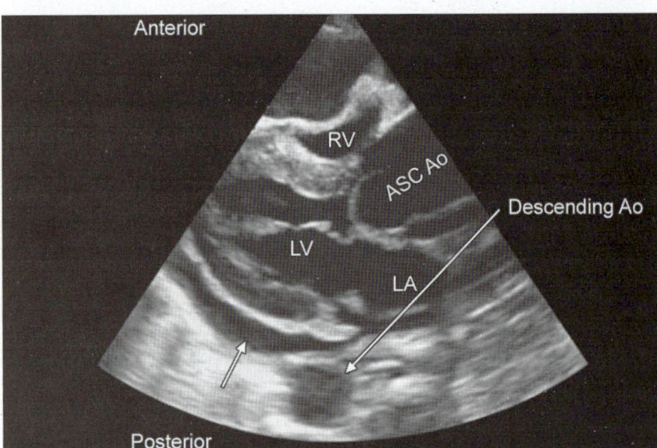

Fig. 24: Pericardial effusion—hypoechoic or anechoic (echo free) space seen around heart denoting blood in pericardial sack. (Ao: aorta; ASC Ao: ascending aorta; LA: left atrium; LV: left ventricle; RV: right ventricle)

Pericardial fluid lies anterior to descending aorta (pleural effusion dorsal). The quantity of pericardial effusion can be gauged from the width of the echo-free space on M-mode scan from the PLAX view.

GRADING THE SIZE OF PERICARDIAL EFFUSION

Small = posterior groove, only in systole, <1 cm; moderate = 1–2 cm, posterior groove ± elsewhere; and large = >2 cm, circumferential.

Remember though, the size of an effusion is not as important as the rate of accumulation. A large effusion which accumulates slowly may not result in any hemodynamic compromise; however, a small or moderate effusion which has accumulated rapidly may result in life-threatening changes to cardiac filling.

A pericardial effusion sometimes needs to be differentiated from a left pleural effusion. Unlike in case of pleural effusion, the echo-free space due to pericardial effusion **(Fig. 25)**:

- Is never more than 4 cm in width
- Terminates abruptly at the AV groove
- Does not extend behind descending aorta

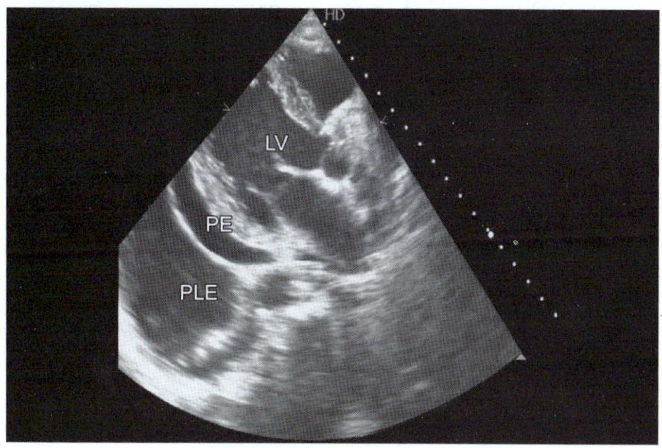

Fig. 25: Combined pericardial effusion (PE) and pleural effusion (PLE). (LV: left ventricle)

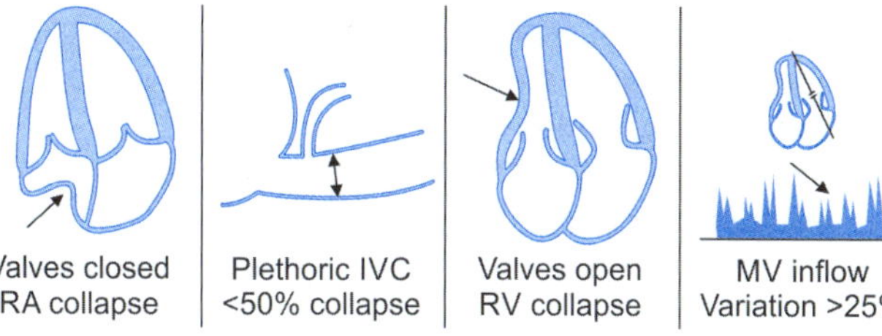

Fig. 26: Echocardiographic signs of tamponade. (IVC: inferior vena cava; MV: mitral valve; RA: right atrium; RV: right ventricle)

CARDIAC TAMPONADE

Whenever a pericardial effusion is imaged, the possibility of tamponade should be considered. When the pressure in the pericardial sac exceeds the pressure within the cardiac chambers, cardiac tamponade occurs with impaired cardiac filling and low cardiac output. 2D-echocardiographic features of cardiac tamponade include right atrial collapse during ventricular systole, right ventricular diastolic collapse, and occasionally there is left atrial collapse **(Figs. 26 and 27)**. Doppler echocardiography demonstrates exaggerated increase in tricuspid and decrease in MV diastolic flow with inspiration.

Pericardiocentesis

Transthoracic echocardiography helps in safe performance of therapeutic echo-guided needle aspiration or pigtail catheter insertion for drainage of pericardial fluid. Parasternal approach is preferred as it has short course, direct visualization of the needle entering the effusion. This approach prevents cardiac laceration, pneumothorax, pneumopericardium, liver lacerations, and trauma to internal mammary artery **(Fig. 28)**.

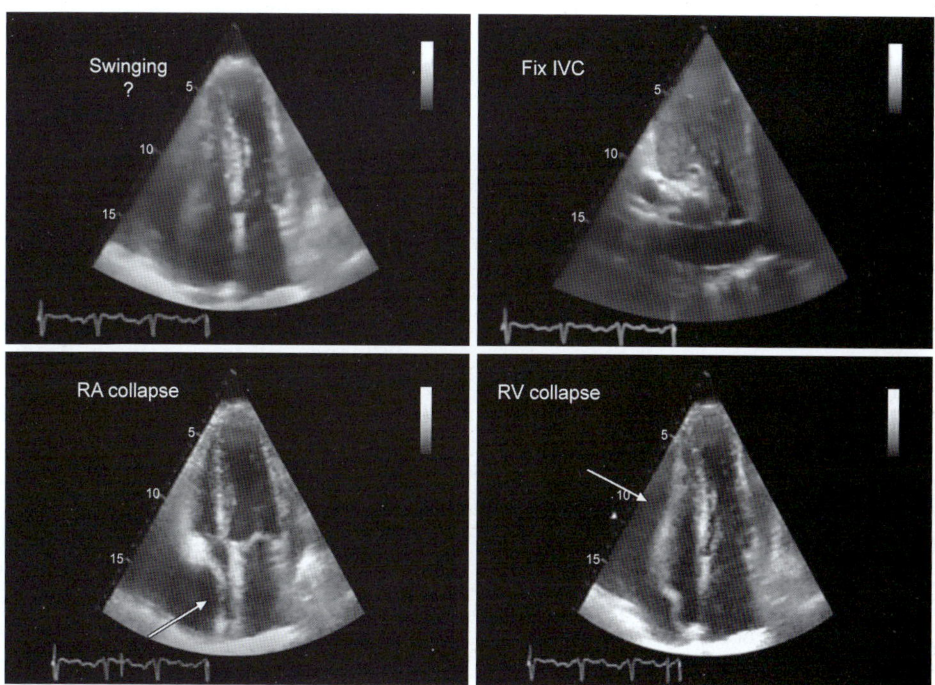

Fig. 27: Four signs of tamponade physiology.

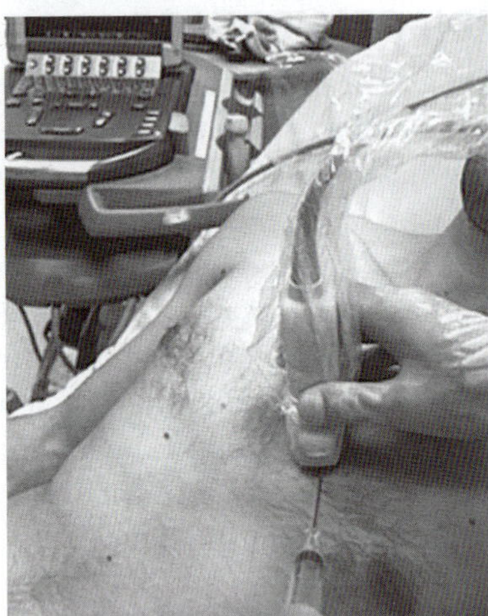
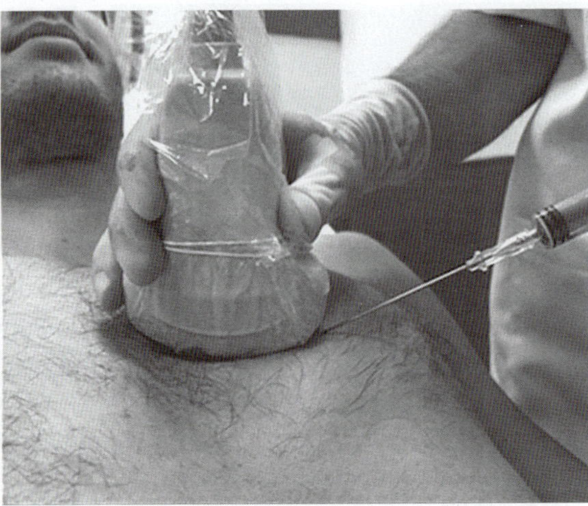

Fig. 28: Parasternal approach for pericardiocentesis *(For color version, see Plate 7)*.

CONCLUSION

Transthoracic echocardiography is a useful, rapid, and noninvasive tool to diagnose pathology and monitor interventional response in the critically ill.

Intensivists should have expertise in assessing LV dysfunction, regional wall motion abnormality, determination of preload responsiveness by real-time measurement of SV variation or passive leg raising, identification and remedies of adverse heart-lung interactions, or integration of lung ultrasonography into echocardiographic findings. Bedside TTE competence has now become a key element of intensive care training.

REFERENCES

1. Dubin J, Wallerson DC, Cody RJ, Devereux RB. Comparative accuracy of Doppler echocardiographic methods for clinical stroke volume determination. Am Heart J. 1990;120:116-23.
2. Baumgartner H, Hung J, Bermejo J, Chambers JB, Evangelista A, Griffin BP, et al. Echocardiographic assessment of valve stenosis: EAE/ASE recommendations for clinical practice. J Am Soc Echocardiogr. 2009;22:1-23.
3. Mayo PH, Beaulieu Y, Doelken P, Feller-Kopman D, Harrod C, Kaplan A, et al. American College of Chest Physicians/ La Société de Réanimation de Langue Française statement on competence in critical care ultrasonography. Chest. 2009;135:1050-60.
4. Rudski LG, Lai WW, Afilalo J, Hua L, Handschumacher MD, Chandrasekaran K, et al. Guidelines for the echocardiographic assessment of the right heart in adults: a report from the American Society of Echocardiography endorsed by the European Association of Echocardiography, a registered branch of the European Society of Cardiology, and the Canadian Society of Echocardiography. J Am Soc Echocardiogr. 2010;23:685-713.
5. Weyman AE, Wann S, Feigenbaum H, Dillon JC. Mechanism of abnormal septal motion in patients with right ventricular volume overload: a cross-sectional echocardiographic study. Circulation. 1976;54:179-86.
6. Lamia B, Teboul JL, Monnet X, Richard C, Chemla D. Relationship between the tricuspid annular plane systolic excursion and right and left ventricular function in critically ill patients. Intensive Care Med. 2007;33:2143-9.
7. Giardini A. Limitations inherent to the simplified Bernoulli equation explain the inaccuracy of Doppler echocardiographic estimates of pulmonary artery pressures in patients with pulmonary hypertension. Chest. 2011;140:270.
8. Narasimhan M, Koenig SJ, Mayo PH. Advanced echocardiography for the critical care physician: part 1. Chest. 2014;145:129-34.
9. De Backer D, Heenen S, Piagnerelli M, Koch M, Vincent JL. Pulse pressure variations to predict fluid responsiveness: influence of tidal volume. Intensive Care Med. 2005;31:517-23.
10. Feissel M, Teboul JL, Merlani P, Badie J, Faller JP, Bendjelid K. Plethysmographic dynamic indices predict fluid responsiveness in septic ventilated patients. Intensive Care Med. 2007;33:993-9.
11. Monnet X, Rienzo M, Osman D, Anguel N, Richard C, Pinsky MR, et al. Passive leg raising predicts fluid responsiveness in the critically ill. Crit Care Med. 2006;34:1402-7.
12. Maizel J, Airapetian N, Lorne E, Tribouilloy C, Massy Z, Slama M. Diagnosis of central hypovolemia by using passive leg raising. Intensive Care Med. 2007;33:1133-8.

CHAPTER

Transesophageal Echocardiography in the Critically Ill

Shilpushp Jagannath Bhosale, Atul Prabhakar Kulkarni

INTRODUCTION

Transesophageal echocardiography (TEE) has been one of the important diagnostic modalities used for a long time in cardiology and cardiac anesthesia and its use is increasing in critical care. TEE is a unique diagnostic tool that provides an accurate and reliable assessment of cardiac intracavitary dimensions, wall motions, valve function, and the great vessels. Transthoracic echocardiography was first described by Elder and Hertz when they used ultrasound to view dynamic cardiac structures. Side and Gosling in 1971 used the color Doppler for cardiac flow, while Frazin and colleagues in 1976 described the M mode, and Hisanaga et al. illustrated the use of cross-sectional real-time imaging in 1977.[1-4] In 1982, with the development of flexible probes, and manipulable tips with phased array transducers, capable of rotating 180° to give the multiplane images, the use of TEE became widespread.[5] Although TEE does have its share of complications, it is still less invasive than other cardiac imaging techniques such as cardiac catheterization. Despite the unique advantages of TEE being less invasive and more reliable, its use is quite limited in critically ill patients. Critical care physicians generally are less familiar with the TEE technique and its potential. They are dependent on the cardiac anesthesiologists or the cardiologists to perform the evaluation, who may not be always available when hemodynamic assessment is needed. Therefore, the onus is on the critical care physicians to acquire the skills needed to perform the TEE. It has been shown that once the intensivist acquires the technical skills to pass the TEE probe and interpret the images, the TEE seems to be quicker and safer than cardiac catheterization techniques.

The issues that limit the use of TEE are that it needs special setup, technique, and preparation, and the instrumentation needs orientation and expertise. Though it is a minimally invasive procedure, there are chances of complications.

Transesophageal echocardiography flexible scope is inserted into the esophagus and the stomach to acquire high-quality images of the heart and blood vessels. The probe has an ultrasound transducer at its tip that can send and receive ultrasound waves. The TEE can acquire two-dimensional (2D) or three-dimensional (3D) images depending on the configuration of the machine. The 2D TEE is used for standard examination while 3D TEE has been used to diagnose complex congenital heart problems, to assess heart valves and the cardiac condition during cardiac surgery. Since the probe remains away from the surgical area, it has been extensively used for intraoperative monitoring in cardiac surgeries.

The advantage of TEE is that since the transducer is positioned in the esophagus right behind the heart with no intervening lung or bone tissue, it allows the use of higher frequency (5 and 7 MHz) transducers to get enhanced image resolution with better signal to noise ratio.[6]

Transthoracic echocardiography is being extensively used in the intensive care unit (ICU) and is minimally invasive however, it does have limitations in terms of frequent poor echo windows due to limited space to acquire images, frequent problems related to patient factors such as surgical tubes, tapes and wires, stickings, emphysematous chest, presence of chest tubes or drains, presence of high PEEP, etc.

Evidence suggests that there are higher interventions after transesophageal than transthoracic echocardiography (TTE) since the structures are better evaluated.

INDICATIONS

Transesophageal echocardiography has been used extensively for various types of clinical indications which are beyond the scope of this discussion. American Society of Anesthesiologists and the Society of Cardiovascular Anesthesiologists recommend the appropriate use of perioperative TEE to improve surgical outcomes. The American Heart Association and the American Society of Echocardiography recommend TEE for diagnostic evaluation of heart function, determining valve size and function, assess postcardiac surgery complications, such as tamponade, conditions such as endocarditis, aortic injury, trauma, evaluation of shock, hemodynamic assessment, and volume responsiveness, in conditions where transthoracic echo is unable to help in reaching the diagnosis. Generally, it is used for the assessment of cardiac function, structural abnormalities such as congenital heart disease, valvular heart disease, and prosthetic valves; diagnosis of infective endocarditis, stroke assessment to look for thrombus, cardiac tumors, septal abnormalities, aortic dissection, coronary artery disease, etc. It is also used during interventional procedures or intraoperative monitoring or to assess volume responsiveness, titrating fluids, inotropes, and vasopressors, in the ICU.[7-9]

CONTRAINDICATIONS

Absolute contraindications for the use of TEE are unevaluated upper gastrointestinal (GI) bleeding, esophageal surgeries, or other esophageal pathologies such as stricture, obstruction, varices or diverticula, cervical spine instability, and presence of bleeding diathesis or presence of surgical anastomosis.

COMPLICATIONS

Transesophageal echocardiography is a relatively safe and minimally invasive procedure however complications with its use have been reported. The majority are minor complications, such as excessive retching or vomiting, sore throat, hoarseness, pharyngeal bleeding, etc.

Major complications reported are arrhythmias, such as supraventricular tachycardia (SVT) or atrial fibrillation (AF), ventricular tachycardia (VT), or bradycardia, transient hypotension or hypertension, angina, congestive heart failure and pulmonary edema, esophageal rupture, and laryngospasm or bronchospasm.[10]

ROLE OF TRANSESOPHAGEAL ECHOCARDIOGRAPHY IN INTENSIVE CARE UNIT

Echocardiography is a standard component of assessment for all patients with hemodynamic instability. TEE is indicated when TTE views are inadequate or limited because of factors such as edema, obesity, heavy musculature, wounds, dressings, or hyperinflation of lungs, thoracotomy or sternotomy incision, and the presence of chest wall devices.

The TEE is a vital tool in critically ill patients for rapid diagnosis and management of structural heart disease. Unexplained hemodynamic instability or heart failure, assessment of volume responsiveness by variation of the superior vena cava (SVC) during mechanical ventilation, unexplained hypoxemia to rule out intracardiac shunt using agitated saline injection and aortic injury such as aortic dissection and in cardiac arrest for assessing the resuscitation quality. It can also be used for pulmonary embolus and during stroke assessment for intracardiac thrombus. It can be used for guidance of procedures such as insertion and positioning of extracorporeal membrane oxygenation (ECMO) cannulas, intra-aortic balloon pump (IABP), or pacemaker placement. Critical care TEE is performed on patients who are intubated and on ventilatory support in an ICU, so the risk of airway complication is low.

Machine Set-up

The TEE probe is similar to a gastroscope except for the ultrasound transducer at the tip. The transesophageal echocardiographic probes are typically 5–7 Mhz frequency with multiplane rotation of the viewing angle. Since the probe is right behind the heart it achieves high-quality resolution images. The monoplane TEE probes provide images in the horizontal plane only while the biplane TEE provides images in a longitudinal plane as well. Nowadays most machines provide multiplane TEE where phased array transducers containing piezoelectric elements (64–256 for 2D and 2,500 for 3D) can be electronically and mechanically rotated in an arc of 180° to produce a continuum of transverse and longitudinal images from a single probe position. It has two rotary control knobs at the handle, the inner knob guides anteflexion and retroflexion, and the outer knob controls medial and lateral movement **(Fig. 1)**. It has a dial to rotate the plane of the viewing angle from 0° to 180° **(Fig. 2)**.

How to perform transesophageal echocardiography and acquire images?

All aseptic precautions need to be taken for performing the procedure. Appropriate written consent and adequate fasting are also important. All ICU TEEs are to be performed on ventilated patients after securing the endotracheal tube. Blind insertion, though commonly done, can cause injury to the hypopharynx, esophageal rupture, bleeding, endotracheal tube dislodgement, etc. Therefore, techniques such as direct laryngoscopy, jaw thrust, mouth guard, and cuff deflation should be used or the patient paralyzed. Routine antibiotic prophylaxis before TEE is not recommended unless it is being done for high-risk patients such as those with prosthetic valves, or those with a past history of infective endocarditis.

Understanding the TEE imaging planes requires orientation concerning both cardiac anatomy and the TEE beam. At its resting position of 0° the beam from the transducer emanates perpendicularly to the long axis of the probe. With the help of the multiplane rotator, the crystals are manipulated and the ultrasound beam is rotated clockwise from 0° to 180° to image different planes of the heart **(Fig. 2)**.

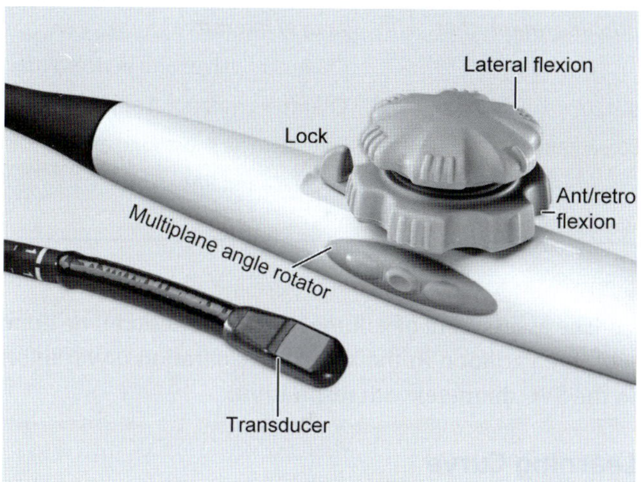

Fig. 1: Transesophageal echocardiography probe showing the transducer at the tip and the dual controls *(For color version, see Plate 7)*.

Transducer Manipulation

The American Society of Echocardiography recommends using designated language for probe manipulation, i.e., advancement or withdrawal (where the probe is pushed or pulled in or out), anteflexion and retroflexion (probe flexed anteriorly or posteriorly), or right and left flexion **(Fig. 3)**.

Probe Position and Standard Views (Table 1)

To achieve standard views the depth of insertion can be guided with the markings on the probe from incisors, i.e. typically for an upper or high esophageal view is about 25–28 cm, for midesophageal is 29–33 cm, for transgastric 38–42 cm and for deep transgastric where a probe is advanced >42 cm. Avoid unduly forcing the probe in the esophagus and abandon the procedure if persistent resistance is encountered.

Basic Echo Views

The American Society of Echocardiography and the Society of Cardiovascular Anesthesiologists describe a set of 20 standard basic and comprehensive TEE views to maintain consistency in examination and training. However, a set of eight basic TEE views are generally practiced for basic TEE examination.[8]

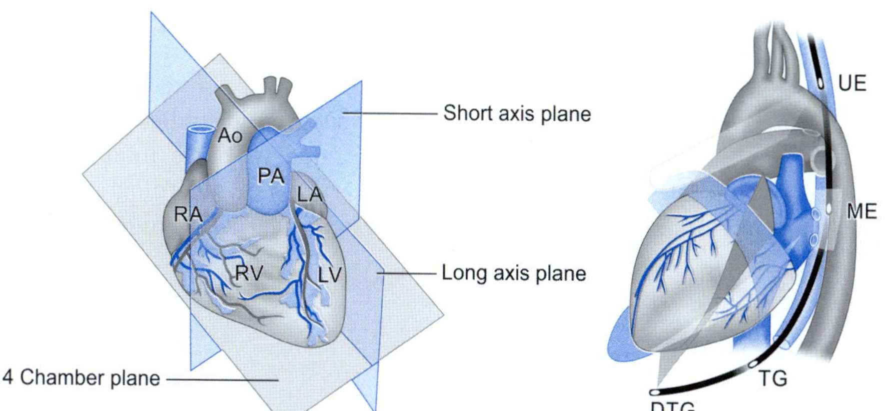

Fig. 2: Various TEE planes of the heart and level of the probe.[7] (Ao: aorta; PA; Pulmonary artery; RA: right atrium; LA: left atrium; RV: right ventricle; LV; left ventricle; UE: upper esophageal; ME: mid esophageal; TEE: transesophageal echocardiography; TG: transgastric; DTG: deep transgastric)

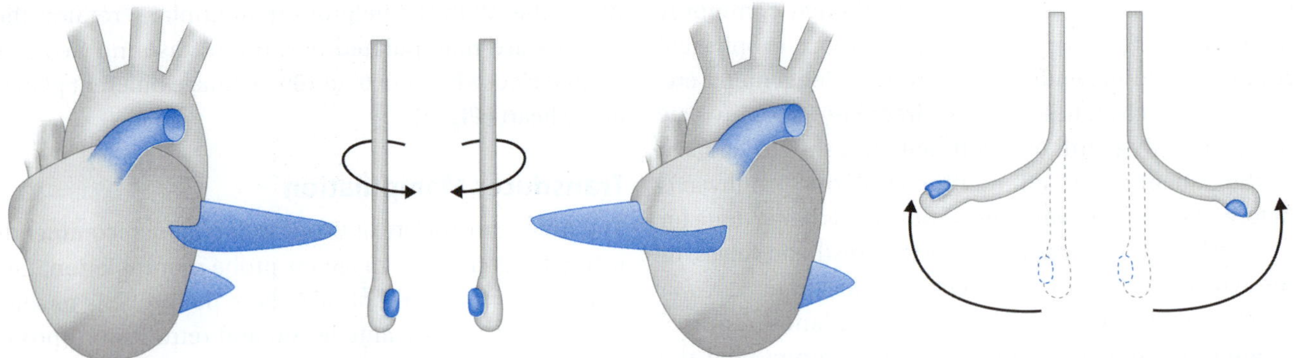

Fig. 3: Basic probe manipulation showing right rotation and left rotation, and anteflexion and retroflexion.

TABLE 1: Probe location and views obtained.[7,9]

Basic view	*Probe location*	*Multiplane orientation*	*Area of interest*
ME 4 chamber	Midesophagus	0°	Chambers, valves and pericardium
ME 2 chamber	Midesophagus	110–120°	Chambers, valves, LA appendage
Transgastric	Stomach	0–90°, anteflexed	Left ventricle short/long axis
Bicaval	Midesophagus	90–100°	SVC, IVC, and RA

(ME: midesophageal; IVC: inferior vena cava; LA: left atrium; RA: right atrium; SVC: superior vena cava)

The University of Toronto algorithm proposed a unique method for probing and plane angle manipulation for optimum image acquisition **(Fig. 4)**. **Figures 5 and 6** depict the schematic for basic image views and the basic transesophageal images.

Assessment of Volume Responsiveness

Assessment of volume responsiveness can be done by looking at changes in LV chamber size and function in the ME view and left ventricular end-diastolic area (LVEDA) in the transgastric midpapillary short-axis (SAX) view before and after fluid bolus.

Quantifying the blood volume ejected through the LVOT with each heartbeat can be acquired using the deep transgastric five-chamber view and calculating the LVOT-VTI to get the stroke volume. LVOT diameter at the aortic valve can be obtained using the midesophageal long-axis (LAX) view.

$$SV = LVOT\ CSA \times LVOT - VTI.$$

The assessment of volume responsiveness can be done with the variation in the VTI with respiration or variation in the SVC diameter with respiration.

Learning Curve

Vieillard-Baron et al. suggested limited-scope, goal-directed TEE in the ICU that included the midesophageal four-chamber view, the transgastric SAX view, and the midesophageal bicaval view for visualization of the SVC, while Benjamin et al. demonstrated competence in limited-scope, goal-directed TEE using four basic views with 10 supervised studies.[11-13] Charron et al. determined that 31 supervised studies would be sufficient to achieve competence in basic image acquisition and about 35 supervised echocardiography studies for advanced transesophageal echocardiographic assessment.[14]

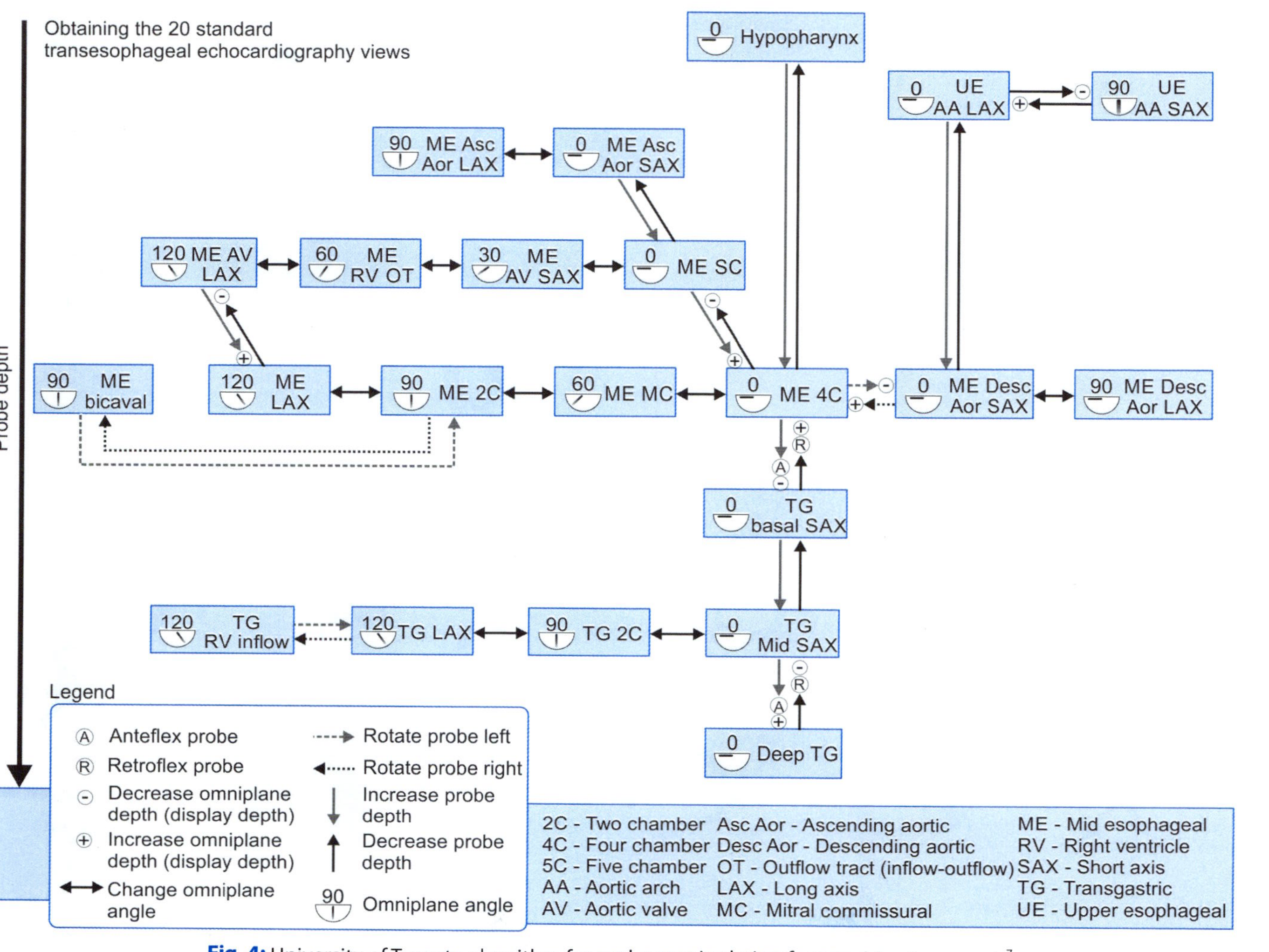

Fig. 4: University of Toronto algorithm for probe manipulation for acquiring image set.[7]

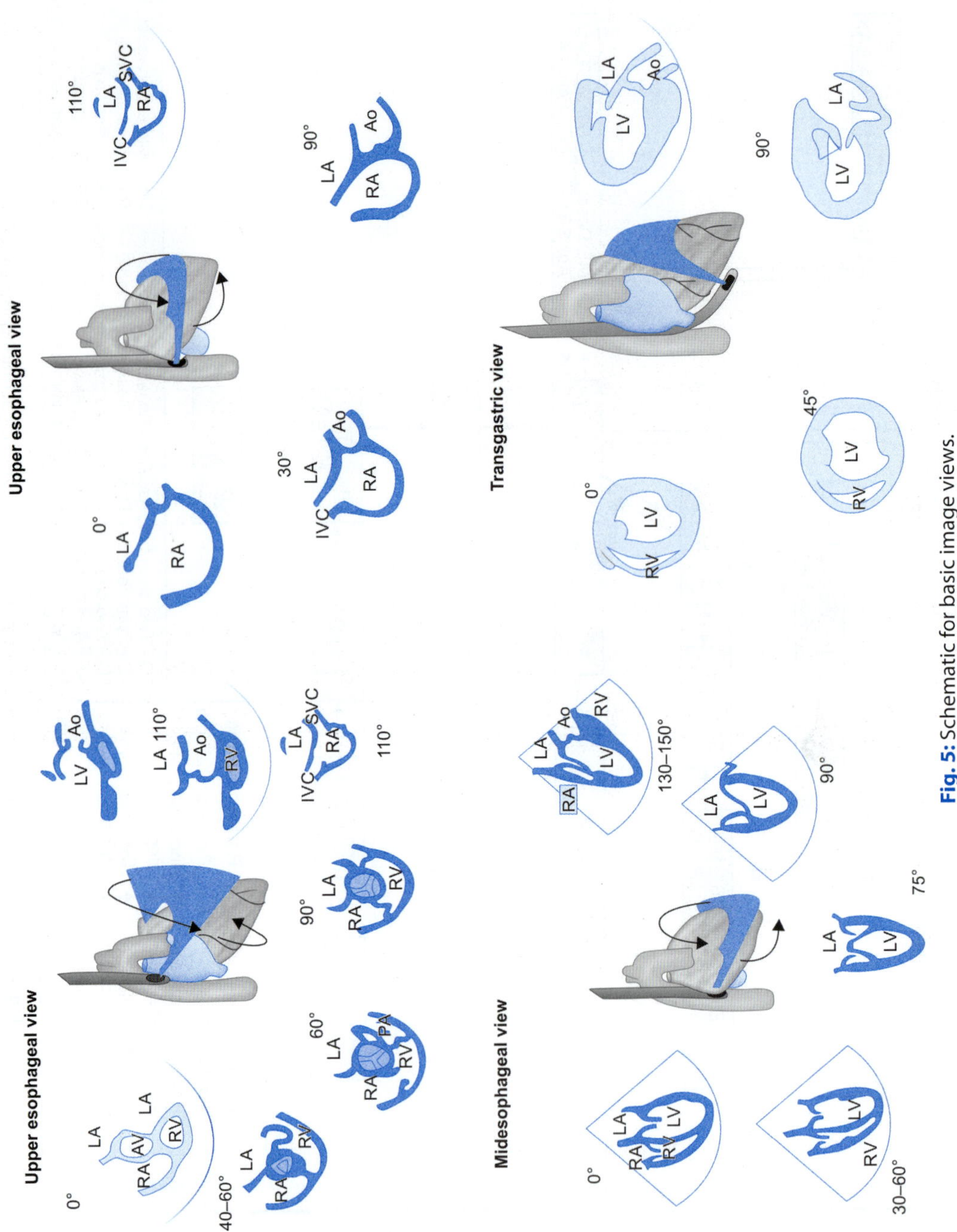

Fig. 5: Schematic for basic image views.

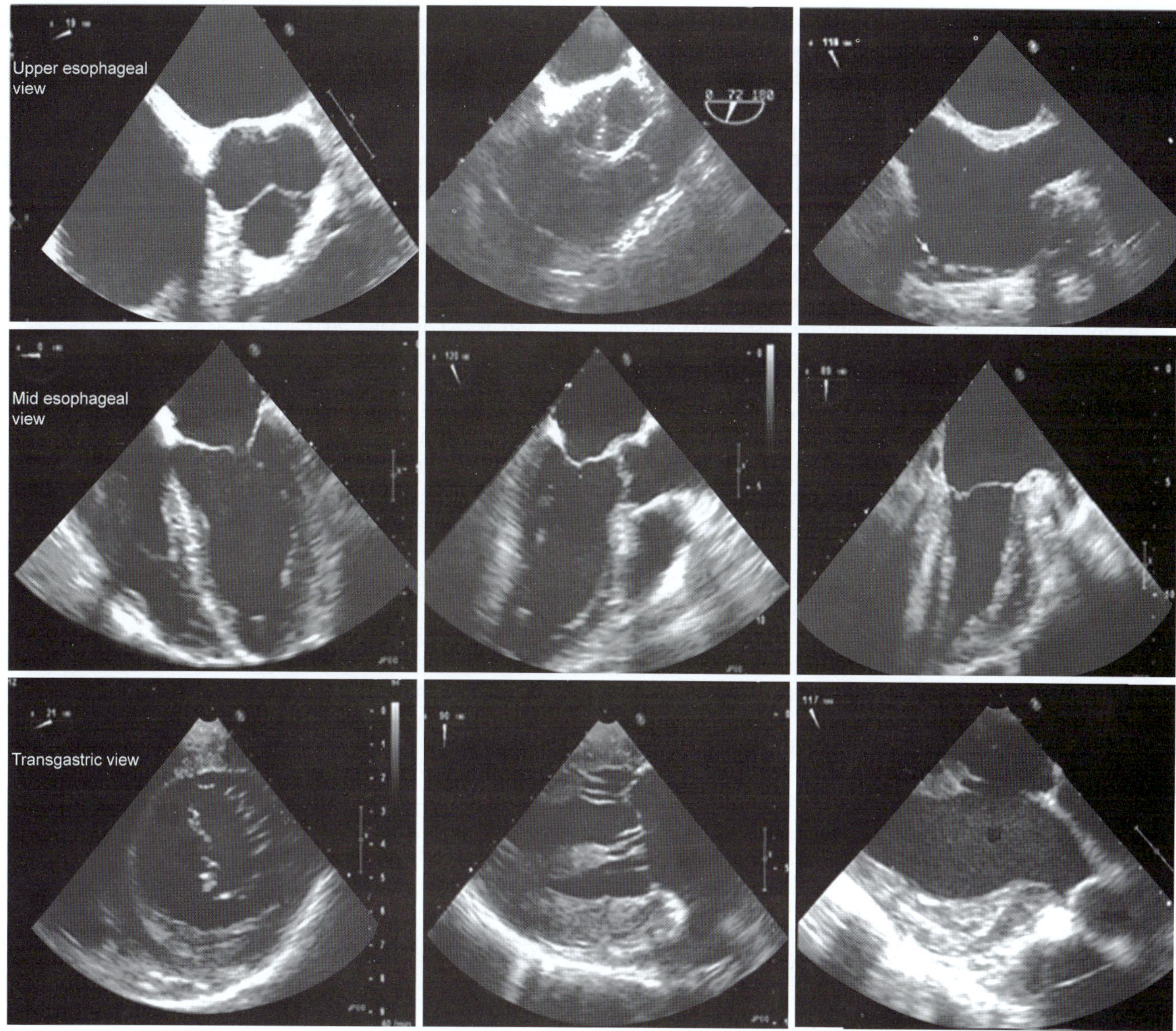

Fig. 6: Basic transesophageal images.

CONCLUSION

Transesophageal echocardiography has increasingly become an important skill for the intensivist to acquire. Though it is more invasive than a TTE, it gives much better image quality since there is minimal or no intervening tissues to obscure the views obtained. A 2D echocardiography is more than sufficient to diagnose and treat the problems routinely faced by the intensivist. A 3D view can be more helpful in diagnosing complex problems but is rarely required in ICU. A systematic approach to the basic examination and the ability to obtain the basic TEE images are of sufficient use at present.

REFERENCES

1. Edler I, Hertz CH. Use of ultrasonic reflectoscope for continuous recording of movement of heart walls. Kung Fysiogr Sallsk Lund Fordhandl. 1954;24:40.
2. Side CD, Gosling RG. Non-surgical assessment of cardiac function. Nature. 1971;232(5309):335-6.
3. Frazin L, Talano JV, Stephanides L, Loeb HS, Kopel L, Gunnar RM. Esophageal echocardiography. Circulation. 1976;54(1):102-8.
4. Hisanaga K, Hisanaga A, Hibi N, Nishimura K, Kambe T. High speed rotating scanner for transesophageal cross-sectional echocardiography. Am J Cardiol. 1980;46(5):837-42.

5. Hisanaga KHA, Nagata K, Yoshida S. A new transesophageal real time two dimensional echocardiographic system using a flexible tube and its clinical application. Proc Jpn Soc Ultrasonics Med. 1977;32:43-4.
6. Dowsett DJ, Kenny PA, Johnstone RE. Ultrasound Principles. In: Dowsett DJ, Kenny PA, Johnstone RE (Eds). The Physics of Diagnostic Imaging, 1st edition. London: Chapman and Hall Medical; 1998. pp. 415-31.
7. Shanewise JS, Cheung AT, Aronson S, Stewart WJ, Weiss RL, Mark JB, et al. ASE/SCA Guidelines for performing a comprehensive intraoperative multiplane transesophageal echocardiography examination: recommendations of the American Society of Echocardiography Council for Intraoperative Echocardiography and the Society of Cardiovascular Anesthesiologists Task Force for Certification in Perioperative Transesophageal Echocardiography. J Am Soc Echocardiogr. 1999;12(10): 884-900.
8. Reeves ST, Finley AC, Skubas NJ, Swaminathan M, Whitley WS, Glas KE, et al. Basic perioperative transesophageal echocardiography examination: a consensus statement of the American Society of Echocardiography and the Society of Cardiovascular Anesthesiologists. J Am Soc Echocardiogr. 2013;26(5):443-56.
9. American Society of Anesthesiologists and Society of Cardiovascular Anesthesiologists Task Force on Transesophageal Echocardiography. Practice guidelines for perioperative transesophageal echocardiography. An updated report by the American Society of Anesthesiologists and the Society of Cardiovascular Anesthesiologists Task Force on Transesophageal Echocardiography. Anesthesiology. 2010;112(5):1084-96.
10. Hilberath JN, Oakes DA, Shernan SK, Bulwer BE, D'Ambra MN, Eltzschig HK, et al. Safety of transesophageal echocardiography. J Am Soc Echocardiogr. 2010;23(11): 1115-27.
11. Vieillard-Baron A, Chergui K, Rabiller A, Peyrouset O, Page B, Beauchet A, et al. Superior vena caval collapsibility as a gauge of volume status in ventilated septic patients. Intensive Care Med. 2004;30(9):1734-9.
12. Vieillard-Baron A, Caille V, Charron C, Belliard G, Page B, Jardin F. Actual incidence of global left ventricular hypokinesia in adult septic shock. Crit Care Med. 2008; 36(6):1701-6.
13. Benjamin E, Griffin K, Leibowitz AB, Manasia A, Oropello JM, Geffroy V, et al. Goal-directed transesophageal echocardiography performed by intensivists to assess left ventricular function: comparison with pulmonary artery catheterization. J Cardiothorac Vasc Anesth. 1998; 12(1):10-5.
14. Charron C, Prat G, Caille V, Belliard G, Lefèvre M, Aegerter P, et al. Validation of a skills assessment scoring system for transesophageal echocardiographic monitoring of hemodynamics. Intensive Care Med. 2007;33(10): 1712-8.

Extended-focused Assessment with Sonography in Trauma

Sachin Gupta, Deeksha Singh Tomar

INTRODUCTION

Blunt abdominal injury is the most common presentation in trauma. The clinical signs and symptoms of patients are varied and hence physical evaluation and physiological assessment are not of much help in documenting the severity of trauma. Abdominal trauma is associated with a high mortality (18–25%).[1] Patients with blunt hollow viscus injury have mortality increased from 6.4 to 12.7% if there is a delay in performing laparotomy of >5 hours.[2] Clarke et al.[3] documented that with every 3-minute delay in performing laparotomy after abdominal injury, increases the mortality by 1%. In earlier days, direct peritoneal lavage (DPL) was done but it was not possible in pregnant patients. Computerized tomography (CT) scan of the abdomen has the highest sensitivity and specificity but it is risky in hemodynamically unstable patients and pregnant patients. Focused assessment by sonography in trauma (FAST) scan is an excellent alternative to DPL and CT scan; as it is a point-of-care bedside imaging test with no risk of radiation and also has high specificity and sensitivity.[4]

The FAST scan is an integral component in the resuscitation of trauma victims and has been incorporated into the advanced trauma life support (ATLS) course.[5]

BASICS OF THE FAST SCAN

The purpose of FAST examination in trauma patients is to detect free fluid, i.e., blood, in potential body spaces like the pleural, peritoneal, and pericardial space. It can be performed in under 5 minutes at the bedside. The advantages of FAST scan are:

- It can accurately detect pneumothorax apart from free fluid in the body spaces.
- Solid organ injury can be determined.
- Serial examinations can be done, to assess the progress of the injury and in pregnant patients, as there is no radiation hazard.
- Safe in hemodynamically unstable patients as do not need to be shifted from the emergency area.
- Rapid
- Very small learning curve as studies have shown that most errors occur during the first 10 examinations only.[6]

TECHNIQUE AND INTERPRETATION

Probe Selection

The curvilinear (convex) transducer probe, with a frequency of 3–5 MHz is ideal as it can be used to scan deep structures, and can easily identify free fluid in the abdomen and pelvis, and solid organ injury. It can also identify the free fluid in the pericardial cavity although the phased array probe (3–4.5 MHz) is the ideal for assessing the pericardial window. Pneumothorax can be identified by the curvilinear probe when placed between the ribs **(Fig. 1)**. For all ultrasound (USG) imaging the marker orientation should be either pointing cephalad in a longitudinal view or toward the right of the patient during the transverse view.

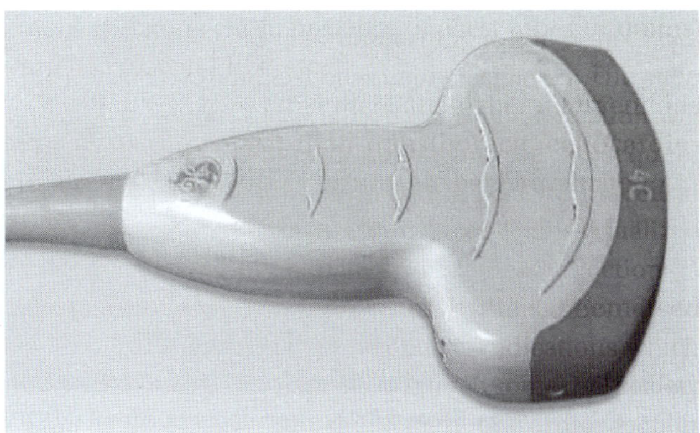

Fig. 1: The curvilinear transducer with a frequency of 3–5 MHz.

Quadrants

The original FAST scan was divided into four quadrants **(Fig. 2)**:

1. Right upper quadrant or the hepatorenal fossa (Morrison's pouch)
2. Left upper quadrant or the splenorenal fossa
3. Suprapubic or the pelvis
4. Subxiphoid view

Later on, the protocol for the detection of pneumothorax/hemothorax by the thoracic window was added to the FAST scan and was named extended FAST (E-FAST).

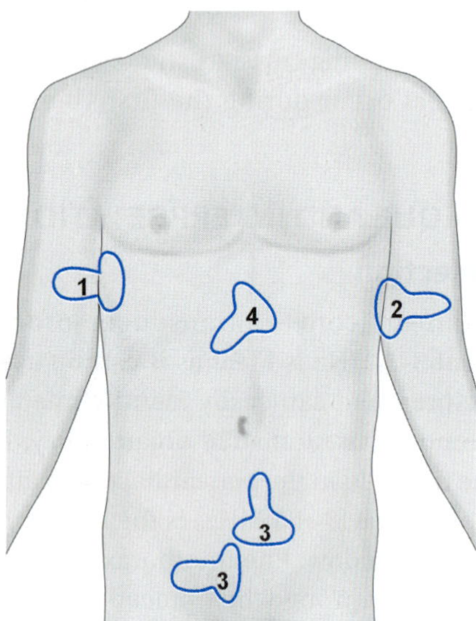

Fig. 2: The four quadrants of FAST. 1 = RUQ or Hepatorenal or Morrison's Pouch; 2 = LUQ or splenorenal; 3 = Suprapubic, transverse, and longitudinal; and 4 = Subxiphoid.

The principle in scanning these quadrants is that blood collects in the most dependent areas. The hepatorenal space is the most dependent area in a paramesocolic area. Similarly, the suprapubic area is the most dependent area in an inframesocolic area.

Right Upper Quadrant View

The transducer is first placed at the anterior axillary line on the right side. The marker on the transducer should be cephalad so that the correct orientation is viewed on the screen. An adequate amount of jelly should be applied to slide the transducer cephalad and caudad. This placement is done to avoid bowel gas by using the liver as an acoustic window **(Figs. 3A and B)**.

The structures that should be visualized in this quadrant are **(Fig. 4)** as follows:

- The space above the diaphragm (pleural space)
- The diaphragm separating pleural and peritoneal space
- Subdiaphragmatic space
- Hepatorenal space or Morrison's pouch
- Inferior pole of the right kidney

The Morrison's pouch is generally visualized at the seventh to ninth rib but one should not waste time in counting the ribs. The transducer is moved cephalad in the pleural space to look for any anechoic collection and absence of mirror image artifact, which is considered blood in trauma patients.[7] It is also done to rule out pneumothorax by identifying the "to and fro" movement of the pleura toward the diaphragm, also known as lung sliding.[8,9]

The presence of hemoperitoneum is confirmed by the appearance of blood as an anechoic collection in the fossa.

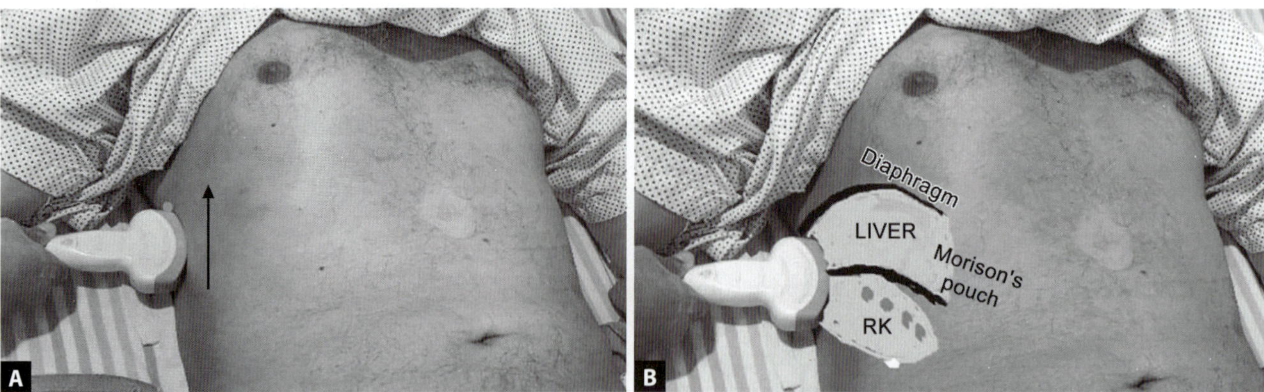

Figs. 3A and B: The right upper quadrant (RUQ) view. (A) The position of the transducer with a marker pointing cephalad; (B) Schematic illustration of structures visible in RUQ. (RK: right kidney)

The inferior pole of the kidney should be visualized to label it as an adequate examination **(Figs. 5A and B)**. The right upper quadrant (RUQ) is the most sensitive view for the presence of hemoperitoneum. In the presence of high clinical suspicion of hemoperitoneum but an absence of free fluid visualization in RUQ view, the patient should be made to lie down in the Trendelenburg position as it would gravitate any free fluid in Morrison's pouch.

The identification of the diaphragm is important to differentiate between pleural and peritoneal space and if the anechoic shadow is above the diaphragm, it is hemothorax. Similarly, the patient can have anechoic shadows both above and below the diaphragm which indicates the presence of hemothorax and hemoperitoenum. Once the blood is detected, it is labeled as RUQ E-FAST positive **(Fig. 6)**.

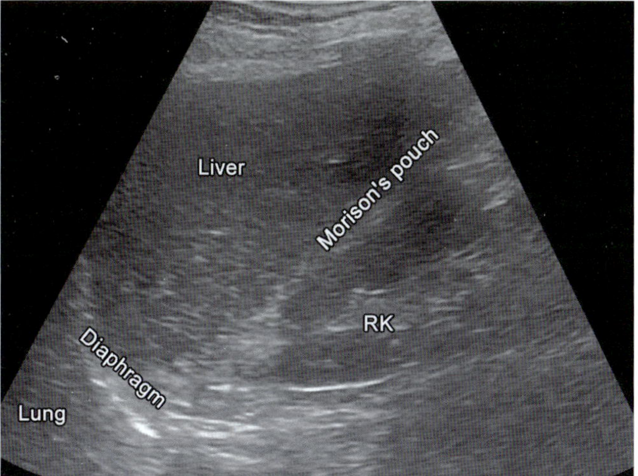

Fig. 4: The ultrasound image of the right upper quadrant (RUQ). (RK: right kidney)

Left Upper Quadrant View

To examine the LUQ, the transducer should be kept in the posterior axillary line almost touching the mattress of the bed. It should be positioned in a manner to use the spleen as an acoustic window to avoid the interference of air-filled bowel. The probe is placed between the sixth and ninth rib **(Figs. 7A and B)** as the left kidney is more posterior to the right kidney due to the smaller size of the spleen as compared to the liver.

The structures to be identified in this view are **(Fig. 8)** as follows:

- Space above the diaphragm (pleural space)
- Infradiaphragmatic and perisplenic area
- Splenorenal fossa

The presence of anechoic collection in these areas should be taken as blood. During the same examination, the probe should be moved cephalad to look for the presence of blood in the left hemithorax which is seen as an anechoic collection or absence of mirror-image artifact. Detection of pneumothorax is done by the presence of a "stratosphere sign" and the absence of lung sliding.[10] If any of the above findings are present, then it is labeled as LUQ E-FAST positive **(Figs. 9A and B)**.

Suprapubic or Pelvic View

The suprapubic examination should be done in both a transverse and longitudinal manner. For the transverse

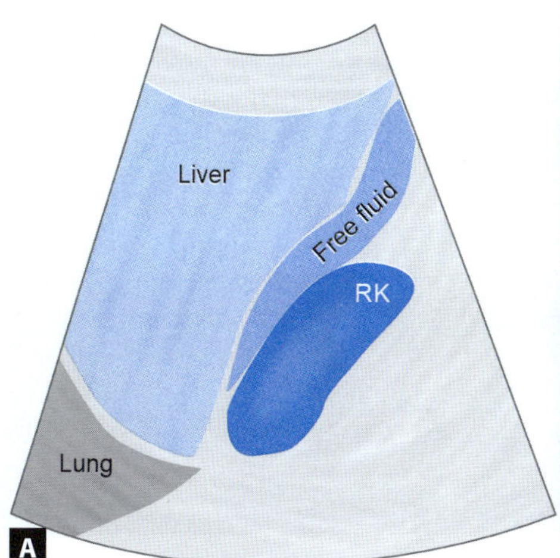

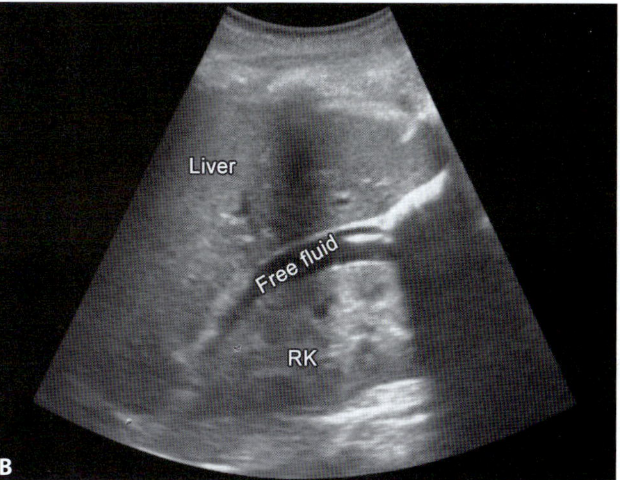

Figs. 5A and B: The right upper-hand quadrant FAST positive view. (A) Schematic illustration of RUQ FAST positive; (B) USG view of RUQ FAST positive. (FAST: focused assessment with sonography for trauma; RK: right kidney; RUQ: right upper quadrant; USG: ultrasound)

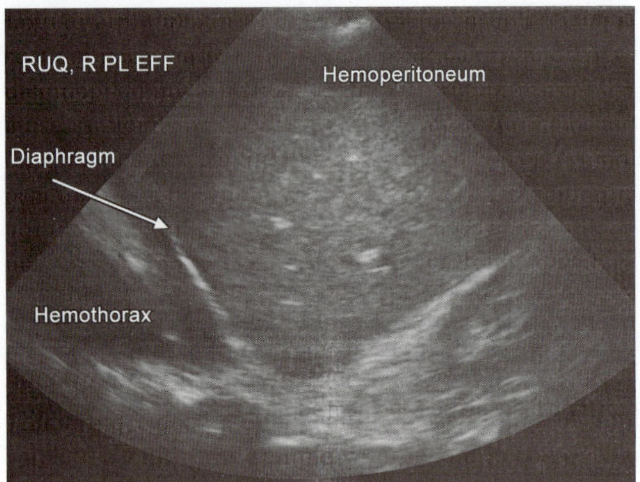

Fig. 6: Hemothorax with hemoperitoneum.

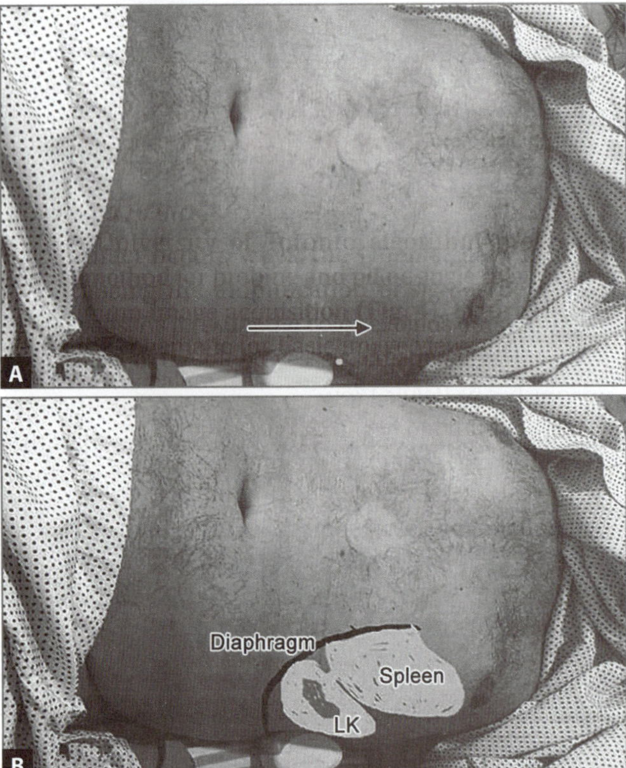

Figs. 7A and B: The left upper quadrant view. (A) The position of the transducer with marker Pointing cephalad; (B) Schematic illustration of structures visible in LUQ [spleen, left kidney (LK), diaphragm are seen].

view, the transducer should be kept just above the pubic symphysis and directed inferiorly toward the pubic bone. The idea is to first identify the urinary bladder and then the free fluid around the bladder. The bladder is best

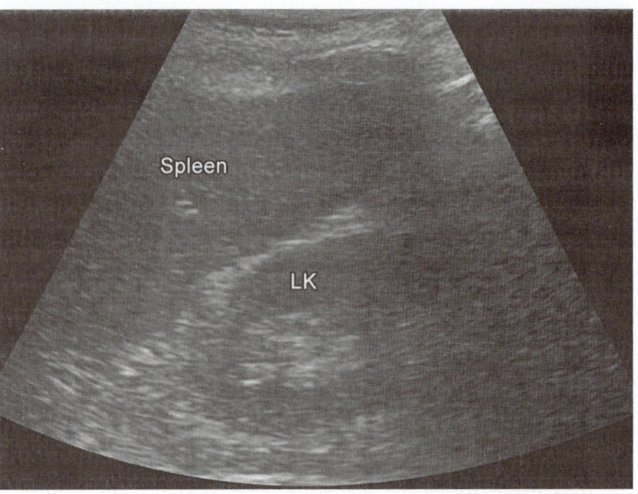

Fig. 8: The ultrasound image of the left upper quadrant (LUQ). (LK: left kidney)

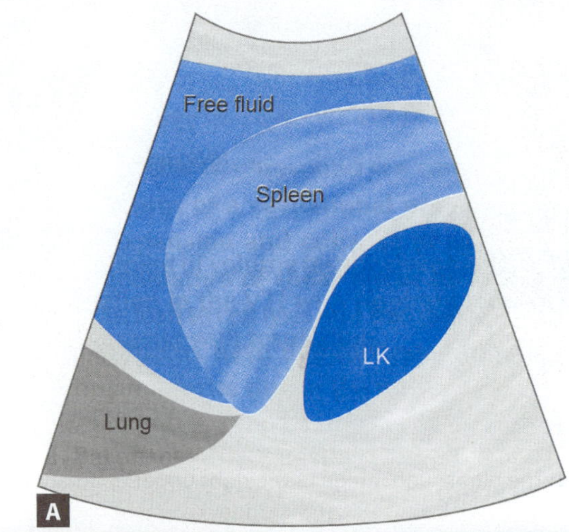

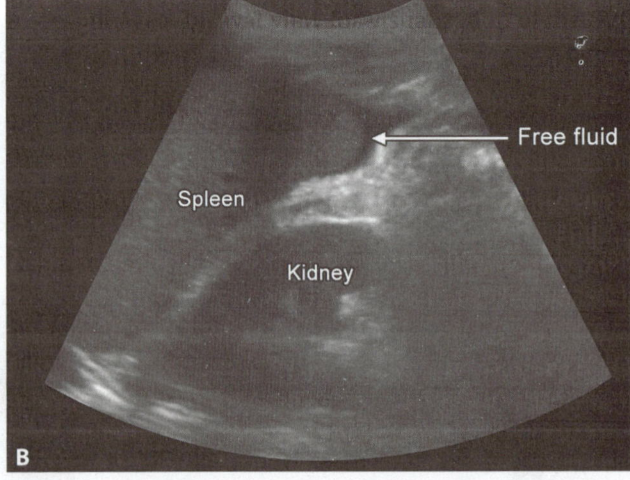

Figs. 9A and B: The LUQ FAST positive view. (A) Schematic illustration of LUQ FAST positive; (B) USG View of LUQ FAST positive. (FAST: focused assessment with sonography for trauma; LUQ: left upper quadrant; USG: ultrasound)

identified when it is full, so the pubic examination should be done before the patient is catheterized. If a urinary catheter has already been placed, try filling the bladder by instilling saline through the catheter for the examination. The marker on the probe should be facing to the right side of the patient **(Figs. 10A and B)**. The bladder may not always be in the midline, so fan the probe on both the right and the left for visualization of the bladder.

The areas to be visualized during this examination are **(Figs. 11A and B)** as follows:

- Urinary bladder
- Recto vesical space in males and rectouterine space (pouch of Douglas) in females
- Seminal vesicles (SV) (in male patients)

Seminal vesicles appear as symmetrical hypoechoic structures just near the posterior wall of the bladder and superior to the prostate. Any free fluid collection would be seen in these spaces as an anechoic shadow **(Figs. 12 and 13)**.

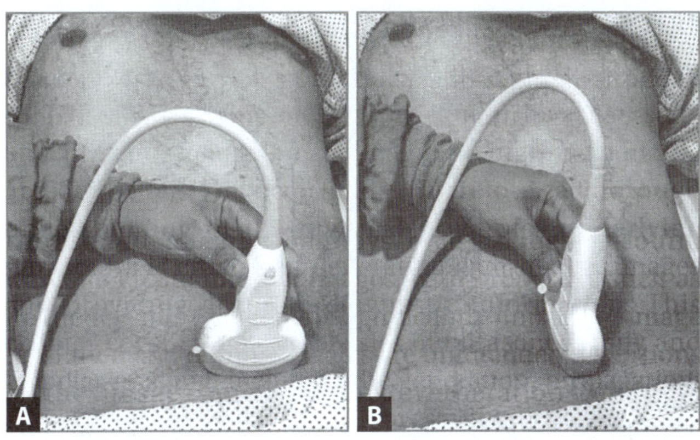

Figs. 10A and B: The suprapubic view. (A) Transverse orientation; (B) Longitudinal orientation.

After the transverse examination, the probe is rotated at 90° in a clockwise direction to obtain the longitudinal view. The marker on the transducer should be facing cranially at this stage. This view is probably better to examine even the smallest amount of fluid collection. The free fluid can be seen in the following **(Fig. 14)**:

- Rectovesical space in males and rectouterine space in females
- Superior, lateral, and posterior to the bladder
- Around the bowel loops

The free fluid in the peritoneum should be differentiated from fluid within the bowel. The bowel exhibits peristalsis, contains gas, and can be seen as a tubular structure whereas free fluid has a pointy appearance. In females of reproductive age, 15 mL of free fluid in a pouch of Douglas is considered normal.[11,12]

In males, the free fluid would be collected just cephalad to seminal vesicles as it is the most inferior part of the peritoneum.

Subxiphoid View

The purpose of this view is to evaluate the presence of free fluid within the pericardial space, which in trauma scenarios should be blood. The choice of view should be a subxiphoid view where the transducer is placed as close as possible to the xiphoid process with the probe pointing toward the patient's left shoulder and the pointer toward the right side of the patient **(Figs. 15A and B)** if curvilinear probe is used for the examination. If a phased array probe

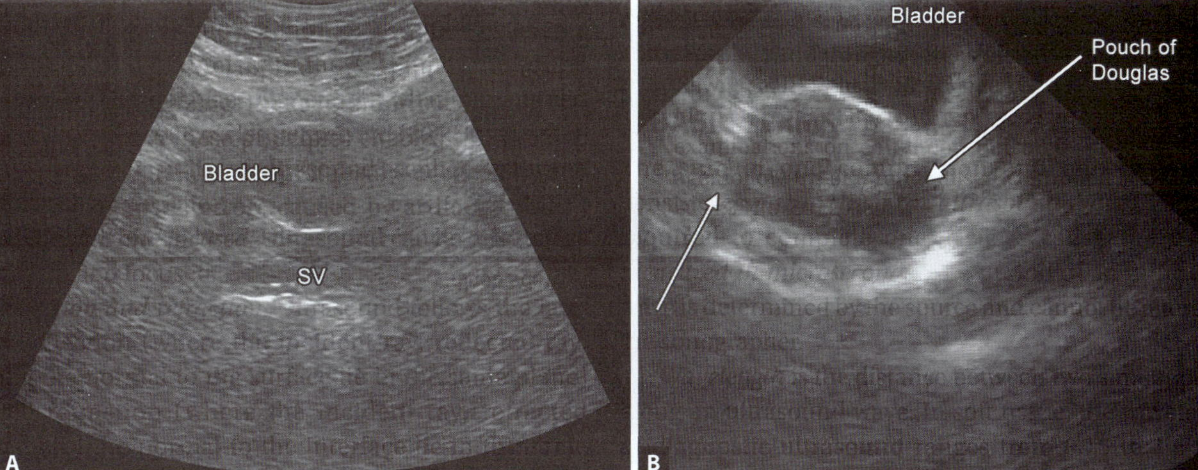

Figs. 11A and B: The ultrasound image of the suprapubic view in transverse orientation for males and females.

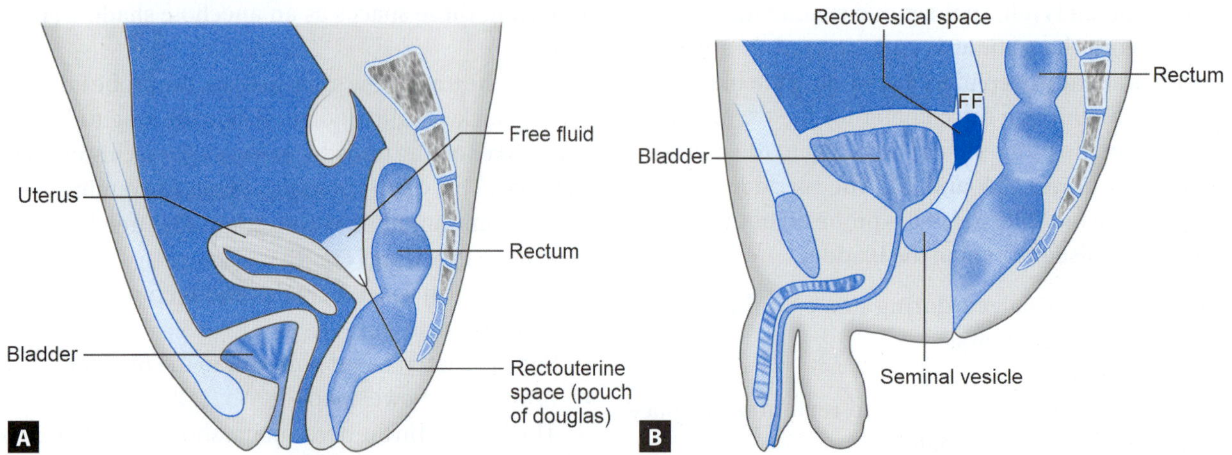

Figs. 12A and B: The schematic representation of a free fluid (FF) collection in suprapubic view in a transverse orientation. (A) Female pelvis; (B) Male pelvis.

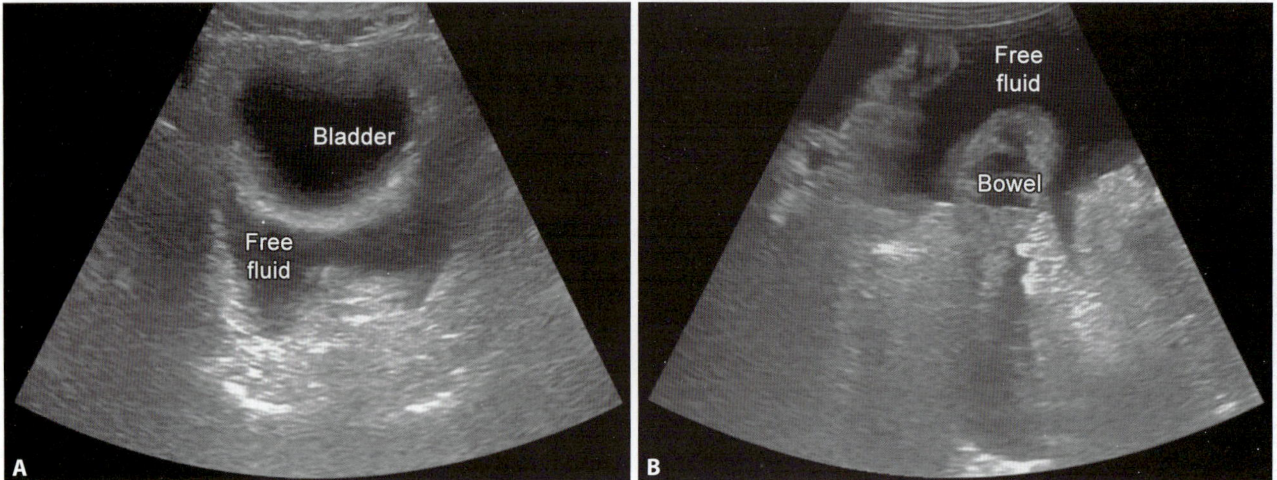

Figs. 13A and B: The ultrasound image of focused assessment with sonography for trauma (FAST) positive suprapubic view.

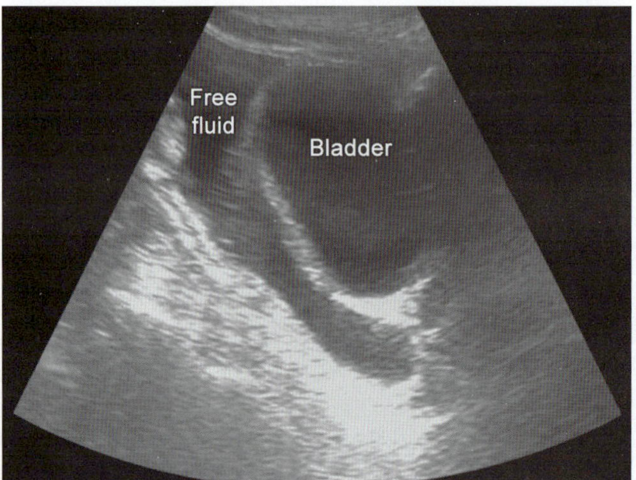

Fig. 14: The USG View of FAST positive suprapubic view, longitudinal orientation. (FAST: focused assessment with sonography for trauma; USG: ultrasound)

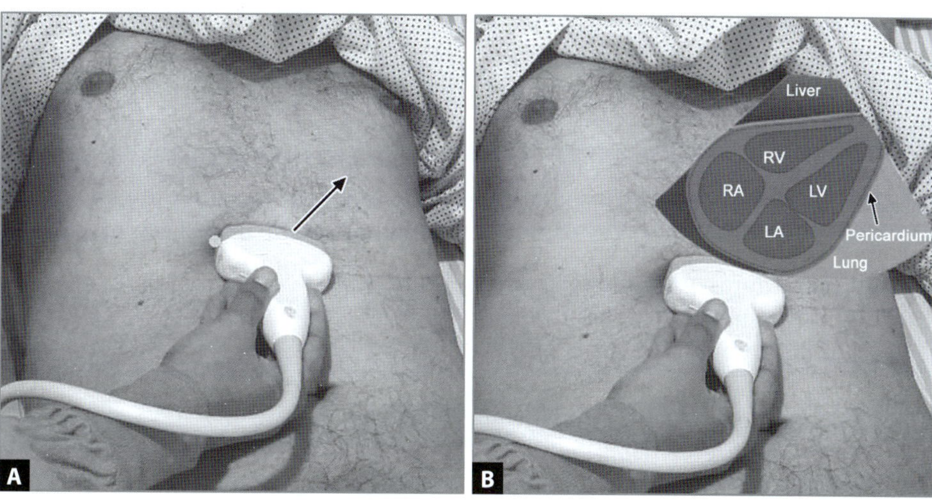

Figs. 15A and B: The subxiphoid view. (A) The position of the Transducer with a marker pointing toward the right shoulder; (B) Schematic illustration of structures visible in subxiphoid view. (LA: left atrium; LV; left ventricle; RA: right atrium; RV: right ventricle)

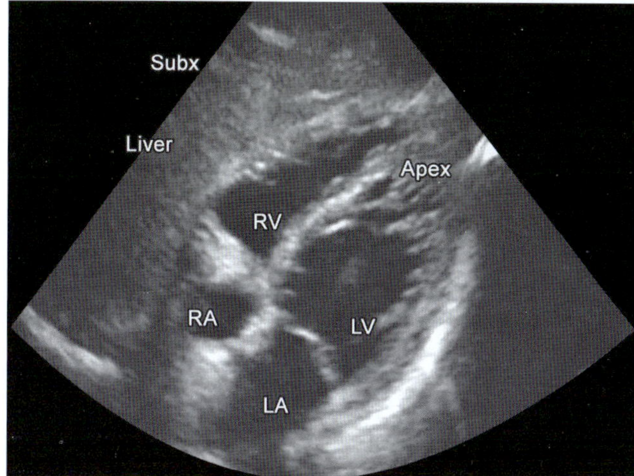

Fig. 16: The normal ultrasound (USG) view of the subxiphoid view. (LA: left atrium; LV; left ventricle; RA: right atrium; RV: right ventricle)

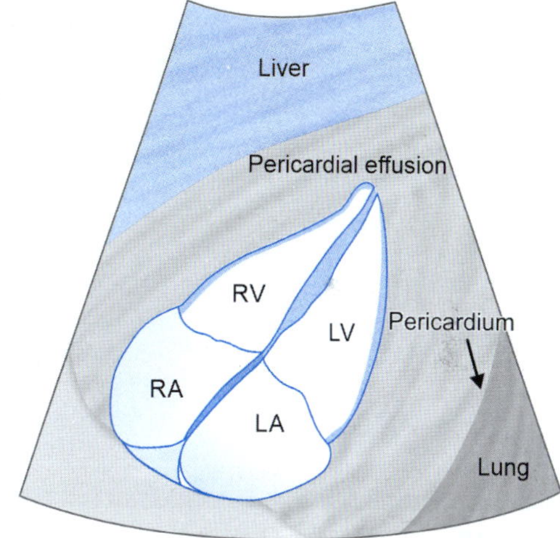

Fig. 17: Schematic representation of pericardial effusion as seen by ultrasound (USG). (LA: left atrium; LV; left ventricle; RA: right atrium; RV: right ventricle)

is used, then the pointer should point toward the left shoulder of the patient.

The structures visualized are **(Fig. 16)** as follows:

- Pericardium attached to diaphragm seen as a white echogenic line
- Four-chamber view of a heart with the right ventricle and right atrium placed more anteriorly (near to the top of the ultrasound screen).
- Liver

If the patient complains of severe abdominal pain and does not allow placing the transducer in the sub-xiphoid area, then a parasternal long-axis view should be done.

The presence of blood is seen as a black (anechoic) strip around the heart. The first point of free fluid collection is posterior to the heart. The fluid accumulates between the visceral and parietal pericardium. Sometimes similar anechoic shadow is visible only anterior to the heart without any evidence of posterior fluid collection. This is due to the presence of epicardial fat **(Fig. 17)**.

The pericardial space can accumulate >1,000 mL of fluid if it collects slowly over a long period of time, without causing any major hemodynamic compromise, in medical conditions such as tuberculosis, malignancy, and uremia.[13] But a rapid accumulation of even as little as 100 mL of blood in trauma gives rise to features of pericardial tamponade. The echocardiographic features of pericardial tamponade such as right ventricular collapse during diastole or right atrium collapse, should be looked for, if there is circumferential collection of fluid **(Figs. 18 and 19)**.

Extended FAST Views

The assessment of the pleural cavity for assessment of pneumothorax and hemothorax was added to the traditional FAST scan and was named extended FAST or E-FAST. There are various studies that have shown the utility of ultrasound in detecting pneumothorax.[14-16] The ultrasound detection of pneumothorax has been discussed in another chapter and so is not being discussed here in detail. Just remember that the salient points about pneumothorax are the absence of lung sliding, absence of lung pulse, absence of B-lines and detection of lung point, and presence of stratosphere sign (appearance of bar-code) on M mode[17,18] **(Figs. 20A and B)**.

The presence of free fluid in the form of anechoic collection in either of the pleural spaces indicates hemothorax. The underlying lung may appear floating in the presence of massive hemothorax. The fluid may be anechoic or may have a hypoechoic appearance depending on the age of the blood collection. **(Fig. 21)**. Similarly, the spine shadow stops at the level of the diaphragm if there is no free fluid in the thoracic cavity or else it appears in the presence of free fluid in the thoracic cavity. This is called a spine sign **(Fig. 22)**.

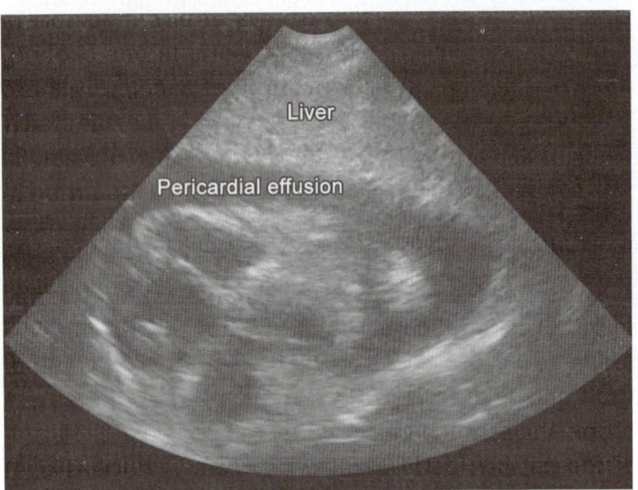

Fig. 18: Circumferential pericardial effusion.

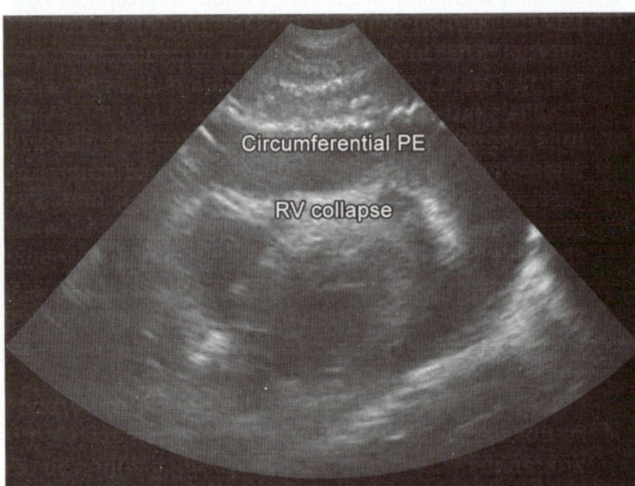

Fig. 19: RV collapse with circumferential PE. These are features of pericardial tamponade. (PV: pericardial effusion; RV: right ventricular)

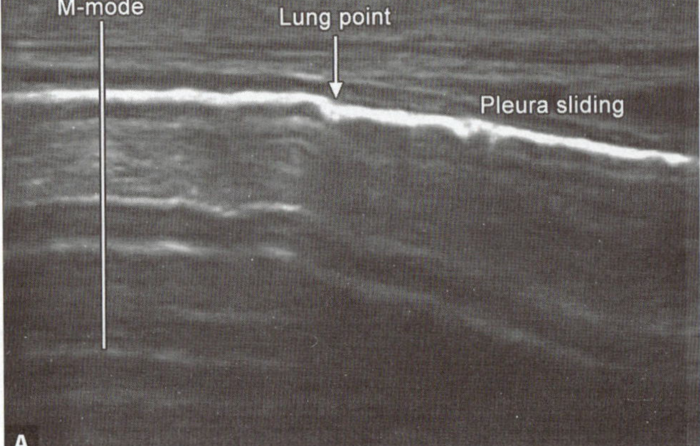

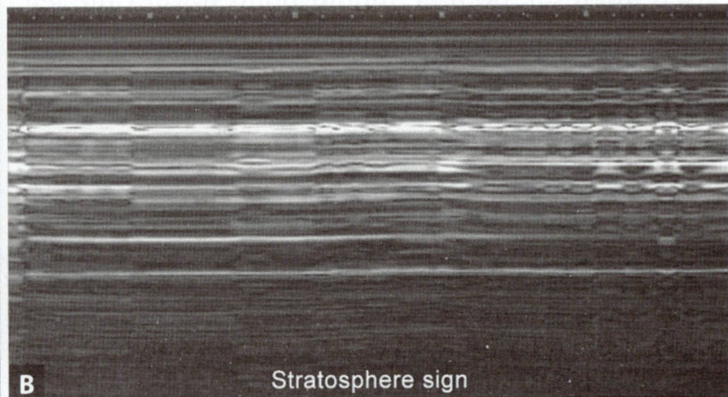

Figs. 20A and B: The USG findings of pneumothorax. (A) Lung point, defined as junction point where the pleura is still attached to the lung; (B) Stratosphere sign, an M-mode finding of pneumothorax.

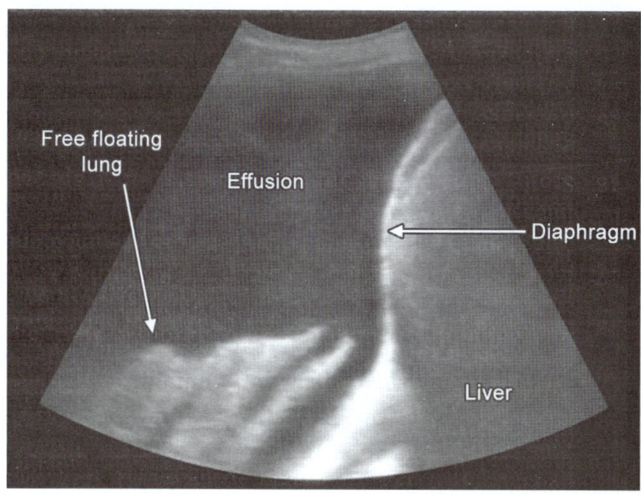

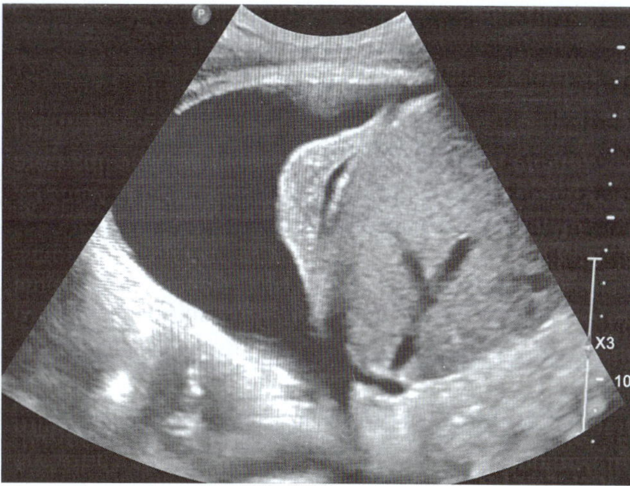

Fig. 21: Massive hemothorax leading to free-floating lung.

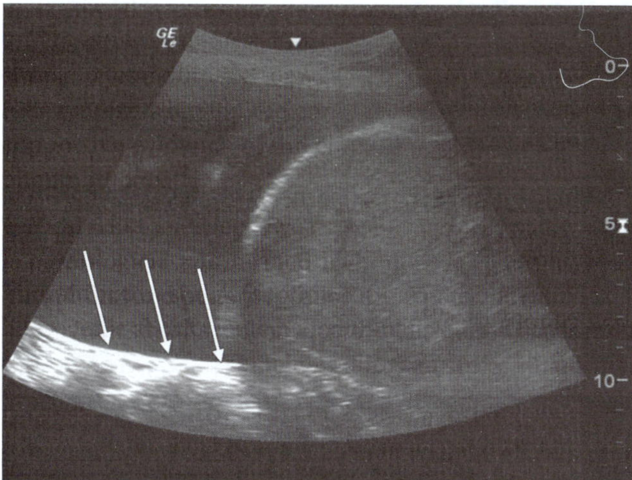

Fig. 22: Spine sign which represents visualization of vertebral bodies above the diaphragm due to the presence of large pleural effusion.

DIAGNOSTIC PERFORMANCE OF FAST SCAN

The performance of the FAST scan varies with the expertise of the operator and also with the quality of equipment but still, the sensitivity and specificity are very good in detecting free fluid in trauma scenarios.[19-21] The average sensitivity of detecting hemoperitoneum in the literature varies from 73 to 100%.[22] In a study by Ollerton et al., FAST scans changed the diagnosis in 32.8% of patients and also led to a decrease in the need for DPL and CT scans.[23] Moylan et al. performed a retrospective analysis in normotensive blunt trauma FAST-positive cases and found a strong correlation with the need for laparotomy.[24] In the study, the sensitivity and specificity of FAST was 75.8 and 97.4%, respectively. The negative predictive value (NPV) was 99.5%.[24]

The performance of FAST in penetrating abdominal injury is excellent and the specificity ranges from 94 to 100%, so FAST-positive cases may warrant a laparotomy. When it comes to diagnosing solid organ injury, the sensitivity of FAST scans is poor and ranges from 32.5 to 82.5%.[25]

Stengel et al. conducted a meta-analysis of 62 studies (over 18,000 patients) and concluded that the FAST scan had a sensitivity of 78.9% indicating that it cannot detect small quantities of free fluid but had a specificity of 99.2% indicating that once detected, FAST scan has a major role in decision making.[26]

The FAST scan can easily detect even <200 mL fluid collection in Morrison's space.[27] For detection of free fluid in the thoracic cavity, a chest X-ray requires at least 175–200 mL whereas an ultrasound chest can detect as little as 50 mL of free fluid in the thoracic cavity.[28]

In a study conducted by Brun et al., the meantime taken to perform a FAST scan was recorded at 3.9 minutes with good specificity and negative predictive value.[29] Similarly in one more study, the skill of emergency medical technician (EMT) in performing FAST scans was compared with the physicians routinely performing ultrasound examinations and it was found that the specificity and negative predictive value were comparable in both the groups, indicating that it has a very small learning curve.[30]

To compile all the data available so far, the specificity of FAST ranges between 95 and 100%, and the sensitivity

TABLE 1: Indications of EFAST.

- Closed chest trauma
- Penetrating chest trauma
- Blunt abdominal trauma
- Penetrating abdominal trauma
- Muti-trauma patient
- Undefined hypotension in a trauma patient

ranges between 69 and 98%. As the specificity is higher, the FAST scan is more useful in ruling in the pathology rather than ruling out.

In emergency and critical care practice, the indications of E-FAST are discussed in **Table 1**.

Limitations

The classical teaching is that RUQ is the first view to be performed to look for intraperitoneal fluid collection and if it is negative then no need to go ahead with the rest of the scan but still one can find fluid in other quadrants despite RUQ FAST negative.[31] LUQ is technically the most challenging view to get due to the more posterior placement of the left kidney. Similarly, fluid collection can be present around the spleen (perisplenic collection) just below the left hemidiaphragm, in the splenorenal fossa, or even in the left paracolic gutter.

Sometimes the clinical signs and the scene raise strong suspicion of intraperitoneal bleed, but the RUQ FAST turns out to be negative. One should look into the pelvic view as fluid <100 mL can be visualized in this quadrant, although it would depend on intraperitoneal adhesions or interloop fluid collection if any.[32] The FAST examination is positive when a minimum critical volume of blood is present in the peritoneal cavity. An average volume of around 668 mL in the supine position and 444 in the Trendelenburg position is required for RUQ FAST positive whereas the volume ranges from 100 to 250 mL for positive CT scans.[33]

The sensitivity of FAST scan for solid organ injury ranges between 55 and 80% and therefore one should perform a CT scan of the abdomen if the suspicion of Grade I-II hepatic or splenic injury is present with a negative FAST examination.[34]

A false negative FAST examination should be considered a nonintraperitoneal injury and has been found to be more in patients with associated head and limb injuries. However, this does not influence the patient outcome, nor does it affect the hospital or ICU length of stay.[6,35] A trauma protocol full body CT scan should be performed in such cases. If the facility of CT scan is not available, the repeat FAST examinations should be performed in negative scans as it increases the sensitivity to up to 85%.[36]

False positive results can be seen in patients with ascites, peritoneal dialysis, ovarian hyperstimulation syndrome, women of reproductive age group, or after massive fluid resuscitation.[37] Similarly the presence of perinephric fat can be misinterpreted as free fluid collection in the hepatorenal or splenorenal fossa. This is called a "double-line sign."[38] Similarly, bullae in the lungs can create a false positive result for pneumothorax.

Another limitation is that FAST cannot detect retroperitoneal blood collection.

E-FAST IN SPECIAL POPULATION

Pediatric Patients

Earlier the use of FAST in the pediatric population was very low as compared to its use in adults but now >93% of pediatric emergency physicians are using this modality in pediatric trauma.[39] This allows for to protection of the children from unnecessary radiation hazards. The sensitivity and specificity of FAST scans in the pediatric population are different from those in adults and are around 80 and 96%, respectively. If both the FAST scan and physical examination are normal, then a conservative strategy can be safely followed. The sensitivity and specificity can be increased further by combining a FAST scan with a CT scan. For chest trauma, NICE does not recommend only FAST scanning but supports the combined use of chest X-ray and ultrasound rather than CT scans.[40]

Patient with Ascites

Patients with preexisting free fluid in the abdomen present a diagnostic dilemma about the specificity of the FAST scan. Clinical history and physical examination play a major role in decision-making. On the FAST scan, the presence of low-intensity echoes within the free fluid and hemodynamics of the patient should guide the decision about laparotomy. Similarly in hemodynamically stable patients, the increase in free fluid in the abdomen on serial examination should give the suspicion of ongoing bleeding and the need for further intervention. But even after this, if there is doubt, then a small diagnostic ascitic sample should be taken to rule out hemorrhage or transudative ascites.

Pelvic Fracture

The utility of FAST scan in identifying hemoperitoneum in patients with pelvic fracture is very low (26%) even if the patients were hemodynamically unstable.[41] Previous studies have also documented that if a FAST scan is negative, the diagnosis should be confirmed with the help of pelvic angiography.[42] If FAST is positive and the patient is hemodynamically unstable, then the need for operative intervention is justified.

Pregnancy

Around 15 mL of free fluid can be found normally in Pouch of Douglas in women of childbearing age. If the presence of free fluid of >50 mL is found in this potential space with signs of shock, then it confirms the diagnosis of hemoperitoneum and the need for surgical intervention. The finding of a clot around the adnexa can also be visible on the scan. The advantage of ultrasound is the protection of the mother and fetus from radiation exposure. The sensitivity and specificity of FAST scanning are similar in both pregnant and nonpregnant patients.[43] For patients with negative FAST, should have continuous fetal heartbeat monitoring for any late-onset bleeding.

Cardiac Arrest

The utility of point-of-care ultrasound (POCUS) during cardiopulmonary resuscitation (CPR) has been validated and accepted in the ACLS guidelines. Detection of reversible factors such as cardiac tamponade, hypovolemia, and tension pneumothorax can be identified and rectified during cardiac arrest in a trauma scenario.

FOCUSED ASSESSMENT WITH SONOGRAPHY FOR TRAUMA ALGORITHM

The FAST scan is not an alternative to a CT scan in patients who are unstable with a FAST negative report. Even patients who have FAST-positive findings but are stable should undergo a CT scan for anatomical localization of the bleeding and for decision-making about surgical intervention.

The FAST scan algorithm developed by the International Consensus Conference is shown in **Flowchart 1**.[44]

As seen in the algorithm, the patient's hemodynamics play a vital role in determining the need for surgical intervention.

Flowchart 1: FAST algorithm.

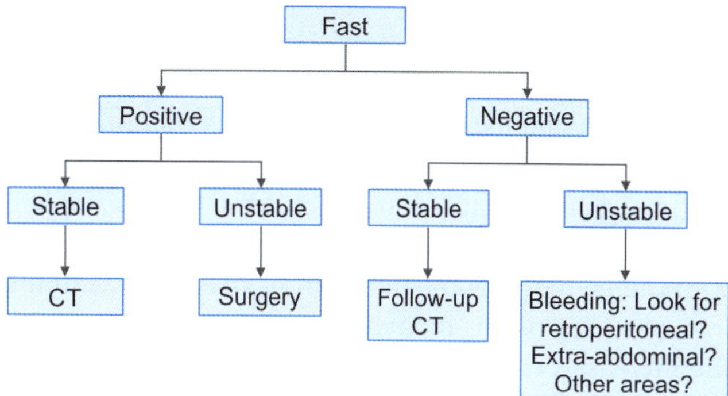

(CT: computed tomography; FAST: focused assessment with sonography for trauma)

Focused Assessment with Sonography for Trauma Positive, Unstable

In such a scenario, the patient is immediately rushed to the operating theater without the need for a CT scan or other radiological diagnostic modality.

Focused Assessment with Sonography for Trauma Positive, Stable

These patients should undergo confirmatory radiological testing such as a CT scan and angiography to determine the site of bleeding or leakage and then further intervention should be planned.

Focused Assessment with Sonography for Trauma Negative, Stable

All trauma patients need not have bleeding, so FAST can be negative. These patients should be observed for 4–6 hours and then the FAST scan can be repeated. If the repeat FAST scan is also negative with stable hemodynamics, then the patient can be safely discharged. Whereas, if the repeat scan becomes positive, the CT scan should be performed to look for the site of bleeding.

Focused Assessment with Sonography for Trauma Negative, Unstable

These are the patients who may be having retroperitoneal bleeding or pelvic fractures and can have FAST negative results. These patients despite being unstable should undergo either a CT scan or pelvic angiography to decide on definitive management of the patient. One should also look for other causes of hypotension in these patients apart from abdominal and thoracic areas.

CONCLUSION

The FAST scan is an excellent diagnostic tool for emergency physicians and can be used for in and out-of-hospital patients. The specificity of the examination is very high and can easily rule in or rule out the diagnosis. Minimal skill is required to perform the FAST scan, and it has a small learning curve. The challenges associated with the pediatric population can be overcome with the increased use of this modality in pediatric trauma. With the increased use of FAST scans, the need for CT scans and DPL has been reduced tremendously. Repeating the FAST scan in hemodynamically stable FAST-negative cases increases the sensitivity of detecting intraperitoneal bleeding.

REFERENCES

1. Gad MA, Saber A, Farrag S, Shams ME, Ellabban GM. Incidence, patterns, and factors predicting mortality of abdominal injuries in trauma patients. N Am J Med Sci. 2012;4(3):129-34.
2. Malinoski DJ, Patel MS, Yakar DO, Green D, Qureshi F, Inaba K, et al. A diagnostic delay of 5 hours increases the risk of death after blunt hollow viscus injury. J Trauma. 2010;69(1):84-7.
3. Clarke JR, Trooskin SZ, Doshi PJ, Greenwald L, Mode CJ. Time to laparotomy for intra-abdominal bleeding from trauma does affect survival for delays up to 90 minutes. J Trauma 2002;52(3):420e5
4. Griffin XL, Pullinger R. Are diagnostic peritoneal lavage or focused abdominal sonography for trauma safe screening investigations for hemodynamically stable patients after blunt abdominal trauma? A review of the literature. J Trauma. 2007;62(3):779-84.
5. Christie-Large M, Michaelides D, James SLJ. Focused assessment with sonography for trauma: the FAST scan. Trauma. 2008;10:93-101.
6. Jang T, Kryder G, Sineff S, Naunheim R, Aubin C, Kaji AH. The technical errors of physicians learning to perform focused assessment with sonography in trauma. Acad Emerg Med. 2012;19(1):98-101.
7. Abu-Zidan FM, Hefny AF, Corr P. Clinical ultrasound physics. J Emerg Trauma Shock. 2012;4(4):501-3.
8. Husain LF, Hagopian L, Wayman D, Baker WE, Carmody KA. Sonographic diagnosis of pneumothorax. J Emerg Trauma Shock. 2012;5(1):76-81.
9. Zhang M, Liu ZH, Yang JX, Gan JK, Xu SW, You ZD, et al. Rapid detection of pneumothorax by ultrasonography in patients with multiple trauma. Crit Care 2006;10(4):R112.
10. Lichtenstein DA, Mezière G, Lascols N, Biderman P, Courret JP, Gepner A, et al. Ultrasound diagnosis of occult pneumothorax. Crit Care Med. 2005;33(6):1231-8.
11. Sirlin CB, Casola G, Brown MA, Patel N, Bendavid EJ, Deutsch R, et al. US of blunt abdominal trauma: importance of free pelvic fluid in women of reproductive age. Radiology 2001;219(1):229-35.
12. Ormsby EL, Geng J, McGahan JP, Richards JR. Pelvic free fluid: clinical importance for reproductive age women with blunt abdominal trauma. Ultrasound Obstet Gynecol. 2005;26(3):271-8.
13. Richards JR, McGahan JP. Focused Assessment with Sonography in Trauma (FAST) in 2017: What Radiologists Can Learn. Radiology. 2017;283(1):30-48.
14. Kirkpatrick AW, Sirois M, Laupland KB, Liu D, Rowan K, Ball CG, et al. Hand-held thoracic sonography for detecting post-traumatic pneumothoraces: the Extended Focused Assessment with Sonography for Trauma (EFAST). J Trauma 2004;57(2):288-295.
15. Rowan KR, Kirkpatrick AW, Liu D, Forkheim KE, Mayo JR, Nicolaou S. Traumatic pneumothorax detection with thoracic US: correlation with chest radiography and CT—initial experience. Radiology. 2002;225(1):210-4.
16. Soldati G, Testa A, Pignataro G, Portale G, Biasucci DG, Leone A, et al. The ultrasonographic deep sulcus sign in traumatic pneumothorax. Ultrasound Med Biol. 2006;32(7):1157-63.
17. Lichtenstein D, Mezière G, Biderman P, Gepner A. The "lung point": an ultrasound sign specific to pneumothorax. Intensive Care Med. 2000;26(10):1434-40.
18. Stone MB. Ultrasound diagnosis of traumatic pneumothorax. J Emerg Trauma Shock. 2008;1(1):19-20.
19. Boulanger BR, McLellan BA, Brenneman FD, Ochoa J, Kirkpatrick AW. Prospective evidence of the superiority of a sonography-based algorithm in the assessment of blunt abdominal injury. J Trauma. 1999;47(4):632-7.
20. Gaarder C, Kroepelien CF, Loekke R, Hestnes M, Dormage JB, Naess PA. Ultrasound performed by radiologists-confirming the truth about FAST in trauma. J Trauma. 2009;67(2):323-7.
21. Verbeek DO, Zijlstra IA, van der Leij C, Ponsen KJ, van Delden OM, Goslings JC. The utility of FAST for initial abdominal screening of major pelvic fracture patients. World J Surg. 2014;38(7):1719-25.
22. Melanson SW, The FAST. Exam: a review of the literature. In: Jehle D, Heller MB (Eds). Ultrasonography in trauma: the FAST Exam. Dallas, TX: American College of Emergency Physicians; 2003. pp. 127-45.
23. Ollerton JE, Sugrue M, Balogh Z, D'Amours SK, Giles A, Wyllie P. Prospective study to evaluate the influence of FAST on trauma patient management. J Trauma. 2006;60(4):785-91.
24. Moylan M, Newgard CD, Ma OJ, Sabbaj A, Rogers T, Douglass R. Association between a positive ED FAST examination and therapeutic laparotomy in normotensive blunt trauma patients. J Emerg Med. 2007;33(3):265-71.

25. Mohammadi A, Ghasemi-Rad M. Evaluation of gastrointestinal injury in blunt abdominal trauma "FAST is not reliable": the role of repeated ultrasonography. World J Emerg Surg. 2012;7:2.
26. Stengel D, Bauwens K, Rademacher G, Mutze S, Ekkernkamp A. Association between compliance with methodological standards of diagnostic research and reported test accuracy: meta-analysis of focused assessment of US for trauma. Radiology. 2005;236(1):102-11
27. Branney SW, Wolfe RE, Moore EE, Albert NP, Heinig M, Mestek M, et al. Quantitative sensitivity of ultrasound in detecting free intraperitoneal fluid. J Trauma. 1995;39(2):375-80.
28. Ma OJ, Mateer JR. Trauma ultrasound examination versus chest radiography in the detection of hemothorax. Ann Emerg Med.1997;29(3):312-5.
29. Brun PM, Bessereau J, Chenaitia H, Pradel AL, Deniel C, Garbaye G, et al. Stay and play eFAST or scoop and run eFAST? That is the question! Am J Emerg Med. 2014;32(2):166-70.
30. Kim CH, Shin SD, Song KJ, Park CB. Diagnostic accuracy of focused assessment with sonography for trauma (FAST) examinations performed by emergency medical technicians. Prehosp Emerg Care. 2012;16(3):400-6.
31. Lobo V, Hunter-Behrend M, Cullnan E, Higbee R, Phillips C, Williams S, et al. Caudal edge of the liver in the Right Upper Quadrant (RUQ) view is the most sensitive area for free fluid on the FAST exam. West J Emerg Med. 2017;18(2):270-80.
32. Von Kuenssberg Jehle D, Stiller G, Wagner D. Sensitivity in detecting free intraperitoneal fluid with the pelvic views of the FAST exam. Am J Emerg Med. 2003;21(6):476-8.
33. Abrams BJ, Sukumvanich P, Seibel R, Moscati R, Jehle D. Ultrasound for the detection of intraperitoneal fluid: the role of Trendelenburg positioning. Am J Emerg Med. 1999;17(2):117-20.
34. Laselle BT, Byyny RL, Haukoos JS, Krzyzaniak SM, Brooks J, Dalton TR, et al. False-negative FAST examination: associations with injury characteristics and patient outcomes. Ann Emerg Med. 2012;60(3):326-334.e3.
35. Tayal VS, Nielsen A, Jones AE, Thomason MH, Kellam J, Norton HJ. Accuracy of trauma ultrasound in major pelvic injury. J Trauma. 2006;61(6):1453-57.
36. Nunes LW, Simmons S, Hallowell MJ, Kinback R, Trooskin S, Kozar R. Diagnostic performance of trauma US in identifying abdominal or pelvic free fluid and serious abdominal or pelvic injury. Acad Radiol 2001;8(2):128-36
37. Slutzman JE, Arvold LA, Rempell JS, Stone MB, Kimberly HH. Positive FAST without hemoperitoneum due to fluid resuscitation in blunt trauma. J Emerg Med. 2014;47(4):427-9.
38. Sierzenski PR, Schofer JM, Bauman MJ, Nomura JT. The double-line sign: a false positive finding on the Focused Assessment with Sonography for Trauma (FAST) examination. J Emerg Med 2011;40(2):188-9.
39. Chamberlain MC, Reid SR, Madhok M. Utilization of emergency ultrasound in pediatric emergency departments. Pediatr Emerg Care. 2011;27(7):628-32.
40. National Institute for Health and Clinical Excellence. Major trauma: assessment and initial management. [Online] Available from: https://www.nice.org.uk/guidance/ng39 [Last accessed October. 2024].
41. Friese RS, Malekzadeh S, Shafi S, Gentilello LM, Starr A. Abdominal ultrasound is an unreliable modality for the detection of hemoperitoneum in patients with pelvic fracture.J Trauma. 2007;63(1):97-102.
42. Ballard RB, Rozycki GS, Newman PG, Cubillos JE, Salomone JP, Ingram WL, et al. An algorithm to reducethe incidence of false-negative FAST examinations in patients athigh-risk for occult injury. J Am Coll Surg. 1999;189(2):145-50.
43. Goodwin H, Holmes JF, Wisner DH. Abdominal ultrasound examination in pregnant blunt trauma patients. J Trauma. 2001;50(4):689-93.
44. Scalea TM, Rodriguez A, Chiu WC, Brenneman FD, Fallon WF Jr, Kato K, et al. Focused assessment with sonography for trauma (FAST): results from an international consensus conference. J Trauma. 1999;46(3):466-72.

CHAPTER

43

Lung Ultrasound: BLUE Protocol and Falls Protocol

Jayant Shelgaonkar

INTRODUCTION

Point-of-care ultrasound is increasingly used in the management of critically ill patients in the critical care and emergency setting. It has become more popular with the introduction of portable machines, which can be taken to the bedside of the patient and used in the diagnosis and management of critically ill patients. Lung ultrasound (LUS) is the most important clinical tool helpful in the diagnosis and management of respiratory failure.

We routinely perform bedside chest X-rays to assess the lung status of the critically ill patient. Bedside chest X-ray has limitations in terms of diagnostic performance.[1,2] The X-ray beam originates anteriorly limiting the correct interpretation of cardiac silhouette, incorrect assessment of pleural effusion, and consolidation. Computed tomography (CT) scan of the chest is the gold standard for the diagnosis of pleural effusion, atelectasis, pneumothorax, lung consolidation, and alveolar-interstitial syndrome. It is also useful for therapeutic procedures in critically ill patients, such as guided drainage of localized empyema, lung abscess, and pneumothorax. However, performing a lung CT scan involves the transfer of a critically ill patient to the CT scanner in the radiology department by a trained doctor. In addition to this, the patients are exposed to substantial radiation,[3] limiting its repeatability. Bedside LUS can easily be performed at the bedside. It can be repeated as and when required and involves no radiation exposure to the patient.

EQUIPMENT

To conduct an LUS examination, a point-of-care ultrasound machine which is easily transportable is required. B-mode (brightness mode) and M-mode (time motion) are used when performing LUS examination.

Probe

- High-frequency probe (7.5–10 MHz) is suitable for detailed examination of chest wall and pleura.
- Curvilinear probe (3–5 MHz) is used to examine deeper structures beneath the pleura **(Figs. 1 and 2)**.
- Microconvex probe (5 MHz), recommended by Lichtenstein et al.,[4] is an ideal single probe for bedside LUS.

The operator should find a good acoustic window in the intercostal space. The probe should be held perpendicular to the skin to obtain a clear image by reducing scattered echoes.

EXAMINATION OF THE LUNG

A complete examination of the lung requires a systematic approach. The patient can be examined satisfactorily in the supine position. One may have to turn the patient in the lateral decubitus position to view the dependent positions of the lung to look for consolidation or pleural effusion commonly seen in this area. For systematic analysis of the

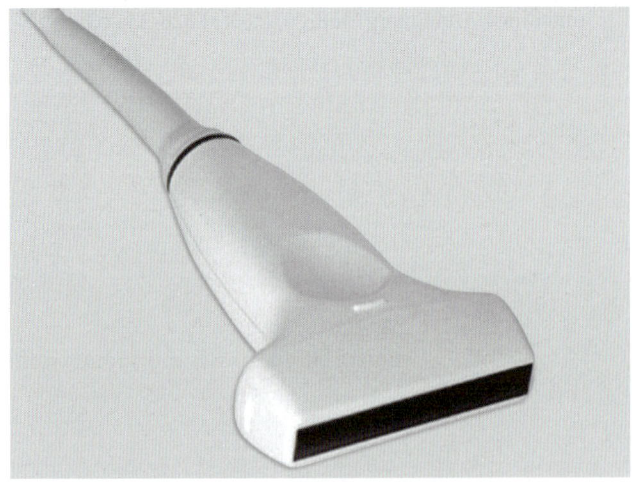

Fig. 1: Linear high-frequency probe.

lung, the chest can be divided into six different regions by using anterior and posterior axillary lines as anatomical landmarks. These two axillary lines divide each lung into upper and lower parts of the anterior, lateral, and posterior

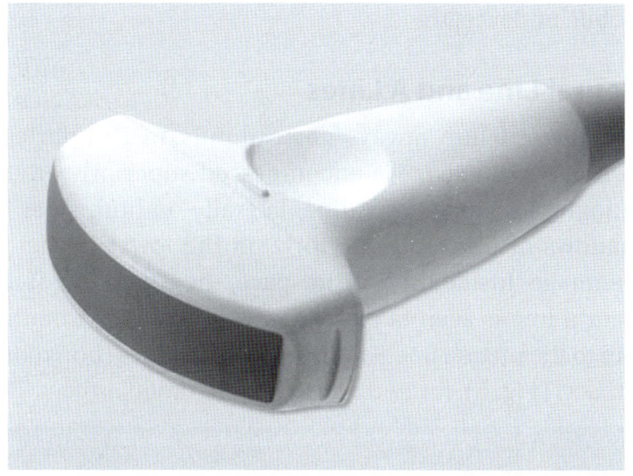

Fig. 2: Curvilinear low-frequency probe.

chest wall **(Fig. 3A)**. The area that cannot be explored by ultrasound is the lung located behind the scapula. The ultrasound examination should cover both lungs just as for auscultation.[5]

Daniel Lichtenstein[6] had described the bedside lung ultrasound in emergency (BLUE) points to standardize the process and to allow reproducible analysis. He has described three points on each side. Two hands are applied to the patient's chest. The little finger of the upper hand should be just below the clavicle, fingertips touching the midline, lower hand just below the upper hand with thumbs excluded. The first point *upper BLUE point* is at the middle of the upper hand. The second point, *lower BLUE point* is at the middle of the lower palm. The third point called the posterolateral alveolar and/or pleural syndrome (PLAPS) point is at the junction of the horizontal line continuing the lower BLUE point and the vertical line continuing the posterior axillary line **(Fig. 3B)**. At this PLAPS point, the user can move the probe

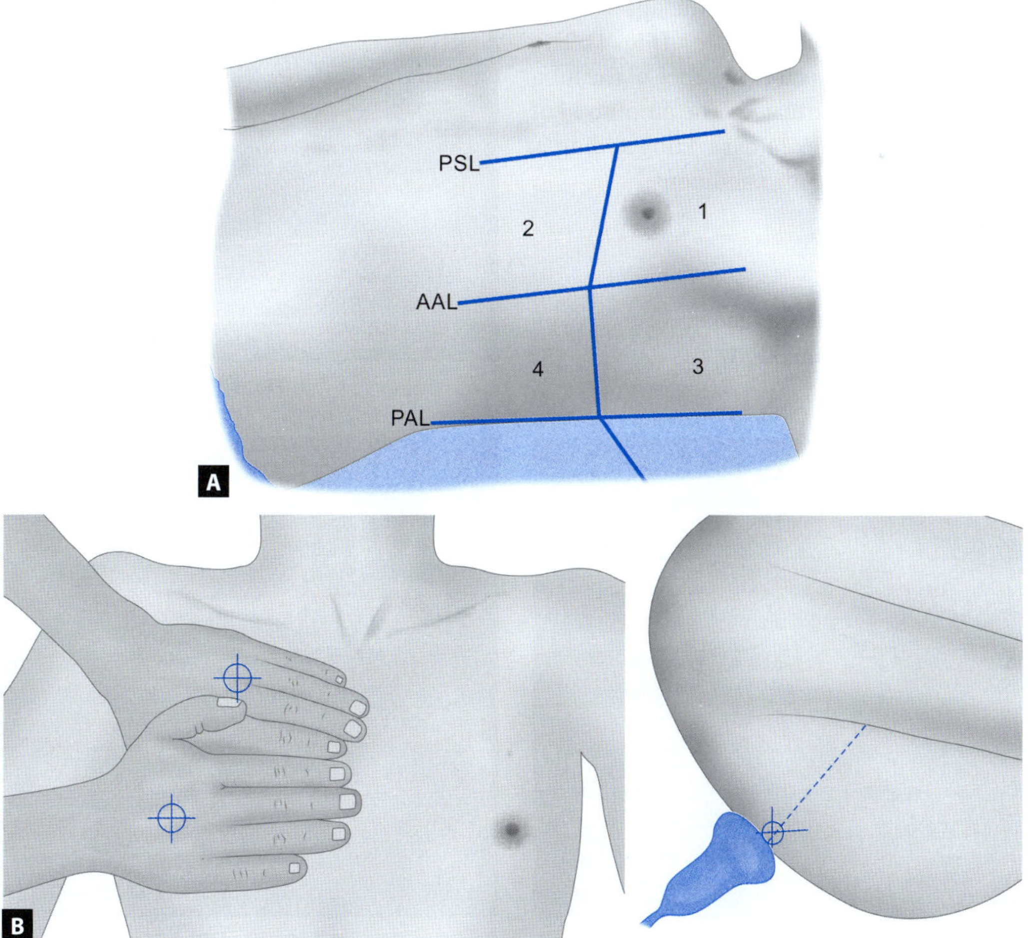

Figs. 3A and B: (A) Six zones; (B) BLUE points. (AAL: anterior axillary line; BLUE: bedside lung ultrasound in emergency; PAL: posterior axillary line; PSL: parasternal line).

posteriorly or downward to look for any pleural effusion or consolidation signs. According to him, these six BLUE points were sufficient for providing 90.5% accuracy of the BLUE protocol.

As ultrasound waves do not travel through the air, it is difficult to examine the lung beyond the pleura. Instead, we see artifacts produced by an interaction between air and fluid-filled lung tissue. This results in specific ultrasound patterns, which are discussed here.

Lung Sliding

In LUS, we usually hold the probe in a position with its marker directed toward the head of the patient and is placed perpendicular to the ribs. With this, we identify the ribs by their posterior shadow. In between two ribs, about 0.5 cm below the rib line, the pleural line is seen as the hyperechoic, sliding line that moves forward and backward with ventilation.[5] This sliding seen is as a result of visceral pleural against the parietal pleura. The sonographic image where you visualize the pleural line between the two rib shadows resembles the appearance of a bat silhouette, hence it is called *Bat sign*[7] **(Fig. 4)**. The presence of lung sliding confirms the presence of the lung which is mobile and getting ventilated. The amplitude of lung sliding decreases from apex to base. Lung sliding is abolished or absent in the following conditions:[8]

- Pneumothorax
- Atelectasis
- Apnea
- Any disorder impairing lung expansion
- Pleurisy, pleurodesis, or pleurectomy
- Inappropriate technique.

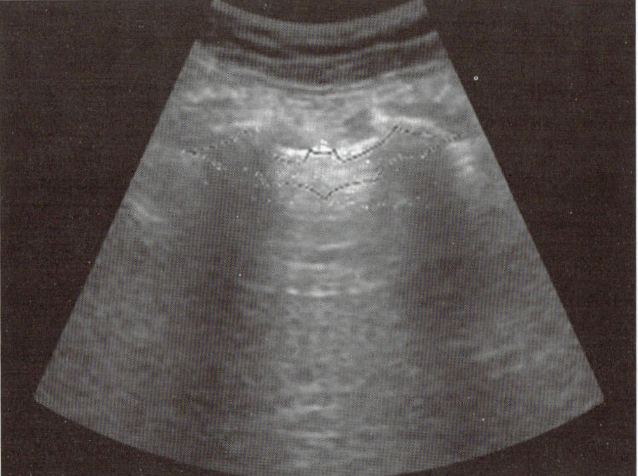

Fig. 4: Bat sign.

If we introduce M-mode here and put a trace in the intercostal space, we see a stratified pattern above the pleural line because of motionless soft tissue. Exactly from the pleural line and below it, the pattern is sandy; hence, it is called *seashore sign*[6] **(Fig. 5)** which confirms the lung is mobile underneath.

Pleural Line and A Lines

The pleural line always corresponds to the parietal pleura. Merlin space is encompassed superiorly on the sonographic image by A line, laterally on both sides by shadows of ribs, and inferiorly on the lower border of the image. Inside the Merlin space, the repetition of the pleural line is seen at a standardized distance from the skin to the pleural line. These are called *A* lines (horizontal artifact) **(Fig. 6)**, formed due to reverberation artifact. The

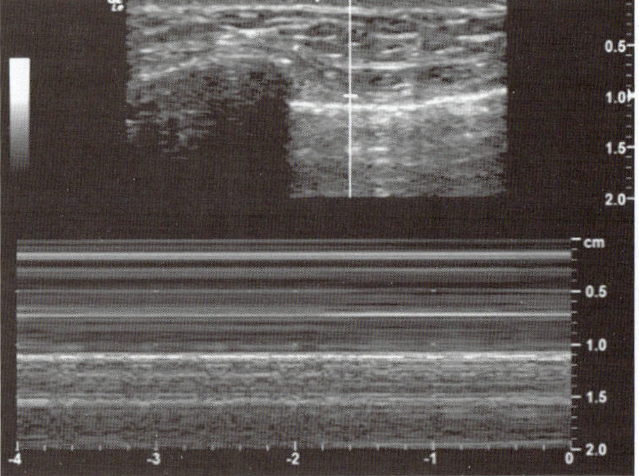

Fig. 5: Seashore sign.

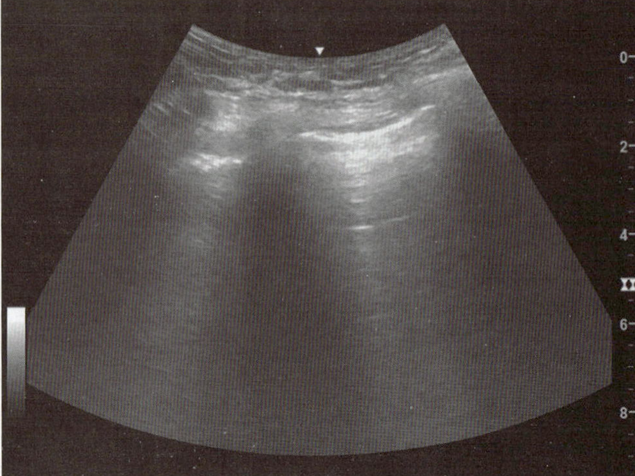

Fig. 6: A lines (horizontal artifact).

presence of A-lines indicates the gas below the pleural line either inside (normal dry lung parenchyma) or outside the lung.[6] A-lines can be complete, traversing across the Merlin space or partially called *O* lines or sometimes invisible. These *O* lines have no pathophysiologic meaning.

B Lines

B lines, now called vertical artifact is a hydroaeric artifacts, and indicate the mingling of fluid and air, having seven characteristic features:

1. A comet tail artifact
2. Arises from the pleural line
3. Always moves with lung sliding
4. Well-defined, laser-like
5. Always long, spreads out without fading to the edge of the screen
6. Always obliterates A lines
7. Always hyperechoic

Ultrasound Interstitial Syndrome

It is seen when there is a loss of lung aeration. This loss of lung aeration leads to the appearance of three or more vertical B lines between two ribs with a loss of A-lines. This is pathological and termed interstitial lung syndrome.[9] This ultrasound pattern is called the B pattern **(Fig. 7)**.

In interstitial syndrome, there is interlobular septal thickening because of increased extravascular lung water in either or both the interstitium or alveolar spaces. The number of vertical B lines has been found to correlate with the degree of aeration loss.[10] Less than three B lines are not consistent with interstitial syndrome. The average distance between two B lines in the septal variant is roughly 6–7 mm. This corresponds to the average size of a lobule. In an adult, between the two ribs, 2 cm of pleural line is visible. It means there is a space for only three or four subpleural interlobular septa. These are called lung rockets when you see more than three B lines in between two ribs. When more than six to seven comet tail artifacts are visible, the distance between each B line is around 3 mm. These ground-glass rockets correlate with CT ground-glass areas.[11]

Pleural Effusion (Quad Sign and Sinusoidal Sign)

The presence of pleural effusion at bases or PLAPS point generates two standard signs, a quad sign, and a sinusoidal sign. It is seen as an anechoic space in the thorax. The presence of echoes in it may be seen in hemothorax, pyothorax, or empyema. We see a pleural line then anechoic space and a line roughly parallel to the pleural line called a lung line, formed by visceral pleura. These two parallel lines (pleural line and lung line) along with two vertical lines formed by shadows of the ribs form a kind of quad. This is called a *quad sign* **(Fig. 8)**.

When the M-mode is placed through the pleural effusion we see a *sinusoidal sign* **(Fig. 9)** formed because of the movement of the lung toward the pleura during inspiration and away from it during expiration. It tells us that the lung is freely moving inside the pleural effusion which is transudative and unloculated. These movements will be reduced in exudative or thick pleural effusion. This sign can be used to calculate the safe distance (15 mm

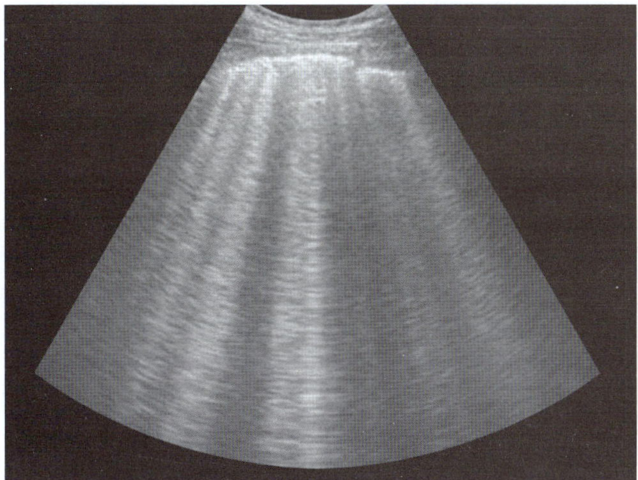

Fig. 7: B lines (vertical artifact).

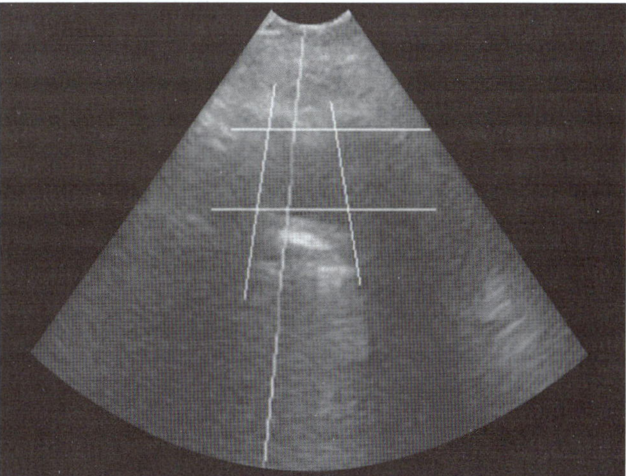

Fig. 8: Quad sign.

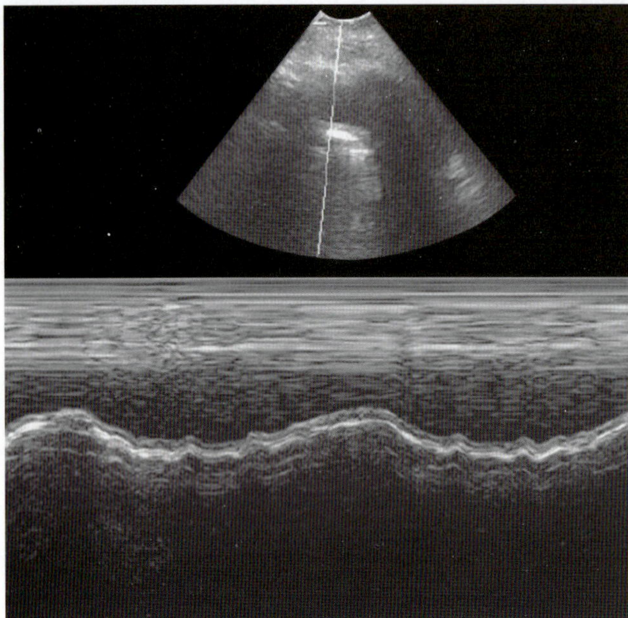

Fig. 9: Sinusoid sign.

minimum during expiration) required for diagnostic and therapeutic procedures.[11]

Consolidation (Shred Sign and Tissue-like Sign)

In consolidation, the air in the alveoli is completely replaced by fluid or inflammatory exudate.

This loss of air allows the transmission of ultrasound through the lung tissue. Subpleural (nonlobar) consolidation ultrasonically appears as poorly defined, wedge-shaped hypoechoic structures, and the deeply seated irregular-shredded boundary between consolidated and aerated lung is called a shred sign.[12] Lobar consolidation appears ultrasonically as a solid organ pattern (image similar to liver/spleen) and is called a tissue-like sign[12] **(Fig. 10)**.

Within the consolidation, air-filled bronchi appear as hyperechoic artifacts within the hypoechoic consolidated lung. This pattern is called an air bronchogram. When an air bronchogram becomes dynamic (movement >1 mm during inspiration), it suggests pneumonia and if static it indicates atelectasis. It has been shown that the dynamic air bronchogram has good specificity (94%), but poor sensitivity (61%) to differentiate pneumonia from atelectasis. In addition, the bronchogram appears as multiple bright dots or branching linear structures in the region of consolidation, whereas it appears as a crowded, parallel running bright line in the region of atelectasis.[13]

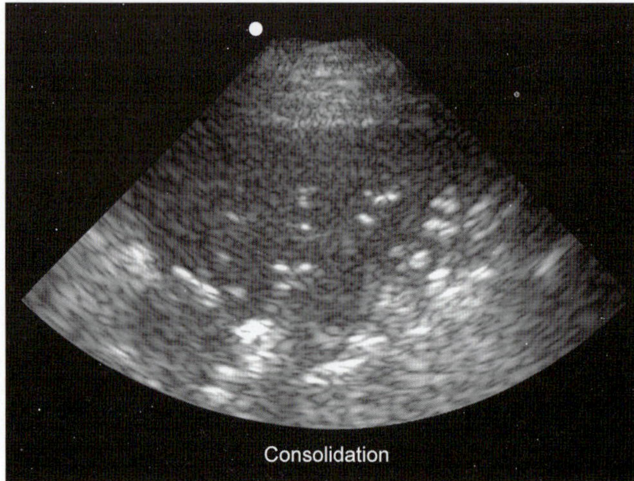

Fig. 10: Tissue-like sign with air bronchogram.

Pneumothorax (Bar Code Sign and Lung Point)

In pneumothorax, the air is present outside the lung parenchyma, between two pleural layers. This is seen as the absent lung sliding on the ultrasound image and the presence of A-lines in the Merlin space. In M-mode ultrasonography, we see a linear pattern in the tissue superficial to the pleural line and a similar linear pattern deep to the pleural line. This is known as the *stratosphere sign* or *barcode sign* **(Fig. 11)**. In the M-mode view, the point where the normal lung pattern (seashore sign) replaces the pneumothorax pattern (stratosphere sign) with inspiration is called the *lung point.* We can even judge the volume of pneumothorax by the position of the lung point. If a lung point is found anteriorly, it is moderate pneumothorax, and a posterior location or absent lung point of it suggests massive pneumothorax.[14] The lung point has a sensitivity of 66%, but specificity of 100%.[14] The lung ultrasound is a better diagnostic tool than a chest X-ray in critically ill patients with suspected pneumothorax.

BLUE PROTOCOL

Lichtenstein et al. have proposed a BLUE protocol for diagnosing the main pathologies causing acute respiratory failure (ARF) (pulmonary edema, pneumothorax, pulmonary consolidation, and pleural effusion), using rapid lung and venous ultrasound.[4] It can be rapidly performed at the bedside. It provides us with step-by-step diagnosis of the main causes of respiratory failure. In this protocol, various signs are combined to form profiles, which are as follows:[11]

- The A profile associate's anterior lung sliding with A-lines.

- The A′-profile is an A-profile with abolished lung-sliding.
- The B-profile associate's anterior lung sliding with lung-rockets.
- The B′-profile is a B-profile with abolished lung-sliding.
- The C-profile indicates anterior lung consolidation regardless of size and number. A thickened, irregular pleural line is an equivalent.

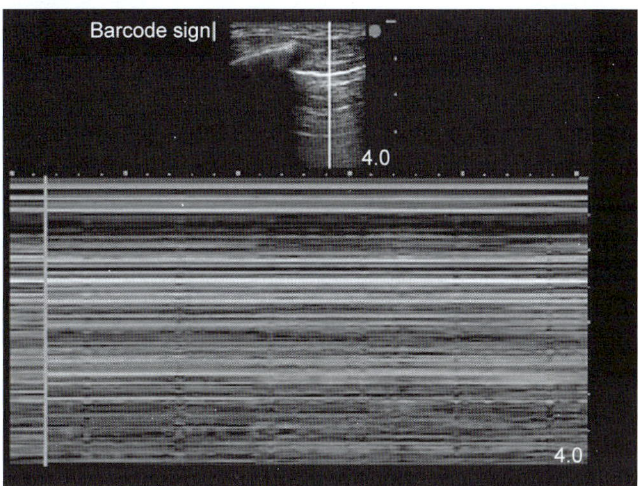

Fig. 11: Barcode or stratosphere sign.

- The A/B profile is a half A-profile at one lung and a half B-profile at another.
- The PLAPS profile designates posterolateral alveolar and/or pleural syndrome.
- A nude profile is A profile without deep vein thrombosis (DVT) or PLAPS.

BLUE ALGORITHM

When the patient is dyspneic and blue, the BLUE protocol is initiated. We check the anterior lung sliding first. The presence of lung sliding rules out pneumothorax in the area examined. After confirming the lung sliding, we seek for A profile or B profile. The presence of the B profile suggests pulmonary edema. B′, A/B and C profiles suggest pneumonia. The presence of A profile prompts the search for venous thrombosis. If present, pulmonary embolism is considered. In the absence of DVT, the PLAPS point is examined. Its presence, i.e., A profile and PLAPS, suggests pneumonia. Only A profile without DVT and PLAPS suggests chronic obstructive pulmonary disease (COPD) and asthma. If the lung sliding is absent, i.e., A′ profile is present then we must look for lung point. A′ profile with lung point is diagnostic of pneumothorax **(Flowchart 1)**.[4]

Flowchart 1: BLUE protocol.

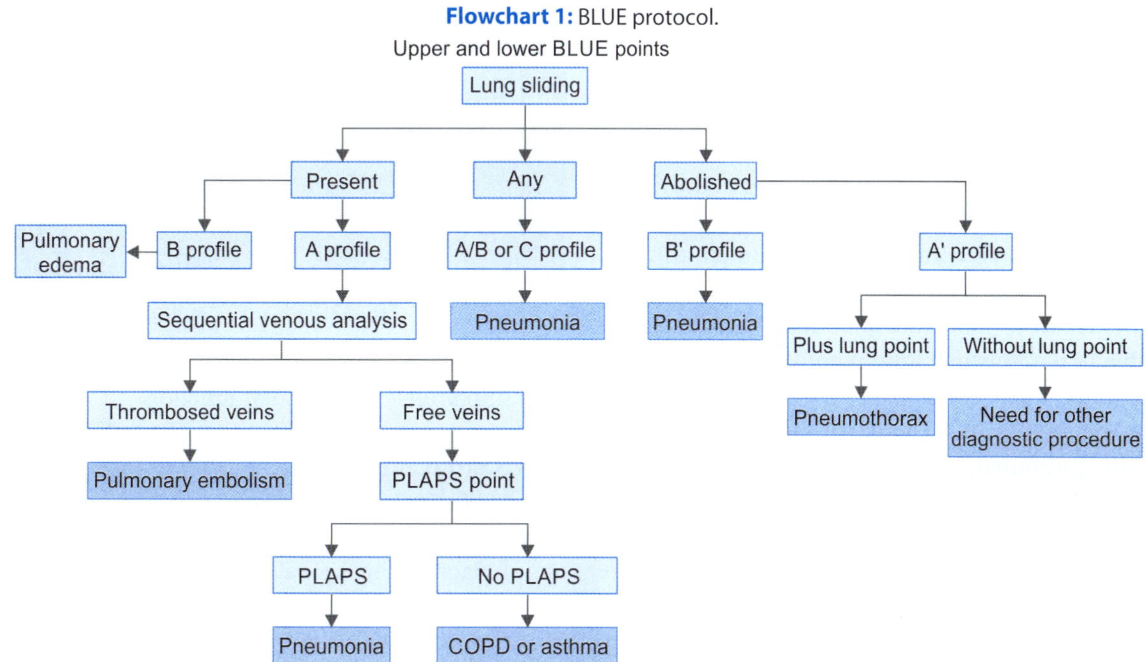

(COPD: chronic obstructive pulmonary disease; PLAPS: posterolateral alveolar and/or pleural syndrome)

FLUID ADMINISTRATION LIMITED BY LUNG SONOGRAPHY PROTOCOL

Fluid administration limited by lung sonography protocol is a helpful tool in dealing with patients with acute circulatory failure. It helps us in knowing the mechanism of shock so that appropriate management can be started. By using ultrasound lung and simple bedside echocardiography, we can rule out the main causes of shock, according to Weil classification. We have seen that ultrasound of the lung is useful and very sensitive in detecting the accumulation of fluid in the lung. A fluid overload or pulmonary edema thickens the interlobular septa. These thickened interlobular septa transmit the ultrasound at its subpleural end generating blue lines. The density or appearance of a number of B lines depends on the severity of pulmonary edema. B lines appear at pulmonary artery occlusion pressure of 18 mm Hg.[15] These B lines erase the A lines which are normally present when the lung is dry in a normovolemic patient **(Box 1)**.

BOX 1: FALLS protocol.

- *Rule out obstructive shock:*
  - *Point-of-care cardiac ultrasound and look for:*
    - Pericardial tamponade
    - Dilatation of right ventricle
  - *BLUE protocol:*
    - Pneumothorax
      - ◊ A' profile with lung point
- *Rule out cardiogenic shock:*
  - *BLUE protocol:*
    - *Pulmonary edema:*
      - ◊ B profile
- *Rule out hypovolemic shock:*
  - *US lung:* A profile
    - Hemodynamic improvement after fluid administration
- *Detecting distributive shock:*
  - No improvement in hemodynamic parameters after fluid therapy
  - Appearance of B profile on US lung (FALLS endpoint)

(FALLS: fluid administration limited by lung sonography; US: ultrasound)

The first step in the FALLS protocol is to look for signs of *obstructive shock*. We use a phased array probe to look at the heart. First, we look for the presence of pericardial effusion in the apical four-chamber view. If it is a large pericardial effusion, look for signs of pericardial tamponade, (1) systolic right atrial inversion, (2) diastolic right ventricular collapse, and (3) plethoric inferior vena cava. In the same view, look for the right atrium and right ventricular enlargement **(Fig. 12)**. If it is difficult to visualize the heart because of a poor cardiac window, a BLUE protocol can be initiated to look for the condition of the lung and inferior vena cava. The next step in the FALLS protocol is for ruling out pneumothorax. The presence of pneumothorax can be confirmed by demonstrating an absence of lung sliding and A lines (A' profile) along with lung point in mild-to-moderate pneumothorax. It may not be possible to demonstrate lung point in case of massive pneumothorax.

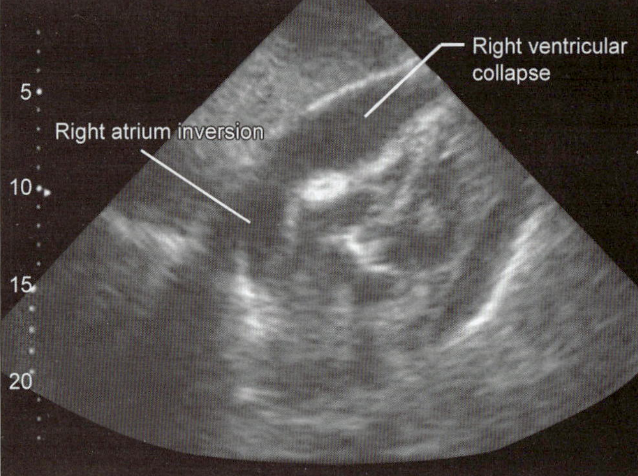

Fig. 12: Pericardial tamponade.

Once the causes of obstructive shock (pericardial tamponade, pulmonary embolism, and pneumothorax) are ruled out, FALLS protocol moves to the next step to look for the US signs of *cardiogenic shock*. On ultrasound lung examination, we would see lung rockets (the presence of three or more lines in one intercostal space) bilaterally, also termed interstitial syndrome. This finding, suggestive of pulmonary edema, is complemented by a demonstration of a hypokinetic heart in the presence of cardiogenic shock. The absence of a B profile rules out pulmonary edema and cardiogenic shock in the presence of unimpaired left ventricular function.

After ruling out obstructive and cardiogenic shocks, FALLS protocol progresses further to look for remaining causes of shock, i.e., *hypovolemic shock* and *distributive shock*. The causes of distributive shock are septic shock, anaphylactic, and spinal shock. The latter two causes are infrequently seen and easy to be diagnosed based on history and clinical examination. The presence of A profile in a shocked patient is considered as a *FALLS responder*. It means we can give fluid to this patient and look for any improvement in cardiac output and blood pressure. If there is no improvement seen after giving volume and B lines, start appearing on the ultrasound lung examination, this step is called the *FALLS endpoint* and fluid therapy should be discontinued. Hypovolemic shock is ruled out if no improvement is seen after fluid therapy. This indicates that the mechanism of shock is distributive, and the position of the heart is now on the flat portion of the Frank–Starling curve. Efforts should be made to bring the heart to an ideal point on the Frank-Starling curve by reducing fluid overload and optimizing blood pressure using vasopressor agents. This is the last step of the FALLS protocol. The main limitation of the FALLS protocol is the presence of B lines on admission. In such a scenario, other criteria (e.g., inferior or superior vena cava variability and cardiac chambers) can be used for fluid administration.

CONCLUSION

Lung ultrasound generates standardized reproducible patterns. It is nearly equivalent to CT in detecting most disorders. It saves time and decreases the need for CT of the chest. CT has its drawbacks like transferring the critically ill patient to a remote location, radiation exposure, cost, cannot being performed repeatedly, and requires keeping the patient in a supine position which may not be possible in some conditions. It helps us in finding out the cause of respiratory failure in >90% of cases. It can be used as a stethoscope in the management of critically ill patients. The advantages of the FALLS protocol are that it is simple, has a steep learning curve, and can be applied at the bedside using a point-of-care ultrasound machine.

REFERENCES

1. Greenbaum DM, Marschall KE. The value of routine daily chest X-rays in intubated patients in the medical intensive care unit. Crit Care Med. 1982;10(1):29-30.
2. Bekemeyer WB, Crapo RO, Calhoon S, Cannon CY, Clayton PD. Efficacy of chest radiography in a respiratory intensive care unit. A prospective study. Chest. 1985;88(5):691-6.
3. Mayo JR, Aldrich J, Muller NL. Radiation exposure at chest CT: a statement of the Fleischner Society. Radiology. 2003;228(1):15-21.
4. Lichtenstein DA, Meziere GA. Relevance of lung ultrasound in the diagnosis of acute respiratory failure: The BLUE protocol. Chest. 2008;134(1):117-25.
5. Bouhemad B, Zhang M, Lu Q, Rouby JJ. Clinical review: Bedside lung ultrasound in critical care practice. Crit Care. 2007;11(1):205.
6. Lichtenstein D. BLUE-protocol and FALLS-protocol: two applications of lung ultrasound in the critically ill. Chest. 2015;147(6):1659-70.
7. Lichtenstein DA, Meziere G, Lascols N, Biderman P, Courret JP, Gepner A, et al. Ultrasound diagnosis of occult pneumothorax. Crit Care Med. 2005;33(6):1231-8.
8. In: Lichtenstein D (Ed). General Ultrasound in the Critically Ill. Berlin Heidelberg: Springer-Verlag; 2002. pp. 108-9.
9. Volpicelli G, Elbarbary M, Blaivas M, Lichtenstein DA, Mathis G, Kirkpatrick AW, et al. International evidence-based recommendations for point-of-care lung ultrasound. Intens Care Med. 2012;38(4):577-91.
10. Lichtenstein D, Meziere G, Biderman P, Gepner A, Barré O. The comet-tail artifact. An ultrasound sign of alveolar-interstitial syndrome. Am J Respir Crit Care Med. 1997;156(5):1640-6.
11. In: Lichtenstein D (Ed). Lung Ultrasound in the critically Ill. Berlin Heidelberg: Springer-Verlag; 2016. pp. 87-91.
12. Lichtenstein DA, Lascols N, Meziere G, Gepner A. Ultrasound diagnosis of alveolar consolidation in the critically ill. Intens Care Med. 2004;30(2):276-81.
13. Lichtenstein D, Meziere G, Seitz J. The dynamic air bronchogram. A lung ultrasound sign of alveolar consolidation ruling out atelectasis. Chest. 2009;135(6):1421-5.
14. Lichtenstein D, Meziere G, Biderman P, Gepner A. The "lung point": An ultrasound sign specific to pneumothorax. Intens Care Med. 2000;26(10):1434-40.
15. Lichtenstein D, Meziere G, Lagoueyte JF, Lagoueyte JF, Biderman P, Goldstein I, et al. A-lines and B-lines: Lung ultrasound as a bedside tool for predicting pulmonary artery occlusion pressure in the critically ill. Chest. 2009;136(4):1014-20.

CHAPTER

Ultrasound and Echocardiography-guided Resuscitation in a Patient with Shock and Cardiopulmonary Arrest

Amol Trimbakrao Kothekar, Anand Vinaykumar Joshi, Vijaya Prakash Patil

"Time is not the main thing. It is the only thing."

—**Miles Davis**

INTRODUCTION

Shock is a life-threatening condition characterized by acute circulatory failure, which leads to inadequate delivery of oxygen to meet tissue demands, ultimately resulting in cellular dysfunction and death. Shock is diagnosed based on clinical and biochemical criteria. In the previous chapter, we discussed how bedside echocardiography aids in the early differentiation of the etiology of shock. In this chapter, we will explore how bedside echocardiography assists in monitoring and titration of therapy during resuscitation.

Resuscitation is a series of timely efforts aimed at the immediate normalization of life-threatening cardiovascular derangements and the restoration of organ perfusion to prevent multiorgan failure and death. Interventions during resuscitation focus on optimizing cardiac preload, contractility, and afterload, with the ultimate goal of normalizing tissue perfusion, as indicated by clinical parameters (mentation, temperature differences, capillary refill, and urine output) and biochemical parameters [such as lactate levels, central venous oxygen saturation ($ScvO_2$), or the partial pressure of carbon dioxide (pCO_2) gap].

Echocardiography can help guide resuscitation by assessing preload and contractility. Historically, a pulmonary artery (PA) catheter was used to monitor these resuscitation parameters. Currently, echocardiography and lesser invasive cardiac output monitors have taken the place of PA catheters. Less invasive cardiac output monitors require setup, expertise, and time for catheter insertion. Echocardiography on the other hand is noninvasive, can be repeated frequently, and provides similar information within minutes. In addition, it also provides valuable insight into the underlying pathology [e.g. hemoperitoneum, myocardial infarction, pulmonary embolism (PE)]. Echocardiography is proposed as the first-line evaluation modality in shock for early differentiation of the types of shock and etiology.[1]

The first part of this chapter discusses echocardiography-guided resuscitation in shock and hemodynamically unstable patients. The second part addresses the role of echocardiography in cardiopulmonary resuscitation (CPR).

ECHOCARDIOGRAPHY FOR RESUSCITATION IN SHOCK OR HEMODYNAMIC INSTABILITY

Echocardiography can be utilized as a resuscitation tool to assess volume status or preload, evaluate cardiac function, and predict fluid responsiveness.

Echocardiography for Measurement of Volume Status or Preload

Preload is defined as the ventricular wall stress at the end of diastole determined by ventricular end-diastolic volume, wall thickness, and end-diastolic pressure. Pulmonary capillary wedge pressure (PCWP) and central venous pressure (CVP) provide the pressure indices of preload. Besides echocardiography, vena cava (inferior and superior) measurements and their respiratory variation are being increasingly used for the assessment of preload. Additionally, the direct measurement of left ventricular end-diastolic area (LVEDA) by echocardiography can also be used as a surrogate of left ventricular (LV) end-diastolic volume and preload.

Inferior Vena Cava Diameter and Its Respiratory Variation

Physiology

The inferior vena cava (IVC) is in a direct continuum with the right atrium (RA) and its intraluminal pressure is a direct reflection of the CVP. The size of IVC depends on the difference between two pressures: the intraluminal pressure (i.e., CVP) and the extraluminal pressure which is the intra-abdominal pressure (IAP).[2] Physiologically, IVC diameter is a function of IVC transmural pressure (IVC_{tp} = CVP – IAP). Hence, in the absence of raised IAP, IVC diameter reflects CVP or right atrial filling pressure.

Respiratory variation of IVC diameter is a function of change in IVC transmural pressure (δIVC_{tp}) and compliance of IVC. Greater variation of IVC diameter can be observed with larger changes in pleural and abdominal pressures. In spontaneous respiration, a larger collapse in IVC diameter can be observed with high inspiratory efforts due to the creation of very high negative pleural pressures. Gignon et al. have observed a significant correlation between diaphragmatic motions and the collapsibility index of inferior vena cava (cIVC) in 52 spontaneously breathing healthy volunteers (r = 0.64).[3] One of the common methods of demonstrating inspiratory collapse in IVC is the sniff test. In controlled ventilation, higher tidal volumes would result in larger distensions in IVC diameter when compared with lower tidal volumes.

Inferior vena cava being a highly compliant structure would distend proportional to the transmural pressure (IVC_{tp}) at smaller volumes. Patients with small and variable IVC can be assumed to be hypovolemic and more likely to be fluid-responsive. At increasing IVC size, compliance of IVC may fall limiting change in IVC diameter. Hence, at higher IVC diameters (higher CVP), further change in CVP may not cause a major change in the IVC diameter. However, the response to volume expansion in these patients will depend on the position of the left ventricle on the Frank–Starling curve.

For the reasons described previously, the respiratory variation of IVC is more likely a reflection of changes in CVP and IAP with respiration, rather than a dynamic index of changes in LV stroke volume (SV) in response to preload.

Techniques of Measurement

The inferior vena cava is visualized using a cardiac or abdominal probe via the subcostal window **(Fig. 1)**. Long-axis (LA) view is preferred over the short-axis (SA) due to higher interobserver reliability.[4] In patients where the subcostal window is inaccessible due to surgical incisions or when a poor subcostal view is caused by bowel gas, the right lateral transabdominal coronal LA (also known as rescue view or transhepatic view) can be helpful **(Fig. 2)**.[4]

The diameter of IVC is commonly measured either close to its entrance to the RA or 1–2 cm caudal to the hepatic vein opening.[5] Measurement of IVC diameter and its respiratory variation can be performed using either M-mode or B-mode. M-mode is commonly used due to its simplicity; however, it has poor interobserver reliability.[4]

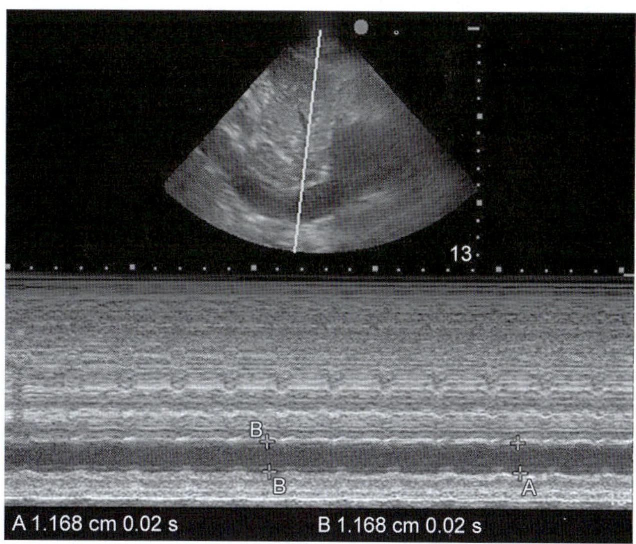

Fig. 1: Measurement of inferior vena cava (IVC) diameter and variability in subcostal view using M-mode.

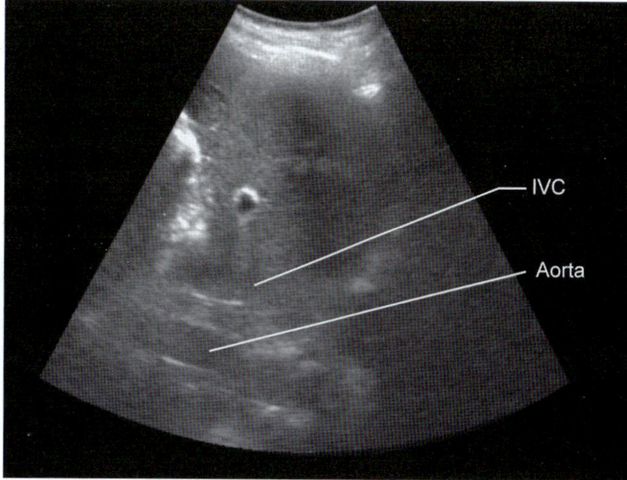

Fig. 2: Measurement of inferior vena cava (IVC) diameter in transhepatic view.

During spontaneous respiration, the magnitude of IVC collapse, known as IVC collapsibility index (IVCc), can be calculated as follows:

IVC collapsibility index (IVCc) = Dmax – Dmin/Dmax.

During controlled mechanical ventilation, IVC distension can be quantified by either IVC distensibility index (dIVC) or delta IVC (ΔIVC) as follows:

Distensibility index (dIVC)
= Dmax – Dmin/Dmin (threshold value of 18%)
Delta IVC (ΔIVC)
= Dmax – Dmin/Dmean (threshold value of 12%)

Evidence

Spontaneous respiration: Airapetian et al. tested the utility of IVC collapsibility in 59 spontaneously breathing patients demonstrating 31% sensitivity and 97% specificity of cIVC >42% for predicting fluid responsiveness.[6] However, further studies in heterogeneous emergency department (ED) patient populations and in spontaneously breathing patients with septic shock, have yielded mixed results.[7,8] A recent pooled analysis of seven studies with 330 spontaneously breathing patients demonstrated 80% sensitivity and 79% specificity with an area-under-the-curve (AUC) of 0.857.[9]

Controlled ventilation: Earlier studies in 2004 by Barbier et al.[10] (dIVC >18%) and Feissel et al.[11] (ΔIVC >12%) have shown a good correlation with fluid responsiveness with positive pressure ventilation using tidal volumes of ≥8 mL/kg. A further study with tidal volumes of 8–10 mL/kg in patients with septic shock showed poor sensitivity (38%) and specificity (61%) with receiver operating characteristics (ROC) AUC of 0.43.[12] A meta-analysis has demonstrated 77% pooled sensitivity and 85% pooled specificity of dIVC >15% in predicting fluid responsiveness.[13] A recent pooled analysis of 13 studies involving 431 mechanically ventilated patients demonstrated 79% sensitivity and 70% specificity with an AUC of 0.75.[9]

Advantages

- Inferior vena cava measurements provide a quick, noninvasive estimation of CVP and volume status **(Table 1)**.[14,15]
- The view for IVC measurement can be easily obtained in most of the patients.

TABLE 1: Correlation of IVC diameter and respiratory variation with CVP.

CVP	IVC diameter[15]	IVC collapsibility index in spontaneously breathing patients[14]
<10	<2 cm	≥50%
>10	≥2 cm	<50%

(CVP: central venous pressure; IVC: inferior vena cava)

- Inferior vena cava measurements require minimum setup compared to actual CVP measurements and repeated measurements also can be done easily.
- Serial measurements of IVC can provide an idea of change in preload status with fluid therapy. Failure of IVC diameter increase in response to adequate fluid therapy or decrease in IVC size should raise suspicion of ongoing losses, such as concealed hemorrhage and third space loss.

Limitations

- Inferior vena cava diameter per se reflects CVP and hence suffers from all the limitations of CVP, which is a static parameter. It is inferior to dynamic indices for the prediction of fluid responsiveness **(Table 2)**. Respiratory variation of IVC has poor sensitivity in identifying fluid-responsive patients. Even the most sensitive cutoff of IVC distensibility will miss one-fourth of the fluid-responsive patients!
- Inferior vena cava diameter cannot provide information about LV preload in the conditions associated with high CVP such as cardiac tamponade, right ventricular failure (RVF), etc.
- Raised IAP can reduce IVC diameter even in the presence of euvolemia or hypervolemia. Therefore, caution should be exercised for the use of IVC diameter for estimation of volume status in these patients.
- Inferior vena cava measurements are highly operator dependent. There is a moderate correlation between ultrasonographic examinations of IVC diameters among the observers (coefficient of correlation κ = 0.56–0.60).[16] Interobserver reliability is poorer with the use of M-mode for IVC measurements.[4]
- There is no consensus on the optimal site and method of measurement. Both LA and SA have been used by researchers.[17] It is generally advised to measure IVC near the heart close to the junction of the hepatic vein. However, measurements at this site in the presence of a saber profile of IVC (bulge near its junction with

hepatic veins) may provide a false sense of normal volume status even in the presence of hypovolemia.[18]

- Relative movement between the transducer probe and IVC due to respiratory mechanics as well as operator drift can result in pseudovariability or *pseudocollapse* of IVC.[17] Blehar et al. have demonstrated 21.7 mm of caudal and 3.9 mm of lateral movement of the IVC during quiet respiration in the subgroup of patients presenting to the ED without acute distress.[17] This would result in an error in the measurement of respiratory variation in SA and LA, respectively. These translational artifacts during inspiration may be incorrectly interpreted as IVC variation.

Summary

- Inferior vena cava diameter and its variation with respiration correlate very well with the CVP **(Table 1)**. In the presence of shock with small and variable IVC, one can safely assume that the patient is likely to be hypovolemic and fluid-responsive. Hence, the presence of small and variable IVC can be reliable in predicting fluid responsiveness. IVC measurement can be done very quickly unlike other cardiac monitors.
- A higher CVP value or a large IVC without respiratory variation might rule out gross hypovolemia; however, they are a poor predictor of fluid responsiveness. In such situations, fluid boluses can be given if the patient is fluid-responsive as demonstrated by other means **(Table 2)**. However, these fluid boluses should be given with caution as large IVC without respiratory variations suggest less compliant IVC, and such patients may be at increased risk of getting fluid overloaded.

Superior Vena Cava Diameter and Respiratory Variation

Physiology

Respiratory variations of superior vena cava (SVC) are exactly opposite of IVC since SVC is an intrathoracic structure and IVC is an extrathoracic structure. During spontaneous respiration, negative intrathoracic pressure increases the size of SVC. During controlled ventilation, positive intrathoracic pressure causes the collapse of SVC.

Techniques of Measurement

Superior vena cava measurements require transesophageal echocardiography (TEE). SVC size and its variation can be quantified like IVC measurements.

Evidence

Vieillard-Baron et al. have demonstrated excellent sensitivity (90%) and specificity (100%) of superior vena cava collapsibility (threshold 36%), in 66 patients getting ventilated with tidal volumes of 8 ± 2 mL/kg.[19] Vignon et al. have demonstrated greater diagnostic accuracy with respiratory variations of SVC diameter (ΔSVC >21%) compared with ΔIVC ≥13% (AUC 0.742 vs. 0.653) in 540 mechanical ventilated patients.[20]

Advantages

- Operator drift error is eliminated in SVC measurement as TEE is used for measurements.
- Based on limited studies, ΔSVC appears to be more accurate than ΔIVC.[20]

TABLE 2: Integrated hemodynamic management plan in clinical situations based on presence or absence of shock or hypovolemia. Shock is diagnosed based on clinical and or biochemical criteria. Hypovolemia or fluid responsiveness can be identified by presence of small IVC (diameter *<1.6–2 cm*) and its respiratory variation *(>40% collapse in spontaneous respiration or >12% distension in controlled ventilation)*.

	Hypovolemia or fluid responsiveness present	***Hypovolemia or fluid responsiveness absent***
Shock present	Fluid boluses are indicated	Patient is at increased risk for fluid overload and pulmonary edema with fluid boluses (low tolerability to fluid boluses) • In the absence of fluid responsiveness, these patients should not receive fluid boluses • Dynamic indices, e.g., LVOT VTI, carotid V-max, PPV, SVV, PLR, etc. should be used for predicting fluid responsiveness • If fluid responsiveness is present, fluids are indicated Monitoring B lines on lung ultrasound can help in the early identification of pulmonary edema
Shock absent	Fluid boluses are not indicated	Fluid restriction ± diuretics may be tried depending on clinical not situation

Limitations

- The measurement of SVC is invasive and needs TEE. Hence, these measurements cannot be obtained easily and quickly compared to IVC measurements.
- Physiologically, SVC variations reflect changes in CVP and intrathoracic pressure. The superiority of SVC variability over IVC variability for predicting fluid responsiveness is backed by limited evidence.

Left Ventricular End-diastolic Area

Physiology

The LVEDA is directly proportional to the LV ventricular end-diastolic volume, one of the indicators of LV preload.

Techniques of Measurement

The LVEDA is measured at a midpapillary level in a parasternal short-axis (PSAX) view. Readers should note that papillary muscles should be included in the LVEDA calculation **(Fig. 3)**. Alternatively, parasternal long-axis view (PLAX) or apical four-chamber view (A4C) can be used for the calculation of ventricular size.

Interpretation of Measurement

The presence of *kissing papillary muscle sign*, in PSAX view generally indicates severe hypovolemia. Significant hypovolemia is likely if the PSAX LVEDA is <10 cm^2 or the LVEDA index [LVEDA/body surface area (BSA)] is <5.5 cm/m^2. The normal range of left ventricular end-diastolic area index (LVEDAI) is between 8 and 12 cm/m.[21,22] Conversely, patients with PSAX LVEDA of >20 cm^2 are likely to have volume overload. However, there are no clear-cut thresholds that can reliably predict fluid responsiveness due to the overlap in values observed in published studies.[5]

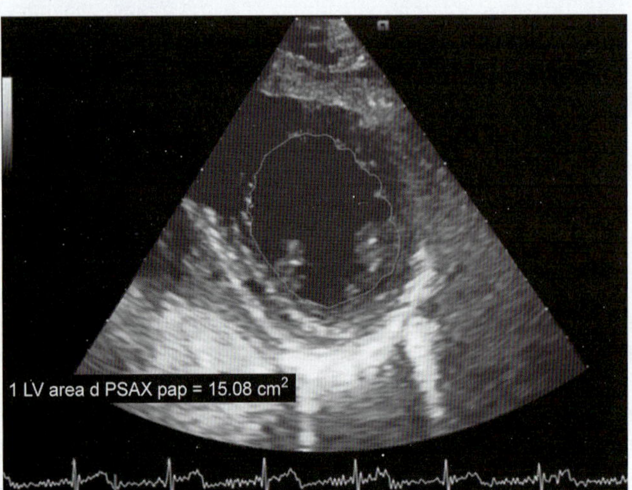

Fig. 3: Measurement of left ventricular end-diastolic area (LVEDA).

Evidence

The LVEDA can be indexed to the BSA similar to the other cardiac parameters. Marik et al., demonstrated ROC AUC of 0.64 in a meta-analysis of five studies examining LVEDAI indicating a poor predictive value.[23]

Advantages

- It provides a direct volume estimate of preload.
- It is not influenced by intrathoracic pressure or IAP where CVP and IVC may be unreliable.

Limitations

- A good acoustic window is required for its assessment.
- There can be individual variation in the calculation of LVEDA.
- LVEDA can be unreliable in patients with severe concentric LV hypertrophy as they can have low LVEDA in the absence of hypovolemia.
- LVEDA is a static marker of preload. LVEDA has failed to predict fluid responsiveness.
- LVEDA is not a reliable indicator of fluid responsiveness in patients.[11,24] Respiratory variations of the internal jugular vein (IJV) diameter during mechanical ventilation at the level of the cricoid cartilage are studied in patients with sepsis and also after cardiac surgery.[25,26] IJV is easily collapsable with slight pressure creating a possibility of error. Respiratory variations of IJV are not routinely used.

ECHOCARDIOGRAPHY FOR ASSESSMENT OF CARDIAC FUNCTION

Cardiac function is assessed either through cardiac output measurements or by measuring LV contractility. LV contractility can be estimated using visual assessment (eyeballing) or by measurement of calculating the area of the ventricular cavity during systole and diastole.

Stroke Volume and Cardiac Output Calculation

Techniques of Measurement

The apical five-chamber view is obtained, and a pulsed-wave Doppler (PWD) gate is placed on the ventricular

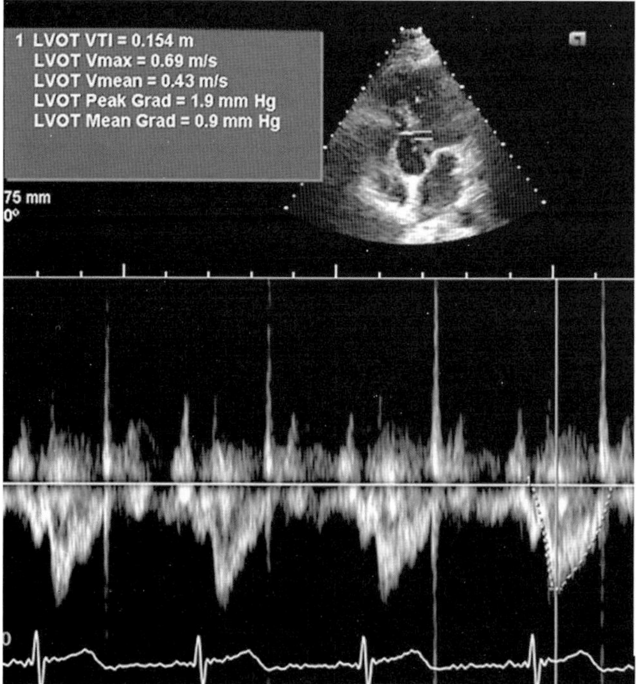

Fig. 4: Measurement of LVOT VTI. Note the presence of a closing click after LV ejection. (LV: left ventricular; LVOT VTI: left ventricular outflow tract velocity time integral)

side of the LVOT, ensuring the ultrasound beam is parallel to the flow through the LVOT. A PWD trace is obtained, and the LVOT ejection waveform is identified below the baseline by the presence of a closing click. Using cardiac measurement software, this waveform is traced to calculate the VTI.

Stroke volume can be calculated by the following formula:[27]

Stroke Volume (SV) = LVOT area × LVOT VTI

Where; LVOT = left ventricular outflow tract, VTI = velocity time integral

Care should be taken to put the sample volume exactly in the LVOT and not in the aorta. This can be identified by the presence of a closing click just after the systolic ejection and the absence of an opening click **(Fig. 4)**. The placement of sample volume in the aorta will provide an inaccurately higher measurement. Secondly, pulse-wave Doppler should be used for measurement as continuous wave Doppler (CWD) would be inaccurate due to the absence of spatial orientation. Doppler should be set for a moderate speed (50–75 mm/s) to allow reliable measurements of VTI.[5]

Left ventricular outflow tract diameter remains fairly constant in a given patient allowing serial measurements of LVOT VTI to serve as a surrogate for changes in cardiac output for LVOT VTI measurement, the operator can trace the ejection graph **(Fig. 4)**. Newer machines can automate this process, reducing human error. Peak aortic flow (Vmax) at LVOT is easy to calculate and can be used instead of VTI for monitoring changes in cardiac output.

Advantages

- It is completely noninvasive.
- It provides a quick assessment of cardiac output in minutes.
- *Absolute LVOT VTI value:* The use of VTI has been extensively used in the rapid ultrasound in shock scanning (RUSH) protocol (discussed further). The reported reference range of LVOT VTI in the healthy population is 18–22 cm for heart rates (HRs) between 55 and 95 beats/min. RUSH VTI protocol targets LVOT VTI > 18 cm. Lower values in the range of 9.5 cm are reported in cardiogenic shock and higher values in the range of 30 cm are reported in septic shock.[27]

Limitations

- Errors in measuring LVOT diameter can be squared in SV calculation, leading to larger inaccuracies.
- Errors in the measurement of VTI can occur due to angulation between the ultrasound beam and the blood flow at LVOT.
- Measurement of cardiac output by echocardiography is not accurate compared with the gold standard (PA catheter) due to errors in calculations of LVOT diameter and VTI.
- Exact calculation of cardiac output with echocardiography is time-consuming and repeated measurements may not be practical.
- *Left ventricular outflow tract obstruction*: In the case of dynamic LVOT obstruction, very high velocities are created in late systole. These velocities exceed the limit of pulse-wave Doppler imaging due to aliasing. Even though continuous wave (CW) Doppler can be used to measure higher velocities, it does not provide accurate measurements due to a lack of spatial resolution.
- The presence of a pathologic LVOT gradient precludes the use of LVOT VTI as a surrogate. Pathologic LVOT gradient can be observed in asymmetric LV septal

hypertrophy, anterior myocardial infarctions with severe hypovolemia, and high inotropic support stimulation in the presence of compensatory hyperdynamic basal segments of the interventricular septum.[27]

- *Aortic regurgitation:* LVOT VTI will not accurately represent forward SV in the presence of moderate-to-severe aortic regurgitation with significant regurgitation volume.
- Echocardiography is not sensitive to identify small changes in the SV. The minimum change in VTI that can be reliably picked up by the single operators is 11% and with different operators, changes <14% may not be accurately identified.[28] Hence, echocardiography is not the ideal monitor of cardiac output measurement during tests of fluid responsiveness such as end-expiratory occlusion (EEO) test and mini fluid challenge that mandate precise detection of small (<10%) changes in cardiac output. These tests are described elsewhere in the textbook.

Summary

The measurement of cardiac output by echocardiography is tedious and not accurate compared with invasive cardiac output monitors. However, it provides a quick and noninvasive estimation of cardiac output. Serial values of LVOT VTI carry more value than a single absolute value. Echocardiography has limited detection of smaller (<11–14%) changes in cardiac output.

Left Ventricular Systolic Function (Contractility) Assessment

Gross Assessment or Eyeballing

Techniques of measurement: Gross categorization of LV systolic function into good, moderate, or poor LV function is done by assessment of the movement of the endocardial border, thickening of the myocardium, movement of the tricuspid annulus, and change in geometry of the ventricle.[29] Use of more than one view can improve the accuracy of estimation. PSAX view at the level of papillary muscle can provide an assessment of LV contractility and regional wall motion abnormality (RWMA). It can also identify severe hypovolemia (kissing papillary muscle sign) pericardial effusion or right ventricle (RV) dilatation.

Advantage: It provides a quick assessment with minimal training.

Eyeballing provides crude but clinically relevant information as management in critically ill patients would not change with minute changes in ejection fraction (EF).

Limitations: It is observer-dependent. It is prone to errors if endocardial borders are not well defined. Dyssynchronous motion (e.g., RWMAs) can make integration of information from several views difficult.

Measurement of Ejection Fraction

Most of the modern ultrasonography (USG) machines have incorporated calculations for EF calculation. The Simpson method is widely followed wherein the A4C view, the volume of the ventricle is calculated during systole and diastole, and EF is calculated. Detailed techniques for EF measurement are beyond the scope of this chapter.

Advantage: It can be used to monitor the response to inotropic therapy.

Limitation:

- Precise measurement of EF is time-consuming. In clinical practice, obtaining exact values during resuscitation is often unnecessary. Categorizing of LV systolic function as good, moderate, or poor is usually sufficient for management during resuscitation.
- The value of EF should be interpreted with caution, as it is a load-dependent variable. The absolute value of EF depends on both LV systolic function and LV afterload.[30] A poorly functioning LV can have a normal value of LVEF in the presence of severe mitral regurgitation (MR) or profound vasoplegia in septic shock. The use of norepinephrine for septic shock is known to unmask global LV hypokinesia with an EF of <45%.[31]
- EF calculation is prone to error due to human factors. EF calculation is inferior to LV global longitudinal peak strain (GLPS) in terms of user dependence and reproducibility.[32]

PREDICTION OF FLUID RESPONSIVENESS USING ECHOCARDIOGRAPHY

Respiratory Variation of Velocity Time Integral or Vmax

Physiology

Stroke volume variation (SVV) is a dynamic index that utilizes the heart-lung interactions to predict fluid responsiveness. LVOT and aortic VTI or Vmax can be used as surrogates of SV. Like SVV, these measures can be used only in patients getting mechanically ventilated with tidal volumes of at least 8 mL/kg and not having arrhythmias or raised abdominal pressure.[33]

Evidence

Respiratory variations in VTI >20% or peak aortic flow (Vmax) >12% predict fluid responsiveness. Feissel et al. have demonstrated that the respiratory variation in the peak velocity (Vpeak) of aortic blood flow accurately identifies patients who are fluid responders.[34] Delta Vpeak threshold value of 12% allowed discrimination between responders and nonresponders with a sensitivity of 100% and a specificity of 89%.

Advantages

It provides a quick and completely noninvasive dynamic index of fluid responsiveness.

Limitations

- *Technical problem:* A good acoustic window and a skilled hand are mandatory for LVOT VTI measurement.
- *Respiratory variation validation:* Respiratory variation in LVOT VTI has limitations similar to the other dynamic parameters of fluid responsiveness like pulse pressure variation (PPV) or SVV. These parameters are validated mainly in patients getting mechanically ventilated with higher tidal volumes (8 mL/kg). There is limited data on patients ventilated with low tidal volumes. Respiratory variation in LVOT VTI is unreliable in patients breathing spontaneously or having arrhythmias.
- *Right ventricle failure:* Caution should be exercised in patients with RVF. Respiratory variations in VTI in this group of patients indicate failing RV rather than fluid responsiveness.[35]

Summary

Respiratory variation of VTI or Vmax can be used such as SVV and PPV for predicting fluid responsiveness in mechanically ventilated patients.

Carotid Artery Velocity Time Integral/Vmax

Physiology

A portion of the SV passing through LVOT reaches the carotid artery. An increase in SV results in increased blood flow through the carotid artery, which can be measured by carotid VTI. Carotid VTI can be used as an alternative to LVOT VTI for surrogate measurements of SV.

Techniques of Measurement

A longitudinal view of the common carotid artery is obtained. The pulsed Doppler sample volume is positioned at the center of the vessel, at 2 cm from the bifurcation, using an angle correction of no. >60° **(Fig. 5)**.

Advantage

Measurement of carotid VTI can be easily performed in most of the patients with a poor cardiac acoustic window, where LVOT VTI cannot be calculated.

Evidence

Estrada et al. have studied respiratory variation in carotid Doppler peak systolic velocity (ΔCDPV) in 19 patients receiving controlled mechanical ventilation with tidal volumes at 6 mL/kg of predicted body weight.[36] ΔCDPV >14% predicted volume responsiveness with 86% sensitivity and specificity (ROC AUC 0.86). In their study, 40% of patients had poor acoustic windows, precluding LVOT VTI measurements. IVC diameter and its respiratory variation (ΔD – IVC) were poor predictors of fluid responsiveness, with ROC AUC 0.52 and 0.54, respectively.

Limitations

Left ventricular outflow tract diameter remains constant over time in a patient; however, the carotid artery diameter

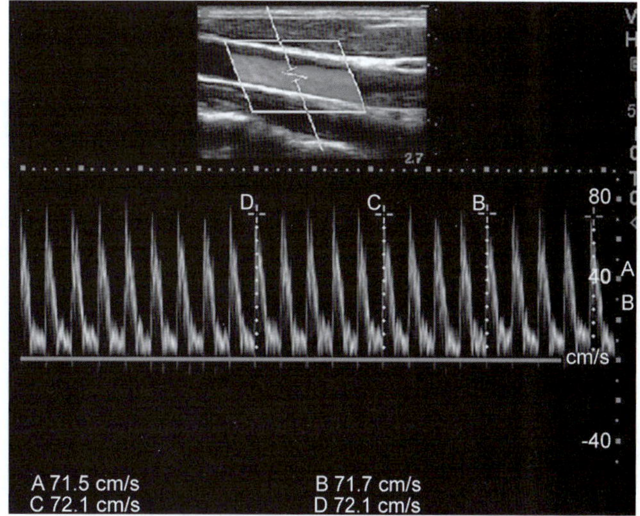

Fig. 5: Measurement of carotid artery VTI/Vmax. (Vmax: variations of maximal velocity; VTI: velocity time integral)

can increase in response to an increase in flow (flow-mediated vasodilatation). This is a significant limitation for the use of carotid VTI as a surrogate for SV. Carotid VTI may track changes in SV in the subset of critically ill septic patients with endothelial dysfunction due to impaired flow-mediated vasodilatation.[37]

Some low-end USG machines do not have software for VTI calculation with a linear probe. These machines provide Vmax instead.

Another limitation of carotid VTI is the orientation of blood flow in relation to the ultrasound beam. While LVOT blood flow is almost parallel to the ultrasound beam, carotid blood flow is nearly perpendicular to it and requires electronic angle correction, which introduces the potential for error.

Summary

Respiratory variations of carotid VTI and Vmax are attractive options due to their ease of calculation. However, their limitations—such as changes in diameter and the need for angle correction—should be considered when interpreting the results. Optimized Sensitivity and Specificity of Dynamic Measurements

Respiratory variations in LVOT VTI, PPV, or SVV are validated in patients receiving mechanical ventilation with higher tidal volumes (8 mL/kg). Low tidal volumes (<6 mL/kg) typically produce smaller variations in SV, leading to decreased accuracy of these parameters. If the cutoff value is reduced, sensitivity increases, allowing more fluid-responsive patients to be identified, albeit at the cost of decreased specificity. These lower cutoffs may be useful in patients with persistent signs of tissue hypoperfusion and a low risk of pulmonary edema. Conversely, increasing cutoff values improves specificity at the expense of sensitivity. These higher cutoffs can be applied in patients for whom unnecessary fluid loading is considered detrimental.

Vignon et al. have identified such differential cutoffs **(Table 3)** based on observations in 540 mechanically ventilated patients, 66% of whom were on tidal volumes <8 mL/kg of predicted body weight.[20] The issue of the low sensitivity with IVC and SVC variation for detecting fluid responsiveness persists even at lower cutoffs. For example, lowering the ΔIVC cutoff to 3% would still miss one-fourth of the patients who are fluid-responsive.

ECHOCARDIOGRAPHY DURING CARDIOPULMONARY RESUSCITATION

Echocardiography can be used to identify reversible causes of cardiac arrest and assist with airway management during CPR.

Identification of Reversible Causes During Cardiopulmonary Resuscitation

Echocardiography can readily identify hypovolemia, cardiac tamponade, or myocardial infarction. It can differentiate between a *true* pulseless electrical activity (PEA) and a pseudo-PEA. Echocardiography is not the modality of choice for diagnosis of PE; however, dilatation of RA and RV is highly suggestive of PE.

Echocardiography performed by a dedicated operator using the subcostal window, within a <10-second interruption, can help identify IVC diameter, mechanical cardiac activity, pericardial effusion, or RV dilatation.

TABLE 3: Threshold values of dynamic parameters to predict fluid responsiveness tailored to risk of fluid overload optimized.

Dynamic indices	*Patients low risk for fluid overload (Need sensitive test of fluid responsiveness)*		*Patients high risk for fluid overload (Need specific test of fluid responsiveness)*	
	Cutoff (%)	*Sensitivity*	*Cutoff (%)*	*Specificity*
ΔIVC, respiratory variations of the diameter of the inferior vena cava	3	74	18	90
ΔSVC, respiratory variations of the diameter of the superior vena cava	4	89	31	90
ΔVmaxAo, respiratory variations of left ventricular outflow tract maximal Doppler velocity	7	90	18	90
ΔPP, pulse pressure variations	4	92	18	89

Current Advanced Cardiac Life Support (ACLS) guidelines suggest considering echocardiography by a qualified sonographer, as long as it does not interfere with the standard cardiac arrest management.[38] If an adequate window is not obtained, echocardiography can be reattempted twice after a gap of 2 minutes.[39]

Breitkreutz et al. have demonstrated that using focused echocardiographic evaluation in life support (FEEL) during prehospital CPR led to changes in management in 78% of cases.[40]

Ultrasonography for Emergency Airway Management

The intensive care unit (ICU) is often considered a challenging *environment* for airway procedures due to the unavailability of specialized equipment a lack of skilled professionals, limited patient access, and inadequate infrastructure.[41] Cricothyrotomy is a rescue strategy for managing "cannot intubate, cannot oxygenate (CICO)" scenarios.[42] Cricothyroid membrane can be palpated and marked prior to the intubation procedure to save some time in an emergency. If the cricothyroid membrane cannot be identified due to poorly defined landmarks, ultrasound can assist in its identification. However, this should be done electively before intubation to avoid delaying airway access during an emergency.

The use of ultrasound during emergencies should be limited to experienced operators with a ready-to-use ultrasound machine near the patient, as long as it does not interfere with oxygenation or airway access procedures.

In addition to identifying the cricothyroid membrane, ultrasound can be used for confirming endotracheal intubation, assessing cuff positioning in relation to the glottis, verifying the tube's placement within the trachea, and performing real-time intubation using ultrasound-guided techniques. In addition to identifying the cricothyroid membrane, ultrasound can be used for confirming endotracheal intubation, assessing cuff positioning in relation to the glottis, verifying the tube's placement within the trachea, and performing real-time intubation using ultrasound-guided techniques.[43]

Advantages and Limitations of Echocardiography-guided Resuscitation

The advantages and limitations of individual parameters have already been discussed in their respective sections. Here, we summarize a few important limitations of using echocardiography during resuscitation.

Advantages

Echocardiography provides a quick assessment of circulatory parameters within minutes. Since time is crucial during resuscitation, every clinician working in the ED or ICU should consider acquiring echocardiography skills. This can aid in the timely resuscitation of critically ill patients. Transthoracic echocardiography is completely noninvasive. It does not require the insertion of catheters in aseptic precautions or correction of coagulopathy. However, echocardiography is not a replacement for invasive monitoring. Patients may still require an arterial line for invasive blood pressure monitoring and frequent lactate measurements. A central line may also be necessary for the infusion of vasoactive agents. Additionally, ultrasound can be helpful in guiding the insertion of these lines, as discussed in Chapter 45: Ultrasonography-guided Procedures in the Critically Ill.

Limitations

- *Observer variability:* Intraobserver and interobserver variations in echocardiographic measurements are well documented.[28,34] Due to this inherent limitation, echocardiography may not be reliable for detecting small changes in measurements.
- *Technically demanding:* Obtaining an echocardiography window for basic assessments, such as IVC diameter or ventricular function is a fundamental skill. However, using echocardiography for more advanced measurements, such as VTI, requires additional training and experience. In contrast, invasive cardiac output devices which require minimal training to generate reliable data.
- *Lack of continuous monitoring:* Echocardiography cannot provide continuous monitoring like less invasive cardiac output monitors. It is also prone to errors if careful attention is not given to sample volume and technique.[44]
- *Limitations as an upstream parameter:* All cardiac output measurements have the limitation of the upstream parameters. It is inappropriate to interpret a cardiac output value without considering tissue demands. For example, a cardiac index of 2 L/min/m^2 may be sufficient for an anesthetized patient who is paralyzed, mechanically ventilated, and

mildly hypothermic. In contrast, a cardiac index of 6 L/min/m^2 may be inadequate for a marathon runner midrace. Cardiac output measurements obtained with echocardiography should be interpreted alongside downstream parameters such as lactate, $ScvO_2$, or pCO_2 gap.

PROTOCOLS

The use of ultrasound during emergencies should follow a comprehensive and protocolized approach to identify the underlying pathology and to avoid missing any abnormality. Various protocols developed for comprehensive and systematic assessment of a shock patient using ultrasound are listed here.[45] It is not necessary to remember all the protocols.

Available Protocols

- *RUSH:* Rapid Ultrasound in Shock scanning
- *FEEL:* Focused Echocardiographic Evaluation in Life Support
- *ACES:* Abdominal and Cardiac Evaluation with Sonography in Shock
- *BEAT:* Bedside Echocardiographic Assessment in Trauma/Critical Care
- *BLEEP:* Bedside Limited Echocardiography by Emergency Physicians
- *EGLS:* Echo-Guided Life Support
- *FALLS:* Fluid Administration Limited by Lung Sonography
- *FAST:* Focused Assessment with Sonography for Trauma
- *FATE:* Focused Assessment with Transthoracic Echocardiography
- *FEER:* Focused Echocardiographic Evaluation in Resuscitation
- *FREE:* Focused Rapid Echocardiographic Examination
- *POCUS:* Point-of-Care Ultrasound

Many of these protocols are not validated in clinical practice. The Rapid Ultrasound in Shock or the RUSH protocol is discussed further. FAST protocol is discussed elsewhere in the textbook.

- *RUSH—The RUSH examination:* Rapid Ultrasound in Shock in the evaluation of critically ill patients was proposed by Perera P et al. in 2010. It has a three-step standardized sequence:
  1. *The pump:* LV contractility, RV strain, and pericardium
  2. *The tank:* IVC, other pleural, pericardial, or abdominal leaks
  3. *The pipes:* Aortic aneurysm, dissection, deep vein thrombosis.

The scanning sequence is remembered with pneumonic—HI-MAP.

- *Heart:* A4C, PLAX, and PSAX views using a cardiac probe
- *Inferior vena cava:* Using the same probe. Change probe to abdominal
- Morrison pouch and bladder
- Aorta and other veins at depth
- *Pleura, pericardium:* Using the same probe to look for any collection

KEY POINTS

- Echocardiography is a rapid and noninvasive diagnostic tool for resuscitation and should be the first-line modality in shock to differentiate between shock types and etiologies early on.
- Inferior vena cava diameter and index are good indicators of preload or volume status. IVC diameter <1.6–2 cm or variability of >40% in spontaneously breathing patients, or >12% in mechanically ventilated patients, indicates hypovolemia in the absence of raised IAP. IVC diameter >2 cm or lack of respiratory variation does not rule out fluid responsiveness. Other parameters can be used to guide fluid therapy as outlined in **Table 2**.
- LVEDA can be measured in PSAX view. *Kissing papillary muscles sign* or LVEDA <10 cm^2 in the absence of severe concentric LV hypertrophy indicates hypovolemia. LVEDA >20 cm^2 is likely to be a volume overload state.
- Velocity time integral or Vmax can be used as surrogate markers of SV as LVOT diameter does not change in a given patient.
- LV function can be qualitatively estimated by visual assessment (eyeballing) of contraction as mild, moderate, and severe LV dysfunction. This needs practice and has high interobserver variability.
- LV function can be quantitatively assessed using the Simpson method for calculating EF.
- Dynamic indices such as respiratory variation in VTI or Vmax can be used to predict fluid responsiveness.
- Echocardiography can identify some of the reversible causes of refractory shock or cardiopulmonary arrest.

- Ultrasonography-guided airway management includes identification of cricothyroid membrane and real-time intubation.
- Echocardiography-guided resuscitation has limitations, including interobserver variability, technical demands, and difficulty correlating with upstream parameters.
- Use of ultrasound during emergencies should follow a comprehensive and protocolized approach to identify the underlying pathology and to avoid missing abnormality.
- Echocardiography and ultrasound are excellent diagnostic tools.[45] However, when used for monitoring, one must recognize their limitations, including dependence on the acoustic window, individual variability, and their constraints as upstream parameters.

CONCLUSION

Echocardiography can be used for rapid bedside assessment of volume status or preload, left ventricular (LV) function, including contractility and cardiac output, as well as fluid responsiveness. Additionally, it can help identify the cause of shock or cardiac arrest. The need for trained personnel, a good echocardiographic window, and intra- and inter-observer variation are important limitations of echocardiography.

REFERENCES

1. Cecconi M, Backer DD, Antonelli M, Beale R, Bakker J, Hofer C, et al. Consensus on circulatory shock and hemodynamic monitoring. Task force of the European Society of Intensive Care Medicine. Intensive Care Med. 2014;40(12):1795-815.
2. Kory P. COUNTERPOINT: Should acute fluid resuscitation be guided primarily by inferior vena cava ultrasound for patients in shock? No. Chest. 2017;151(3):533-6.
3. Gignon L, Roger C, Bastide S, Alonso S, Zieleskiewicz L, Quintard H, et al. Influence of diaphragmatic motion on inferior vena cava diameter respiratory variation in healthy volunteers. Anesthesiology. 2016;124(6):1338-46.
4. Finnerty NM, Panchal AR, Boulger C, Vira A, Bischof JJ, Amick C, et al. Inferior vena cava measurement with ultrasound: what is the best view and best mode? Western J Emerg Med. 2017;18(3):496-501.
5. De Backer D, Fagnoul D. Intensive care ultrasound: VI. Fluid responsiveness and shock assessment. Ann Am Thorac Soc. 2014;11(1):129-36.
6. Airapetian N, Maizel J, Alyamani O, Mahjoub Y, Lorne E, Levrard M, et al. Does inferior vena cava respiratory variability predict fluid responsiveness in spontaneously breathing patients? Crit Care. 2015;19:400.
7. Corl K, Napoli AM, Gardiner F. Bedside sonographic measurement of the inferior vena cava caval index is a poor predictor of fluid responsiveness in emergency department patients. Emerg Med Australas. 2012;24(5):534-9.
8. Lanspa MJ, Grissom CK, Hirshberg EL, Jones JP, Brown SM. Applying dynamic parameters to predict hemodynamic response to volume expansion in spontaneously breathing patients with septic shock. Shock. 2013;39(2):155-60.
9. Das SK, Choupoo NS, Pradhan D, Saikia P, Monnet X. Diagnostic accuracy of inferior vena caval respiratory variation in detecting fluid unresponsiveness: A systematic review and meta-analysis. Eur J Anaesthesiol. 2018;35(11):831-9.
10. Barbier C, Loubières Y, Schmit C, Hayon J, Ricôme JL, Jardin F, et al. Respiratory changes in inferior vena cava diameter are helpful in predicting fluid responsiveness in ventilated septic patients. Intensive Care Med. 2004;30(9):1740-6.
11. Feissel M, Michard F, Faller JP, Teboul JL. The respiratory variation in inferior vena cava diameter as a guide to fluid therapy. Intensive Care Med. 2004;30(9):1834-7.
12. Charbonneau H, Riu B, Faron M, Mari A, Kurrek MM, Ruiz J, et al. Predicting preload responsiveness using simultaneous recordings of inferior and superior vena cavae diameters. Crit Care. 2014;18(5):473.
13. Bentzer P, Griesdale DE, Boyd J, MacLean K, Sirounis D, Ayas NT. Will this hemodynamically unstable patient respond to a bolus of intravenous fluids? JAMA. 2016;316(12):1298-309.
14. Kircher BJ, Himelman RB, Schiller NB. Noninvasive estimation of right atrial pressure from the inspiratory collapse of the inferior vena cava. Am J Cardiol. 1990;66(4):493-6.
15. Prekker ME, Scott NL, Hart D, Sprenkle MD, Leatherman JW. Point-of-care ultrasound to estimate central venous pressure: a comparison of three techniques. Crit Care Med. 2013;41(3):833-41.
16. Akkaya A, Yesilaras M, Aksay E, Sever M, Atilla OD. The interrater reliability of ultrasound imaging of the inferior vena cava performed by emergency residents. Am J Emerg Med. 2013;31(10):1509-11.
17. Blehar DJ, Resop D, Chin B, Dayno M, Gaspari R. Inferior vena cava displacement during respirophasic ultrasound imaging. Crit Ultrasound J. 2012;4(1):18.
18. In: Lichtenstein DA (Ed). Inferior vena cava. General Ultrasound in the Critically Ill. Berlin: Springer; 2005. pp. 82-6.
19. Vieillard-Baron A, Chergui K, Rabiller A, Peyrouset O, Page B, Beauchet A, et al. Superior vena caval collapsibility as a gauge of volume status in ventilated septic patients. Intensive Care Med. 2004;30(9):1734-9.
20. Vignon P, Repessé X, Bégot E, et al. Comparison of echocardiographic indices used to predict fluid responsiveness in ventilated patients. Am J Respir Crit Care Med. 2017;195(8):1022-32.

21. Beaulieu Y, Marik PE. Bedside ultrasonography in the ICU: part 1. Chest. 2005;128(2):881-95.
22. Vermeiren GL, Malbrain ML, Walpot JM. Cardiac ultrasonography in the critical care setting: a practical approach to asses cardiac function and preload for the "non-cardiologist". Anaesthesiol Intensive Ther. 2015;47:s89-104.
23. Marik PE, Cavallazzi R, Vasu T, Hirani A. Dynamic changes in arterial waveform derived variables and fluid responsiveness in mechanically ventilated patients: a systematic review of the literature. Crit Care Med. 2009;37(9):2642-7.
24. Tavernier B, Makhotine O, Lebuffe G, et al. Systolic pressure variation as a guide to fluid therapy in patients with sepsis-induced hypotension. Anesthesiology. 1998;89:1313-21.
25. Guarracino F, Ferro B, Forfori F, Bertini P, Magliacano L, Pinsky MR. Jugular vein distensibility predicts fluid responsiveness in septic patients. Crit Care. 2014;18(6):647.
26. Ma GG, Hao GW, Yang XM, Zhu DM, Liu L, Liu H, et al. Internal jugular vein variability predicts fluid responsiveness in cardiac surgical patients with mechanical ventilation. Ann Intensive Care. 2018;8(1):6.
27. Blanco P, Aguiar MF, Blaivas M. Rapid ultrasound in shock (RUSH) velocity-time integral: A proposal to expand the RUSH protocol. J Ultrasound Med. 2015;34(9):1691-700.
28. Jozwiak M, Mercado P, Teboul JL, Gimenez J, Dépret F, Richard R, et al. What is the lowest change in cardiac output that transthoracic echocardiography can detect? Crit Care. 2019;23:116.
29. Sonography. (2019). 3.2.3 Left ventricular function. [online] Available from https://www.123sonography.com/ ebook/left-ventricular-function [Last accessed October, 2024].
30. Vieillard-Baron A. Septic cardiomyopathy. Ann Intensive Care. 2011;1(1):6.
31. Vieillard-Baron A, Caille V, Charron C, Belliard G, Page B, Jardin F. Actual incidence of global left ventricular hypokinesia in adult septic shock. Critical Care Med. 2008;36(6):1701-6.
32. De Geer L, Oscarsson A, Engvall J. Variability in echocardiographic measurements of left ventricular function in septic shock patients. Cardiovasc Ultrasound. 2015;13:19.
33. Charron C, Fessenmeyer C, Cosson C, Mazoit JX, Hebert JL, Benhamou D, et al. The influence of tidal volume on the dynamic variables of fluid responsiveness in critically ill patients. Anesth Analg. 2006;102(5):1511-7.
34. Feissel M, Michard F, Mangin I, Ruyer O, Faller JP, Teboul JL. Respiratory changes in aortic blood velocity as an indicator of fluid responsiveness in ventilated patients with septic shock. Chest. 2001;119(3):867-73.
35. Mahjoub Y, Pila C, Friggeri A, Zogheib E, Lobjoie E, Tinturier F, et al. Assessing fluid responsiveness in critically ill patients: false-positive pulse pressure variation is detected by Doppler echocardiographic evaluation of the right ventricle. Crit Care Med. 2009;37(9):2570-5.
36. Ibarra-Estrada MA, Lopez-Pulgarin JA, Mijangos-Mendez JC, Díaz-Gómez JL, Aguirre-Avalos G. Variation in carotid peak systolic velocity predicts volume responsiveness in mechanically ventilated patients with septic shock: A prospective cohort study. Crit Ultrasound J. 2015;7(1):29.
37. Becker L, Prado K, Foppa M, Martinelli N, Aguiar C, Furian T, et al. Endothelial dysfunction assessed by brachial artery ultrasound in severe sepsis and septic shock. J Crit Care. 2012;27:316.e9-14.
38. Link MS, Berkow LC, Kudenchuk PJ, Halperin HR, Hess EP, Moitra VK, et al. Part 7: Adult Advanced Cardiovascular Life Support: 2015 American Heart Association Guidelines Update for Cardiopulmonary Resuscitation and Emergency Cardiovascular Care. Circulation. 2015;132(18 Suppl 2):S444-64.
39. Chardoli M, Heidari F, Rabiee H, Sharif-Alhoseini M, Shokoohi H, et al. Echocardiography integrated ACLS protocol versus conventional cardiopulmonary resuscitation in patients with pulseless electrical activity cardiac arrest. Chin J Traumatol. 2012;15(5):284-7.
40. Breitkreutz R, Price S, Steiger HV, Seeger FH, Ilper H, Ackermann H, et al. Focused echocardiographic evaluation in life support and peri-resuscitation of emergency patients: a prospective trial. Resuscitation. 2010;81(11):1527-33.
41. Cook TM, Woodall N, Frerk C; Fourth National Audit Project. Major complications of airway management in the UK: results of the Fourth National Audit Project of the Royal College of Anaesthetists and the Difficult Airway Society. Part 1: anaesthesia. Br J Anaesth. 2011;106(5):617-31.
42. Frerk C, Mitchell VS, McNarry AF, Mendonca C, Bhagrath R, Patel A, et al. Difficult Airway Society 2015 guidelines for management of unanticipated difficult intubation in adults. Difficult Airway Society Intubation Guidelines Working Group. Br J Anaesth. 2015;115(6):827-48.
43. Fiadjoe JE, Stricker P, Gurnaney H, Nishisaki A, Rabinowitz A, Gurwitz A, et al. Ultrasound-guided tracheal intubation: a novel intubation technique. Anesthesiology. 2012;117(6):1389-91.
44. Porter TR, Shillcutt SK, Adams MS, Desjardins G, Glas KE, Olson JJ, et al. Guidelines for the use of echocardiography as a monitor for therapeutic intervention in adults: a report from the American Society of Echocardiography. J Am Soc Echocardiogr. 2015;28(1):40-56.
45. Seif D, Perera P, Mailhot T, Riley D, Mandavia D. Bedside ultrasound in resuscitation and the rapid ultrasound in shock protocol. Crit Care Res Pract. 2012;2012:503254.

CHAPTER

Ultrasonography-guided Procedures in the Critically Ill

Tineesh Mathew, Amol Trimbakrao Kothekar

"The only thing worse than being blind is having sight but no vision."

—**Helen Keller**

INTRODUCTION

Ultrasonography has been used in interventional procedures for over 40 years.[1] The earliest work describing the use of sonographic needle guidance can be traced back to 1961 when Berlyne used an A-mode apparatus to identify the needle tip during renal biopsy.[2] In 1967, Joyner and associates described the use of ultrasonography for selecting the site for aspiration of pleural fluid.[3] In 1978, Ullman and Stoelting were the first to describe central venous catheterization using Doppler imaging guidance.[4] In 1986, Yonei et al. introduced real-time, two-dimensional ultrasonography for cannulation of the internal jugular vein (IJV).[5] Advances in ultrasound machine portability and sonographic imaging techniques have ushered in a new era of point-of-care ultrasound-guided interventional procedures.

LIMITATIONS OF LANDMARK (BLIND) TECHNIQUE

The traditional landmark (blind) technique for vascular cannulation relies on external anatomical landmarks for vessel localization. However, there is often a lack of correlation between these external landmarks and the actual location of the vessel. For example, IJV is not always in the typical anterolateral position relative to the carotid artery.[6] Anatomical variations in the relative positions of the vein and artery are also common. The femoral vein can be overlapped by the femoral artery in 8–10% of the cases.[7,8] Vessel thrombosis, which is particularly common in oncologic and critically ill patients, further complicates cannulation. Veins with a diameter of 7 mm or smaller (cross-sectional area 0.4 cm^2) are associated with a higher failure rate.[9] These factors contribute to an unacceptably high failure rate using the external landmarks technique, with failure rates of 7.0–19.4% for the first attempt and 25% for subsequent attempts.[10,11] Increased number of attempts can lead to a higher incidence of complications, delays in monitoring and treatment, and can cause patient discomfort.

ADVANTAGES OF ULTRASONOGRAPHY-GUIDED PROCEDURES

Ultrasonography enhances the ability to safely and successfully perform cannulation by revealing anatomical details and increasing the likelihood of success. It helps identify the most suitable site for vessel cannulation by assessing the depth of the skin and the relationship with adjacent structures, such as arteries or the pleura. Additionally, ultrasonography can detect conditions that may preclude cannulation, such as overlapping or very small vessels (<7 mm) and thrombus **(Figs. 1A to D)** in the vessel. These anatomical challenges are not identifiable with the "blind" technique, even by experts. In other words, experience alone cannot replace the advantages of using ultrasonography for many vascular cannulations. Ultrasonography is particularly beneficial in patients with severe hypotension and circulatory arrest, where pulses are not palpable.

Ultrasound guidance is the recommended technique and standard of care for most central venous cannulations.[12] Moreover, there is high-level evidence supporting an increased success rate for radial artery cannulation in both adult and pediatric populations when performed under ultrasound guidance.[13] Ultrasonography is also valuable for many other procedures. For example, thoracentesis performed with ultrasound guidance has a lower risk of pneumothorax and bleeding complications.[14] Currently, all pericardiocentesis procedures are conducted under

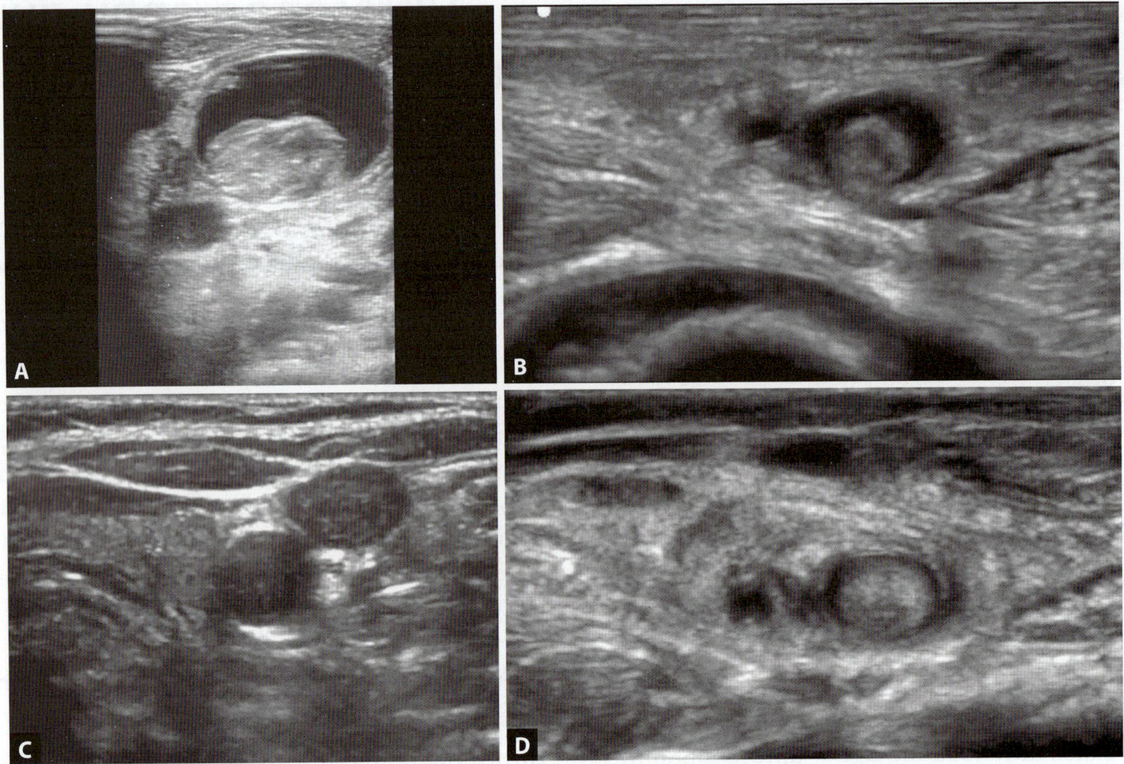

Figs. 1A to D: Venous thrombus with partial (A and B) and complete (C and D) occlusion.

ultrasound guidance. Historically, attempts at blind percutaneous pericardial drainage were associated with an exceedingly high mortality rate (8.5%).[15] Additionally, ultrasound guidance for catheter insertion is part of a multifaceted strategy that has been shown to reduce the risk of catheter-related blood-stream infection (CRBSI).[16]

MULTILEVEL APPLICATION OF ULTRASONOGRAPHY IN VASCULAR CANNULATIONS

Ultrasonography can be used at various stages during vascular cannulation, some of which are discussed here:

- Identification of the most appropriate vessel for cannulation
- Site of injection of local anesthetic
- Needle puncture
- Guidewire insertion
- Troubleshooting of difficult guidewire insertion
- Confirmation of guidewire in the vessel of interest
- Identifying guidewire malposition by scanning adjacent vessels
- Confirmation of catheter tip position by saline injection contrast echocardiography
- Diagnosis of postprocedure complications, such as pneumothorax.

It is crucial to confirm the guidewire position in the vessel of interest **(Figs. 2A and B)** with ultrasonography to avoid accidental dilatation of the artery during venous cannulation.

PHYSICS AND TECHNICAL ASPECTS OF ULTRASONOGRAPHY-GUIDED PROCEDURES

The physics of ultrasonography is described in detail elsewhere in this textbook. Here, we highlight the key technical points relevant to ultrasonography-guided cannulations:

- Higher frequency linear transducer probes >7 MHz (10–15 MHz) offer excellent resolution at the cost of reduced penetration.[9] Commercially available linear probe generally allow visualization of structures up to 6 cm deep (exact maximum depth depends on the frequency of the probe) which facilitates cannulation of most vessels, including internal jugular, femoral, and subclavian veins. For structures deeper than 6 cm, a small curvilinear probe or microconvex probe may be used.

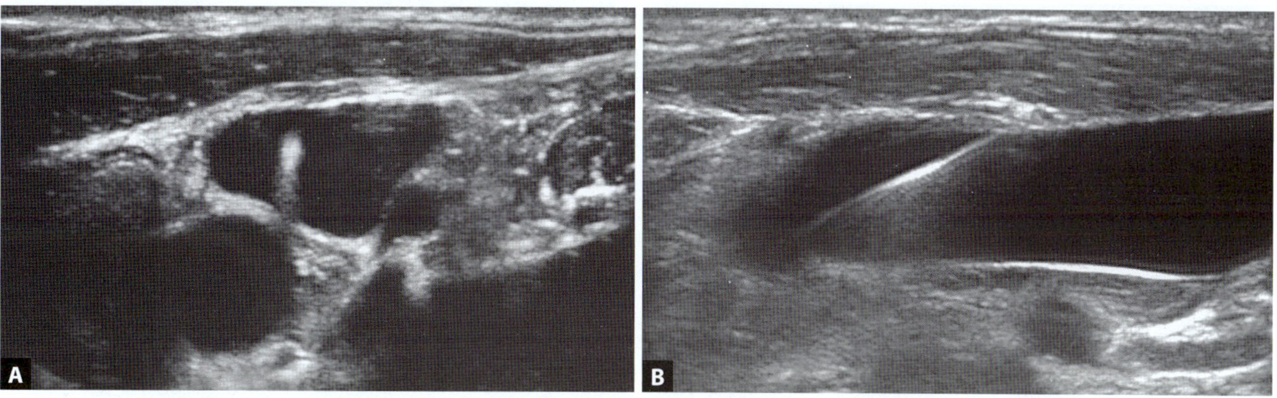

Figs. 2A and B: Ultrasound images of a guidewire in the internal jugular vein in (A) short- and (B) long-axis views.

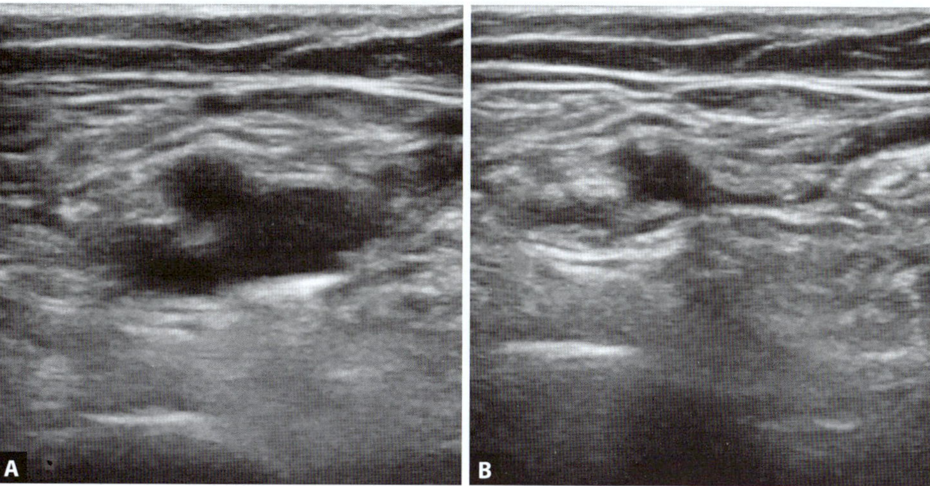

Figs. 3A and B: Ultrasound image showing compressibility of the vein: (A) Without compression; (B) With compression.

- The imaging capability of the ultrasonography machine can be optimized by selecting the highest possible frequency or a minimum depth that visualizes all structures of interest. Image quality can be further improved by "fine-tuning" the gain. Once any thrombus in the vessel is ruled out **(Figs. 1A and B)**, compression ultrasonography **(Figs. 3A and B)** can be done to differentiate the artery from the vein. Color flow or pulse wave Doppler can be used to confirm the artery and vein **(Figs. 4A and B)**. When using color flow Doppler, the focus should be on the flow pattern (pulsatile vs. continuous flow) rather than the color alone. The blue color on Doppler does not necessarily indicate venous blood flow!
- It is crucial to understand that conventional ultrasonography is a two-dimensional modality, visualizing a very thin slice of tissue at one time (about as thick as a credit card). Failure to account for this may result in the unintentional puncture of another structure if the ultrasonography beam is not aligned to visualize the needle tip. This issue is commonly encountered during the initial stages of learning the ultrasound-guided cannulation of IJV. Remedies for this are described in detail further in the section on approaches.
- Successful ultrasound-guided procedures rely on clear visualization of the needle. Ultrasonography depends on the angle of insonation **(Fig. 5)**. The needle is best visualized at an angle of insonation close to 90°. Needle visibility diminishes as the angle of insonation approaches zero. This issue is commonly encountered during cannulation of the deeper vessels, which require a steeper angle of insertion and thus a lesser angle of insonation. Solutions for this issue using alternative probes are also described in detail further in the section on approaches.

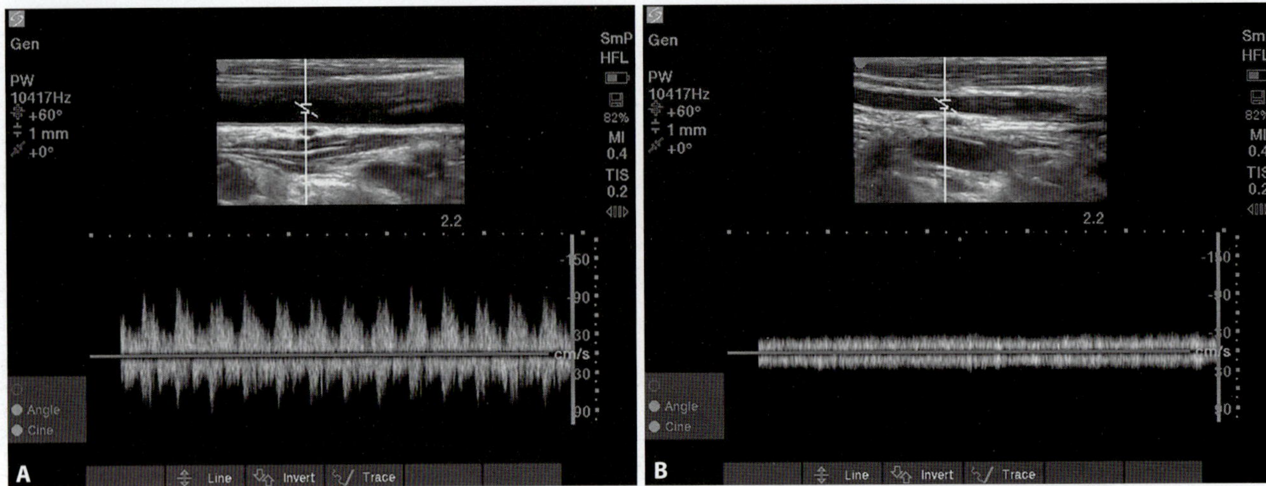

Figs. 4A and B: Doppler ultrasound images showing different flow patterns in vascular structures: (A) Pulsatile show in the artery; (B) Continuous/nonpulsatile flow in the vein.

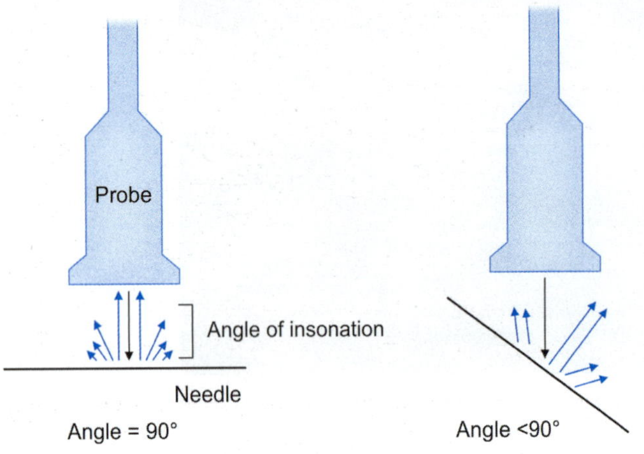

Fig. 5: The angle of insonation between the ultrasound beams and the needle.

- *Ultrasonography* does not replace the need for appropriate patient positioning. *Trendelenburg position* may still be required to promote venous engorgement by gravitating the blood toward the head end, making the vein more prominent. This position can also help prevent air embolism during the procedure. *Valsalva maneuver* can be used to increase vessel diameter;[9] but it may also increase the risk of pneumothorax if the needle puncture is too close to the pleura.
- Excessive pressure from the probe should be avoided. This issue is common during the initial learning phase. Excessive pressure can collapse the veins, making identification and cannulation more difficult. Beginners should be trained to develop the skill of maintaining adequate probe-skin contact with minimal pressure.

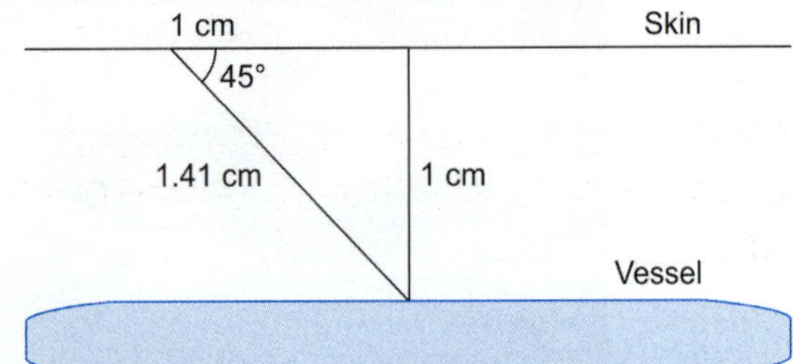

Fig. 6: Estimation of needle depth using Pythagorean theorem.

- The *Pythagorean theorem* can be used to estimate the distance a needle must travel through the tissues to puncture a vessel **(Fig. 6)**, for example, if the vessel is at a depth of 1 cm, the needle can enter the skin 1 cm away from the probe at 45° angle to the skin. The needle needs to travel a distance of $1 \times \sqrt{2}$ cm which is approximately 1.4 cm **(Fig. 6)**. Depth measured by the ultrasound probe might be slightly less than the actual depth due to tissue displacement caused by the probe. To calculate the actual depth, the measured depth can be multiplied by a correction factor. A correction factor of 1.2–1.4 has been reported for the use of a microconvex probe.[17] If this factor is considered, the actual needle distance could be roughly 2 cm for a vessel that is 1 cm deep. When using a linear probe, it may be safer to assume a needle distance that is 1.5–2 times the depth from the skin.
- Since the needle is not exactly perpendicular to the skin, needle entry in the vessel is proximal to the skin

puncture. This is important to consider, especially if compression is needed for accidental arterial injury.

- The needle puncture can create a skin indentation, leading to loss of probe-skin contact. This may result in a significant loss of view. The probe can be readjusted once the needle has passed through the tougher outer layers of skin, which are typically no deeper than 2–3 mm (not cm), in a controlled manner. Alternatively, the needle can be advanced through the previous skin puncture.
- Central vein diameter can decrease during inspiration in spontaneously breathing patients. Complete inspiratory collapse of the vein increases the risk of air embolism and may complicate cannulation.[18] To address this, procedures to increase central venous diameter such as placing the patient in the Trendelenburg position, using the Valsalva maneuver, or administering fluid infusion, may be considered.

APPROACHES AND VIEWS OF ULTRASONOGRAPHY-GUIDED VASCULAR CANNULATIONS

Two approaches to ultrasound-guided procedures are described based on the relationship between the ultrasound beam and the needle path: The "out-of-plane" and "in-plane" approaches. For ultrasound-guided vascular cannulations, three views are defined based on the relationship between the ultrasound beam and the vessel axis, namely the short axis, long axis, and oblique axis (OAX) views **(Table 1)**.

TABLE 1: Comparison of the three approaches.

	Transverse	*Longitudinal*	*Oblique*
Vessel section	Cross-section	Long-axis	Oblique
Needle and ultrasound plane orientation	Out-of-plane	In-plane	In-plane
Operator skill	Minimum	High level	High level
Lateral discrimination of vein from artery	Yes	No	Yes
The entire needle path is seen in a single view	No	Yes	Yes
Space requirement for probe position	Requires less space	Requires more space	Requires more space

Short-axis View/Transverse View/ Out-of-Plane Approach

In this approach, the probe is positioned at a 90° angle to the course of the vessel **(Fig. 7A)**. In this view, the vessel appears in cross-section **(Fig. 7B)**, hence, the name short-axis (SAX). Additionally, in this view, the needle is not within the plane of the ultrasound beam giving rise to the term, "*out-of-plane*" technique **(Figs. 7C and D)**.

Advantages

- All the relevant structures including both the artery and vein are visible in a single view. Additionally, there is minimal change in view of the image with small, inadvertent movements or shakes of the probe, making this approach generally recommended for beginners.
- Lateral wall punctures and vessel wall damage during guidewire insertion are minimized, as the vessel can be punctured at the 12 o'clock position.
- The SAX approach results in faster cannulation times compared to the long-axis (LAX) approach.[9]
- Novice operators tend to find the SAX approach easier to use than the LAX approach.[9]

Disadvantages

- *Lack of visualization of the entire needle path:* This is one of the major disadvantages of this approach. As previously mentioned, ultrasonography is a two-dimensional imaging modality and can only visualize a very thin slice of tissue at any given time. Since both the needle tip and the shaft produce similar images on ultrasonography, there is a risk of the operator mistaking the needle shaft for the needle tip. This misinterpretation can lead to the unintentional puncture of adjacent structures, as the operator may have a false sense of security due to the ultrasound image of the needle shaft. Utilizing dynamic needle tip positioning (discussed further) can help mitigate this complication.
- *Higher incidence of posterior wall injury:* The SAX approach is associated with a higher risk of posterior wall injury, particularly during subclavian cannulation.[19]

Dynamic Needle Tip Positioning for Short-axis View

The technique involves the repetition repetitions of three basic steps, ensuring constant monitoring of the needle tip until the vessel is successfully punctured **(Fig. 8)**.

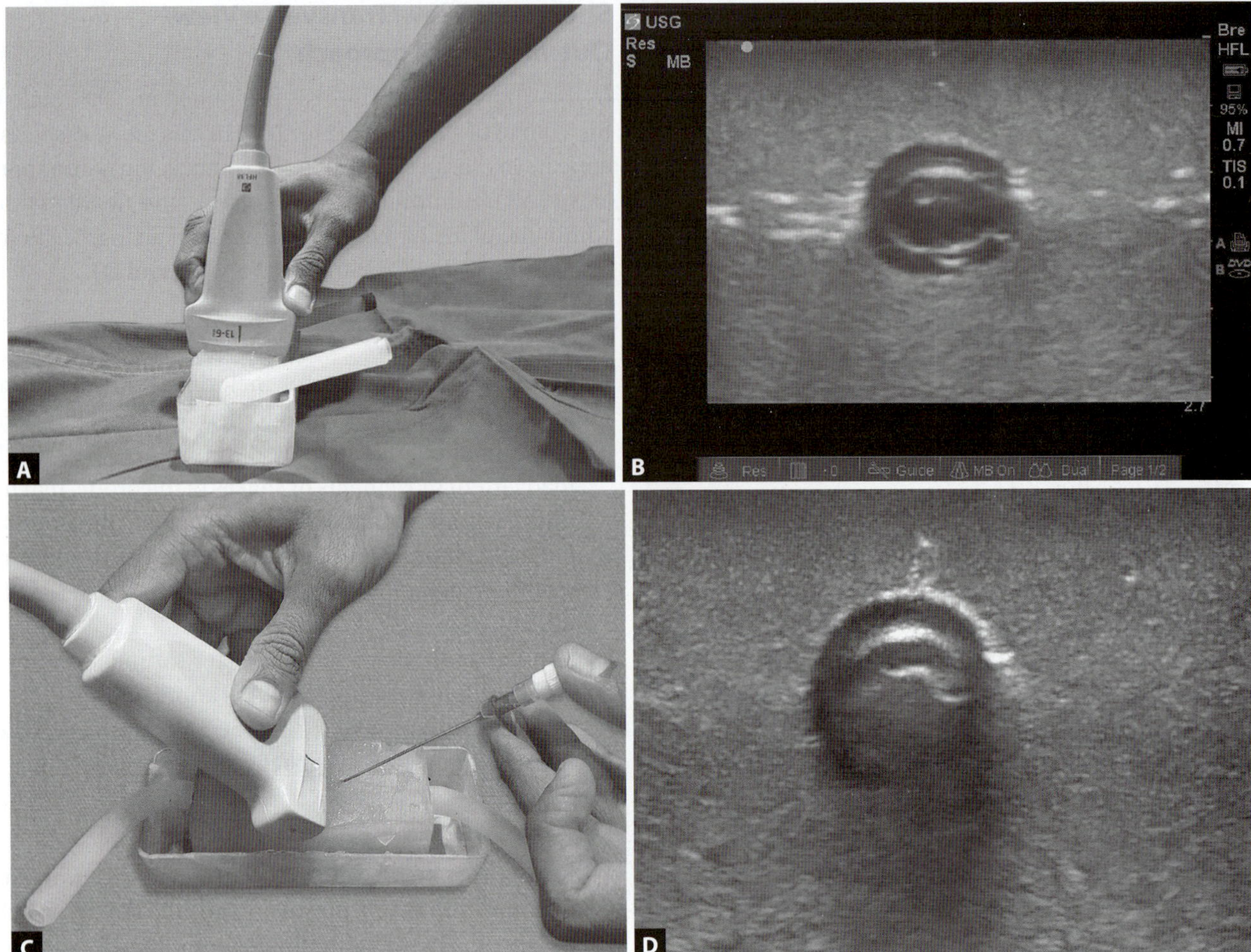

Figs. 7A to D: Images of short-axis view: (A) Relationship of the probe and the vessel; (B) Ultrasonography image of the vessel showing a cross-section of the vessel; (C) Relationship of liner probe, vessel, and needle; and (D) Ultrasonography image of the vessel showing needle as a dot and the vessel in the short axis. (All the images are for representative purposes only. Readers are strictly advised to follow aseptic precautions including sterile gloves) *(For color version, see Plate 7)*.

- *Step 1:* Visualize the vessel in the SAX view. Puncture the skin with the needle at a 45° angle, slightly away from the probe.
- *Step 2:* While keeping the probe stationary, advance the needle until the needle tip appears as a hyperechoic dot on the monitor, located between the skin and the vessel.
- *Step 3:* Hold the needle steady, then shift or tilt the probe slightly away from the operator just until the needle tip disappears from view.
- *Step 4:* Without moving the probe, advance the needle until the needle tip reappears on the monitor.

Repeat *steps 3* and *4* until the needle tip punctures the vessel and blood can be aspirated into the syringe. Alternatively, instead of moving the probe, it can be tilted or fanned in place, especially when there is limited room for probe movement.

Clemensen et al.[20] demonstrated a higher success rate with the SAX view using dynamic needle tip positioning compared to the LAX in-plane needle tip approach.

Long-axis View/Longitudinal View/In-plane Approach

The LAX view, also known as the longitudinal view, is obtained when the probe is aligned parallel to the LAX of the vessel **(Fig. 9A)**. In this view, the vessel appears tubular, hence the name LAX **(Fig. 9B)**. In this view, the needle within inserted in the plane of the ultrasound beam, giving this approach, the name "in-plane" **(Figs. 9C and D)**.

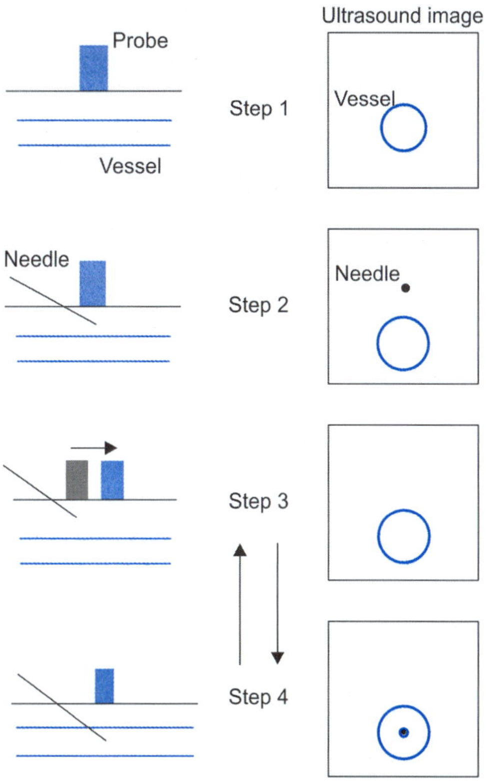

Fig. 8: Steps of dynamic needle tip positioning in short-axis view.

Advantages

- *Visualization of the entire needle path:* The LAX view allows for the visualization of the entire needle path. Direct observation of the needle's full course into the vessel can help prevent puncturing the posterior vessel wall.
- *Troubleshooting guidewire insertion:* This view is beneficial during guidewire insertions, as it helps in troubleshooting difficult insertions.
- *Cannulation of the supraclavicular subclavian vein:* For cannulating the supraclavicular subclavian vein, the LAX view may be the only practical approach.

Disadvantages

- *Challenges with probe stability:* Keeping the probe steady to maintain constant alignment of the thin ultrasound beam with the needle can be challenging. Beginners may find this approach more difficult. Various needle guides (described further) have been developed to assist with needle-beam alignment.[10]
- *Lack of lateral resolution:* In the longitudinal approach, it is often difficult to view both the IJV and the carotid artery in a single image, even if they are close together. The underlying vessel may shift with slight movements or drifts of the probe, potentially leading to accidental puncture of the carotid artery. This limitation makes the approach less suitable for beginners.
- *Difficulty in visualizing the needle:* During cannulation of deeper structures, reduced angle of insonation can make visualization of the needle challenging. Several solutions to address this issue are described underneath.
  - *Needle guides:* In the longitudinal approach, maintaining the needle within the thin ultrasound beam is crucial. In-plane needle guides **(Fig. 10)** can assist in directing the needle into the imaging plane, which is especially helpful for beginners.
  - *Alternative probes:* The needle surface acts as a reflector similar to a mirror. When the angle between the needle and the ultrasound beam (angle of insonation) is close to 90°, a greater number of echoes are reflected, improving needle visibility **(Fig. 5)**. Conversely, if the angle of insonation is less than 55°, needle visibility decreases.[21]
  - The probe with a curved footprint (curvilinear or microconvex probe) emits diverging ultrasound waves, which increases the angle of insonation for a given needle insertion angle, thereby improving needle visualization **(Fig. 11)**. However, the curvilinear probe is not ideal due to its poorer resolution. A pediatric microconvex probe offers a better balance between needle visualization and resolution, especially for deeper structures when using the in-plane technique. This modification is particularly useful in the "in-plane technique."
  - *Enhancement software:* Modern ultrasonography machines are equipped with software that enhances needle visualization, even at steeper angles. One such commercially available enhancement software utilizes the principle of phase inversion harmonics **(Figs. 12A and B) (Figs. 13A and B)**. Similar to the use of the curvilinear probe, the benefits of enhancement software are limited to the in-plane technique.

Oblique Axis View

This approach combines the advantages of both the SAX and LAX views while minimizing their limitations. Initially, the vessel is located using LAX followed by the rotation of the probe midway between the SAX and LAX views to

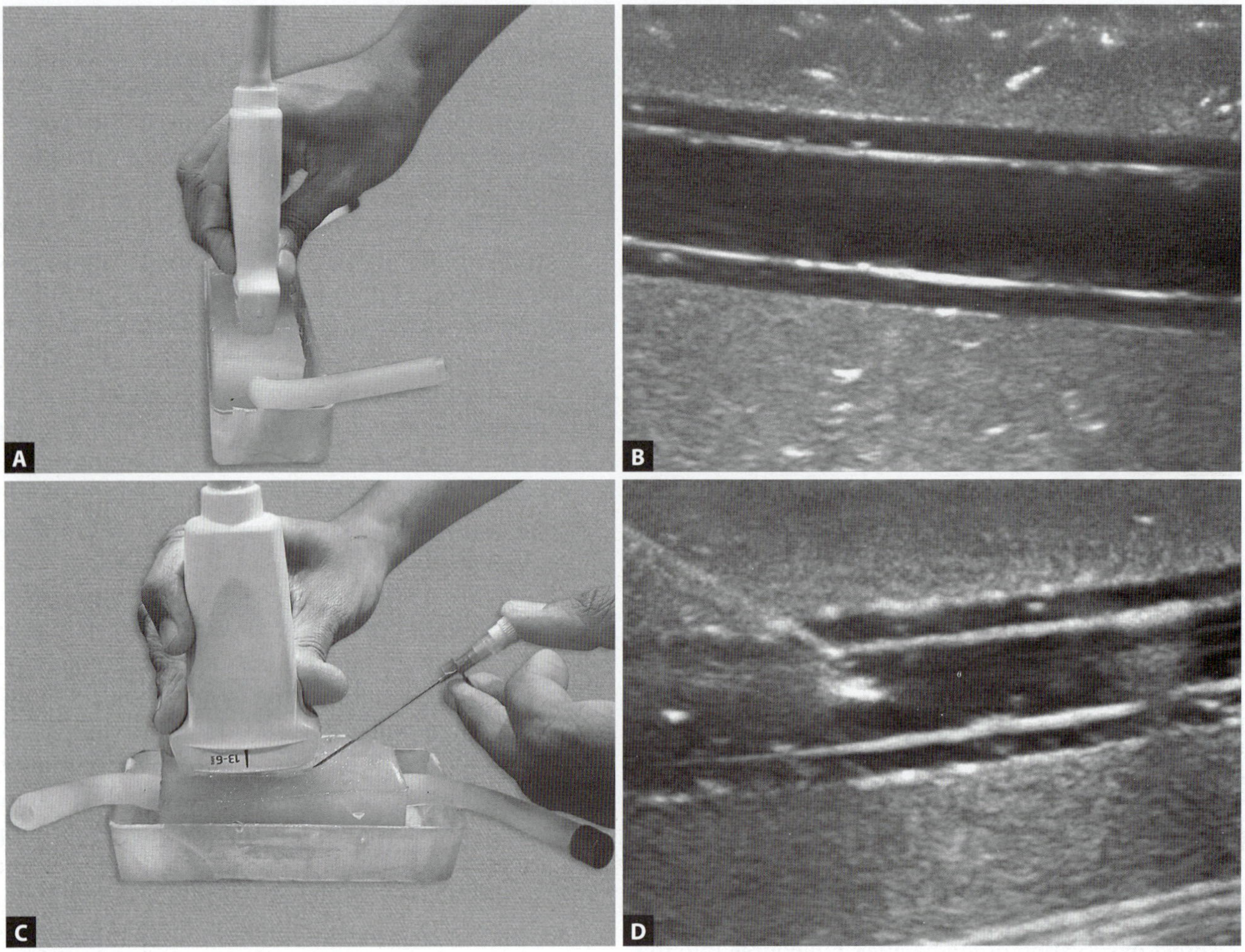

Figs. 9A to D: Images of long-axis view: (A) Relationship of the probe and the vessel; (B) Ultrasonography image of the vessel showing a longitudinal section of the vessel; (C) Relationship of liner probe, vessel, and needle; and (D) Ultrasonography image of the vessel showing needle and vessel in the long axis, in-plane approach. (All the images are for representative purposes only. Readers are strictly advised to follow aseptic precautions including sterile gloves) *(For color version, see Plate 8)*.

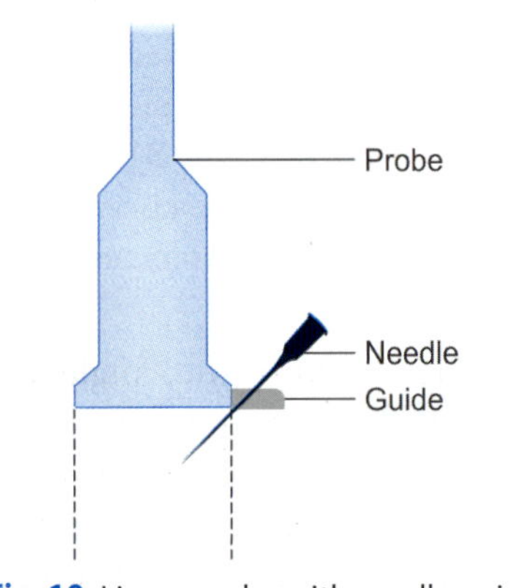

Fig. 10: Linear probe with needle guide.

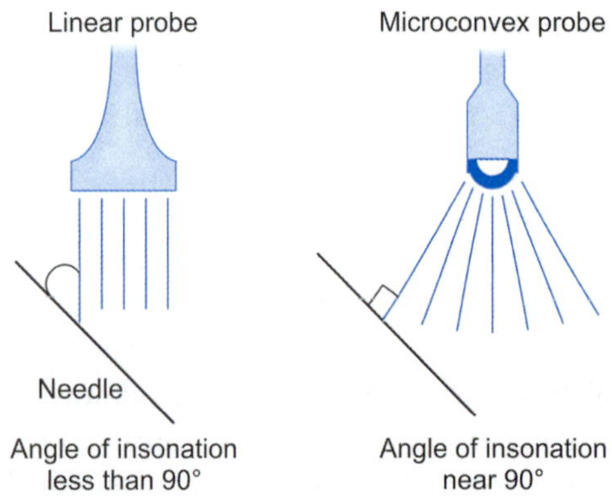

Fig. 11: Comparison of angle of insonation in a linear probe and microconvex probe.

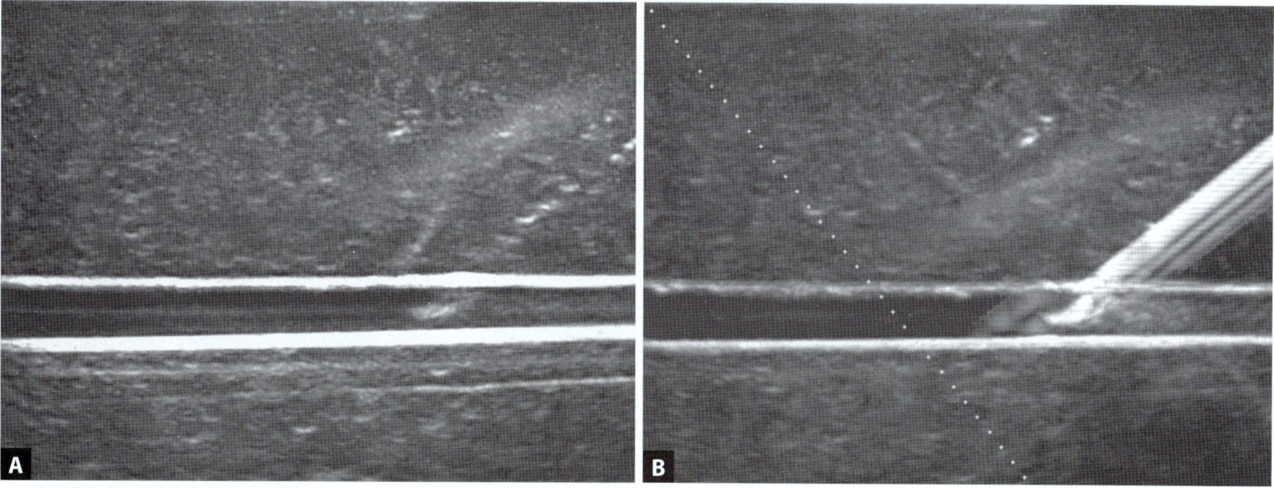

Figs. 12A and B: In-plane needle visualization in a simulator (A) without any enhancement and (B) with enhancement software.

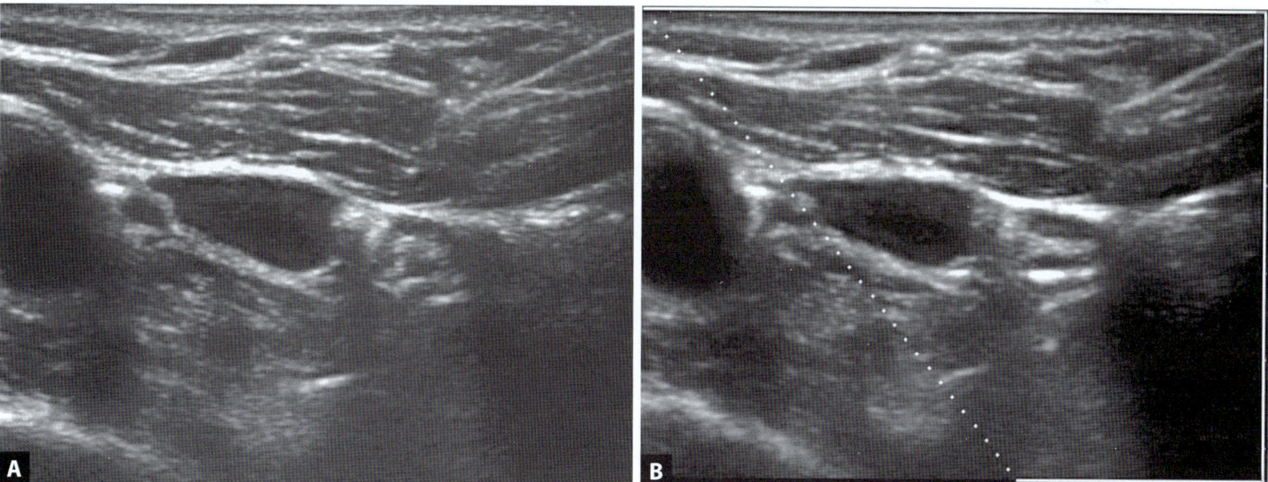

Figs. 13A and B: In-plane needle visualization in a patient (A) without any enhancement and (B) with enhancement software.

provide an oblique cross-section of the vessel. The needle is advanced within the plane of the ultrasound beam, making this an in-plane technique. This approach allows for complete visualization of the complete needle path, similar to the LAX view, while also visualizing adjacent structures similar to the SAX view[22] **(Figures 14A to D)**. For internal jugular cannulation, OAX is associated with the highest success rate on the first needle pass, though it has a slightly higher rate of mechanical complications compared with the LAX approach.[23] Additionally, the OAX approach for radial artery cannulation has been shown to improve both first-attempt and overall success rates.[24] This approach should be considered an additional option rather than a replacement for SAX and LAX approaches.[22]

PROCEDURE FOR ULTRASOUND-GUIDED CANNULATION[12]

Both static and real-time ultrasonography can be employed to guide vascular cannulation.

- *Static or indirect technique:* This technique is used before cannulation to assess the vessel for thrombus and to identify its anatomy. This information helps in deciding the puncture site, angle, and depth of insertion. When only the static technique is used, the procedure is referred to as "ultrasound-assisted" cannulation.
- *Real-time or direct technique:* In this approach, the needle is advanced under continuous ultrasound

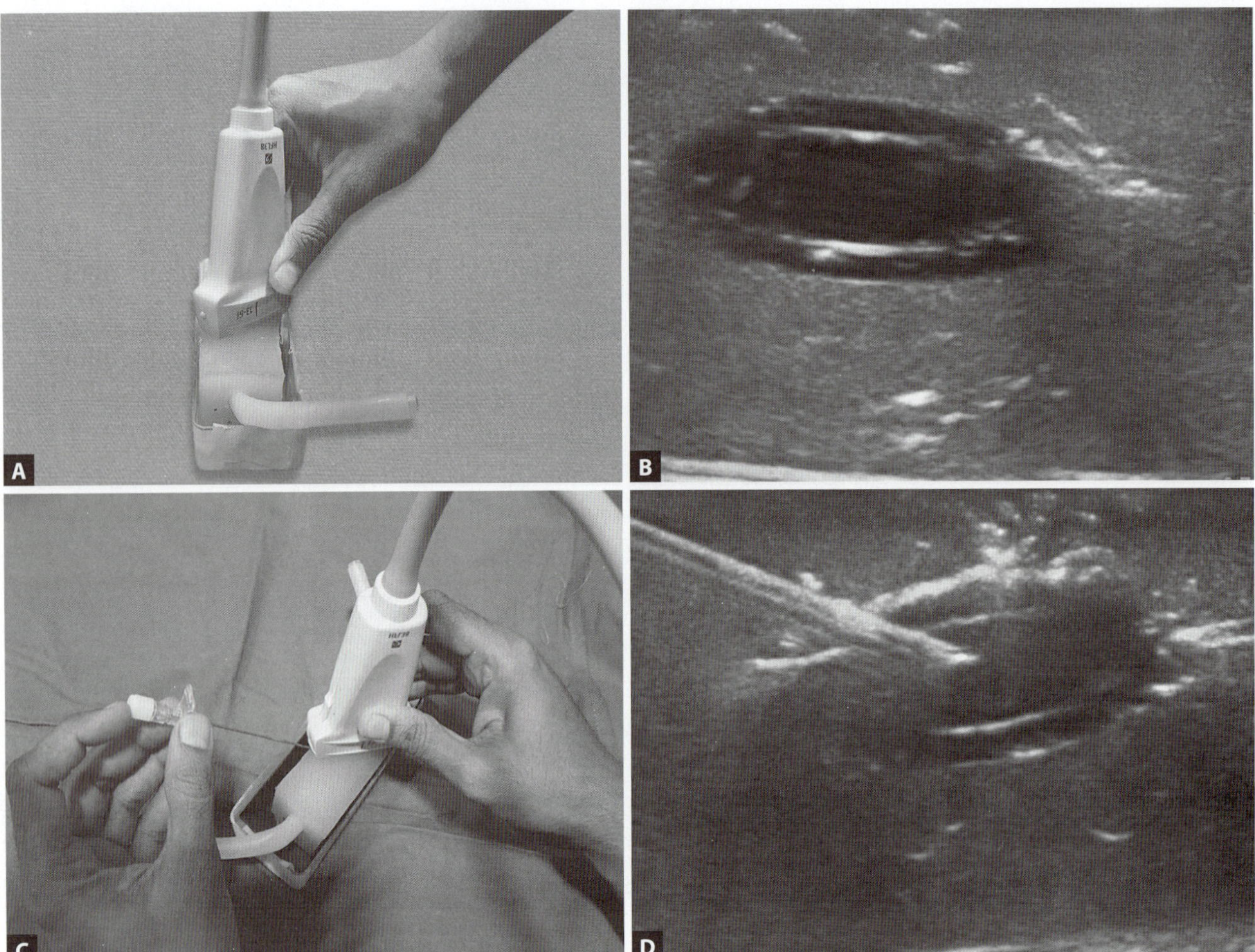

Figs. 14A to D: Images of oblique-axis view: (A) Relationship of the probe and the vessel; (B) Ultrasonography image of vessel in oblique view; (C) Relationship of liner probe, vessel, and vessel in oblique approach; and (D) Ultrasonography image of the vessel showing needle and vessel in the oblique view. (All the images are for representative purposes only. Readers are strictly advised to follow aseptic precautions including sterile gloves) *(For color version, see Plate 8).*

visualization, which is known as "ultrasound-guided" cannulation.

One major limitation of the static technique is that the underlying anatomy of the vessel can change with the patient's position. Additionally, it cannot be used for guidewire insertion and confirmation. Therefore, the real-time technique is preferred and most effective for ultrasound-guided vascular access.[9]

For ultrasound-guided peripherally inserted central catheter (PICC) insertion, both two-person and one-person methods are described.[25] Beginners may find the two-person method easier to use. However, for central venous cannulation, we recommend the one-person method for both beginners and experts. In this approach, the probe is held with the nondominant hand while the needle is advanced with the dominant hand. Various training modules and simulators are available to practice ultrasound-guided cannulation, helping to build and refine hand-eye coordination for the one-person method.

Internal Jugular Vein

We are using ultrasound-guided cannulation of the right IJV as a prototype for description.

Anatomic Considerations

The IJV extends from the external jugular foramen at the base of the skull to the clavicle **(Fig. 15)**. In clinical practice, location of the IJV is typically located anterolateral to the carotid artery in most patients; however, it can be medial to the carotid in approximately 2% of cases or outside the predicted path based on landmarks in 5.5% of patients.[9]

The IJV is relatively easy to cannulate due to its superficial location. The right IJV is particularly preferred because of its direct course to the superior vena cava **(Figs. 16A and B)**.

Cannulation Technique

All prerequisites for cannulation, such as explaining the procedure to the patient, obtaining consent, correcting coagulation abnormalities, and positioning the patient, should be performed similarly to the landmark technique. Ultrasonography does not replace the need for proper patient positioning. The Trendelenburg position can help enlarge the IJV, particularly in hypovolemic patients, and reduce decreases the risk of air embolism. Hyperextension of the neck using a pillow under the shoulder blades is generally not required.

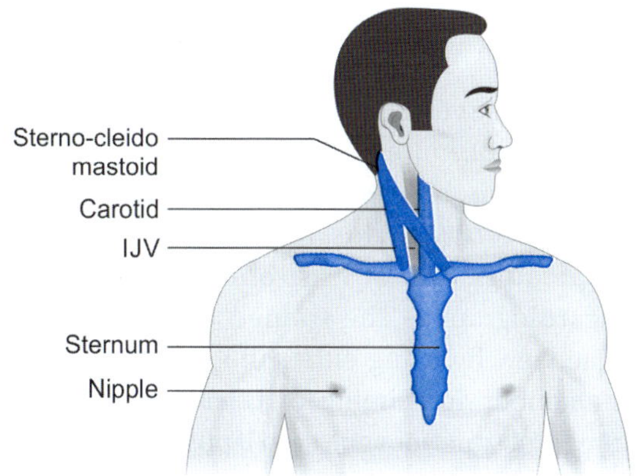

Fig. 15: Demonstrating anatomic relationship of internal jugular vein (IJV).

Before scrubbing the patient and the operator, the operator, positioned at the head end, performs a static ultrasonography and Doppler examination to identify the relevant anatomy. This involves assessing the distance of the IJV from the skin, its relative position with respect to the carotid artery and pleura, and identifying any anatomical variations or abnormalities, such as a thrombus. If a hyperechoic structure within the vessel suggests a thrombus, avoid applying pressure, as this could dislodge the thrombus and potentially cause a pulmonary embolism. If the vein appears uniformly hypoechoic, its patency can be assessed by compression. Additionally, identifying the thyroid gland and trachea is advisable to orient the operator towards the midline.

Static ultrasonography helps identify potential difficulties with cannulation, allowing the user adequate time for further preparation or site adjustment.

An aseptic technique, adhering to maximal sterile barrier precautions as recommended by the Infectious Diseases Society of America (IDSA) should be universally followed during central line cannulation.[26] The ultrasound probe should also be covered with a sterile cover. The footprint of the probe can be covered with a sterile glove, sterile camera cover, or a sterile transparent dressing **(Figs. 17A and B)**. Sterilized jelly or normal saline can be

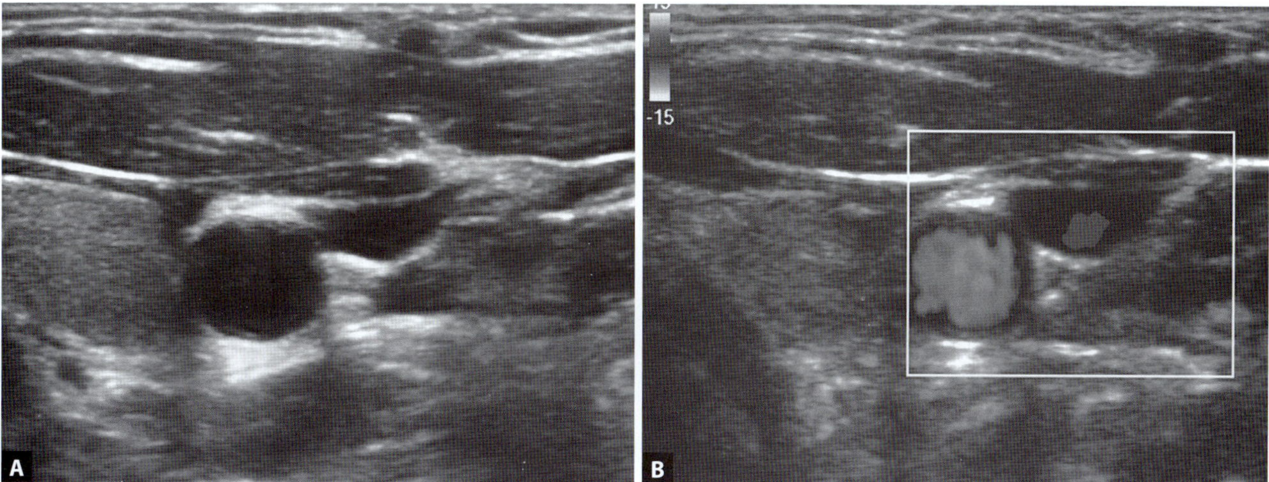

Figs. 16A and B: Ultrasound images demonstrating the anatomic relationship of the internal jugular vein: (A) B-mode ultrasound image of the internal jugular vein and carotid artery; (B) Color mode ultrasound image of the internal jugular vein and carotid artery *(For color version, see Plate 8)*.

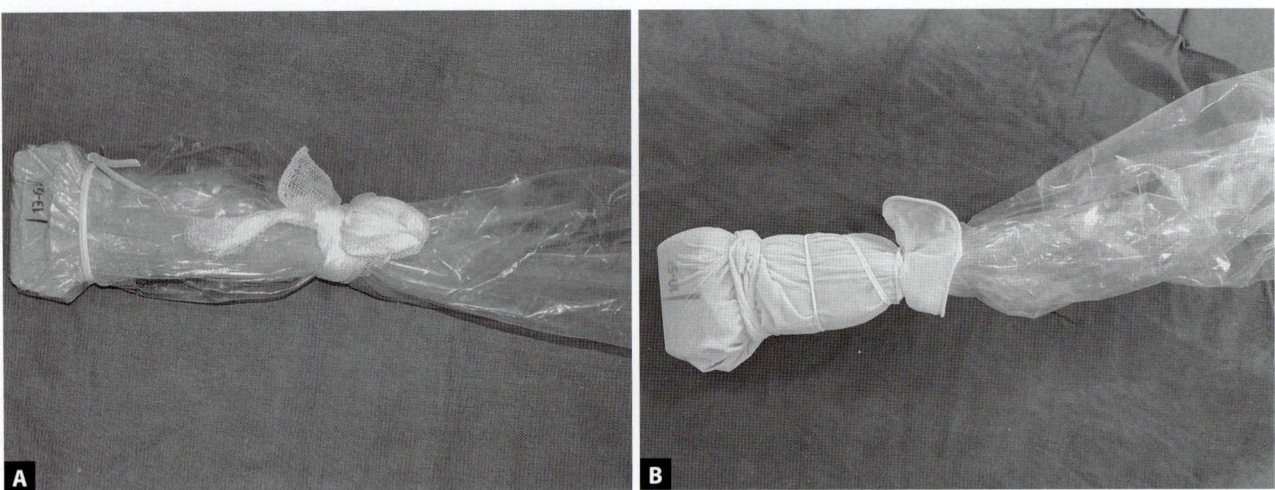

Figs. 17A and B: Image of ultrasound probe covered with (A) sterile camera cover and (B) sterile gloves *(For color version, see Plate 9).*

used as the conducting medium between the sterile probe and the skin.

Readers are strongly advised to follow the manufacturer's recommendations for cleaning and sterilization of the probe. Generally, alcohol-based solutions should not be used for sterilization or disinfection, as they can damage the transducer probe.

Probe orientation should be reconfirmed before needle puncture. It is good practice to reorient to the midline by visualizing the thyroid gland and trachea again. For cannulation of right IJV, the thyroid and trachea are on the left side of the vessels. The left side of the screen should correspond to the left side of the patient. The point of infiltration of the local anesthetic can be selected using ultrasound guidance. Air bubbles are eliminated from the local anesthetic, as they can impair vessel visualization.

The vessel can be cannulated using real-time ultrasonography guidance within one of the previously described approaches. The use of real-time ultrasonography is not limited to guiding the vein puncture; it can also be used to confirm the position of needle, guidewire, and catheter in the vein.[12]

Postcannulation Ultrasonography

A quick postcannulation ultrasonography can be performed immediately after guidewire insertion, as described here:

- *Identifying guidewire malposition:* Occasionally, the guidewire may be malpositioned in the right or left subclavian vein or the left IJV. This can be identified by scanning these vessels with the same linear probe used during the procedure.
- *Confirmation of central line tip with contrast echocardiography:* This requires the presence of two operators with at least one trained in focused echocardiography. The trained operator obtains a cardiac view by using either the subcostal or apical four-chamber view aiming for a clear image of the right atrium (and superior vena cava if possible).[27] The other operator injects 10 mL of normal saline through the distal hub of the central venous catheter. Opacification of the right atrium within 2 seconds of injection indicates correct placement **(Figs. 18A and B)**. Delayed or absent opacification suggests malposition. Occasionally, the catheter tip may be seen in the right atrium on a postprocedure echocardiogram **(Fig. 19)**.
- *Diagnosis of postprocedure complications like pneumothorax:* For instance, pneumothorax can be quickly identified by scanning the lungs with the same probe used for the procedure; however, pneumothorax may develop later. Diagnosis of pneumothorax is discussed elsewhere in this textbook.

Subclavian Vein Cannulation

Many intensivists prefer subclavian vein cannulation because it enhances patient comfort and reduces the incidence of infections. The presence of coagulopathy is not an absolute contraindication; however, it should be avoided as the location of the subclavian artery below the clavicle makes it a noncompressible site.[28]

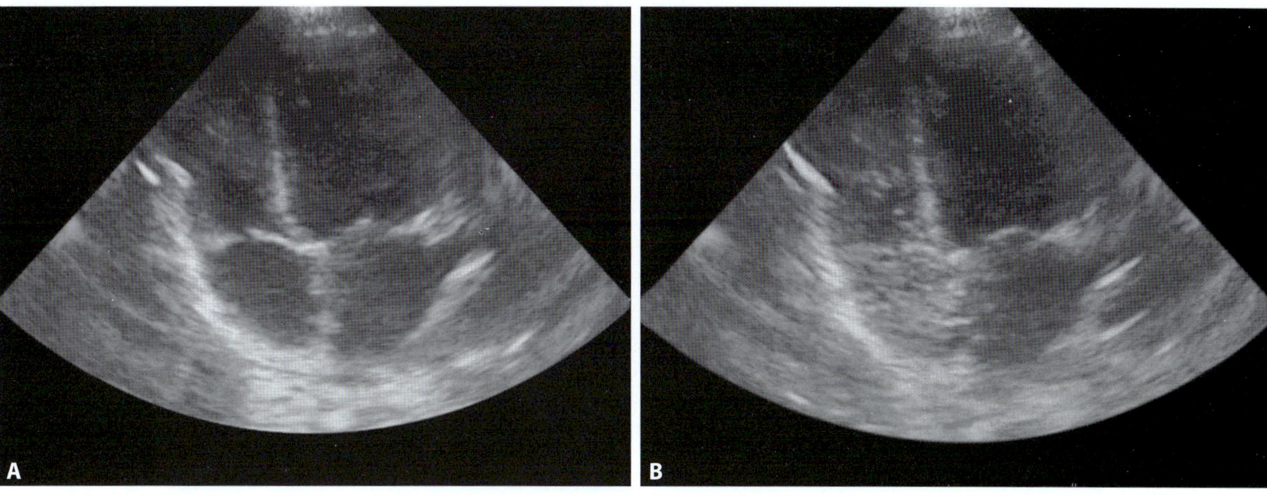

Figs. 18A and B: Contrast echocardiography for confirmation of central line tip: (A) The right atrium with no contrast; (B) The right atrium getting clouded after the injection of saline.

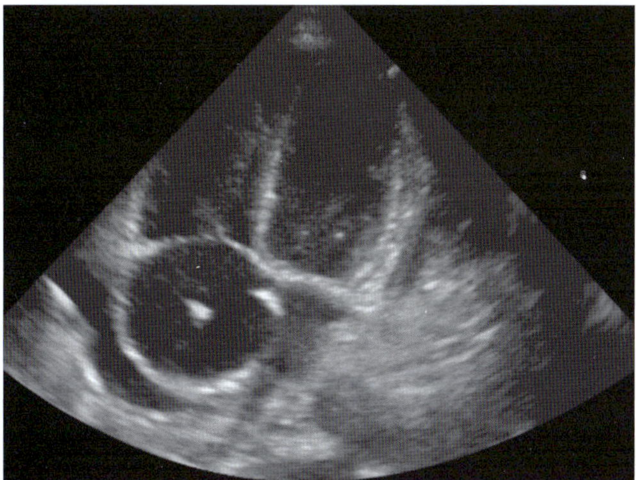

Fig. 19: Apical four-chamber view showing the catheter tip is seen in the right atrium.

Anatomic Considerations

The subclavian vein **(Figs. 20A and B)** is situated beneath the clavicle, continuing laterally to the outer border of the first rib as an axillary. The subclavian vein can be accessed via either a supraclavicular or an infraclavicular approach.

Cannulation Technique

The supraclavicular approach offers a shorter and more direct path to the subclavian vein compared to the infraclavicular approach, which involves puncturing through the pectoralis major muscle and may increase the risk of catheter malpositioning. In the supraclavicular approach, maintaining probe-skin contact can be challenging when using a transverse approach. Due to the limited space, cannulation is often performed in the longitudinal approach using either a linear probe with a smaller footprint or a microconvex probe. Mallin et al. have described using an endocavitary probe for this purpose; however, this probe is not typically available in the intensive care unit (ICU).[29]

For the infraclavicular approach, both longitudinal and transverse techniques can be employed. Ultrasonography in this approach allows visualization of the subclavian and axillary vein in the clavipectoral triangle and pleura below and the needle entry into the vessel is lateral to the landmark method.[30] Ultrasonography also helps in the identification of pleura.

Cannulation of Femoral Vessels (Vein and Artery)

Anatomic Considerations

The common femoral artery and femoral vein are located within the femoral triangle in the inguinal-femoral region **(Fig. 21)**. The superior border of this triangle is formed by the inguinal ligament, the medial border by the adductor longus muscle, and the lateral border by the sartorius muscle. The femoral artery is situated at the midpoint of the inguinal ligament, which extends from the anterior superior iliac spine to the pubic tubercle, while the common femoral vein is typically located medial to the common femoral artery **(Figs. 22A and B)**.[9] In 8–10% of individuals, the femoral vein can be completely overlapped by the femoral artery.[8]

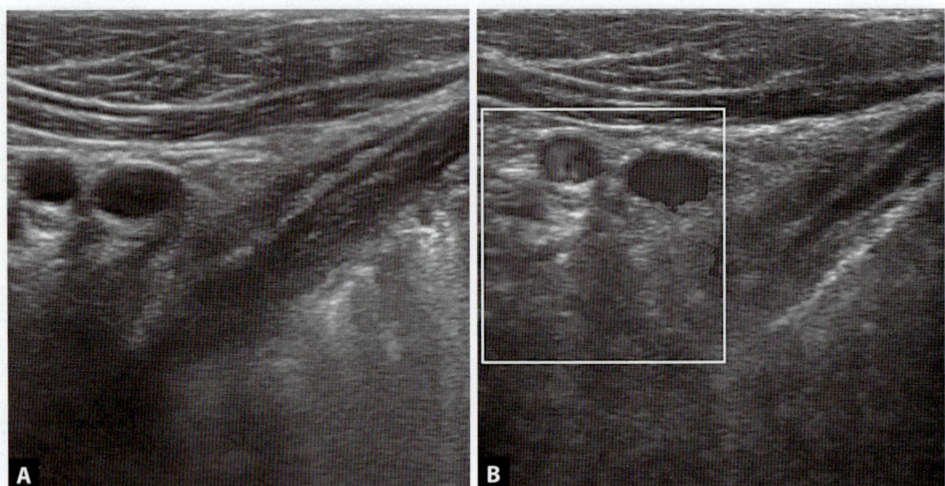

Figs. 20A and B: Ultrasound images demonstrating the anatomic relationship of the subclavian vein: (A) B-mode ultrasound image of subclavian vein and artery; (B) Color mode ultrasound image of subclavian vein and artery *(For color version, see Plate 9)*.

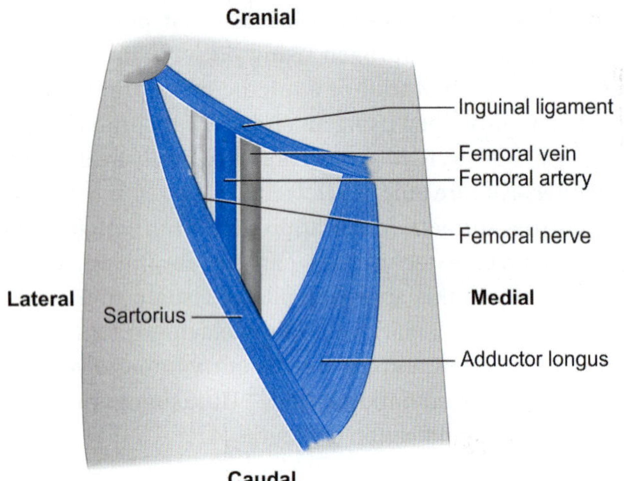

Fig. 21: The anatomic relationship of the femoral vein.

Cannulation Technique

The procedure requires positioning the patient positioning with the hip either in a neutral position or with slight hip abduction and external rotation. The reverse Trendelenburg position increases the cross-sectional area of the femoral vein by 50%.[9] Abduction and external rotation improve the accessibility of the common femoral vein from 70–83% in adults and increase the vessel diameter in children compared with a straight-leg approach.[9] On ultrasonography, the femoral vein is easily identified medial to the common femoral artery and receives the great saphenous vein. In the SAX, these structures create the "Mickey Mouse" sign.[31] The femoral vein is typically a larger, compressible structure, anteromedial to the femoral artery, which is noncompressible, pulsatile femoral artery. Using real-time imaging, the femoral vein is punctured in either the SAX or LAX view. The needle tip should be centered in the vein before introducing the guidewire. The remaining steps follow those of IJV cannulation: using the Seldinger technique, the catheter is inserted into the vein and the final position is confirmed by ultrasonography. Occasionally, resistance to guidewire insertion may occur after smooth initial passage due to acute vessel angulation in propped up position. Aligning the bed straight can resolve this issue.

Radial Artery Cannulation

The radial artery is smaller in size compared to the femoral artery and central veins. On two-dimensional ultrasonography, it appears as a pulsating black circle against a static tissue background **(Figs. 23A and B)**. This can be further confirmed with the color Doppler, which identifies pulsatile flow patterns. The positioning of the patient and operator is similar to the landmark technique. Both LAX and SAX approaches have been described. Spasm of radial artery during cannulation is known and various agents such as topical or subcutaneous local anesthetic, injection of nitroglycerine, and verapamil have been used to prevent it.[13,32-34]

A recent meta-analysis indicates a clear benefit of ultrasonography guidance for radial artery catheterization compared to the traditional palpation method.[33]

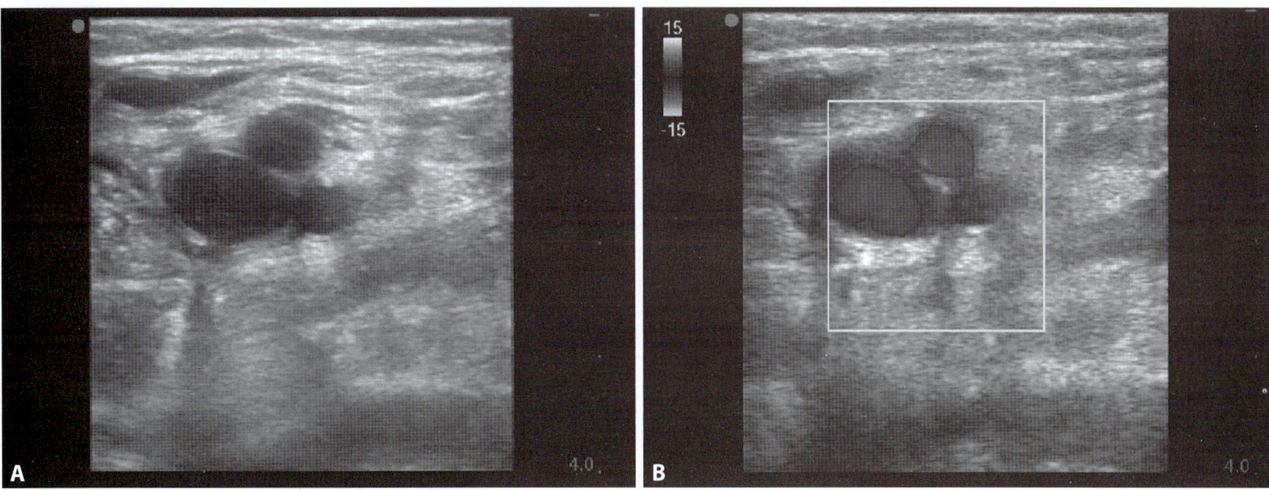

Figs. 22A and B: Ultrasound images demonstrating the anatomic relationship of femoral vessels: (A) B mode ultrasound image of femoral vessels; (B) Color mode ultrasound image of femoral vessels *(For color version, see Plate 10)*.

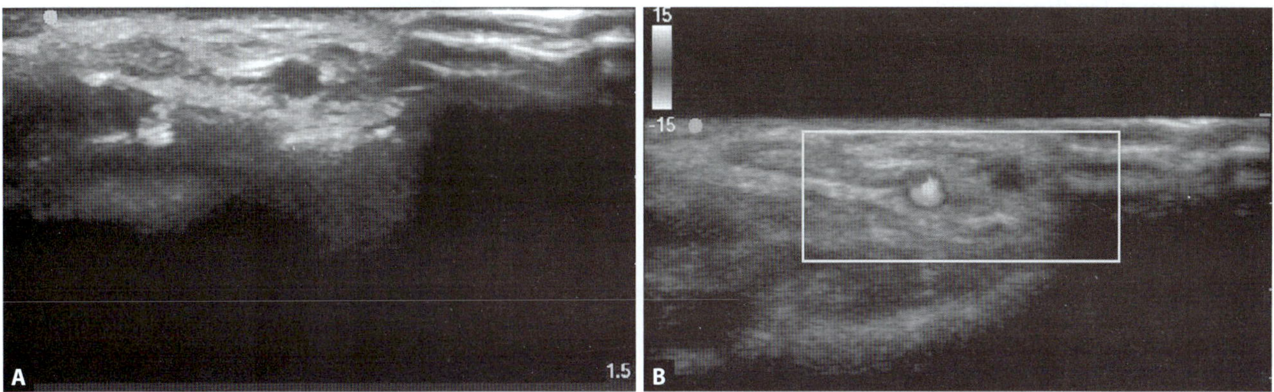

Figs. 23A and B: Ultrasound images of the radial artery: (A) B mode ultrasound image of the radial artery; (B) Color mode ultrasound image of the radial artery *(For color version, see Plate 10)*.

Ultrasonography guidance significantly improves the first-attempt success rate in both adult and pediatric populations.[13]

Compared to standard landmark-based cannulation, ultrasonography-guided cannulation of the radial, ulnar, brachial, and femoral arteries is generally easier and faster, particularly when the artery's pulsation is difficult to detect or when the artery is small. It is recommended to use ultrasonography routinely in adults when trained operators are available.[35]

Applications of Ultrasonography Beyond Vascular Cannulation

Apart from vascular cannulation, ultrasonography can also be used for other procedures described further.

Confirmation of Endotracheal Tube Placement

While capnography is considered the gold standard for confirming endotracheal tube placement, it may be inaccurate in conditions with compromised pulmonary blood flow, such as massive pulmonary embolism and cardiac arrest. In such situations, ultrasonography can effectively confirm tube placement in the trachea.

Thoracentesis with ultrasound guidance has become the standard of care for thoracentesis. The success rate of thoracentesis for small pleural effusions increases from 66 to 90% with the use of ultrasound.[36] Ultrasonography allows measurement of the distance from the skin to the parietal and visceral pleura, helping to determine the safety of the procedure and guiding the selection of an appropriate needle length.

Pericardiocentesis

Cardiac ultrasonography (echocardiography) aids in selecting the needle puncture site based on the thickness of the effusion and its proximity to the thoracic wall.[37]

Pacing

Ultrasonography can serve as a safe alternative to fluoroscopy for the insertion of a temporary transvenous pacemaker.[38]

Extracorporeal Membrane Oxygenation

Ultrasound and echocardiography can assist in the positioning of extracorporeal membrane oxygenation (ECMO) cannula to avoid recirculation. A detailed discussion of this is beyond the purview of this chapter.

Percutaneous Tracheostomy

Ultrasonography can identify critical structures such as the cricothyroid membrane, tracheal cartilage, vessels, thyroid gland, and isthmus, as well as a high-riding brachiocephalic (innominate) artery. Real-time ultrasonography enhances the accuracy of needle l puncture and reduces complications during the procedure.

PITFALLS OF ULTRASONOGRAPHY

- *Subcutaneous emphysema:* Ultrasonography can be limited in the presence of subcutaneous emphysema which is identified clinically by the presence of palpable crepitus and radiologically by radiolucent shadows in the subcutaneous space **(Fig. 24)**. The ultrasonographic appearance of subcutaneous emphysema **(Fig. 25)** resembles B-lines seen in lung ultrasonography but originates from subcutaneous tissue rather than the pleura **(Fig. 26)**.
- *Deeper structures >6 cm:* Most of the commercially available linear probes have a maximum depth of approximately 6 cm. Imaging deeper structures requires low-frequency probes, which offer poorer resolution.
- *Experience of the operator:* Successful use of ultrasonography depends on the operator's experience. Inexperienced operators might find ultrasonography more challenging than landmark methods. *Key principles must be followed:* In the out-of-plane approach, the needle tip must be closely monitored, while in the in-plane approach, both the needle and

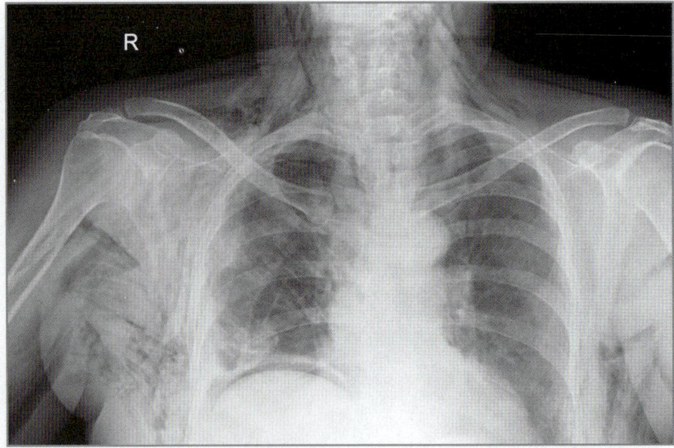

Fig. 24: Chest radiograph showing subcutaneous emphysema. (Note the gas under the diaphragm.)

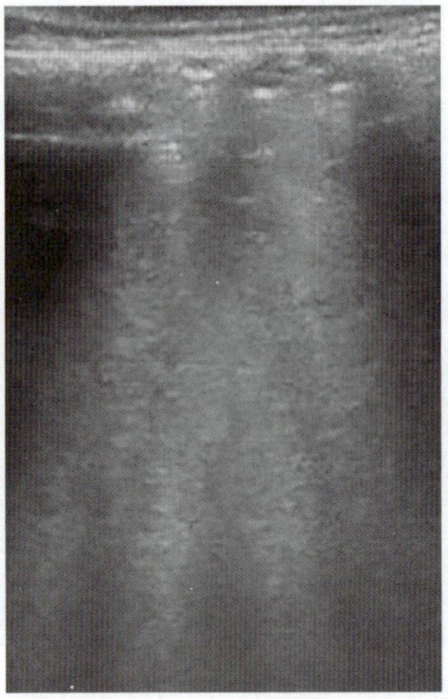

Fig. 25: Ultrasound image of subcutaneous emphysema.

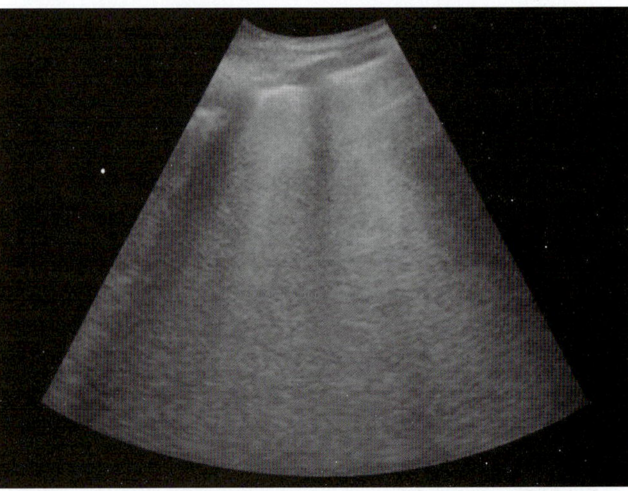

Fig. 26: Ultrasound image of B lines in a case with interstitial edema.

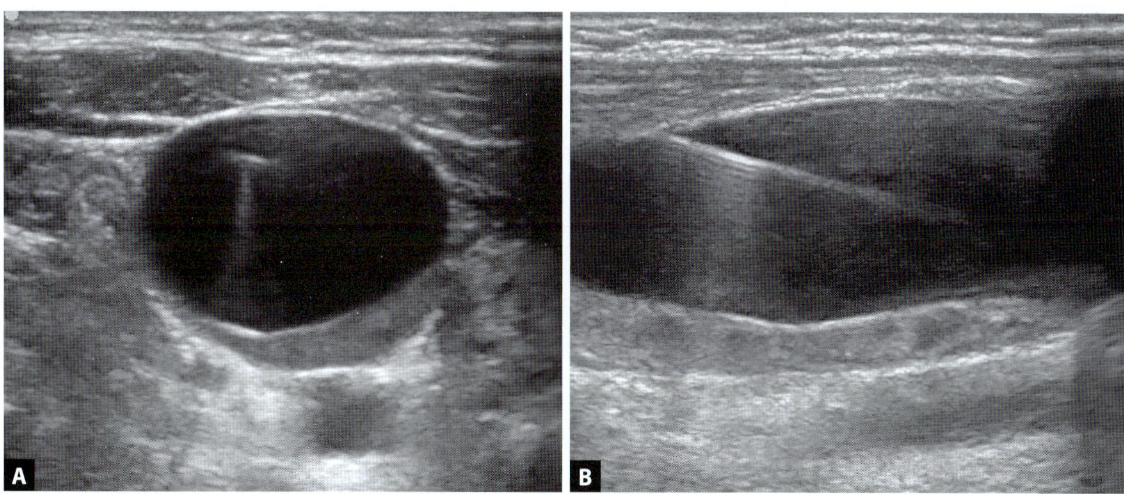

Figs. 27A and B: Ultrasound image of vessel after cannulation showing posterior wall injury in (A) short- and (B) long-axis views. Note the guidewire in the vessel.

probe must be stabilized to ensure full visualization of the needle path. Therefore, ultrasonography should initially be used in elective cases to build proficiency before applying it in emergencies.

- *Injury to the posterior wall:* Despite real-time ultrasonography, posterior wall penetration can occur **(Figs. 27A and B)**. The prevalence of posterior wall penetration was reported as follows: Internal jugular SAX 25%, internal jugular LAX 21%, subclavian SAX 64%, and subclavian LAX 39%.[19]
- *Legal prerequisites and mandates:* Depending on local laws, there may be legal requirements for the procurement, maintenance, and usage of ultrasonography machines. It is essential for institutions to ensure compliance with these regulations.
- *Deskilling of blind techniques:* Frequent reliance on ultrasonography for vascular access and other procedures may lead to the deskilling of traditional blind techniques, which are still useful in cases where ultrasound equipment is unavailable.

GUIDELINES AND RECOMMENDATIONS

- *Real-time ultrasonography for internal jugular cannulation:* Real-time ultrasonography-guided cannulation of the IJV is highly recommended by various medical societies due to its superior accuracy and safety.[9]
- *Subclavian vein cannulation:* Societies offer differing recommendations for real-time ultrasonography use in subclavian vein cannulation. Traditional blind cannulation targets the subclavian vein below the clavicle, a region typically inaccessible to ultrasound. However, ultrasound-guided cannulation in the infraclavicular approach targets the axillary vein, a continuation of the subclavian vein. Static ultrasonography is particularly advised in obese and coagulopathic patients. Although real-time ultrasonography is not uniformly recommended as the initial technique for subclavian cannulation, it is advised as a rescue technique.[9]
- *Femoral venous access in adults:* Ultrasonography is generally advised to identify anatomical challenges, such as vessel overlap and thrombus, to ensure safer cannulation.
- *Radial artery cannulation:* The use of ultrasonography has been shown to improve first-pass success rates for radial artery cannulation, especially in difficult cases.[13,33,34]
- *Pediatric populations:* In pediatric patients, real-time ultrasonography is strongly recommended during both internal jugular and femoral vein cannulation to enhance precision and reduce complications.[9]

ACKNOWLEDGMENT

I sincerely appreciate Dr Tineesh Mathew for his invaluable assistance in writing the previous edition of this chapter.

CONCLUSION

The limitations of landmark-based blind techniques for vascular cannulation have driven the development of real-time ultrasound-guided procedures. Ultrasound can be employed at various stages of cannulation, including vessel identification, needle puncture, guidewire confirmation, and post-procedure complication assessment. Higher-frequency linear transducer probes are generally preferred for these procedures.

As ultrasonography is a two-dimensional modality, various approaches have been described for its use. The choice of approach depends on vessel anatomy and the operator's experience. Adherence to sterile aseptic precautions and universal barrier precautions is essential.

Real-time ultrasound-guided cannulation of the internal jugular vein (IJV) is highly recommended, and other vessels can also be effectively cannulated under ultrasound guidance.

REFERENCES

1. McGahan JP. The history of interventional ultrasound. J Ultrasound Med. 2004;23(6):727-41
2. Berlyne GM. Ultrasonics in renal biopsy: an aid to determination of kidney position. Lancet. 1961;2(7205): 750-1.
3. Joyner CR Jr, Herman RJ, Reid JM. Reflected ultrasound in the detection and localization of pleural effusion. JAMA. 1967;200(5):399-402.
4. Ullman JI, Stoelting RK. Internal jugular vein location with the US Doppler blood flow detector. Anesth Analg. 1978;57(1):118.
5. Yonei A, Nonoue T, Sari A. Real-time ultrasonic guidance for percutaneous puncture of the internal jugular vein. Anesthesiology. 1986;64(6):830-1.
6. Gallieni M. Central venous catheterization of dialysis patients with real time ultrasound guidance. J Vasc Access. 2000;1(1):10-4.
7. Hughes P, Scott C, Bodenham A. Ultrasonography of the femoral vessels in the groin: implications for vascular access. Anaesthesia. 2000;55(12):1198-202.
8. Warkentine FH, Pierce MC, Lorenz D, Kim IK. The anatomic relationship of femoral vein to femoral artery in euvolemic pediatric patients by ultrasonography: implications for pediatric femoral central venous access. Acad Emerg Med. 2008;15(5):426-30.
9. Troianos CA, Hartman GS, Glas KE, Skubas NJ, Eberhardt RT, Walker JD, et al. Guidelines for performing ultrasound guided vascular cannulation: recommendations of the American Society of Echocardiography and the Society of Cardiovascular Anesthesiologists. J Am Soc Echocardiogr. 2011;24(12):1291-318.
10. Sznajder JI, Zveibil FR, Bitterman H, Weiner P, Bursztein S. Central vein catheterization. Failure and complication rates by three percutaneous approaches. Arch Intern Med. 1986;146(2):259-61.
11. Troianos CA, Jobes DR, Ellison N. Ultrasound-guided cannulation of the internal jugular vein. A prospective, randomized study. Anesth Analg. 199;72(6):823-6.
12. Saugel B, Scheeren TWL, Teboul JL. Ultrasound-guided central venous catheter placement: a structured review and recommendations for clinical practice. Crit Care. 2017;21(1):225.
13. White L, Halpin A, Turner M, Wallace LM. Ultrasound-guided radial artery cannulation in adult and paediatric populations: a systematic review and meta-analysis. Br J Anaes. 2016;116(5):610-7.
14. Soni NJ, Franco R, Velez MI, Schnobrich D, Dancel R, Restrepo MI, et al. Ultrasound in the diagnosis and management of pleural effusions. J Hosp Med. 2015;10(12): 811-6.
15. Callahan JA, Seward JB, Nishimura RA, Miller FA Jr, Reeder GS, Shub C, et al. Two-dimensional echocardiographically guided pericardiocentesis: experience in 117 consecutive patients. Am J Cardiol. 1985;55(4):476-9.
16. O'Grady NP, Alexander M, Burns LA, Dellinger EP, Garland J, Heard SO, et al. Guidelines for the prevention of intravascular catheter-related infections. Clin Infect Dis. 2011;52(9):e162-93.
17. Lichtenstein DA. Interventional ultrasound. In: Lichtenstein DA (Ed). General Ultrasound in the Critically Ill. Berlin: Springer; 2007. pp. 170-74.
18. Lichtenstein DA. Upper-extremity central veins. In: Lichtenstein DA (Ed). General Ultrasound in the Critically Ill. Berlin: Springer; 2007. pp. 70-81.
19. Vogel JA, Haukoos JS, Erickson CL, Liao MM, Theoret J, Sanz GE, et al. Is long-axis view superior to short-axis view in ultrasound-guided central venous catheterization? Crit Care Med. 2015;43(4):832-9.
20. Clemmesen L, Knudsen L, Sloth E, Bendtsen T. Dynamic needle tip positioning – ultrasound guidance for peripheral vascular access. A randomized, controlled and blinded study in phantoms performed by ultrasound novices. Ultraschall Med. 2012;33(7):E321-5.
21. Chin K, Perlas A, Chan V, Brull R. Needle visualization in ultrasound-guided regional anesthesia: challenges and solutions. Reg Anes Pain Med. 2008;33(6):532-44.
22. Phelan M, Hagerty D. The oblique view: an alternative approach for ultrasound-guided central line placement. J Emerg Med. 2009;37(4):403-8.
23. Batllori M, Urra M, Uriarte E, Romero C, Pueyo J, López-Olaondo L, et al. Randomized comparison of three transducer orientation approaches for ultrasound guided internal jugular venous cannulation. Br J Anaes. 2016; 116(3):370-6.
24. Abdalla UE, Elmaadawey A, Kandeel A. Oblique approach for ultrasound-guided radial artery catheterization vs transverse and longitudinal approaches, a randomized trial. J Clin Anes. 2017;36:98-101.
25. Shiono M, Takahashi S, Kakudo Y, Takahashi M, Shimodaira H, Kato S, et al. Upper arm central venous port implantation: a 6-year single institutional retrospective analysis and pictorial essay of procedures for insertion. PLoS One. 2014;9(3):e91335.

26. Marschall J, Mermel LA, Fakih M, Hadaway L, Kallen A, O'Grady NP, et al. Strategies to prevent central line-associated bloodstream infections in acute care hospitals: 2014 update. Infect Control Hosp Epidemiol. 2014;35(7): 753-71.
27. Korsten P, Mavropoulou E, Wienbeck S, Ellenberger D, Ellenberger D, Vasko R, et al. The "rapid atrial swirl sign" for assessing central venous catheters: performance by medical residents after limited training. PLoS One. 2018;13(7):e0199345.
28. Schulman PM, Gerstein NS, Merkel MJ, Braner DA, Tegtmeyer K. Ultrasound-guided cannulation of the subclavian vein. N Engl J Med. 2018;379(1):e1.
29. Mallin M, Louis H, Madsen T. A novel technique for ultrasound-guided supraclavicular subclavian cannulation. Am J Emerg Med. 2010;28(8):966-9.
30. Rezayat T, Stowell JR, Kendall JL, Turner E, Fox JC, Barjaktarevic I. Ultrasound-guided cannulation: time to bring subclavian central lines back. West J Emerg Med. 2016;17(2):216-21.
31. Mumoli N, Cei M. The "Mickey Mouse" sign. BMJ Case Rep. 2009;2009:bcr2007054080.
32. Rigatelli G, Zuin M, Dell'Avvocata F, Vassiliev D. Topical anaesthesia before transradial approach for supraoartic vessels angiography and stenting in the elderly: a feasible alternative. J Geriatr Cardiol. 2017;14(10):644-8.
33. Tang L, Wang F, Li Y, Zhao L, Xi H, Guo Z, et al. Ultrasound guidance for radial artery catheterization: an updated meta-analysis of randomized controlled trials. PLoS One. 2014;9(11):e111527.
34. Levin PD, Sheinen O, Gozal Y. Use of ultrasound guidance in the insertion of radial artery catheters. Crit Care Med. 2003;31(2):481-4.
35. Lamperti M, Bodenham AR, Pittiruti M, Blaivas M, Augoustides JG, Elbarbary M, et al. International evidence-based recommendations on ultrasound-guided vascular access. Intensive Care Med. 2012;38(7):1105-17.
36. Havelock T, Teoh R, Laws D, Gleeson F; BTS Pleural Disease Guideline Group. Pleural procedures and thoracic ultrasound: British Thoracic Society Pleural Disease Guideline 2010. Thorax. 2010;65 suppl 2:ii61-ii76.
37. Tsang TS, Enriquez-Sarano M, Freeman WK, Barnes ME, Sinak LJ, Gersh BJ, et al. Consecutive 1127 therapeutic echocardiographically guided pericardiocenteses: clinical profile, practice patterns, and outcomes spanning 21 years. Mayo Clin Proc. 2002;77(5):429-36.
38. Ferri LA, Farina A, Lenatti L, Ruffa F, Tiberti G, Piatti L, et al. Emergent transvenous cardiac pacing using ultrasound guidance: a prospective study versus the standard fluoroscopy-guided procedure. Eur Heart J Acute Cardiovasc Care. 2016;5(2):125-9.

Index

Page numbers followed by *b* refer to box, *f* refer to figure, *fc* refer to flowchart, and *t* refer to table.

A

B

C

J

K

L

M

N

O

Q

R

S

T

U

V

W

X

Y